Developmental

Neuroimaging

Developmental Neuroimaging

MAPPING THE DEVELOPMENT OF BRAIN AND BEHAVIOR

Edited by

Robert W. Thatcher

College of Medicine
University of South Florida
Tampa, Florida

G. Reid Lyon

Human Learning and Behavior Branch Center for Research for Mothers and Children
National Institute of Child Health and Human Development
National Institutes of Health
Bethesda, Maryland

J. Rumsey

National Institutes of Mental Health
National Institutes of Health
Bethesda, Maryland

N. Krasnegor

Human Learning and Behavior Branch Center for Research for Mothers and Children
National Institute of Child Health and Human Development
National Institutes of Health
Bethesda, Maryland

Academic Press

San Diego   London   Boston   New York   Sydney   Tokyo   Toronto

Academic Press, Inc.
525 B Street, Suite 1900, San Diego, California 92101-4495, USA
http://www.apnet.com

Academic Press Limited
24-28 Oval Road, London NW1 7DX, UK
http://www.hbuk.co.uk/ap/

Library of Congress Cataloging-in-Publication Data

Developmental neuroimaging : mapping the development of brain and
    behavior / edited by Robert W. Thatcher ... [et al.].
        p.   cm.
    Includes index.
    ISBN 0-12-686070-X (alk. paper)
    1. Developmental neurobiology.   2. Brain--Imaging.   I. Thatcher,
Robert W.
QP363.5.D475   1996
612.8'2--dc20   96-3067
                                                  CIP

PRINTED IN THE UNITED STATES OF AMERICA
96 97 98 99 00 01 EB 9 8 7 6 5 4 3 2 1

Contents

I

NEUROIMAGING OF STRUCTURAL BRAIN DEVELOPMENT

1

The Developing Human Brain: A Morphometric Profile

Verne S. Caviness, Jr., David N. Kennedy, Julianna F. Bates, Nikos Makris

2

Modeling Morphometric Changes of the Brain during Development

Arthur W. Toga, Paul Thompson, Bradley A. Payne

3

Structural Morphometry in the Developing Brain

David N. Kennedy, Nikos Makris, Julianna F. Bates, Verne S. Caviness, Jr.

4

Measurement and Analysis Issues in Neurodevelopmental Magnetic Resonance Imaging

Eric Courchesne, Elena Plante

II

NEUROIMAGING OF PERCEPTUAL AND COGNITIVE DEVELOPMENT

5

Spatio-Temporal Modeling of Brain Waves

Peter C. M. Molenaar, Hilde M. Huizenga,
Han L. J. van der Maas

6

PET and fMRI in the Detection of Task-Related Brain Activity: Implications for the Study of Brain Development

Guinevere F. Eden, Thomas A. Zeffiro

7

Neuroimaging of Cyclic Cortical Reorganization during Human Development

Robert W. Thatcher

8

Nuclear Magnetic Resonance Spectroscopic Studies of Cortical Development

Nancy J. Minshew, Jay W. Pettegrew

9

Multimodal Assessments of Developing Neural Networks: Integrating fMRI, PET, MRI, and EEG/MEG

Robert W. Thatcher

III

NEUROIMAGING OF ABNORMAL DEVELOPMENT

10

Functional Neuroimaging of Language in Children: Current Directions and Future Challenges

Susan Y. Bookheimer, Mirella Dapretto

11

Functional Magnetic Resonance Imaging as a Tool to Understand Reading and Reading Disability

Bennett A. Shaywitz, Sally E. Shaywitz, Kenneth R. Pugh, Pawel Skudlarski, Robert K. Fulbright, R. Todd Constable, Richard A. Bronen, Jack M. Fletcher, Alvin M. Liberman, Donald P. Shankweiler, Leonard Katz, Cheryl Lacadie, Karen E. Marchione, John C. Gore

12

Structural Variations in Measures in the Developmental Disorders

Pauline A. Filipek

13

Neuroimaging of Developmental Nonlinearity and Developmental Pathologies

Harry T. Chugani

14

Event Related Potential Correlates of Glucose Metabolism in Normal Adults during a Cognitive Activation Task

Frank B. Wood, Amy S. Garrett, Lesley A. Hart, D. Lynn Flowers, John R. Absher

15

Structural Variation in the Developing and Mature Cerebral Cortex: Noise or Signal?

Christiana M. Leonard

IV

NEUROIMAGING DEVELOPMENT OF BRAIN–BEHAVIOR RELATIONSHIPS

16

Conceptual and Methodological Issues in the Interpretation of Brain–Behavior Relationships

F. Gonzalez-Lima, A. R. McIntosh

17

Measurement Issues in the Interpretation of Behavior–Brain Relationships

Jack M. Fletcher, Karla K. Stuebing, Bennett A. Shaywitz,
Michael E. Brandt, David J. Francis, Sally E. Shaywitz

18

Dynamic Growth Cycles of Brain and Cognitive Development

Kurt W. Fischer, Samuel P. Rose

19

Functional Specialization and Integration in the Brain: An Example from Schizophrenia Research

Karl J. Friston

20

Self-Regulation and Cortical Development: Implications for Functional Studies of the Brain

Phan Luu, Don M. Tucker

Contributors

Numbers in parentheses indicate the pages on which the authors' contributions begin.

John R. Absher (197) Section on Neuropsychology, Bowman Gray School of Medicine, Wake Forest University, Winston-Salem, North Carolina 27157

Julianna F. Bates (4, 29) Department of Neurology, Massachusetts General Hospital, Harvard Medical School, Boston, Massachusetts 02114

Susan Y. Bookheimer (143) Division of Brain Mapping, School of Medicine, University of California, Los Angeles, Los Angeles, California 90095

Michael E. Brandt (255) Departments of Psychiatry and Behavioral Sciences and Pediatrics, Houston Medical School, University of Texas, Houston, Texas 77030

Richard A. Bronen (157) Department of Diagnostic Radiology, Yale University School of Medicine, New Haven, Connecticut 06510

Verne S. Caviness, Jr. (4, 29) Department of Neurology, Center for Morphometric Analysis, Massachusetts General Hospital, Harvard Medical School, Boston, Massachusetts 02114

Harry T. Chugani (187) Positron Emission Tomography Center, Children's Hospital of Michigan, Wayne State University School of Medicine, Detroit, Michigan 48201

R. Todd Constable (157) Department of Diagnostic Radiology, Yale University School of Medicine, New Haven, Connecticut 06510

Eric Courchesne (43) Department of Neurosciences, School of Medicine, University of California at San Diego, La Jolla, California 92093, and Autism and Brain Development Research Laboratory, Children's Hospital Research Center, San Diego, California 92097

Mirella Dapretto (143) Division of Brain Mapping, School of Medicine, University of California, Los Angeles, Los Angeles, California 90095

Guinevere F. Eden (77) Section of Functional Brain Imaging, National Institutes of Health, Bethesda, Maryland 20892

Pauline A. Filipek (169) Departments of Pediatrics and Neurology, University of California, Irvine, College of Medicine, Irvine, California 92717

Kurt W. Fischer (263) Department of Human Development and Psychology, Harvard University, Cambridge, Massachusetts 02138

Jack M. Fletcher (157, 255) Department of Pediatrics, University of Texas Medical School, Houston, Texas 77030

D. Lynn Flowers (197) Section on Neuropsychology, Bowman Gray School of Medicine, Wake Forest University, Winston-Salem, North Carolina 27157

David J. Francis (255) Department of Psychology, University of Houston, Houston, Texas 77004

Karl J. Friston (281) The Wellcome Department of Cognitive Neurology, Institute of Neurology, London WCIN 3B6, United Kingdom

Robert K. Fulbright (157) Department of Diagnostic Radiology, Yale University School of Medicine, New Haven, Connecticut 06510

Amy S. Garrett (197) Section on Neuropsychology, Bowman Gray School of Medicine, Wake Forest University, Winston-Salem, North Carolina 27157

F. Gonzalez-Lima (235) Institute for Neuroscience and Department of Psychology, University of Texas, Austin, Texas 78712

John C. Gore (157) Department of Diagnostic Radiology, Yale University School of Medicine, New Haven, Connecticut 06510, and Department of Ap-

ix

plied Physics, Yale University, New Haven, Connecticut 06510

Lesley A. Hart (197) Section on Neuropsychology, Bowman Gray School of Medicine, Wake Forest University, Winston-Salem, North Carolina 27157

Hilde M. Huizenga (69) Department of Psychology, University of Amsterdam, 1018 WB Amsterdam, The Netherlands

Leonard Katz (157) Haskins Laboratories, New Haven, Connecticut 06510

David N. Kennedy (4, 29) Departments of Neurology and Radiology, Massachusetts General Hospital, Harvard Medical School, Boston, Massachusetts 02114

Cheryl Lacadie (157) Department of Diagnostic Radiology, Yale University School of Medicine, New Haven, Connecticut 06510

Christiana M. Leonard (207) Department of Neuroscience, University of Florida, Gainesville, Florida 32610

Alvin M. Liberman (157) Haskins Laboratories, New Haven, Connecticut 06510

Phan Luu (297) Department of Psychology, University of Oregon, Eugene, Oregon 97403

Nikos Makris (4, 29) Department of Neurology, Massachusetts General Hospital, Harvard Medical School, Boston, Massachusetts 02114

Karen E. Marchione (255) Department of Pediatrics, Yale University School of Medicine, New Haven, Connecticut 06510

A. R. McIntosh (235) Rotman Research Institute of Baycrest Centre, University of Toronto, Toronto, Ontario M6A 2E1 Canada

Nancy J. Minshew (107) Departments of Psychiatry and Neurology, University of Pittsburgh School of Medicine, Pittsburgh, Pennsylvania 15213

Peter C. M. Molenaar (69) Department of Psychology, University of Amsterdam, 1018 WB Amsterdam, The Netherlands

Bradley A. Payne (15) Laboratory of Neuro Imaging Department of Neurology, Division of Brain Mapping, UCLA School of Medicine, Los Angeles, California 90024

Jay W. Pettegrew (107) Departments of Psychiatry, Neurology, and Health Services Administration, University of Pittsburgh School of Medicine, Pittsburgh, Pennsylvania 15213

Elena Plante (43) Center for Childhood Language Disorders, Scottish Rite/University of Arizona, Tucson, Arizona 85701, and Department of Speech and Hearing Sciences, University of Arizona, Tucson, Arizona 85701

Kenneth R. Pugh (157) Department of Pediatrics, Yale University School of Medicine, and Haskins Laboratories, New Haven, Connecticut 06510

Samuel P. Rose (263) University of Colorado, Denver, Colorado

Donald P. Shankweiler (157) Haskins Laboratories, New Haven, Connecticut 06510

Bennett A. Shaywitz (15, 255) Departments of Pediatrics and Neurology, Yale University School of Medicine, New Haven, Connecticut 06510

Sally E. Shaywitz (157, 255) Department of Pediatrics, Yale University School of Medicine, New Haven, Connecticut 06510

Pawel Skudlarski (157) Department of Diagnostic Radiology, Yale University School of Medicine, New Haven, Connecticut 06510

Karla K. Stuebing (255) Department of Pediatrics, Houston Medical School, University of Texas, Houston, Texas 77030

Robert W. Thatcher (91, 127) Departments of Neurology and Radiology, University of South Florida College of Medicine, Tampa, Florida 33612

Paul Thompson (15) Laboratory of Neuro Imaging, Department of Neurology, Division of Brain Mapping, UCLA School of Medicine, Los Angeles, California 90024

Arthur W. Toga (15) Laboratory of Neuro Imaging Department of Neurology, Division of Brain Mapping, UCLA School of Medicine, Los Angeles, California 90024

Don M. Tucker (297) Department of Psychology, University of Oregon, Eugene, Oregon 97403, and Electrical Geodesics, Inc., Eugene, Oregon 97403

Han L. J. van der Maas (69) Department of Psychology, University of Amsterdam, 1018 WB Amsterdam, The Netherlands

Frank B. Wood (197) Section on Neuropsychology, Bowman Gray School of Medicine, Wake Forest University, Winston-Salem, North Carolina 27157

Thomas A. Zeffiro (77) Laboratory of Diagnostic Radiology Research, National Institutes of Health, Bethesda, Maryland 20892

Foreword

One hundred years ago, the ability of human beings to understand the development and function of their own brain was not only questionable but generally thought to be impossible. In the intervening decades, development of the multidisciplinary field of neuroscience research and its associated neurotechnologies has forever turned the impossible into the probable. A watershed in the evolution of these events occurred in the early 1980s when the tools of brain imaging became available to both basic and clinical research, providing entirely new and unanticipated windows of opportunity for understanding the human brain. The increasing sophistication and refinement of these powerful tools has culminated in research methodologies with the capability of simultaneously—and noninvasively—examining the relationships between brain structure and brain function in living, behaving human beings.

The advances of this century have not, of course, been defined by imaging alone, but by a progression of knowledge in the growing array of disciplines that constitute neuroscience. Today approximately 35,000 neuroscientists work around the clock, on a global basis, producing an overwhelming amount of raw data. Seeking to harness these data and the knowledge that is synthesized there from is informatics. Informatics currently includes elements from the fields of information science, engineering, mathematics, and computer science. Combining the field of informatics with all that is now subsumed within the field of neuroscience creates neuroinformatics and, potentially, a worldwide electronic capability for collecting, storing, accessing, and analyzing the comprehensive arsenal of basic and clinical research findings. In the United States this effort is called the Human Brain Project (HBP), and it is sponsored by 16 federal research organizations (including 12 institutes and centers of the National Institutes of Health). Efforts to expand the HBP to an international level are currently being pursued by leading researchers in all parts of the world.

Nothing has contributed to, and will benefit more from, developments in neuroinformatics than the burgeoning field of neuroimaging; nowhere is it more critical to readily visualize, integrate, translate, and manipulate data than in this highly promising field. The reader of this volume will be truly awed by the range and the depth of issues addressed in developmental neuroimaging. Used both alone and in combination with other noninvasive research techniques, neuroimaging technology applied to development issues and disorders can do more to further our theoretical and applied understanding of human brain dysfunction than any other branch of neuroscience. The studies reported in this monograph are stellar examples of this potential.

Stephen H. Koslow

Preface

Recent and dramatic advances in the techniques and applications of neuroimaging have given rise to this edited volume. The development of functional and structural neuroimaging methodologies has allowed scientists, for the first time, to visualize and quantify human cognitive and perceptual activities. Until recently, however, human neuroimaging technologies have been limited primarily to use in normal adults and adult patients with various neurological disorders. This is largely due to reliance on radioactive isotopes in positron emission studies such as in PET and SPECT, which preclude their use in normal children. As a consequence, these techniques have been used in a very limited and restricted manner in children with confirmed neurological disorders. Further, in both children and adults these techniques have traditionally been used well after the onset of symptoms. There have been virtually no neuroimaging studies of normal human development or the development of neurological and psychiatric disorders such as schizophrenia and dyslexia.

Developmental neuroimaging, however, has now reached a level of maturity where it is possible to apply noninvasive and comprehensive imaging methodologies to normal human brain development as well as to the study of the development of brain pathologies. This new stage of neuroimaging has come about largely because of two factors: (1) the development of noninvasive magnetic resonance spectroscopy (MRS) and functional magnetic resonance imaging (fMRI); and (2) the development of methodologies for the coregistration of noninvasive electrophysiological (EEG) and magnetoencephalography (MEG) measures to the MRI and fMRI. These new advances in neuroimaging technologies make possible the creation of data bases of the anatomical structure of human brain development in addition to cognitive and perceptual development over the entire human lifespan. By comparison to normal development, the new imaging technologies also provide important diagnostic and prognostic tools for studying the development of childhood neurological and psychiatric disorders.

This volume recognizes the development of these new noninvasive neuroimaging technologies. The book is divided into four sections which represent some of the most important areas of development in this burgeoning field. The goal of each section is to address and expound on both basic science and clinical issues in developmental neuroimaging. Section I is dedicated to new developments in the quantitative analysis of the anatomical development of the human brain. Although emphasis is placed on structural imaging technologies, these same mathematical and quantitative methods can be applied to fMRI and EEG/MEG studies. The chapters in Section I also provide new and important anatomical information about human brain development. The chapter by Caviness et al. presents new perspectives and methods of the analysis of male versus female brain development and the histogenesis of brain growth. Toga et al. provide quantitative methods for cortical surface modeling and image warping as a way to visualize brain development. Kennedy provides new perspectives and methodologies for structural morphometry of the developing brain. Finally, Courchesne and Plante discuss the importance of experimental design and the interplay between quantitative MRI methodologies and the developmental research questions under review. Section II is dedicated to both the theoretical foundations (Molenaar et al.) and the practical applications of magnetic resonance spectroscopy (Minshew and Pettegrew) and multimodal registration of EEG, MRI, and fMRI (Eden and Zeffiro, Thatcher) to the study of human cognitive and perceptual development. Unfortunately, as of the publication of this book, there are very few fMRI studies of human brain development. Nonetheless, the methods for the application of fMRI are nearly identical to those developed in PET and

SPECT studies. Therefore, these more traditional imaging technologies are presented in Section II. This section also addresses deeper issues involved in the dynamics of neural development, which may help guide the design of future neuroimaging studies.

Section III is dedicated to some of the clinical issues which may be addressed through the application of neuroimaging technologies. The chapters by Bookheimer and Dapretto, Shaywitz et al., and Filipek and Wood all discuss developmental disorders. Crucial questions concerning whether brain development is linear or nonlinear are addressed specifically in the chapter by Chugani. The application of fMRI to the study of dyslexia and normal brain development is also discussed in Section III. Finally, Section IV addresses some of the critical conceptual issues that will help guide the future applications of neuroimaging technologies. Understanding of brain and behavior relationships requires a careful interplay of practical and theoretical approaches, as discussed by Gonzalez-Lima and McIntosh and by Fletcher et al. The chapters by Fischer and Rose and by Luu and Tucker deal with the issues of nonlinear versus linear developmental processes. The clinical implications of these technologies as they relate to nonlinear developmental disorders, such as schizophrenia, are addressed by Friston.

At the earliest planning stages of this book, the editors discussed some of the critical issues in the study of human brain development and asked the authors to consider these issues as they wrote their respective chapters, although as editors we understood the difficult nature of these issues and did not expect each and every author to specifically address them. Nonetheless, we were pleased to find that many of these issues were discussed either directly or in the context of the experimental designs and scientific questions that were addressed. Among the most important issues was determining which imaging technology may be optimal for different developmental questions—for example, the issue of linear versus nonlinear rates of development, the presence or absence of critical periods, or the best techniques to measure the development of neural connections. Dr. Minshew's chapter in Section II reviews the important success of magnetic resonance spectroscopy (MRS) in the quantification of the development of synapses in the human brain. This is an important chapter because functional MRI is not capable of such direct measurements as MRS. Similarly, quantitative EEG and MEG studies are suitable for the noninvasive study of large populations of children over the entire lifespan, which is crucial for the neuroimaging of nonlinearities in cortical development. EEG and MEG, however, are primarily limited to cortical development and lack spatial precision without coregistration to MRI or fMRI. Another critical issue that the authors considered was whether interpretations from adult neuroimaging are similar and appropriate for the interpretations of neural functioning in children. For example, do the same structures have different functions at different ages or does the development of neural network connections result in the emergence of new functions? Although these are critical issues, the answers must await the future application of these new neuroimaging technologies.

Finally, the issue of nonlinear models of synaptic proliferation and synaptic pruning versus linear models of continuous and stable synaptogenesis is addressed by several authors (see the chapters by Molenaar et al., Thatcher, Fischer and Rose, and Luu and Tucker). This again is not a simple subject and will require time and effort to understand the presence or absence of regionally specific synaptogenesis or sudden changes in the strength of synaptic coupling. Nevertheless, it is exciting to realize that some of these most crucial and fundamental issues may some day be answered by and within the domain of developmental neuroimaging. It is hoped that this book may help stimulate thought and guide the efforts necessary to find the answers.

Robert W. Thatcher

List of Color Plates

I

NEUROIMAGING OF STRUCTURAL BRAIN DEVELOPMENT

1

The Developing Human Brain: A Morphometric Profile

Verne S. Caviness, Jr., David N. Kennedy, Julianna F. Bates, and Nikos Makris

Department of Neurology, Massachusetts General Hospital, Harvard Medical School, Boston, Massachusetts 02114

How large is the human brain? What is the rate of brain growth across the life progression from fetus through adolescence? These questions are central to cognitive neuroscience and the expectations of cognitive development. This is because each neural processing element of the brain is finite in size, and the number of processing elements is specified by the finite size of the brain (Cherniak, 1990, 1994; Ringo, 1991). Whereas it is inevitable that the processing capacity of the brain will be constrained by its volume, little is known about the arrangements and attributes of processing elements within the volume and the contributions of discrete processing operations to cognition and overt behavior (Goldman-Rakic, Isseroff, Schwartz, & Bugbee, 1983; Goldman-Rakic, 1987; Thatcher, Walker, & Giudice 1987; Fischer and Rose, 1994; Rakic, Bourgeois, & Goldman-Rakic, 1994). Our present knowledge is insufficient to support any coherent theory interrelating fundamental structural brain science and cognitive neuroscience. Yet the pace of advancements in the technology of functional brain imaging and the increasing analytic power of behavioral paradigms adapted to this technology are gradually bridging this gap. One current strategy of such investigations is to define elementary processing functions by behavioral paradigms and to map the brain locale where these functions are performed. The mapping process specifies location, but cannot at present specify the volume occupied by processing components. Furthermore, the mapping process implies an as-yet-unspecified quantitative relationship between the activity of discrete numbers of neurons and of synaptic transmissions in the realization of processing functions.

Thus, brain morphometry, though integral and necessary to an evolving theoretical and observational fabric of cognitive neuroscience, has not yet realized its full potential. For the time being, while its more analytical applications must wait, the challenge is to achieve a usefully complete and coherent observational database. Our present concern is to answer the questions phrased at the outset: How large is the brain and its component parts? What are the characteristics of brain growth across the developmental interval? Emerging brain imaging technology and computer assisted methods of image analysis place in hand the means to approach these questions.

The present essay has two specific objectives, which anticipate increasing integration of volumetric morphometry into cognitive neuroscience. The first is to provide, in volumetric terms, an overview of the growth profile of the human brain. The second is to interpret the growth profile in terms of the development of cellular and subcellular processing elements. The volumetric data is drawn from two general sources: volumetric analyses in living subjects based upon magnetic resonance imaging (MRI) with computer assisted image analysis methodology, and brain weights obtained postmortem. Presently, MRI-based volumetric studies have been extended only to the brain of the young adult and to that of the school age child. The data

DEVELOPMENTAL NEUROIMAGING

set for the young adult presents the brain just beyond the end of its growth cycle, when it is at full volume. The data set for the school age child provides the perspective of the brain in its terminal phase of growth, where volumetric increments, though modest, will be of paramount significance for adaptive behavior.

Substantial gaps in our volumetric profile of human brain development are left by these MRI-based studies. The gap in volumetric characterization between school age and the completion of the growth cycle is relatively small. The gap antecedent to school age is great; in fact, it is more than 90% of the growth trajectory of the brain. Thus, published values for brain weight obtained postmortem, our second source of data relating to brain growth, must for the present complete our general profile of overall brain growth.

Brain tissue obtained postmortem has also been the basis for analyses of cellular histogenesis in the human brain. Although of considerable value, these are of limited scope. For this reason, we will complement the view of histogenesis based upon analysis of human brain tissue with data derived from comprehensive histogenetic investigations in the developing monkey brain.

I. The Human Brain at the End of the Growth Cycle

The human brain completes its growth cycle and is at maximum volume by the middle of the second decade of life (Fig. 1; Lemire, Loeser, Leech, & Alvord, 1975; Dekaban and Sadowsky, 1978; Kretschmann, Kammradt, Krauthausen, Sauer, & Wingert, 1986). The mean volume of the entire brain of young adults, where male and female brains are equally represented, is 1380 cc^3 (Fig. 2) (Filipek, Kennedy, Caviness, Sprag-

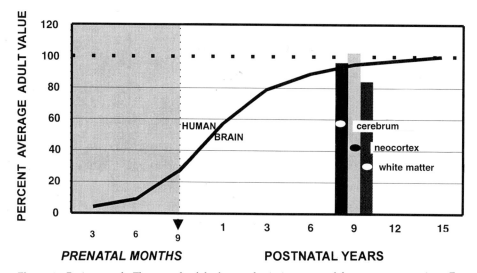

Figure 1 Brain growth. The growth of the human brain is presented from two perspectives. For both perspectives brain weight or volume is expressed as a percentage of the mean adult volume or weight (ordinate: 1 g = 1 centimeter^3), where 100 corresponds to the mean adult value. Age (abscissa) is expressed in months for fetal life and in years for postnatal life. (1) Curve: The first perspective is that of the full profile of brain growth, based upon brain weights obtained postmortem. This is expressed as a continuous change with growth continuing through the fetal months and the first 15 years of postnatal life (adapted from Lamire *et al.*, 1975). (2) Histograms: The second perspective is based upon volumetric analyses of magnetic resonance images. This perspective is the size of the cerebrum, the neocortex, and the cerebral central white matter taken from a cross-sectional analysis in the school age child. We have taken the mean volume for the full series where values for males and females were averaged (*n* = 30, including 15 male and 15 female brains) over an age range of 6–11 years, mean age 9 years, and have placed the histograms for the mean volumes at the mean age. At school age the overall cycle of growth is approximately completed (histogram in relation to curve; histograms adapted from Caviness *et al.*, 1996). Cerebral volume of the school age child, mean age 9 years, is scaled to overall brain size. That is, cerebral volume at school age, mean age 9 years, like total brain volume, is approximately 95% of the corresponding adult volume. By contrast, the neocortex is a relatively greater, while the cerebral central white matter is a relatively smaller, percentage of the corresponding adult values. This format for illustrating the profile of brain growth and the volumetric values for cerebrum, neocortex, and central white matter at school age, mean age 9 years, is also adapted to Figs. 8–10.

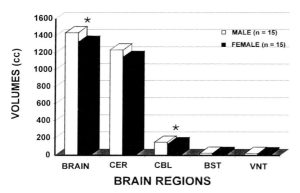

Figure 2 Volumes of principal brain regions of the adult male and female. The principal brain regions are cerebrum (CER), cerebellum (CBL), brain stem (BST), and ventricular system (VNT). (Adapted from Filipek *et al.*, 1994.) These structures are placed in relation to total brain volume (BRAIN). Significant (*p* < .05) gender effects are indicated with an asterisk.

gins, Rossnick, & Starewicz, 1989; Filipek, Richelme, Kennedy, & Caviness, 1994). This volume, computed from three-dimensional T1-weighted magnetic resonance image data sets, is concordant with that predicted from brain weights obtained postmortem (gram = cc^3) (Wessely, 1970; Paul, 1971; Zilles, 1972). The cerebrum is nearly 90% of the volume of the entire brain (Filipek et al., 1994). The volume of this region is 8 times that of the cerebellum and more than 50 times that of the brain stem. The cerebrum, in turn, is dominated by its gray matter components which represent more than 60% of the total volume, with less than 40% of cerebral volume represented by white matter.

More than 90% of cerebral gray matter is neocortex (Fig. 3), a proportion that highlights the central and

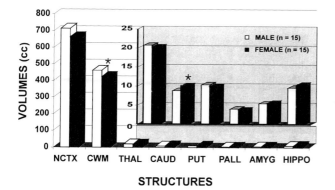

Figure 3 Volumes of cerebral structures of the adult male and female brain. The cerebral structures are neocortex (NCTX), central white matter (CWM), diencephalon (THAL), caudate nucleus (CAUD), putamen (PUT), globus pallidus (PALL), amygdaloid nucleus (AMYG), and hippocampus (HIPPO). The insert presents the volumes of smaller structures at a magnified scale. Significant (*p* < .05) gender effects are indicated with an asterisk. (Adapted from Filipek *et al.*, 1994.)

dominant role that neocortex plays in virtually all fully-integrated functions of the central nervous system. Other gray matter structures of the cerebrum, including diencephalon, basal ganglia, amygdala, and hippocampus, variably represent less than 1% to nearly 2% of the other gray matter of the cerebrum. In terms of neocortical volume relative to other gray matter structures, the approximate ratios vary from 128 times for the amygdala, to 70 times for caudate and hippocampus, 50 times for lenticulate nucleus, and 35 times for the thalamus.

A. Symmetry of Bilaterally Represented Structures

The volumes of bilaterally represented structures are symmetric or nearly so. Statistically significant asymmetries, favoring the structure in the right hemisphere, were noted only for neocortex (3.7%) and amygdala (9%). Particularly with respect to the neocortex, this close matching of right–left volumes could not have been predicted. Asymmetries are known to occur in neocortical gyral patterns, which are particularly conspicuous in the peri-sylvian region (Geschwind and Levitsky, 1968; Galaburda, Sanides, & Geschwind, 1978; Cheverud, Fall, Vanier, Konigsberg, Helmkamp, & Hildebolt, 1990; Ono, Jubik, & Abernathy, 1990; Rademacher, Galaburda, Kennedy, Filipek, & Caviness, 1992; Rademacher, Caviness, Steinmetz, & Galaburda, 1993). At present our measures (Filipek et al., 1994) apply only to overall neocortical volume and do not consider regional asymmetries, which may be correlated with the known local asymmetries in gyral patterns and lobular prominence.

B. Sexual Dimorphism

The brain volume of the adult female is about 93% that of the male brain (Filipek et al., 1994). Approximately 70% of this difference is attributable to the greater volume of central white matter in the male cerebrum, with the remainder of the difference attributable to a larger cerebellar volume in the male (Fig. 2). There is uniform female-to-male scaling of about 93% of volumes of major regions of the brain as well as of the separate structures within the cerebrum. Exceptions to this uniform female-to-male volumetric scaling are encountered with both caudate (absolute volume larger in female), and hippocampus (volume relative to cerebral volume greater in female). In terms of absolute volumetric differences, the structure most significantly smaller in the female forebrain is the cerebral central white matter. The absolute volume of the caudate nucleus and the volume of the hippocampus as a proportion of total cerebral volume are actually larger in the female than in the male brain.

II. Human Brain Growth

The foregoing volumetric analysis of the young adult brain characterizes the human brain at the end of its growth cycle when its volume will be maximum. The brain reaches its maximum size in the course of a developmental interval which extends over 1.5 decades of life. For a profile of the overall growth of the human brain across the full developmental interval, we resort to published weights of normal brains obtained postmortem (Lemire *et al.*, 1975; Dekaban and Sadowsky, 1978; Gilles, Leviton, & Dooling, 1983; Kretschmann *et al.*, 1986). The increase in brain volume, or weight, with development time is a non-linear function. Conventionally depicted, brain weight ascends continuously and smoothly (Fig. 1). The rate of brain growth is greatest during fetal and early postnatal life. A weight of approximately 100 g at 20 weeks gestation becomes 400 g at term. The absolute rate of growth is maximum (6% of the adult weight/month) in the several weeks bracketing term birth. This rate of growth decelerates by a factor of 2 by 10 months and by a factor of 4 by 18 months postnatal age (Dobbing and Sands, 1979). Substantial growth is to be expected after 18 months. The brain weight at that age, 800 g, is only 60% of the projected weight of 1100 g at 3 years, and the weight at 3 years is still only 80% of the projected weight at the end of the growth cycle. The asymptote is finally reached during the late grade-school years with approach of puberty (Lemire *et al.*, 1975; Kretschmann *et al.*, 1986).

Observation of the brain postmortem has also provided an overview of the emergence of brain shape in relation to developmental age and brain growth (Lemire *et al.*, 1975). The general shape of gray and white matter structures emerges early in the course of brain growth. All cortical and nuclear structures of the brain and the principal axonal pathways form during the first half of gestation, when brain growth is gradual (Sidman and Rakic, 1982). The appearance of gyri and sulci of the cerebral surface follows during the second half of gestation as the rate of brain growth accelerates. The sylvian fissure, the principal landmark of the lateral cerebral surface, is already evident by the end of the second trimester. Asymmetries in the configuration of this fissure and the adjacent opercular region and temporal plane are already evident as early as the fifth gestational month (Witelson and Pallie, 1973; Wada, Clarke, & Hamm, 1975; LeMay, 1976; Chi, Dooling, & Gilles, 1977). The general pattern of sec-

ondary fissures is evident at birth, and the full cerebral gyral pattern, including the tertiary fissures, is established by the end of second postnatal year of life (Larroche 1966–1967; Yakovlev and Lecours, 1967).

A. The Developing Brain: A View from the Asymptote of Growth

A volumetric analysis of the developing human brain which is sufficiently comprehensive and methodologically suitable for comparison with volumetrics taken at the end of the growth cycle has been accomplished only in children of grade school age (Caviness, Kennedy, Filipek, & Rademacher, 1995). The range of age in this childhood series, in which boys and girls are equally represented (15 males and 15 females), is 6–11 years with a mean age of 9.2 years. These children were normal with respect to gestational and postnatal history, school performance, neurological examination, and extensive psychometric testing (see Caviness *et al.*, 1995 for details of ascertainment of these "normal" criteria). The analysis is a cross–sectional survey, so that it carries no implications with respect to whether brain growth is stepwise or smoothly continuous with time. The average brain volume is 1312 cc^3 (Fig. 4). The cerebral hemispheres contribute 86% (1137 cc^3), the cerebellum is 11% (140 cc^3), while the brain stem and total ventricular system are only 2% (21 cc^3) and 1% (15 cc^3) respectively of total brain volumes. The total cerebral volume is approximately 67% gray matter and 33% white matter structures. The neocortex, mean volume 700 cc^3, is 62% of the total volume of the cerebrum (Fig. 5). The neocortex constitutes 92% of the total gray matter volume of the cerebrum. It is some 60 times the volume of the diencephalon, the second largest of the cere-

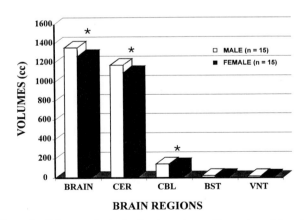

Figure 4 Volumes of principal brain regions of the male and female school age child. The principal brain regions are cerebrum (CER), cerebellum (CBL), brain stem (BST), and ventricular system (VNT). Significant ($p < .05$) gender effects are indicated with an asterisk. (From Caviness *et al.*, 1996).

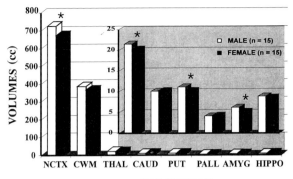

Figure 5 Volumes of cerebral structures of the male and female school age child. The cerebral structures are neocortex (NCTX), central white matter (CWM), diencephalon (THAL), caudate nucleus (CAUD), putamen (PUT), globus pallidus (PALL), amygdaloid nucleus (AMYG), and hippocampus (HIPPO). The insert presents the volumes of smaller structures at a magnified scale. Significant ($p <$ .05) gender effects are indicated with an asterisk. (From Caviness *et al.*, 1996.)

bral gray matter structures, and 165 times the volume of the amygdala, the smallest of the other cerebral gray matter structures. Thus, with the exception of the diencephalon, (about 3% of the total cerebral gray matter) none of the other cerebral gray matter structures distinguished in this analysis contributed more than 1% of the total cerebral gray matter. The ratio of total gray matter (neocortex, hippocampus, basal ganglia, amygdala, and thalamus) to central white matter in the cerebrum is 2:1. As with the brain as a whole (at the end of its growth cycle), bilaterally represented structures taken in their entirety are either symmetric or differ in their volumes by no more than a few percent.

B. Volumetric Comparison: Male and Female Brains

The brain of the school age female child is approximately 93% of the volume of the brain of the male child at this age (Fig. 4). This difference in volume of the entire brain is uniformly scaled among the major brain regions: cerebrum, cerebellum, and brain stem. That is, each of these principal regions in the female child's brain is variably 93–95% of its volume in the male child's brain. Within the cerebrum, the neocortex, thalamus, putamen (collectively 94% of the cerebral gray matter), and the central white matter of the female brain are also variably 92–95% of their volumes in the male brain (Fig. 5). Exceptions to this pattern of uniform scaling are the caudate, hippocampus, pallidum, and amygdala. The caudate, hippocampus, and pallidum are indistinguishable in size in male and female; that is, they are disproportionately large in the

female brain. The volume of the amygdala in the female, by contrast, is only 84% its volume in the male brain; that is, the amygdala is disproportionately small in the female brain.

This analysis documents a substantial dissociation in the relative stages of growth of gray matter and white matter in the school age brain. This implies that in the years of development leading up to school age, the modes of growth for gray and white matter are different, but both are approaching their terminal phases in the transition through childhood. The volumes of the collective gray matter structures of the forebrain of the child are already at their adult values (Fig. 6, 7). Certain subcortical gray matter structures, such as the caudate, putamen, and amygdala in the male child and the pallidum in the female child, are measured at greater volumes in the school age brain than in the adult brain. The only cerebral gray matter structures larger in adults than in children are the hippocampus in both males (not statistically significant) and females (statistically significant), and the amygdala (statistically significant) in females. The central white matter of the cerebrum, in contrast to the gray matter, is only approximately 85% of its anticipated volume in the adult brain (Filipek *et al.*, 1994). However, the hippocampus, as parcellated in this analysis, includes white matter fiber systems (fimbria, fornix, commissure) which are probably volumetrically large relative to the actual size of the hippocampal "gray matter" or cortex proper. Thus, the gray matter component of the "hippocampus," as with other gray matter structures of the cerebrum, may also be larger than the adult counterpart, though this was not detected here.

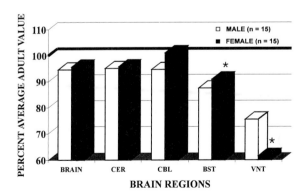

Figure 6 Volumes of principal brain regions of the male and female school age child as percent of adult values. (From Filipek *et al.*, 1994.) The heavy dark line at 100% corresponds to the mean value for the young adult brain regions. The principal brain regions are cerebrum (CER), cerebellum (CBL), brain stem (BST), and ventricular system (VNT). Significant ($p <$ .05) gender effects are indicated with an asterisk. (From Caviness *et al.*, 1996.)

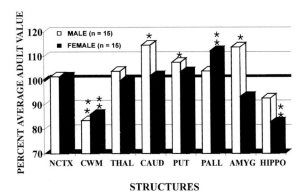

Figure 7 Volumes of cerebral structures of the male and female brain of the school age child as percent of adult values. (From Filipek *et al.*, 1994.) The heavy dark line at 100% corresponds to the mean value for the young adult cerebral regions. The cerebral structures are neocortex (NCTX), central white matter (CWM), diencephalon (THAL), caudate nucleus (CAUD), putamen (PUT), globus pallidus (PALL), amygdaloid nucleus (AMYG), and hippocampus (HIPPO). Significant ($p < .05$) gender effects are indicated with an asterisk and ($p < .002$) with two asterisks. (From Caviness *et al.*, 1996.)

Dissociation in the relative stages of growth of gray matter and white matter over the first 9 years, as revealed in the volumetric analysis of the brain of the school age child, is reflective of a fundamental strategy of histogenesis known to be general to central nervous system development in mammals. Thus, the development of the neuronal elements of the central nervous system advances through a "progressive" mode which is succeeded by a "regressive" mode of development. The progressive mode is marked by increase in neuronal numbers and by growth and differentiation of dendritic, axonal, and somatic components of the neuron. In contrast, the regressive mode is marked by elimination of large numbers of neurons. There is also redirection of axons and pruning back of axonal and dendritic arbors.

As will be seen in the subsequent comparative presentation of cellular development in the monkey and the human brain, the neuronal population of the brain at school age may be inferred to be in transition between progressive and regressive modes of development. This is explicit with respect to gray matter which is principally "neuronal" (predominantly neuronal somata, dendrites, and local axonal circuits) in composition. The monkey-to-human comparison suggests that the transition between progressive and regressive modes of growth occurs well before school age with respect to axons. In children of school age, the determinants of volumetric growth of central white matter are, presumably, enlargement and proliferation of glial elements with formation of myelin.

III. Beyond Volumetrics: The Cellular Structure of the Brain

The gray and white matter structures of the brain are distinguished by their different signal intensities in magnetic resonance images (Caviness, Filipek, & Kennedy, 1993). For volumetric morphometry of gray and white matter structures, their boundaries are defined by computer assisted "segmentation" methods (Caviness *et al.*, 1993). The spatial resolution of this magnetic resonance-based method of morphometry is some 1–2 mm, which is several orders of magnitude less than the resolution required for visualization of the cellular processing elements of neural circuits. We must also remind ourselves that the segmentation lines which distinguish gray and white matter imply an artificial separation between the neuronal cell body and the axon, which transmits an action potential from that cell body to its synaptic destinations.

A. The Neuronal Component of Gray Matter

Gray matter volumes of neocortex, and probably also of other forebrain gray matter structures, allow useful inferences about the densities of cellular processing elements in these structures. This is because the cellular processing elements are distributed at relatively uniform density within gray matter structures of the forebrain in the mammalian central nervous system (Schüz and Palm, 1989; Cherniak, 1990). For reference, we review very briefly the set of principal neuronal elements of the neocortex. Neuronal elements, strictly speaking, represent only about 30% by volume of the cerebral cortex, the remainder of the volume being taken by glial and non-neuroglial elements (Schüz and Palm, 1989; Cherniak, 1990). Of the strictly "neuronal" volume, 8% corresponds to neuronal somata while only 22% is given to "neuropil," (dendrites, axons, and synapses), the actual contact points for systems operation. Only some 10% of the somata belong to Golgi type I neurons, which are the source of the cortical efferent axons that descend and exit the cortex (Globus and Scheibel, 1967; Braitenberg, 1978, 1989; Szentagothai, 1978). Interneurons, the predominant interneuronal class, give rise to axons involved only in local circuitry within the cortex (Braitenberg, 1978). Collectively, the synapses of the local cortical circuitry probably constitute as much as 80% or more of the total cortical synapses. The remaining synaptic complements are contributed by the terminals of cortical afferents, including those arising subcortically and those arising from other cortical regions of the same or opposite hemisphere (Braitenberg, 1978, 1989; Szentagothai, 1978).

B. The Neuronal Component of White Matter

The axon of the Golgi type I neuron, upon exiting the cortex, enters the central white matter of the cerebrum. This compartment is largely composed of axons mediating excitatory connections between neocortical regions, separated from each other by millimeters to centimeters (Krieg, 1963; Braitenberg, 1978, 1989; Szentagothai, 1978). Approximately 95% of these fibers interconnect cortical regions of the same hemisphere, while an estimated 2–4% cross the corpus callosum and interconnect regions in the two hemispheres (Nunez, 1989; see also Lamantia and Rakic, 1990, for comparable estimates for rhesus). No more than 1–2% of the fibers of the cerebral central white matter are thought to constitute neocortical afferents from the thalamus or cortical efferents directed to subcortical structures.

IV. Histogenesis as an Engine of Brain Growth

The strictly neuronal composition of gray and white matter structures becomes established in the course of an extended series of complex overlapping cellular events. The brain of the school age child, we have inferred, is in transition between opposing modes of histogenesis when the vigorous progressive processes become supplanted by the fine tuning of regressive processes. Extensive analyses of histogenetic events in the rhesus monkey brain, marked by state-of-the-art cytological and statistical treatments, provide a framework from which to deduce the course of less well-characterized histogenetic events of human brain development.

The histogenetic interval in monkey brain growth continues for a only a fraction of the time required for brain histogenesis in the human brain. In order to use the sequence of histogenetic events in monkey as a model for those in human, we have "normalized" the rhesus developmental time line to that of the human. To do this, we have designated a series of "timemarks" of equivalence to act as fixed points for "stretching" the time line in monkey to fit the longer time line in human. The time line in monkey has been stretched by a factor increasing from 2 during early gestation, to 3 for the prepubertal years, and to 4 for puberty and beyond. For example, neocortical cytogenesis, completed at 3 months gestation in monkey, continues until nearly 6 months in the human cerebrum. Term occurs at 5.5 months in monkey, but at 9 months in human. Puberty, occurring at 3 years in monkey, is to be matched by puberty at 12 years in human. Finally, the end of the histogenetic cycle, accepted to be 5 years in monkey, is here taken to be 20 years in man. In the account of neocortical histogenesis to follow, we transfer the pattern of the progression of cellular events as experimentally determined in monkey upon the profile of brain growth in man, where the progression of events in monkey and brain growth in man are normalized as percentiles of total development. Reflecting the emphasis upon these structures in cytological studies in man and monkey, our emphasis here is upon the cellular events of cerebral development; in particular, its the development of neocortex and central white matter.

A. Cerebral Histogenesis

1. Neocortex

Reliable measurements of the path of developmental change of neocortical volume in the human are not available. However, by extrapolation from analyses in the monkey, the volume of human neocortex may be expected to attain, or even exceed, the adult volume in early postnatal life (Fig. 8). The prefrontal cortex of the rhesus reaches its maximum thickness 2 months after birth (Bourgeois, Goldman-Rakic, & Rakic, 1994). The width of the cortex declines only slightly over the next 2 years as the animal approaches puberty. After puberty and beyond the third year of life, cortical width (and volume) drops steadily over several years. The width of the cortex at the end of the growth cycle in monkey is only approximately 60–70% the maximum value observed at 2 months (Bourgeois et al., 1994). Neocortical volume in the human brain is projected by extrapolation from monkey to be still-sustained at maximum values through school age years, but with gradual regression occurring afterwards to puberty.

By the time that maximum cortical width is achieved in the human, just as in the monkey neocortex, both the cycle of neuronal formation and that of neuronal elimination by histogenetic cell death have run their overlapping courses and the number of neocortical neurons has become fixed. Surviving neocortical neurons will have completed their cycles of elaboration and pruning of dendritic arbors, so that the configuration of their dendritic arbors will have become fixed (Fig. 8; Becker, Armstrong, Chan, & Wood, 1984; Mrzljak, Uyling, Kostovic, & van Eden, 1992; Huttenlocher, 1994). Correspondingly, the neuropil in monkey reaches its maxi-

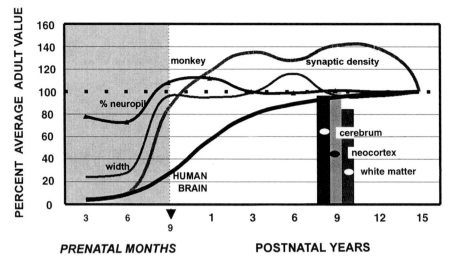

Figure 8   Developmental profile of cellular elements of neocortex. Measures in the developing monkey include neuropil as percent cortical volume (% neuropil), cortical width (width), and synaptic density, each illustrated as a separate curve. (Adapted from Bourgeois et al., 1994.) These measures are placed in relation to the profile of human brain growth as illustrated in Fig. 1. These values are expressed as a percentage of adult values (ordinate) as normalized to the human developmental time interval (abscissa) by conventions set forth in text. The format for representing human brain growth and volumes of cerebrum, neocortex, and cerebral central white matter in the school age child is described in the legend for Fig. 1.

mum proportion of neocortex, 84%, at the second postnatal month (Fig. 8). The principal afferent systems of the forebrain will have established their general patterns of distribution with respect to the neocortical map long before cortical width becomes maximum, (during the latter half of gestation) (Goldman and Galkin, 1978; Goldman-Rakic, 1981; Schwartz and Goldman-Rakic, 1991; Schwartz, Dekker, & Goldman, 1991), and the fundamental columnar organization characteristic of the interhemispheric and neocortical associational systems will have been established (Goldman-Rakic, 1981; Schwartz and Goldman-Rakic, 1984). In the human neocortex, enlargement of neuronal somata and dendritic arbors continues minimally for an uncertain time after the third postnatal year and is no longer detectable by the sixth year of life (Conel, 1939–1967).

The profile of human and monkey neocortical synaptogenesis surges in the early postnatal period to attain densities which are as much as 150% of those characteristic of the end of the growth cycle (Bourgeois, Jastreboff, & Rakic, 1989; Bourgeois and Rakic, 1993; Bourgeois et al., 1994; Huttenlocher, de Courten, Garey, & Van der Loos, 1982; Huttenlocher, 1987) (Fig. 8). The surge in synaptogenesis is delayed somewhat, relative to the profile of increase in width of cortex and the progression of neuropil as a percentage of cortical volume (Fig. 8). In the occipital region, the maximum total number of synapses is also 150% greater than the number at the end of the growth cycle (Huttenlocher et al., 1982; Huttenlocher, 1990). The advance of synapto-

genesis in the prefrontal cortex, as reflected in synaptic density, is closely parallel in man and monkey after normalization for differences in the developmental time scale (Huttenlocher, 1979; Bourgeois et al., 1994). Synaptic density in the rhesus prefrontal cortex ascends in parallel with that of the overall neuropil (Zecevic, Bourgeois, & Rakic, 1989; Bourgeois et al., 1994), and parallels that of cortical width and of neuropil as a percent of total cortical volume, with maximum values sustained through puberty. Synaptic density then declines gradually through puberty and adolescence (Bourgeois et al., 1994; Huttenlocher, 1994; Rakic et al., 1994) to the adult levels, which are approximately 50% of the maximum values registered in the early postnatal period (Bourgeois et al., 1994). General neocortical glucose utilization in the human brain, determined from birth through adult life by positron emission tomography (PET) scanning (and taken to be an index of synaptic activity), follows closely the profile of prefrontal synaptic density. Thus, maximum signal intensities, twice those of the adult brain, are achieved in the first 2 years of life. These high values are sustained through age 9 and then decline gradually to adult values through adolescence (Chugani and Phelps, 1986; Chugani, Phelps, & Mazziotta, 1987; Chugani, 1994).

2. Central White Matter

The corpus callosum is the only major cortico-cortical fiber system of the cerebral central white matter for which the developmental events in the brains of human and monkey have been worked out in detail (Clarke, Kraftsik, Van der Loos, & Innocenti, 1989; Lamantia and Rakic, 1990). The corpus callosum in the human brain is assumed here to follow the same sequence of cellular developmental events that is characteristic of callosal development in rhesus and other callosal species (Innocenti, 1991). The human commissure enlarges in its cross-sectional area in late fetal life, reaching a maximum area for the fetal phase of development late in the third trimester (Clarke *et al.*, 1989). A secondary phase of areal enlargement is initiated in the early months of postnatal life and continues rapidly through 5 years of age, at which time the callosal area is some 80–90% of the adult value. The residual areal growth of some 10–20% occurs between 5 and 14 years of age. This normalized pace of enlargement of the commissure in the monkey brain corresponds generally to that in the human, though the maximum area and length of the commissure are approached somewhat earlier, relatively speaking, than in the human brain (Fig. 9).

In monkey, this general developmental profile of the corpus callosum has been considered in terms of numbers of axons traversing the commissure at the cerebral midline and axonal density in the commissure (Fig. 10). The initial axons to cross the midplane, in the dorsal septal massa commissuralis (Rakic and Yakovlev, 1968), do so before midgestation. The rate of decussation accelerates and the maximum number of callosal axons, achieved by birth, is 3.5 times the number to cross the commissure in the adult animal. At this point, where the number of crossing axons is maximum, the cross-sectional area of the commissure is only about half that of the adult (Fig. 9). In the early postnatal period, there follows a process of elimination of callosal axons which continues rapidly through the first postnatal weeks and then more slowly through puberty, until the final number is reached in early adult life. This system of axons in the human brain, by extrapolation from the observations in monkey, should reach its maximum numbers in the perinatal period, with subsequent sharp decline to approach the adult values between the third and fifth years of life (Fig. 10). Thus, there is the paradox that the period of rapid reduction in the number of callosal axons roughly parallels the interval of most rapid growth in the cross-sectional area of the commissure.

Whereas a portion of the population of eliminated axons must arise from neurons of layers V and VI (Lamantia and Rakic, 1990), or even from neurons of the subplate (Kostovic and Rakic 1980; Chun, Nakamura, & Shatz, 1987), most of the pruning involves reduction of an axonal contingent arising from the neocortical association neurons of the supragranular layers (Lamantia and Rakic, 1990; Innocenti, 1991). We have assumed that the sequence and timing of cellular events of callosal development are approximately representative of the much-greater mass of associational neurons of the cerebral hemisphere. In support of this general assumption, it has been observed in the cat

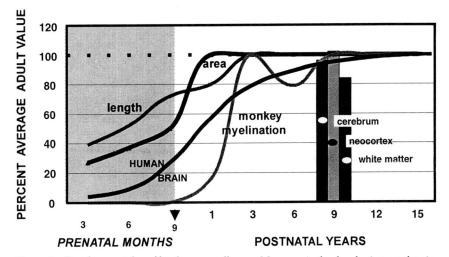

Figure 9 Developmental profile of corpus callosum. Measures in the developing monkey include callosal length (length), callosal area (area), and the percentage of callosal axons which are myelinated (myelination). (Adapted from Lamantia and Rakic, 1990.) These measures are placed in relation to the profile of human brain growth illustrated in Fig. 1. These values are expressed as a percentage of adult values (ordinate) as normalized to the human developmental time interval (abscissa) by conventions set forth in text. The format for representing human brain growth and volumes of cerebrum, neocortex, and cerebral central white matter in the school age child is described in the legend for Fig. 1.

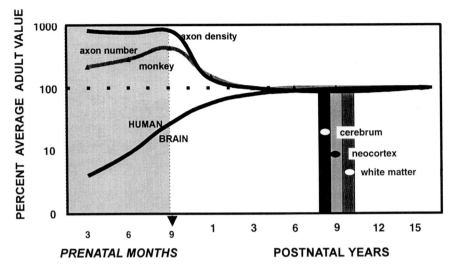

Figure 10 Developmental profile of corpus callosum. Measures in the developing monkey are callosal axon density and total number of callosal axons (axon number). (Adapted from Lamantia and Rakic, 1990.) These measures are placed in relation to the profile of human brain growth illustrated in Fig. 1. These values are expressed as a percentage of adult values (ordinate) as normalized to the human developmental time interval (abscissa) by conventions set forth in text. The format for representing human brain growth and volumes of cerebrum, neocortex, and cerebral central white matter in the school age child is described in the legend for Fig. 1.

that pruning of callosal axons arising from neurons of the auditory region is coordinated with the formation of associational connections within the same hemisphere (Innocenti, 1986, 1991).

The apparent paradox of callosal development—that the commissure enlarges most rapidly as its axons are most rapidly eliminated—reflects the preeminent contribution of myelination to the volume of the cerebrum. In monkey, only a relatively small fraction of callosal axons becomes myelinated in fetal and early postnatal life (Lamantia and Rakic, 1990), that is, during the period of axonal elaboration and the most rapid period of axonal elimination. The pace of myelination picks up only in the fourth postnatal week, when the process of axonal elimination is already proceeding swiftly, and continues strongly through the end of the first postnatal year (Fig. 9). The staggered phasing of axonal elimination and myelination suggests that the myelinated axons are not those which are eliminated (Lamantia and Rakic, 1990). The total area of the commissure continues to increase and reaches its maximum value near puberty. This continued increase beyond the first year of life in monkey, and by extrapolation during the prepubertal years in human, represents enlargement of axons and expansion of the glial composition of the commissure, and not further modification of the number of axonal elements of which it is constituted (Lamantia and Rakic, 1990). Thus, the augmentation in volume of central

white matter in the human brain, to be expected beyond school age, probably reflects the advance of myelination without revision of the axonal population itself.

MRI-based morphometry, in conjunction with other technological modes of analysis, is presently in a state of methodological development. This prolonged stage of methodological development will ultimately give way to a substantially larger emphasis upon application in human brain science. The organizing goals will remain the definition and mapping within the brain of the elementary processing components of neural systems that contribute to cognitive operations and generation of overt behavior. Coordinated behavioral and imaging methods will become increasingly reliable. Invariant mapping patterns will emerge, and these will support an increasingly coherent theoretical synthesis relating to the nature of the cognitive process. Obviously, much depends upon the analytic force of cognitive and behavioral paradigms. Much also depends upon the efficiency and reliability of tools and procedures of analysis which, for the present, are highly constrained by the environment imposed by functional imaging systems. Advances will depend upon the suitability of quantitative methods. We anticipate that morphometry will be indispensable in this overall program of human brain science, both as a mode of mapping and as basis for a quantitative denominator for foci of activation.

Acknowledgments

Supported by NIH Grant PO1 NS27950 and a grant from the Fairway Trust.

References

Becker, L. E., Armstrong, D. L., Chan, F., & Wood, M. M. (1984). Dendritic development in human occipital cortical neurons. *Developmental Brain Research, 13*, 117–124.

Bourgeois, J., Goldman-Rakic, P. S., & Rakic, P. (1994). Synaptogenesis in the prefrontal cortex of rhesus monkeys. *Cerebral Cortex, 4*, 78–96.

Bourgeois, J. P., Jastreboff, P. J., & Rakic, P. (1989). Synaptogenesis in visual cortex of normal and preterm monkeys: Evidence for intrinsic regulation of synaptic overproduction. *Proceedings of the National Academy of Sciences, USA 86*, 4297–4301.

Bourgeois, J., & Rakic, P. (1993). Changes of synaptic density in the primary visual cortex of the macaque monkey from fetal to adult stage. *Journal of Neuroscience, 13*, 2801–2860.

Braitenberg, V. (1978). Cortical architectonics: general and areal. In M. Brazier & H. Petsche (Eds.), *Architectonics of the cerebral cortex* (pp. 442–465). New York: Raven.

Braitenberg, V. (1989). Some arguments for a theory of cell assemblies in the cerebral cortex. In L. Nadel, L. Cooper, P. Culiocover, & M. Harnish (Eds.), *Neural connections, mental computation* (pp. 137–145). Cambridge, MA: MIT.

Caviness, V. S., Jr., Kennedy, D. O., Filipek, P. A., & Rademacher, J. (1996). The brain of the school age child: A volumetric analysis based upon magnetic resonance images. *Cerebral Cortex*, in press.

Caviness, V. S., Jr., Filipek, P. A., & Kennedy, D. N. (1993). Longitudinal research and a biology of human brain development and behavior. In C. P. Magnuson (Ed.), *Longitudinal research: Present status and future perspectives (pp. 60-74)* Cambridge, UK: Cambridge Univ. Press.

Cherniak, C. (1990). The bounded brain: Toward quantitative neuroanatomy. *Journal of Cognitive Neuroscience, 2*, 58–68.

Cherniak, C. (1994). Component placement optimization in the brain. *Journal of Neuroscience, 14*, 2418–2427.

Cheverud, J., Fall, D., Vanier, M., Konigsberg, L., Helmkamp, R. C., & Hildebolt, C. (1990). Heritability of brain size and surface features in rhesus macaques *(Macaca mulatta). Journal of Heredity, 81*, 51–57.

Chi, J., Dooling, D., & Gilles, F. (1977). Left–right asymmetries of the temporal speech areas of the human fetus. *Archives of Neurology, 34*, 346–348.

Chugani, H. (1994). Development of regional brain glucose metabolism in relation to behavior and plasticity. In G. Dawson & K. W. Fischer (Eds.), *Human behavior and the developing brain* (pp. 153–175). New York: Guilford.

Chugani, H. T., & Phelps, M. E. (1986). Maturational changes in cerebral function in infants determined by 18FDG positron emission tomography. *Science, 231*, 840–843.

Chugani, H. T., Phelps, M. E., & Mazziotta, J. C. (1987). Positron emission tomography study of human brain functional development. *Annals of Neurology, 22*, 487–497.

Chun, J. J., Nakamura, M. J., & Shatz, C. J. (1987). Transient cells of the developing mammalian telencephalon are peptide–immunoreactive neurons. *Nature (London), 325*, 617–620.

Clarke, S., Kraftsik, R., Van der Loos, H., & Innocenti, G. (1989). Forms and measures of the adult and developing corpus callosum: Is there sexual dimorphism. *Journal of Comparative Neurology, 280*, 213–230.

Conel, J. L. (1939–1967). *The postnatal development of the human cerebral cortex*. Cambridge, MA: Harvard.

Dekaban, A., & Sadowsky, D. (1978). Changes in brain weight during the span of human life: Relation of brain weights to body heights and body weights. *Annals of Neurology, 4*, 345–356.

Dobbing, J., & Sands, J. (1979). Comparative aspects of the brain growth spurt. *Early Human Development, 3*, 79–83.

Filipek, P. A., Kennedy, D. O., Caviness, V. S., Jr., Spraggins, T. A., Rossnick, S. L., & Starewicz, P. M. (1989). MRI-based morphometry: Development and applications to normal controls. *Annals Neurology, 25*, 61–67.

Filipek, P. A., Richelme, C., Kennedy, D. N., Caviness, V. S., Jr. (1994). The young adult human brain: An MRI-based morphometric analysis. *Cerebral Cortex, 4*, 344–360.

Fischer, K. W., & Rose, S. P. (1994). Dynamic development of coordination of components in brain and behavior: A framework for theory and research. In G. Dawson & K. W. Fischer (Eds.), *Human behavior and the developing brain* (pp. 3–66). New York: Guilford.

Galaburda, A. M., Sanides, F., & Geschwind, N. (1978). Cytoarchitectonic left-right asymmetries in the temporal speech region. *Archives of Neurology, 35*, 812–817.

Geschwind, N., & Levitsky, W. (1968). Human brain: Left–right asymmetries in temporal speech region. *Science, 161*, 168–187.

Gilles, F. H., Leviton, A., & Dooling, E. C. (1983). *The developing human brain*. Boston, MA: John Wright, PSG Inc.

Globus, A., & Scheibel, A. B. (1967). Pattern and field in cortical structure: The rabbit. *Journal of Comparative Neurology, 131*, 155–172.

Goldman, P. S., & Galkin, T. W. (1978). Prenatal removal of frontal association cortex in the fetal rhesus monkey: Anatomical and functional consequences in postnatal life. *Brain Research, 152*, 451–485.

Goldman-Rakic, P. S. (1981). Development and plasticity of primate frontal association cortex. In F. O. Schmit, F. G. Worden, S. G. Dennis, & G. Adelman (Eds.), *The organization of cerebral cortex*. (pp. 69–97) Cambridge, MA: MIT.

Goldman-Rakic, P. S. (1987). Development of cortical circuitry and cognitive function. *Child Development, 58*, 601–622.

Goldman-Rakic, P. S., Isseroff, A., Schwartz, M. L., & Bugbee, N. M. (1983). The neurobiology of cognitive development. In P. Mussen (Ed.), *Handbook of child psychology: Biology and infancy development* (pp. 281–344). New York: Wiley.

Huttenlocher, P. R. (1979). Synaptic density in human frontal cortex. Developmental changes and effects of aging. *Brain Res. 163*, 195–205.

Huttenlocher, P. R. (1987). The development of synapses in striate cortex of man. *Human Neurobiology, 6*, 1–9.

Huttenlocher, P. R. (1990). Morphometric study of human cerebral cortex development. *Neuropsychologia, 28*, 517–527.

Huttenlocher, P. R. (1994). Synaptogenesis in human cerebral cortex. In G. Dawson & K. W. Fischer (Eds.), *Human behavior and the developing brain* (pp. 137–152). New York: Guilford.

Huttenlocher, P. R., de Courten, C., Garey, L. J., & Van der Loos, H. (1982). Synaptogenesis in the human visual cortex—evidence for synapse elimination during normal development. *Neuroscience Letters, 33*, 247–252.

Innocenti, G. M. (1986). General organization of callosal connections in the cerebral cortex. In E. G. Jones & A. Peters (Eds.), *Cerebral cortex: Sensory-motor areas and aspects of cortical connectivity* (pp. 291–354). New York: Plenum.

Innocenti, G. M. (1991). The development of projections from cerebral cortex. *Progress in Sensory Physiology, 12*, 65–114.

Kostovic, I., & Rakic, P. (1980). Cytology and time of origin of interstitial neurons in the white matter in infant and adult human and monkey telencephalon. *Journal of Neurocytology, 9,* 219–242.

Kretschmann, H. J., Kammradt, G., Krauthausen, I., Sauer, B., & Wingert, F. (1986). Brain growth in man. In H. J. Kretschmann (Eds.), *Brain growth* (pp. 1–26). Basel: Karger.

Krieg, W. J. S. (1963). *Connections of the cerebral cortex.* Chicago: Brain Books.

Lamantia, A. S., & Rakic, P. (1990). Axon overproduction and elimination in the corpus callosum of the developing rhesus monkey. *Journal of Neuroscience, 10,* 2156–2175.

Larroche, J. C. (1966–1967). Development of the nervous system in early life, In F. Falkner (Ed.), *Human development* (pp. 257–276). Philadelphia: Saunders.

LeMay, M. (1976). Morphological cerebral asymmetries of modern man, fossil man, and nonhuman primate. *Annals of the New York Academy of Sciences, 280,* 349–366.

Lemire, R. J., Loeser, J. D., Leech, R. W., & Alvord, E. C., Jr. (1975). *Normal and abnormal development of the human nervous system.* Hagerstown, MD: Harper & Row.

Mrzljak, L., Uylings, H. B., Kostovic, I., & van Eden, C. G. (1992). Prenatal development of neurons in the human prefrontal cortex. II. A quantitative Golgi study. *Journal of Comparative Neurology, 316,* 485–496.

Nunez, P. (1989). Generation of human EEG by a combination of long and short range neocortical interactions. *Brain Topography, 1,* 199–215.

Ono, M., Jubik, S., & Abernathy, C. D. (1990). *Atlas of the cerebral sulci.* New York: Thieme Verlag.

Paul, F. (1971). Biometrische Analyse der Firschvolumina des Grosshirnrinde und des Prosencephalon von 31 menschlichen, adulten Gehirnen. *Zeitschrift für Anatomie und Entwicklungs-Geschichte, 133,* 325–368.

Rademacher, J., Caviness, V. S., Jr., Steinmetz, H., & Galaburda, A. M. (1993). Topographical variation of the human primary cortices: implications for neuroimaging, brain mapping and neurobiology. *Cerebral Cortex, 3,* 313–329.

Rademacher, J., Galaburda, A. M., Kennedy, D. N., Filipek, P. A., & Caviness, V. S., Jr. (1992). Human cerebral cortex: Localization, parcellation, and morphometry with magnetic resonance imaging. *Journal of Cognitive Neuroscience, 4,* 352–374.

Rakic, P., Bourgeois, J., & Goldman-Rakic, P. S. (1994). Competitive interactions during neural and synaptic development. *Progress in Brain Research 102,* 227–243.

Rakic, P., & Yakovlev, P. I. (1968). Development of the corpus callosum and cavum septi in man. *Journal of Comparative Neurology, 132,* 45–72.

Ringo, J. L. (1991). Neuronal interconnection as a function of brain size. *Brain Behavior and Evolution, 38,* 1–6.

Schüz, A., & Palm, G. (1989). Density of neurons and synapses in the cerebral cortex of the mouse. *Journal of Comparative Neurology, 286,* 442–455.

Schwartz, M. L., Dekker, J. J., & Goldman, R. P. S. (1991). Dual mode of corticothalamic synaptic termination in the mediodorsal nucleus of the rhesus monkey. *Journal of Comparative Neurology, 309,* 289–304.

Schwartz, M. L., & Goldman-Rakic, P. S. (1984). Callosal and intrahemispheric connectivity of the prefrontal association cortex in rhesus monkey: Relation between intraparietal and principal sulcal cortex. *Journal of Comparative Neurology, 226,* 403–420.

Schwartz, M. L., & Goldman-Rakic, P. S. (1991). Prenatal specification of callosal connections in rhesus monkey. *Journal of Comparative Neurology, 307,* 144–162.

Sidman, R. L., & Rakic, P. (1982). Development of the human central nervous system. In W. Haymaker & R. D. Adams (Eds.), *Histology and histopathology of the nervous system* (pp. 3–145). Springfield, IL: Thomas.

Szentagothai, J. (1978). The neural network of the cerebral cortex: A functional interpretation. *Proceedings of the Royal Society, London, 201,* 219–248.

Thatcher, R. W., Walker, R. A., & Giudice, S. (1987). Human cerebral hemispheres develop at different rates and ages. *Science, 236,* 1110–1113.

Wada, J. A., Clarke, R., & Hamm, A. (1975). Cerebral hemispheric asymmetry in humans: Cortical speech zones in 100 zones adult and 100 infant brains. *Archives of Neurology, 32,* 239–246.

Wessely, W. (1970). Biometrische Analyse der Frischvolumina des Rhombencephalon des Cerebellum und der Ventrikel von 31 adulten, menschlichen Gehirnen. *Journal Für Hirnforschung, 12,* 11–28.

Witelson, S. F., & Pallie, W. (1973). Left hemisphere specialization for language in the newborn: neuroanatomical evidence of asymmetry. *Brain, 96,* 641–646.

Yakovlev, P. I., & Lecours, A. R. (1967). The myelogenetic cycles of regional maturation of the brain. In A. Minkowski (Ed.), *Regional development of the brain in early life* (pp. 3–70). Oxford, U. K.: Blackwell.

Zecevic, N. Bourgeois, J. P., & Rakic, P. (1989). Changes in synaptic density in motor cortex of rhesus monkey during fetal and postnatal life. *Developmental Brain Research, 50,* 11–32.

Zilles, K. (1972). Biometrische Analyse der Frischvolumina verschiedener prosencephaler Hirnregionen von 78 menschlichen adulten Gehirnen. *Gegenbaurs Morphologisches Jahrbuch 118,* 234–273.

2

Modeling Morphometric Changes of the Brain during Development

Arthur W. Toga, Paul Thompson, and Bradley A. Payne

Laboratory of Neuro Imaging, University of California, Los Angeles, California 90024

I. Introduction

The anatomic and cellular organization of the fetal brain have been well-characterized for several species at different developmental stages, on the basis of both clinical scanning (Damasio, 1994) and *postmortem* histologic studies (Schambra, Lauder, & Silver, 1992). Modeling morphometric changes during brain development provides a means for quantitating and visualizing the rate and extent of the complex growth processes taking place throughout the system. As with any spatial measurement, the geometry of the system being analyzed must be clearly defined in order to understand its shape. Three-dimensional (3D) reconstruction techniques for representing the internal and external geometry of the brain provide an excellent resource for modeling the dynamic changes in the cellular architecture during development. Manipulation of the morphometric models with image warping techniques provides a mathematical representation of the changes observed in a developing biological system.

Numerous biological explanations for the developmentally driven changes that occur in the brain have been suggested. For example, developmental models describe the radial architecture which guides cell migration in the vertebrate brain (Rakic, 1972). Others provide explanation for the emergence of folding patterns in the cortical surface on the basis of the mechanical properties and thickness of its component layers (Richman, Stewart, Hutchison, & Caviness, 1975), or as the result of biphasic growth within individual gyri (Smart and McSherry, 1986). In several of these models, a link is effected between the gross anatomy of the fetal brain and the microstructure of the cerebrum, which constrains the cellular processes occurring within it. Some models rely on restrictive assumptions about the geometry and elasticity of the embryonic brain, modeling it as a triaxial ellipsoid (Todd, 1982), or as possessing cortical layers which are homogeneous and uniformly stressed, making uniform growth implicit (Richman et al., 1975). However, none of these models incorporates computerized representations to help substantiate, quantitate, and visualize the effects of the hypothesized explanations. A more sophisticated analysis of the internal and external topological and geometric changes of the fetal brain and its substructures requires 3D digital data, together with algorithms capable of modeling and quantitating the internal volume and surface dynamics of the system, at a local level.

This chapter describes the use of 3D reconstruction and warping techniques to model the geometry of the brain at different stages of development. The modeling transformations are biologically constrained and result in a quantitative visual representation of morphological changes during development. The chapter is organized into four parts. First, we examine three dynamic components of the embryonic process in the vertebrate brain. The emphasis is on the geometric transforma-

DEVELOPMENTAL NEUROIMAGING

tions which these processes induce in key substructures of the brain. Second, we review previous models of fissuration in the cerebral cortex, and the light these models shed on the differential growth regimes responsible for producing convolutions in the surface. Third, we outline computational models for representing the surfaces of key structures in the developing brain. Finally, we present and evaluate methods for warping into correspondence images of the brain acquired at different developmental time-points. These are used in the generation of synthetic representations and simulations of development.

II. Gross Brain Changes

Gross morphological changes in the developing human brain result from the complex interaction of several concurrent processes. For modeling purposes, we review the *radial* proliferation of the cerebral hemispheres, the *arching* of the brain and many of its sub-

structures into a characteristic C-shape, and the *fissuring and folding* of the cerebral cortex into the intricate labyrinths of gyri and sulci, which penetrate deep into the brain.

A. Radial Proliferation of the Cerebral Hemispheres

The development of the human cerebral cortex is a highly stereotyped process in which onset occurs around embryonic day 23. In vertebrates, the entire brain is generated by the proliferation of the embryonic neural tube (Purves and Lichtman, 1985). Different rates of growth and proliferation within the sheath of cells that make up the tube produce ongoing geometric deformations of its inner and outer surfaces.

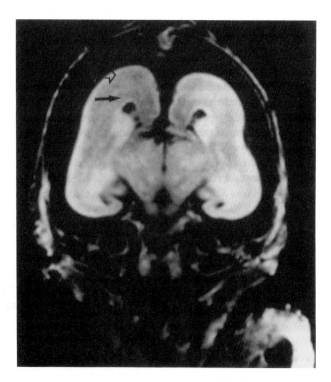

Figure 1 Formalin-fixed fetus, estimated at 16 weeks gestational age by crown-rump length. Coronal T_1-weighted MRI shows a smooth brain surface; a wave of migratory neurons can be seen, coursing from the germinative zone at the ventricular surface *(black arrow)* to the cortical plate at the brain surface *(white arrow)*. Images of this quality may be obtainable by MR imaging *in utero.* (J. Kucharchyk, M. Moseley, and A. J. Barkovich (eds.), 1994. Reprinted by permission of CRC Press, Boca Raton, Florida.)

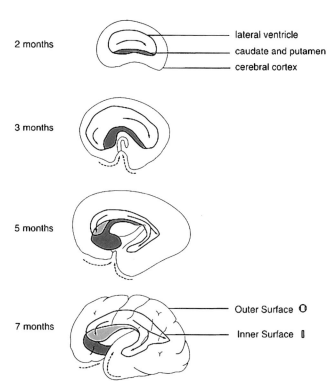

Figure 2 Development of the human brain at 2, 3, 5, and 7 months of embryonic age. Due to cellular proliferation during development, the chief structures of the brain are distorted into a characteristic C-shape. The lateral ventricles are continuously transformed *(arrows)* into an arched shape in synchrony with many other structures. These include a major functional unit, located on the floor of the lateral ventricles *(shaded)*, consisting of the *caudate* and *putamen*. The *hippocampal formation*, and the *parahippocampal* and *cingulate gyri* of the limbic system are similarly transformed (not shown). The *hippocampus* arches under the temporal horn of the ventricles (q.v., Fig. 3, *arrow* 6). The two aforementioned *gyri* are formed on the medial surface of each cerebral hemisphere. [Adapted from Kandel et al. (1991) and F. Hochstetter (1929).]

The formation of the cerebral hemispheres begins as neuronal precursors divide at the inner surface of the neural tube. The inner surface surrounds a central canal, which starts to branch out to form two outward cavities at its anterior end. These two pockets of fluid, at the front end of the embryo, are destined to become the lateral ventricles at maturity. A system of radial fibers connects these primitive ventricles to the *pia mater*, which serves to guide the migration of postmitotic ventricular cells to the outer cortex, preserving their topographic relationships as they are projected from the inner surface to the exterior surface. The inner germinal surface for each hemisphere becomes the respective lateral ventricle at maturity. Once the fluid-filled precursors of the lateral ventricles have protruded out from the central canal of the neural tube, one on each side, the evolution of the cortical surface is constrained medially by an equal and opposing pressure exerted by the growing tissue of the other hemisphere. The division and migration of cells on each side of the ventricular system results in the two cerebral hemispheres, separated by the midsagittal fissure. This configuration is apparent in Figure 1. The six-layered cortical plate is gradually assembled as migrating populations of cells arrive at the exterior surface in successive waves, the later ones forming more superficial layers, after traversing the layers of cells already assembled (Rakic, 1972).

B. Arching of Neural Substructures into Characteristic C-Shape

The lateral ventricles are useful landmarks for understanding the regional anatomy of the cerebral hemispheres. During development, the proliferation of cells in the cerebral hemispheres forces the lateral ventricles and many other major structures of the brain into a characteristic C-shape (Kandel, Schwartz, & Jessell, 1991). This process is illustrated in Figure 2. Since this dramatic growth causes different regions of the tissue around the ventricular cavities to physically expand at different rates, the inner and outer limiting surfaces of the cavity and cortex are continuously deformed until they become irregular. In later developmental stages, however, four stereotypical features on the lateral ventricles become distinct and are readily identified—the *atrium*, and the frontal, occipital, and inferior horns (Fig. 3). The caudate and the hippocampus lie on the inner and outer banks of the ventricles, and deform the ventricular surface as they grow.

Since the caudate nucleus runs along the *lateral wall* of the lateral ventricle, its shape in both development and maturity largely parallels that of the ventricular surface. The hippocampus starts to form a shallow surface depression in the ventricle's medial surface, and soon sends out efferent fibers, in the form of the fornix, which project around the ventricles. These fibers then

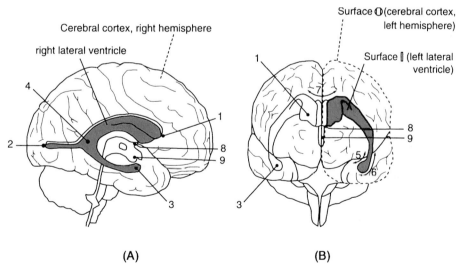

(A) **(B)**

Figure 3. The mature morphology of the lateral ventricles and the cerebral cortex. (A) represents the human brain as seen from the right hand side, with the right lateral ventricle shaded. When viewed from the front (B), the lateral ventricle ▯ *(shaded)* and cerebral cortex ◌ *(dashed lines)* in each hemisphere (here, the left) are seen as nested closed surfaces. The frontal, occipital, and temporal extremities *(arrows 1, 2, 3)* and *atrium (4)* of the lateral ventricles are shown; the tail of the *caudate (5)* and the foot of the *hippocampus (6)* project to form the roof and floor of the temporal horn, and the *corpus callosum* roofs over the *atrium (7)*.

arch forward and upward, and finally descend into the mammillary bodies of the hypothalamus (Gray, 1989). This internal arching of the caudate and the fornix induces a similar geometric arching in the structures which surround them, including the cingulate and parahippocampal gyri of the limbic system. The cerebrum, anchored to this dynamically evolving foundation, also sustains changes in its surface geometry as a result. The arching structures are also responsible for producing an emerging pattern of indentations at the internal, ventricular surface.

C. Formation of Gyri and Sulci

One of the most striking changes in the geometry of the developing primate brain is the formation of fissures in the cerebral surface. There has been some controversy over what exactly determines this folding pattern, and what are the chief mechanical factors and dynamic processes, at the cellular level, responsible for producing these deepening fissures in the cortex.

In 1986, Smart and McSherry published a detailed investigation of the internal histologic changes which occur during the folding sequence in the cerebral cortex. Both the radial "scaffolding" (Rakic, 1972) of projections down from the cortical surface, and the tangential banding of the six cortical layers, were apparent in stained serial sections of developing ferret cortex. Together, these sharply-defined tissue lines provided a curvilinear mesh whose deformation during development gave a detailed indication of the differential growth occurring within a gyrus. By examining the transformation of this coordinate system over time, it is clear that a spreading of the radial tissue lines occurs in

the gyral crown as increasing amounts of proliferating cortical tissue are enclosed between the diverging lines. This process is illustrated in Figure 4.

III. Models of Fissure Formation

Since the major growth and migratory processes in cerebral tissue take place in the context of a radially and tangentially organized cellular architecture (Rakic, 1972; Smart & McSherry, 1986), it seems logical to resolve the local differential growth and deformation, at any one time, into components along these principal directions. Earlier models tended to impose an idealized (usually Cartesian) geometric structure on the developing cortex. In contrast, a *curvilinear mesh*, first advanced as a developmental model in Smart & McSherry (1986) not only allows the tissue lines themselves to indicate the dynamic changes taking place in the system, but also makes allowances for the influences on migration and expansion in the brain exerted by its intrinsic fiber structure. Thus, there are potential advantages to deriving a material *coordinate* system which is consonant with the intrinsic radial and tangential fiber structure of the brain.

The dramatic folding characteristics of the cortex have prompted several explanatory models specifically based on these intrinsic structural forces. Richman et al. (1975) proposed a mechanical model for the development of tertiary convolutions in the human cortex, driven by stresses created by differential elasticity between an outer stratum (layers I, II, and III) and an inner stratum (layers IV, V, and VI). An analogous model (Smart & McSherry, 1986) of local patterns of migration and differential growth in the developing brain suggests that a strong influence may be exerted on these processes by the brain's inherent radial and tangential fiber structure.

The structural expansion and dilation in the gyral crown may be decomposed geometrically (Smart & McSherry, 1986) into components of radial and tangential spreading of local mature tissue. The site of the future sulcal bed, on the other hand, remains relatively quiescent during this phase; deferring its rapid tangential spreading to a later stage. Such a biphasic model of cortical growth is attractive theoretically, since it describes a time-varying pattern of differential cubical dilation within an intrinsic curvilinear mesh. It improves on earlier models (Bok, 1929), which consider the effect of folding a layered system with a radial structure which retains a *constant volume* during the folding process. Since the cortex increases significantly in both depth and area during development, the inclusion of an internal growth component is therefore

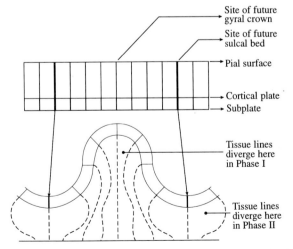

Figure 4. Suggested model of differential growth during the formation of the coronal gyrus in the embryonic ferret. [Adapted from Smart and McSherry, 1986, p. 38.]

an essential component of any model of gyrogenesis.

In a different interpretation of models of the intrinsic curvature of the cerebral cortex, Griffen (1994), using fractal dimension measurements, argued that the high degree of intrinsic curvature that accompanies cortical sheet development could be the result of evolutionary pressures. The developmental sequence of fissuration in the cortex was shown to decrease the *mean geodesic* of the surface, a measure which is defined to be the average distance separating any two points on the surface. Any introduction of intrinsic curvature into a surface, (e.g., during the formation of sulci), will usually reduce the required length of a projection within the surface connecting two given points. For this reason, fissuration is hypothesized to be favored by evolutionary selection, because it reduces the theoretical cost of wiring two cortical areas together using a minimum of white matter, which in turn increases the metabolic efficacy and speed of signal transduction in cortical neural networks.

The models discussed thus far provided primarily theoretical, biologically focused explanations for the morphological changes that occur during development. None of them have been extended to include computerized *simulations* to these hypotheses. The use of digital geometric representations to quantitate and visualize the changing morphometry can greatly enhance the value of biologically based hypotheses. Computerized simulations can help explain the forces responsible for the chief developmental changes outlined so far. With this goal in mind, we now turn to examine several algorithms which are effective in modeling and rendering surfaces in 3D images of the brain.

IV. Surface Modeling

In many brain mapping applications, surface models are used to represent anatomic or functional units in the brain. They provide explicit definitions of the geometry at specific time-points, and can be viewed quickly using well known algorithms (Foley, Van Dam, Feiner, & Hughes, 1992).

Techniques for surface modeling can be divided into outline-based and volumetric-based approaches. Outline-based methods (Levinthal & Ware, 1972; Christian & Sederberg, 1978) work by assembling contours corresponding to the intersection of the desired object with a set of sampling planes. Most commonly, as in Fuchs, Kedem, and Uselton (1977), these planes are parallel, and the reconstruction process works by creating triangular tiles connecting consecutive pairs of planes (Boissonnat, 1988; Ekoule, Peyrin, & Odet, 1991; Shinagawa & Kunii, 1991; Shinagawa, Kunii, &

Kergosien, 1991; Payne & Toga, 1994). Surface models can also originate with direct volumetric techniques such as "Marching Cubes" (Lorenson & Cline, 1987). These methods bypass the complexity of reconstruction from planar samples, working directly in the volumetric data grid. Generally, they are only applicable where the surface can be found by an automatic process; thus, the constant-density isosurface of a volume can be modeled by volumetric techniques, but subtle anatomic or functional features cannot. The need for identification of homologous points at different developmental stages may make outline-based methods more appropriate.

Regardless of construction method, properly constructed surface models have common properties, many of which are useful in developmental applications. They partition space into an interior and exterior region, retaining local spatial features that provide considerable morphometrically relevant information. From these models, any information that can be derived from adjacency, such as point neighborhoods or geodesics, can be efficiently derived by following the appropriate informational links.

V. Cortical Flattening Algorithms

Flattening a biological surface with intrinsic curvature may elucidate potential differential growth regimes responsible for producing the surface in question. Geometrically, it is important to appreciate the fundamental theoretical distinction between folding and intrinsic curvature of a surface (Van Essen & Maunsell, 1980). Intuitively, *folding* represents a type of curvature which can be reduced without distorting the surface; an *intrinsically* curved surface, however, such as a sphere, cannot be flattened without introducing discontinuities, or without stretching some areas at the expense of others. A crumpled-up sheet of newspaper, for example, exhibits folding alone; ironing it out would not distort the distances, measured within the sheet, between pairs of words on the page. The earth's surface, by contrast, like that of the brain, is intrinsically curved, and any method for displaying its geography in 2D will misrepresent, to some degree, the metrical relations between pairs of points on the surface.

Several research groups have developed flattening algorithms in an attempt to generate 2D maps of distinct functional regions and cytoarchitectonic boundaries in the cerebral cortex (Van Essen & Maunsell, 1980; Schwartz & Merker, 1986). The technique, in a sense, represents the reversal of the normal developmental process of fissuration in the cortex. Before flattening techniques were originated, the wide variations in gyral configuration and in the intrinsic curvature of the cortical surface had bedeviled attempts to represent and analyze the spatial relations of adjacent functional regions within the cortex.

After introducing their method for flattening the visual cortex in the cat and the *macaque* monkey, Van Essen and Maunsell (1980) suggested that the developmental basis for convolutions in the cortical surface probably results from a folding process accompanied by small changes in intrinsic curvature (*cf.* Schwartz & Merker, 1986, p. 39). Unfortunately, it is anticipated that higher levels of distortion, (or the introduction of additional discontinuities), will be necessary to create equivalent maps of the human cortex, in which the majority of the cortical surface is hidden within developmentally significant folds (Griffen, 1994, p. 267).

VI. Image Warping

Any comprehensive approach to modeling brain development must draw upon methods for quantitating its material transformation between pairs of images acquired at successive developmental timepoints. The complexity of such a task is considerable, since it requires repeated acquisitions, possibly averaging across subjects, and tracking homologous landmarks over a series of 3D data sets.

Since the advent of high-resolution medical imaging, modeling shape changes of a biological system under deformation has been the subject of intense research. (See Kambhamettu & Goldgof 1992, p. 222, for a review.) Algorithms for recovering, modeling, and tracking structures in complex nonrigid motion have been used effectively in producing high-resolution surface animations of the beating heart (Kambhamettu & Goldgof, 1992; Chen, Huang & Arrott, 1994), white blood cell motility (Bartels, Bovik, & Griffen, 1994), and optical flow algorithms (Horn, 1986; Denney & Prince, 1992). Common to these approaches is a technique known as image warping.

Warping is a method for calculating the distortion of a 3D image volume which would be required to map it onto a target volume, such as another 3D image set—of the same or of a different brain—at a later timepoint. The transformation must be calculated to bring the internal and external anatomic boundaries of the object in the first data set into register with their structural counterparts in the second image set. For each anatomic point in the first set, the warping algorithm specifies a displacement vector which would take it onto its structural counterpart in the second.

The warp is a model. It specifies the displacement of every anatomic point in the brain across the developmental stage spanned by the two images. As such, it permits complete morphometric quantitation of the dynamic effects of the embryonic process on the geometry of the brain and its substructures. It allows points, surfaces, and curved anatomic interfaces to be matched up in pairs of image sets. As a result, changes in volumes, surface areas, orientations, distances, and metrical relations between substructures—as well as measures of dilation rates, contraction rates, and rates of shearing and divergence of the cellular architecture—may be computed locally, for all structures, directly from the warping field. Since the warping field assigns a displacement for every anatomic point across a developmental phase, curves, surfaces, and volumes in an early image may be reidentified in a later one. This enables relative areas, lengths, and volumes to be compared over time. Temporal derivatives of these quantities allow rates of growth to be quantified locally for any structure; spatial derivatives of the warping field allow shearing and dilation to be measured locally, and compared for different substructures.

Determining accurate homologous point correspondences between two images is essential in modeling the process which transforms one image to the next in the sequence. One apparent difficulty is the emergence of new structures during the embryonic process. It may not be feasible to distort an early-stage fetal image and produce a later one, due to the more detailed anatomic configuration at later developmental time-points. This is, however, only a logistic difficulty, since it is readily overcome by first warping the later image onto the earlier one (i.e., allowing structures to disappear) and then reversing the displacement field to reconstruct the desired warp in the forward direction. For the moment, though, we will restrict ourselves to analyzing some of the more effective techniques for warping brain images, in conditions where essentially the same structures are represented in both the first and second data sets.

The methods for warping brain images fall into two main categories: density-based and fiducial-based approaches. Density-based techniques utilize regional patterns in intensity. These patterns are compared to find optimal matches between the two data sets. Since these approaches require extraction of point correspondences between two images, without *ad hoc* guidance from a user, their mathematical form is more complex than that of fiducial-based strategies. Fiducial-based methods usually require specification of a set of point correspondences (e.g., between easily identifiable anatomic landmarks) to constrain the warping field.

A. Density-Based Techniques

Density-based warping techniques often utilize algorithms that model the human brain under deformation as an elastic solid (Broit, 1981; Bajcsy & Kovacic, 1989; cf. Gee, Reivich, & Bajcsy, 1993). This elastic solid is distorted by a system of forces associated with the target image. The mathematical form of the force field is specifically chosen to bring the edges of similar structures in the two data sets into correspondence. The material is chosen to be elastic in order to penalize severe structural reorganization of the model, which could occur in cases where structures in the two were incorrectly matched. The warp can be represented as a displacement field $W(x)$, which specifies a 3D displacement vector to be applied to each point, or voxel, x, in the template to deform it onto its structural counterpart in the target.

All density-based approaches compute the displacement of each voxel in the template by searching the target volume for intensity motifs which correspond to the neighborhood of the voxel in the template. Edges of substructures, for example, can often be warped into correspondence, appealing to the fact that the local gradient in image intensity is often similar in both scans at the same structural interface. Nevertheless, for any given region in the template, similar motifs may be fairly abundant in the target image, so the matching problem is ill-posed and, in general, permits several possible candidate matches for each voxel in the template (Bartels et al., 1994, p. 111).

Consequently, to encourage transformations which match motifs using only small local displacements of the template, an approach based on *energy functionals* is often implemented. Although the positional variation of brain structures is considerable across individuals, (or across consecutive developmental time-points), this variation occurs within limits. When searching for point matches between images, a penalty is assigned against matches which would cause a severe distortion of the template. Therefore, approaches based on energy functionals tend to model the template as a 3D material body whose energetics can be stipulated as linearly *elastic* (Broit, 1981; Bajcsy & Kovacic, 1989), *viscous* (Miller, Christensen, Amit, & Grenander, 1993; Christensen, Rabbitt, & Miller, 1993), and described by *metric tensors* (Bartels et al., 1994) or by a more complex operator (Gee, Haynor, Reivich, & Bajcsy, 1994). The role of the energetics operator is to limit the degree of structural reorganization of the template, by associating an internal energy value with every distorted version of the template. The energy is defined to be high when the template is severely distorted, and the optimal warp is one that minimizes the energy of the system. By penal-

izing excessive reorganization of the template, the internal energy functional reduces the likelihood of accidental registration of inappropriate motifs in the template and target. This is especially likely to happen in cases where recurrent motifs occur in the target image, or where the geometric structure of the anatomy is highly tessellated.

Additional energy constraints such as *data-driven* energy terms can be designed to favor the matching of points with similar curvature (Gourdon & Ayache, 1993; Benayoun, Ayache, & Cohen, 1994), similar intensity profiles in their neighborhoods (Broit, 1981; Bajcsy & Kovacic, 1989), or other geometric criteria. The energy approach can be used to derive a set of three partial differential equations (PDEs) describing the appropriate displacement for each voxel. The optimum displacement creates a global minimum of the energy of the reorganized template, when both data-driven and internal material energy terms are combined. This displacement field, $x \rightarrow x + u$, is given by the set of Navier-Stokes equations for a fixed point in the template, x:

$$\mu \nabla^2 u_i(x) + (\lambda + \mu)\{\partial \theta / \partial x_i\} + F_i(u) = 0, \quad i = 1,2,3.$$

(1)

Here the u_i are the three components of the displacement vector for voxel x, Lamé's elastic constants λ and μ refer to the elastic properties of the body, and $\theta \equiv \partial u_1/\partial x_1 + \partial u_2/\partial x_2 + \partial u_3/\partial x_3 = \nabla \cdot u(x)$ is the cubical dilation of the medium. For any vector field describing the deformation of the medium, θ and $\nabla^2 u_i(x)$ can be approximated numerically, by convolving kernels with small regions of the 3D arrays which contain u's components (Bartels, Bovik, Aggarwal, & Diller, 1993). Finally, the data-driven term, $F(x) \equiv (F_1, F_2, F_3)^T$, is the force applied to each point x before deformation. The geometric criterion of structural correspondence depends on the cross-correlation of local intensity patterns, with a force term proportional to $\nabla S(x,u)$. $S(x,u)$ is the normalized correlation value given by the formula

$$S(x,u) := \int_{r \in B(0;R_c)} \{T(x+r) - \mu(T)\}\{S(u+r) - \mu(S)\}\, dr /$$
$$[\int_{r \in B(0;R_c)} \{T(x+r) - \mu(T)\}^2\, dr]^{1/2} \cdot [\int_{r \in B(0;R_c)} \{S(u+r) - \mu(S)\}^2\, dr]^{1/2}.$$

In this formula, (1) r takes all values in a search space described by the cubical box $B(0;R_c)$, of side R_c and center the origin; (2) $T(p)$ and $S(p)$ are the image intensities at position vector p in the template and target scans, respectively; and (3) $\mu(T)$ and $\mu(S)$ are the mean template and target intensities inside boxes $B(x;R_c)$ and $B(u;R_c)$, respectively. The resulting set of differential equations (Eq. 1), whose solution gives the optimal displacement field, can then be solved iteratively by finite difference (Bartels et al., 1993) or finite element (Gee et al., 1994) methods.

Boundary conditions on the displacement field (or an assumption that displacements are small), are necessary to prevent the optimization routine from converging to a displacement field which creates merely a local minimum of the combined energy functional defined on the distorted template. In view of this issue, some research groups have been led to refine the *data-driven term*, in hope that a more comprehensive set of geometric criteria will serve to determine point correspondences unambiguously, between any two anatomic images. A *curvature-based* approach has recently been implemented, which produces results of superior accuracy (Ayache, 1993). Technical remarks on this approach can be found in the appendix to this chapter.

In contrast, other researchers have attempted to refine the *energetics* operator still further, in the hope of accurately representing the statistics of natural biological variation at each point in the template. In an energy functional approach, this prior information on anatomic variability would be used to limit the search space in the target, when looking for corresponding motifs, reducing the chance of accidental misregistration. Instead of characterizing the energetics of the brain under deformation as that of a uniform medium, the deformation of those tissue regions which are most prone to natural variation would be favored over comparatively invariant substructures. The estimation of an appropriate continuum mechanics operator for the human brain under deformation is currently being attempted, using massively parallel connection machines to tackle this high-dimensional optimization problem (Miller & Grenander, 1994).

In warping brain data from distinct developmental time-points or individuals, the operator stipulating the energetics of different brain substructures could incorporate statistical information on the morphometric variability of each anatomic point. Morphometric changes in the developing brain can be resolved locally into components along the curvilinear mesh produced by its inherent fiber structure. Energetics operators which favor displacements of anatomic structures along the radial fiber tracts of the developing system might therefore be used in the warping model. This resource would, very likely, facilitate the recovery of the material warp of the brain from one developmental time-point to the next.

In spite of the preceding arguments, it remains an important strategy to develop warping algorithms based on *simple* control criteria, including approaches which exploit the biological information inherent in each data set. Control criteria can be simplified, if the variations of biological substructures across various data sets can be shown to bear an underlying topological (or even metrical) relation to an optimally efficient set of fiducial points, curves, and surfaces. Ideally, these fiducials should mark biological structures that have a crucial role in guiding the morphological development of the brain during the embryonic process. They must also be identifiable in all data sets.

B. Fiducial-Based Techniques

Fiducial-based approaches avoid several of the difficulties inherent in the density-based formulation. A fiducial is an anatomical landmark which can be easily identified, either manually or automatically, in each data set, and the point correspondences which result can be used to constrain the warping field. Ideally, a large fiducial set should be available, in order to allow the displacement field to be adequately interpolated into all regions of the volume. Previous research on warping images has tended to concentrate on using *point* fiducials, in view of the difficulty in assigning one-to-one point correspondences between general curves and surfaces in data sets (Bookstein, 1989). All fiducials fall into four basic categories: (1) *anatomically-defined features*, such as those lying at the interface of two or more anatomically-defined substructures; (2) *geometrically-defined features*, such as the extrema of substructures, or structural interfaces, in any arbitrary direction; (3) *extrinsic fiducials*, such as external markers mechanically introduced into tissue, or stereotaxic frame elements applied to the exterior of the skull during a clinical scan; and (4) *intensity motifs*, such as edge points (with high intensity gradient), crest lines (with high curvature), or regions with high cross-correlation to some explicit pattern. Such "fiducials" are, in essence, what is tacitly used to drive the density-based technique.

The first step in creating a fiducial-based developmental warp is to select *control manifolds*, which are present in images acquired at each successive developmental stage, and use the displacement field that brings them into correspondence to constrain the transformation from one image volume to the next in the sequence. A manifold, in an image data set or in any other 3D space, is a general name for any point, curve, or surface lying in the space. In fiducial-based approaches, a warp is often derived from a set of point correspondences on a set of manifolds that is subsequently interpolated to the full volume. For example, Chen, Huang, and Arrott, (1994), tracked a number of bifurcations in the coronary artery across a sequence of 16-cine angiographs captured at a uniform frequency during the cardiac cycle, and produced a surface animation of the beating heart. Here, the method of tracking the position of fiducial points on the surface, through a series of images, enabled surfaces to be fitted through the data in each successive frame by spherical harmonic interpolation.

C. Ventricular and Cortical Fiducials

In an earlier section, we suggested that the first step in characterizing the neuroanatomical variations between two scans in a developmental series might be to analyze the differences in the surface geometry of the ventricles and cerebral cortex. These structures are displayed in Plates 1A and 1B. The cortical and ventricular surfaces are fundamental developmentally, since their geometry dynamically reflects the processes of accretion, arching, and differential growth taking place in the structures which lie between them. Moreover, these morphometric changes occur in the context of a radially organized cellular architecture, which exerts a strong influence on the migration, expansion, and differential growth processes in the fetal brain. Since this radial architecture is essentially interposed between the cortical and ventricular surfaces in each hemisphere, the cellular events effectively take place within an evolving material coordinate system, which radially connects these two nested surfaces in each cerebral hemisphere.

Several stereotypical features can be extracted from the ventricles and cortex [using Canny–Deriche image filters and Voronoi segmentation (Kruggel, Horsch, Mittelhaüsser, & Schnabel, 1989)]. The most obvious of these are primary sulci, which are formed early in development and remain relatively stable, in both their topological configurations and metrical relations, into old age (Kruggel et al., 1989, p. 218). Once these sulcal beds and the ventricular surface have been extracted, the transformation which maps each of them onto their counterparts in the next image of the developmental sequence can be found, by interpolating known values of the displacement field at extremal points across the entire manifold (Moshfeghi, Raganath, & Nawyn, 1994). Although there is no guarantee of the accuracy of point-to-point registration within these manifolds (since this requires a complete, consistent parametrization of each manifold in both template and target images) several methods have been used successfully in the past to interpolate displacement fields across biological surfaces (see Chen et al., 1994). A warp of brain images, defined from one image to the next on a set of manifolds including ventricles and cortical sulci, could be interpolated into the full template volume (Plate 2). This would be sufficient to completely define the transformation which takes one image volume to the next in a developmental sequence, and could serve as the basis for a manifold-based model of the geometry of the developing brain. Additional remarks on using control manifolds to constrain warping fields for the developing brain can be found in Appendix B.

All warping approaches perform best when the warps transforming one image to the next involve only small displacements. This not only requires a large set of images, acquired at short intervals in the developmental process, but also a method for standardizing these images so that the differences reflect brain development in general, particularly when homologous points are difficult or impossible to identify.

D. Distance Fields

Distance fields (Payne & Toga, 1992) allow surface manipulation without regard to topology or homology. A distance field is a volume in which each scalar voxel value encodes the distance from that point to the nearest point on the surface. This distance is signed, with points interior to the surface having a positive distance.

The distance field of a polyhedral model can be computed by taking the minimum distance over all polyhedra in the model, then combining it with the sign (Plate 3). In practice, the computation can be streamlined using a hierarchical data structure to prevent unnecessary distance computations (Payne & Toga, 1992).

The distance field has several useful properties that make it preferable to direct utilization of surface models in certain cases. These include computations which model solid geometry, surface averaging, interpolation, and statistical characterization of multiple surfaces, including developmental surfaces at specific time-points.

The sign of the distance field of a model provides a voxel-level map of which points are inside and which points are outside the model. This map can be used for derivation of statistical variability measures of multiple models. The first approximation of this is a derived volume containing a count of the number of overlapping models for each point in the volume. This type of volume allows isosurfaces to be created, indicating the statistical surface containing a given number m out of n sample surfaces. The use of integer counts makes the derived surfaces vulnerable to aliasing; an alternative is to derive a continuous m-of-n object field by sorting the n input values at each point and taking the mth value in reverse sorted order.

Other types of solid model computation can also be carried out voxel-by-voxel. Typical operations in computational solid modeling include computing the complement of a given surface, forming the union of two surfaces, and forming the intersection of two surfaces. Making such computations with surfaces directly is necessary for modeling with arbitrary precision, but is implementationally very expensive. With distance fields, these same operations correspond to simple functions of the input distances: negation for complement, minimum for intersection, and maximum for union. (Note that the latter two are special cases of the statistical surfaces previously described.)

Distance fields support a simple method for interpolating and averaging between arbitrary surfaces. Given two surfaces $s(t_0)$ and $s(t_1)$, representing the desired state at times t_0 and t_1, distance fields $f_0 = dfld(s_0)$ and $f_1 = dfld(s_1)$ are derived. The interpolation of the surfaces is accomplished by weighted averaging of the volumes followed by isosurface extraction. The average of the two surfaces can be derived, with both weights equal to one-half. Plate 4 shows frames from an animation sequence created by the weighted average technique.

Interpolation of surfaces via interpolation of distance fields is computationally straightforward, but it lacks some desirable properties. Since no point homologies are established, there is no guarantee that corresponding points will be correctly represented during the interpolation, or indeed that the intermediate surface models will be biologically reasonable at all. Since the interpolation does not involve computing a transformation of the enclosing space, the surface interpolation does not allow any corresponding transformation of densitometric data within the surface.

These limitations will motivate the more powerful (though costly) technique of distance field volume warping. Surfaces can be incorporated as constraints in a volume warp by using surface distance fields as a form of derived density data. From a full volume warp, transformation and interpolation of both surfaces and volumes can be computed in a way that is sensitive to homology.

VII. Atlasing

Traditional approaches to comparing data sets from different time-points or different individuals involve atlases. The imposition of standardized coordinate systems and their relationship to anatomic nomenclature is particularly difficult when potentially drastic morphological differences exist among the data sets. The spatial positioning scheme described by Talairach and Tournoux (1988) bases its registry and scaling on the bicommissural line in an attempt to equilibrate disparate data sets. Since this approach is so dependent on the selection of specific, and presumably consistent,

anatomic landmarks, similarly based atlas methods may not work when applied to developmentally different data sets. More extreme deformations could be imposed to fit all stages of development into a standard atlas, but this would hardly meet the primary requirement of atlasing, which is to provide a standard coordinate framework for localizing and classifying structures present in developing brains, at arbitrary time-points. There are two potential ways to overcome this difficulty. One approach would be to base the coordinate system of the atlas on a purely intrinsic framework such as the control manifolds described in earlier sections. This, of course, reduces the functionality of the atlas for making comparisons between developmental stages and precludes comparisons between subjects of a single stage.

Alternatively, a different atlas and coordinate system for several discrete stages of development might be used. Numerous anatomic features, due to their emergence and disappearance during development, could be used to place individual brains into the coordinate system of an appropriate atlas in the set. The warps described previously could then be applied to the coordinate systems themselves as a basis for comparison and quantitation of development. Temporal interpolation between atlases in the set could also be used to generate additional anatomical templates, representing brains at any state of maturity in between those stages represented in the initial inventory. Atlases of brains earlier and later than the brain in question (in terms of maturity) could be identified, and by referring to the warping field which maps the first atlas onto the second, a fixed fraction of this field could be applied to the prior atlas to generate an intermediate one. This type of temporal interpolation between atlas templates would greatly extend the range of applicability of the initial atlas sequence, by representing brains at arbitrary developmental stages. Ultimately, such atlasing approaches can be used in conjunction with the warping techniques outlined above, to comprehensively characterize the morphology of brains at different stages of development.

VIII. Conclusion

Modeling the changes that occur in the brain during development requires both biological and mathematical considerations. In order to adequately explain the morphological changes observed during development, mechanical, genetic, and experiential forces must be incorporated. This chapter has reviewed some of the biologically-based models of development and proposed the use of geometrically-based digital models to illustrate and simulate these changes. The use of image warping methods to relate one anatomic image to the next in a sequence will be highly relevant in modeling the way in which the geometry of the developing brain changes. Density-based approaches to the problem, which model the material energetics of the system under deformation, might allow anatomic points to be tracked satisfactorily through a sequence of developing images. Fiducial-based models, however, aim to extract a set of fundamental control curves and surfaces in the brain, whose evolution during development dynamically reflects, and can be used to characterize, the geometric evolution of the system. Distance field-based warping, constrained by developmentally significant control manifolds, provides interpolative capabilities that are useful in the simulation and visualization of the morphological changes. By combining these warping strategies with an inventory of atlases from several developmental stages, intermediate atlases can be created for a comprehensive description of the developing brain.

Appendix A:
Curvature-Based Image Warping

As stated in the main text, the aim of the curvature-based image warping technique (Benayoun et al., 1994; Ayache, 1993) is to bias the warping field to favor the matching of points with similar *Euclidean curvature*, as well as points with similar intensity gradient norm (as before). The curvature paradigm is an extension of an earlier collaboration (Gourdon & Ayache, 1993), which produced a way of registering curves on surfaces by exploiting their shared differential properties; this involved bringing their Frenet and Darboux frames into register by equating the geodesic torsion and curvature of each manifold.

In Benayoun et al. (1994), the warp registering the template T onto the target image was designed to be optimal with respect to a weighted sum of energy functionals E_{gradient}, $E_{\text{curvature}}$, and E_{internal}, where $E_{\text{internal}} \equiv \int_T \|\nabla f\|^2$, f being the correspondence function $x \Rightarrow W(x)$; they also defined

$$E_{\text{gradient}} + E_{\text{curvature}} \equiv \int_T w_c(f_c,x)f_c(x) + w_g(f_g,x)f_g(x)dx,$$

where

$$f_c(x) \equiv \{C(x) - C[W(x)]\}^2,$$

C being the Euclidean curvature, and

$$f_g(x) \equiv \{\|\nabla I(x)\| - \|\nabla I(W(x))\|\}^2,$$

I being the intensity function.

The w_i are high-pass polynomial filters, with

$$w_c(f_c,x) \equiv -2\gamma(f_c,x)^3 + 3\gamma(f_c,x)^2,$$

where

$$\gamma(f_c,x) \equiv \frac{\{f_c(x) - \min_{x \in T}(f_c(x))\}}{\{\max_{x \in T}(f_c(x)) - \min_{x \in T}(f_c(x))\}}$$

$w_g(f_g,x)$ and $\gamma(f_g,x)$ are similarly defined.

This technique represents a viable alternative to the basic elastic approach, without appealing to fluid dynamics for the template. This is because the high-pass weighting of energy functionals allows the attenuation of the internal energy term, in cases where this hinders the complete warping of the template onto the target.

Appendix B:
Warping Using Control Curves and Surfaces

As described in the text, feature extraction and surface interpolation techniques allow us, in principle, to specify a displacement field which brings into register a set of curves and surfaces, such as the sulcal beds and ventricular surface in each cerebral hemisphere, in the template and target image. For more details on this type of approach, please see Moshfeghi et al. (1994).

The task is to find an interpolation scheme which adequately extends this displacement field into the full template volume, and therefore completely specifies the volumetric transformation $W(x)$ which takes points x in one brain image onto their anatomic counterparts in the next image. The method outlined here exploits the distance field and surface rendering algorithms outlined in the text. It allows us to weight the contribution of each control manifold to the displacement of an arbitrary point x in the template volume, depending on the distance of x, namely $d_i(x)$, from its nearest point np_i on that manifold.

Let the set of n curves in the template and target images be homogeneously parametrized as free curves $\{T_i(t)\}_{i=1 \text{ to } n}$ and $\{S_i(t)\}_{i=1 \text{ to } n}$ with $t \in [0,1]$. Let the direction of increase of t be consistent in both image volumes. For $x \in \{T_i(t)\}$, we define $W_i(x) \equiv S_i(t) - T_i(t)$, for each $i=1$ to n, and assume $W(x)$ to be already specified on the free curves $\{T_i(t)\}_{i=1 \text{ to } n}$ and on the ventricular surface as $W_V(x)$ in that hemisphere. We aim to write $W(x) = \Sigma_{i=1 \text{ to } n+1} w_i(x)D_i(x)$, where the $w_i(x)$ are normalized weights (i.e., $\Sigma_{i=1 \text{ to } n+1} w_i(x) = 1$), and the D_i are distortion functions due to each manifold. Let x be an arbitrary point in the volume; let the distance of x from its near point on each of the manifolds $\{T_i(t)\}_{i=1 \text{ to } n}$ be $d_i(x)$. As x approaches the manifold $T_i(t)$ for a fixed i, we require the displacements defined on the other manifolds to have a contribution to $W(x)$ which tends to zero.

Therefore, consider the set of $n+1$ functions

$$\gamma_i(x) \equiv \{\Sigma_{j=1 \text{ to } n+1} d_j(x)\}/d_i(x).$$

Each γ_i becomes infinite as x approaches T_i. Then the associated $n+1$ weight functions

$$w_i(x) \equiv \gamma_i(x)/\{\Sigma_{j=1 \text{ to } n+1} \gamma_j(x)\}$$

can be used to weight the influence of control points inversely with their distance from x, the point for which the displacement is to be calculated. (*Note:* The weight functions serve to control the relative influence of different members of a set of control manifolds; the way in which each manifold affects the transformation at x, however, is described by the distortion functions $D_i(x)$, and is independent of the choice of weight functions.) So if we define $D_i(x) \equiv W(np_i(x))$, where $np_i(x)$ is x's near point on T_i, then the formula:

$$W(x) \equiv \Sigma_{i=1 \text{ to } n+1} w_i(x)D_i(x), \text{ for all } x,$$

defines a simple volume warp taking one volume onto the next. Of course, more refined approaches would define the $D_i(x)$ to let points other than the nearest point on each manifold to x influence the contribution of the ith manifold to the warp of anatomic point x, from one image to the next in the developmental sequence.

Acknowledgments

The authors wish to thank colleagues in the Laboratory of Neuro Imaging and Division of Brain Mapping for their assistance. Special thanks go to Andrew Lee for his digital figure work. This work was supported in part by the National Institutes of Health (RR05956) and the Human Brain Project funded jointly by the National Institute of Mental Health, the National Institute on Drug Abuse (P20 MH52176), and the National Science Foundation (BIR-9322434). P.T. was supported by grant G-1-00001 of the United States Information Agency, Washington, D.C., by a Fellowship of the Howard Hughes Medical Institute, and by a Fulbright Scholarship from the U.S.–U.K. Fulbright Commission, London. Thanks also go to the Brain Mapping Medical Research Organization, the Pierson–Lovelace Foundation, and The Ahmanson Foundation.

References

Ayache, N. (September 1993). Volume image processing: Results and research challenges. *INRIA Report No. 2050*.

Bajcsy, R., & Kovacic, S. (1989). Multiresolution elastic matching. *Computer Vision, Graphics, and Image Processing, 46*, 1–21.

Bartels, K. A., Bovik, A. C., Aggarwal, S. J., & Diller, K. R. (1993). The analysis of shape change from multi-dimensional dynamic images. *Journal of Computerized Medical Imaging and Graphics, 17*(2):89–99.

Bartels, K. A., Bovik, A. C., & Griffen, C. E. (1994). Spatio-temporal tracking of material shape change via multi-dimensional splines. *Proceedings 1994 IEEE Workshop on Biomedical Image Analysis, Cat. No. 94TH0624-7*, 110–116.

Benayoun, S., Ayache, N., and Cohen, I. (May 1994). An adaptive model for 2D and 3D dense non-rigid motion computation. *INRIA Internal Report No. 2297*.

Boissonnat, J. D. (1988). Shape reconstruction from planar cross sections. *Computer Vision, Graphics and Image Processing, 44*, 1–29.

Bok, S. T. (1929). Der Einfluss in den Furchen und Windungen auftretenden Krummungen der Grosshirnrinde aur die Rindenarchitektur. *Zeitschrift für die gesamte Neurologie und Psychiatrie, 121*, 682–750.

Bookstein, F. L. (1989). Principal warps: Thin-plate splines and the decomposition of deformations. *IEEE Transactions on Pattern Analysis and Machine Intelligence, 11*(6), 567–585.

Broit, C., (1981). *Optimal registration of deformed images.* Unpublished doctoral dissertation, University of Pennsylvania, Philadelphia, PA.

Chen, C. W., Huang, T. S., and Arrott, M., (1994). Modeling, analysis and visualization of left ventricle shape and motion by hierarchical decomposition, *IEEE Transactions on Pattern Analysis and Machine Intelligence, 16*(4), 342–356.

Christensen, G. E., Rabbitt, R. D., & Miller, M. I. (1993). A deformable neuroanatomy text-book based on viscous fluid mechanics. *Proc. of the 27th Annual Conference on Information Sciences and Systems*, 211–216.

Christian, H. N., & Sederberg, T. W. (1978). Conversion of complex contour line definitions into polygonal element mosaics. *Computer Graphics, 12*(3), 187–192.

Damasio, H. (1994). *Human brain anatomy in computerized images.* New York: O.U.P.

Denney, T. S., Jr., & Prince, J. L. (March 1992). On optimal brightness functions for optical flow. *Proceedings IEEE ICASSP-92*.

Ekoule, A. B., Peyrin, F. C., & Odet, C. L. (1991). A triangulation algorithm from arbitrary shaped multiple planar contours. *ACM Transactions on Graphics, 10*(2), 182–199.

England, M., & Wakely, J. (1991) *Atlas of the human brain and spinal cord* (pp. 26, 71). St. Louis, MO: Mosby-Yearbook, Inc.

Foley, J., Van Dam, A., Feiner, S., & Hughes, J., (1992). *Computer graphics principles and practice.* 2nd Ed., Reading, MA: Addison–Wesley.

Fuchs, H., Kedem, Z. M., & Uselton, S. P. (1977). Optimal surface reconstruction from planar contours. *Communications, ACM, 20*(10), 693–702.

Gee, J. C., Haynor, D. R., Reivich, M., & Bajcsy, R. (1994). Finite element approach to warping of brain images. *SPIE, 2167* (Image Processing), 327–337.

Gee, J. C., Reivich, M., & Bajcsy, R. (1993). Elastically deforming 3D atlas to match anatomical brain images. *Journal of Computer Assisted Tomography 17*(2), 225–236.

Gourdon, A., & Ayache, N. (December 1993). Registration of a curve on a surface using differential properties. *INRIA Internal Report No. 2145*.

Gray, H. (1989). P. Williams *et al.* (Eds.), *Gray's anatomy* (pp. 139–140). Edinburgh, U. K., and New York: Livingstone.

Griffen, L. D. (1994). The intrinsic geometry of the cerebral cortex. *Journal of Theoretical Biology, 166*, 261–273.

Horn, B. K. P. (1986). *Robot Vision.* Cambridge, MA: MIT.

Kambhamettu, C., & Goldgof, D. (1992). Point correspondence recovery in non-rigid motion. *Proceedings 1992 Comp. Soc. Conference on Comp. Vision and Pattern Recognition, Cat. No. 92CH3168-2*, 222–227.

Kandel, E. R., Schwartz, J. H., & Jessell, T. M. (1991). Functional anatomy of the central nervous system. *Principles of neural science,* (3rd ed., Part 4, pp. 305–308). Amsterdam: Elsevier.

Kruggel, F., Horsch, A., Mittelhaüsser, G., & Schnabel, M. (1994). Image processing in the neurologic sciences. *Proc. IEEE Workshop on Biomedical Image Analysis, Cat. No. 94TH0624-7,* 214–223.

Kucharchyk, J., Moseley, M., & Barkovich, A. J., eds. (1994). *Magnetic resonance neuroimaging,* p. 189. Boca Raton, FL: CRC Press.

Levinthal, C., & Ware, R. (1972). Three-dimensional reconstruction from serial sections, *Nature (London), 236,* 207–210.

Lorenson, W. E., & Cline, H. E. (1987). Marching cubes: A high resolution 3D surface construct algorithm. *Computer Graphics, 21*(3), 163–169.

Miller, M. I., Christensen, G. E., Amit, Y., & Grenander, U. (1993). Mathematical textbook of deformable neuroanatomies. *Proceedings of the National Academy of Sciences, U.S.A., 90,* 11944–11948.

Miller, M. I., & Grenander, U. (1994). Representations of knowledge in complex systems. *Journal of the Royal Statistical Society, 4,* 574–575.

Moshfeghi, M., Raganath, S., & Nawyn, K. (1994). Three-dimensional elastic matching of volumes. *IEEE Transactions on Image Processing, 3*(2), 128–138.

Payne, B. A., & Toga, A. W. (1992). Distance field manipulation of surface models. *IEEE Computer Graphics and Applications, 12*(1), 65–71.

Payne, B. A., & Toga, A. W. (1994). Surface reconstruction by multiaxial triangulation. *IEEE Computer Graphics and Applications, 14*(6), 28–35.

Purves, D., & Lichtman, J. W. (1985). *Principles of neural development.* Sunderland, MA: Sinauer.

Rakic, P. (1972). Mode of cell migration to the superficial layers of fetal monkey neocortex. *Journal of Comparative Neurology, 145,* 61–84.

Richman, D. P., Stewart, R. M., Hutchison, J. W., & Caviness, V. S. (1975). Mechanical model of brain convolutional development. *Science, 189,* 18–21.

Schambra, V. B., Lauder, J. M., & Silver, J. (1992). *Atlas of the Prenatal Mouse Brain.* San Diego: Academic Press.

Schwartz, E. L., & Merker, B. (April 1986). Computer-aided neuroanatomy: Differential geometry of cortical surfaces and an optimal flattening algorithm, *IEEE Computer Graphics,* 36–44.

Shinagawa, Y., & Kunii, T. L. (1991). Constructing a Reeb graph automatically from cross sections. *IEEE Computer Graphics and Applications, 11*(5), 44–51.

Shinagawa, Y., & Kunii, T. L., & Kergosien, Y. L. (1991). Surface coding based on Morse theory. *IEEE Computer Graphics and Applications, 11*(5), 66–78.

Smart I. H. M., & McSherry, G. M. (1986). Gyrus formation in the cerebral cortex in the ferret. II. Description of the internal histological changes. *Journal of Anatomy, 147,* 27–43.

Talairach, J., & Tournoux, P. (1988). M. Rayport (transl.), *Co-planar Stereotaxic Atlas of the Human Brain.* New York: Thieme Medical.

Todd, P. H. (1982). A geometric model for the cortical folding pattern of simple folded brains. *Journal of Theoretical Biology 97,* 529–538.

Van Essen, D. C., & Maunsell, J. H. R. (1980). Two-dimensional maps of the cerebral cortex. *Journal of Comparative Neurology, 191,* 255–281.

3

Structural Morphometry in the Developing Brain

David N. Kennedy, Nikos Makris, Julianna F. Bates,
and Verne S. Caviness, Jr

*Center for Morphometric Analysis and MGH-NMR Center, Massachusetts General Hospital,
Charlestown, Massachusetts 02129*

I. Introduction

Morphometry is the measurement of morphologic properties such as size, shape, location, and physical composition of the component structures of an object.

A. Anatomic and Functional Brain Structures

By definition, a *structure* is any spatially contiguous region with a homogeneous representation in some descriptor which establishes a means of distinction, or contrast, between the region and its neighborhood. Structure contrast can arise, for example, from differential distribution of neuronal cell bodies versus axons, (resulting in gray matter versus white matter), gyral topography, cyto- and myelo-architecture, and patterns of connectivity. These classes of substructure form classic neuroanatomic description of the brain. Equally important is the identification of structure defined by contrasts arising from functional considerations such as neurotransmitter receptor distribution or activation patterns. These functional *structures* are equally amenable to morphometric description. At the heart, therefore, of understanding how the brain works, is the establishment of a complete understanding of anatomic and functional mapping of all of the tasks which the brain subserves; a determination of *where* functionally specific sites are located, *what* operations are performed, and *how* distributed processing is organized (Zeki, Watson, Lueck, Friston, Kennard, & Frackowiak, 1991). This is indeed a tall order, the solution to which may, in fact, only be approached asymptotically.

It has been summarized by Mountcastle that "the brain is a complex of widely and reciprocally interconnected systems and its function springs-out of the dynamic interplay of neural activity within these systems" (Edelman and Mountcastle, 1978). To accomplish this, there is a hierarchy of spatial scales which span the relevant anatomic structures. From the finest to the grossest spatial scale, one can consider neurons, cortical columns, architectonic areas, systems-level networks, gyral pattern, lobes, hemispheres, and the brain as a whole. Similarly, there is a hierarchy in the functional domain: the neuron, (the basic, unitary functional subset of the brain), is part of a local network of neurons, which, in turn, is part of a network of distributed, reciprocally interconnected networks, which ultimately compose the functioning being (Churchland and Sejnowski, 1988). These anatomic and functional descriptions form two distinct, yet interconnected means of characterizing the brain.

B. Brain Morphometry

Given that anatomic and functional *structures* exist in the brain, what makes these structures *morphometrically interesting?* In other words, what is the precedence for size, shape, location, and compositional characteristics of these structures to be biologically meaningful? One can easily identify numerous broad domains over which this question can be answered.

- The anatomy and function of the brain undergoes dramatic change over time from conception through birth, childhood, adolescence, and adulthood. Each specified morphometric characteristic can be expressed as a function of time over the life cycle of the organism (Jernigan, Press, & Hesselink, 1990; Pfefferbaum, Mathalon, Sullivan, Rawles, Zipyrsky, & Lim, 1994). These temporal changes characterize the rate of growth and development of the structure in terms of size, shape, location, and composition. When making multiple measurements over time, additional quantitative measures can then be derived to characterize the time rate of change (first and second temporal derivatives) of the parameters to evaluate "velocity" and "acceleration" of these changing structures (Filipek, Kennedy, & Caviness, 1991).
- Specific brain functions are carried out at anatomically distinct locations. Evidence for this assertion has been mounting over the past century through lesion deficit correlation, and more recently through cognitive activation studies. The location of functional structures may not be static. Reorganization can be shown in response to insult, as well as developmental factors. Indeed, some evidence exists that functional organization is dynamically modulated at the neural network level (Van Essen and Anderson, 1990). The degree and extent to which reorganization occurs is also strongly coupled to the developmental state of the system. It is known that children demonstrate a greater potential for reorganization than adults (Kimura, 1975). This neural plasticity highlights the dynamic qualities of functional localization.
- The brain is functionally and anatomically lateralized. Aphasias provided the initial and most robust evidence for a functional asymmetry of the human brain and legitimized the claim that language is lateralized in the left hemisphere in the majority of right-handed individuals (Bear, Schiff, Saver, Greenberg, & Freeman, 1986). In addition, historically, the right cerebral hemisphere has been thought to have greater influence in emotional functions, whereas the left cerebral hemisphere plays a more dominant role in analytic functions (Goodglass and Butters, 1984; Sperry, 1985). Morphometric parameters can be used to provide quantitative characterization to laterality measurements of size,

shape, location, and composition of brain structures. Besides direct comparison of morphometric parameters between hemispheres, the measures of bilateral structures can be combined to derive a single "lateral asymmetry" index which reflects that structure's overall asymmetry. (See, for example, Galaburda, Lemay, Kemper, & Geschwind, 1978.)
- The brain is functionally and anatomically sexually dimorphic. Numerous authors have reported volumetric differences in global brain volume and specific substructures between male and female subjects (Filipek, Richelme, Kennedy, & Caviness, 1994; Zatz, Jernigan, & Ahuada, 1982; Swaab and Hofman, 1984). There are also reports of functional organization and lateralization differences between the sexes (de Lacoste, Horvath, & Woodward, 1990; Zilles, 1990; Knox and Kimura, 1970). These anatomic and functional data highlight the differential effect that gender plays in the development of the brain.
- Pathology affects structure. The results of gross pathologic insult, such as stroke and tumor, as well as developmental abnormalities, have been shown to result in altered anatomic and functional structure. Pathologies can be classified as progressive (i.e. tumor or infection), related to anomalous development or aging (i.e. Alzheimer's disease), or the result of a local destructive process (i.e. stroke or injury).

The aforementioned domains are not independent; in fact, there is a combinatorial effect as each of the domains interact or coexist. The quantification of morphometric parameters enables testing of (or search for) structural correlates of cognitive, behavioral, developmental, and functional attributes of the subject. The morphometric measures are not typically an endpoint itself, but a characteristic which may (or may not) bear some relationship to specific behaviors or functions. For example, the morphometric observation of the asymmetry of the planum temporale in normal right-handed subjects, (left is larger than right), is not particularly interesting without the "discovery" of the correspondence of the asymmetry with language lateralization; (language is predominantly lateralized in the left hemisphere in this population) (Geschwind and Galaburda, 1987; Geschwind and Levitsky, 1968; Galaburda, LeMay, Kemper, & Geschwind, 1978; Habib, Robichon, Levrier, Khalil, & Salanon, 1995). Specifically, morphometric measures of anatomic and functional structures permit issues like sexual dimorphism, lesion deficit correlation, and structural–functional correlation to be studied.

II. Methods

A. Morphometric Parameters and Classes of Measurements

As previously indicated, a structure can be characterized by its size, shape, location, and physical composition. In general, these measures are potentially independent, and each has a distinct measurement methodology (see Fig. 1). Since the brain is a three-dimensional object, the morphometric parameters can be characterized with one-, two- and three-dimensional representations (see Table 1). Take *size* for example. The linear, (one-dimensional) size of the brain can be expressed at the anterior–posterior length; the areal, (two-dimensional) size of the brain can be expressed at a particular cross-sectional location or projection; and the volumetric, (three-dimensional) size can be expressed for the structure in its entirety. The one- and two-dimensional measurements of a three-dimensional object provide an approximate representation of the desired morphometric parameter. Measuring the "size" of the brain by making a one- or two-dimensional measurement relies on an implicit assumption regarding the relationship of the measure and the desired property of the true three-dimensional object. The one-dimensional size, shape, and location measurements of a three-dimensional object are not unique. The linear distance measure can be interpreted to relay information regarding size, shape, or location, depending upon the underlying assumptions and hypothesis in question.

Shape can be described by decomposing an arbitrary shape into its constituent component standard (ortho-normal) shapes (Kennedy, Filipek, & Caviness, 1990; Ehrlich and Weinberg, 1970). Examples of the basis shape functions in two dimensions include the circular and elliptical harmonics (Ehrlich and Weinberg, 1970). Spherical harmonics, for example, can be used as a three-dimensional shape basis set (Sacks, Kennedy, Filipek, & Caviness, 1990). Each of these types of measurements requires the identification of an appropriate structural feature. These features are typically points (landmarks), lines, and surfaces in one, two, and three dimensions, respectively. The analysis of *location* requires the identification of a suitably chosen coordinate system (origin and axes) with which to measure a vector quantity in the appropriate dimension.

Once a structure has been identified in the desired number of dimensions (1, 2, or 3), the intensity distribution of the imaged quantity over defined structure can be observed, yielding a measurement of tissue *composition*. The interpretation of the measure of composition depends upon assumptions relating the imaged intensity to the underlying compositional features of interest.

B. Image Acquisition

Virtually all practical applications of morphometry require the acquisition of an image. The image may be formed optically, and viewed by the observer (optical microscopy), or it may be generated electronically, and

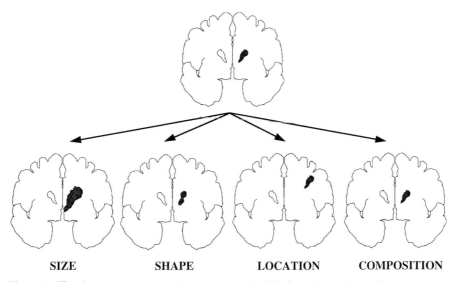

SIZE **SHAPE** **LOCATION** **COMPOSITION**

Figure 1 This figure represents a schematic example of the four classes of morphometric parameters discussed: size, shape, location, and composition. The examples shown attempt to illustrate the potential independence of each of these measures.

Table 1: Size, Shape, and Location Morphometric Parameters
for a Three-dimensional Object

Dimension	Size	Shape	Location
1D	Linear Distance	Linear Distance	1D Vector (relative to reference location)
2D	Area	2D Shape Analysis	2D Vector (relative to reference location)
3D	Volume	3D Shape Analysis	3D Vector (relative to reference location)

detected and stored by computer. The complete details of numerous contemporary structural and functional imaging techniques are explored in other chapters in this book (see chapter by Le Bihan). It is important, in the context of morphometric analysis, to review a number of particularly significant features of these imaging techniques here.

1. Structural Anatomic Imaging

In early brain–behavior correlational studies, clinical observations were matched with autopsy findings. This resulted in a powerful combination documenting a strong relationship between cerebral structures and behavioral phenomena. These postmortem analyses can potentially capture structural detail at the microscopic level. Pathological analyses, for obvious reasons, are limited to individual and cross-sectional population studies.

More recent technologies enabled these relationships to be evaluated in the living brain. Detailed anatomical descriptions can now be obtained by us-ing x-ray computed tomography and magnetic resonance imaging (MRI). *In vivo* studies are more versatile for cross-sectional or longitudinal follow-up studies, structural–functional coregistration, multipurpose volumetric assessments, and for intersubject (population) statistical studies (Caviness, Filipek, & Kennedy, 1989). State-of-the-art MRI provides a degree of anatomic detail that enables both the identification of structures of the brain and the measurement of their volumes (Filipek, Kennedy, & Caviness, 1992). Due to its relative noninvasiveness and anatomic resolution, MRI has become the method of choice for neuroanatomic evaluation and morphometric analysis. Part of MRI's success in neuroimaging results from the wide variety of tissue properties to which the MRI acquisition can be made sensitive. For the most part, clinical MR imaging is designed to take advantage of the differences in T_1 (longitudinal relaxation time), T_2 (transverse relaxation time), and intrinsic proton density found between gray matter, white matter, and cerebrospinal fluid (CSF). (See Figure 2.)

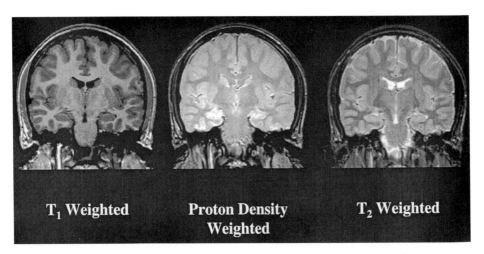

T₁ Weighted   **Proton Density Weighted**   **T₂ Weighted**

Figure 2 Example coronal MR images demonstrating T_1, T_2, and proton density weighting. Note the contrast differences between gray matter, white matter and CSF-filled spaces.

2. Functional Imaging

Changes in neuronal activity are accompanied by focal changes in cerebral blood flow (Fox and Raichle, 1986), blood volume (Fox and Raichle, 1986; Belliveau, Kennedy, McKinstry, Buchbinder, Weisskoff, Cohen, et al., 1991), blood oxygenation (Fox and Raichle, 1986), and metabolism (Phelps, Kuhl, & Mazziotta, 1981; Prichard, Rothman, Novotny, Petroff, Kuwabara, Avison, et al., 1991; Fox, Raichle, Mintun, & Dence, 1988). Brain function can be detected with techniques such as positron emission tomography (PET), functional magnetic resonance imaging (fMRI), electroencephalography (EEG), and magnetoencephalography (MEG). These physiological changes can be used to produce functional maps of component mental operations. Coregistration of functional and structural images provides a platform for the study of human behavior in relation to its neurobiological background. Moreover, developmental neuroimaging extends this analysis to include the temporal evolution of structure and its subserved function from conception to adulthood, as well as alterations which occur due to pathological or environmental influences.

III. Conflicting Constraints in Image Acquisition

The following properties are desirable for image data to be used in morphometric analysis: high spatial resolution, high structural contrast, and low total imaging time. High spatial resolution, (all other things being equal), is desirable in order to make as precise a measurement as possible, enhancing the potential sensitivity and specificity of the analysis. High structural contrast, or high "segmentability" alludes to the fact that someone (or something) must be able to *perceive* the tissue characteristics which enable the demarcation of the morphometric property, (landmarks, structural borders, etc.). The easier this identification task is, the quicker, more precise and more sensitive the resulting measurement will be. There are numerous reasons why imaging time needs to be minimized. First, time is money. The longer the imaging time, the more expensive the imaging session will be. Second is the issue of subject compliance. It is essential that the subject remain motionless during the complete image acquisition in order to obtain high quality images. The less cooperative a subject is, (as is typically true with patients and younger children), the shorter the duration of cooperative motionlessness that can be maintained without sedation. Hence the dilemma: increasing spatial and anatomic resolution typically requires increases in

imaging time, which has adverse effects on subject compliance. Thus, for every study a tradeoff is made regarding the overall precision and sensitivity, difficulty of analysis, and degree to which subjects can participate in the study.

A. Image Segmentation

Image data acquisition must be followed by a measurement protocol. This can range from making physical measurements on the hardcopy output itself to fully automatic computerized characterization of structures present at each image location. The term *segmentation* is used to represent the act of dividing an image into its structural components. In general, the structural components may be defined by tissue type, texture, functional characteristics, and so forth. Anatomic segmentation requires two steps: first, the *classification* of tissue type at each image voxel (volume element), (i.e., a given voxel is composed of gray matter, white matter, or CSF); and second, the assignment of a *label* (or name) to spatial distributions of the tissue classes (i.e., some groups of gray matter voxels constitute cortex, others subcortical nuclei).

The first step for structural morphometry is the delineation of regions of interest. Once structural borders have been defined, subsequent morphometric analysis of volume, shape, localization, and composition can be performed on the results of the segmentation. A comprehensive comparison of segmentation methods is outside the scope of this review (see Haralick & Shapiro, 1985), but it is useful to reiterate a number of the most common classes of segmentation methods currently found in the literature.

The difficulties found in practical image data make segmentation of an arbitrary MR brain slice very difficult. However, traditional segmentation techniques can often be tuned to work for specific images. These methods include edge-based methods (Rosenfeld & Kak, 1982), region growing, spatial clustering and morphological operations (Olhander, Price, & Reddy, 1978; Minor and Sklansky, 1981; Bowmans, Mersereau, Eisner, & Lewine, 1990; Brummer, 1991), heuristic methods (Bister, Cornelis, & Taeymans, 1991; Dawant, Zijdenbos, & Margolin, 1992; Ozkan, Sprenkels, & Dawant, 1990), and rule- and model-based methods (Raya, 1990; Bhanu and Holben, 1990). Using high quality multidimensional data (T_1, T_2, and proton density), good results can be produced using multispectral clustering techniques (Hall, Bensaid, Clarke, Velthuizen, Silbiger, & Bezdez, 1992). Some promising recent segmentation techniques that share a common framework include anisotropic diffusion and constrained optimization methods. Anisotropic diffusion reduces high frequency noise using a diffusion operation modulated by boundaries detected in the image (Cohen and Grossberg, 1984; Grossberg and Todorovic, 1988; Perona and Malik, 1990). Gerig et al. (Gerig, Martin, Kikinis, Kobler, & Jolesz, 1991) apply anisotropic diffusion as a preprocessing technique to increase the separability of clusters for a supervised classification technique. In constrained optimization methods, an objective or energy function is defined which imposes constraints such that the minimization of the energy function leads to the segmentation of the image (Geman, Geman, Graffigne, & Dong, 1990; Hertz, Krogh, & Palmer, 1991; Snyder, Logenthiran, Santago, Link, Bilbro, & Rajala, 1991; Amartur, Piraino, & Takefuji, 1992; Wang, Zhuang, & Xing, 1992; Worth, Lehar, & Kennedy, 1992).

B. Limitations to Current Approaches in Segmentation

There are a number of technical limitations applicable to the segmentation methods introduced in the preceding section. These include:

- Intensity is not an absolute measure. In magnetic resonance imaging, as opposed to x-ray computed tomography, the absolute value of an image pixel can be affected by many sources of variation in addition to those intrinsic to the object itself. The problem is compounded by intensity gradients across an image.
- Not all intensity-based borders are sharp edges. A major contribution to this problem is the partial volume blurring which occurs when multiple regions contribute to the signal in a given pixel. In these situations, techniques which require edge information to bound the formulation of a region will tend to either develop a discontinuous edge or merge the two regions. Edge-based segmentation methods alone are not sufficient to automatically segment brain images, because anatomical borders do not necessarily correspond with sharp changes in intensity at a given scale.
- Generalizability. Many of the segmentation systems which appear in the literature tend to be quite domain specific and often involve the use of "tricks" in order to successfully accomplish each specific task. There is no automatic system that is effective on practical image data. A synergistic system with a rigorous framework is needed to combine the multiple (possibly conflicting) constraints that must be satisfied to produce a valid segmentation.

Numerous tradeoffs exist between the level of user interaction required for analysis, the complexity and accuracy of the measurements, and the total amount of analysis time required for the analysis. Invariably, the analysis systems which provide the greatest degree of automation, and hence minimize user interaction, also have significant restrictions or requirements on type and quality of data necessary.

In our laboratory, we predominantly use intensity contour mapping and differential intensity contour mapping algorithms on each planar MR image for anatomic segmentation (Kennedy, Filipek, & Caviness, 1989). Anatomic structures are delineated by primary borders, corresponding to signal intensity transitions at brain–CSF or at gray–white matter interfaces; and secondary borders, knowledge-based anatomic subdivisions within a gray or white matter field which are not defined by signal intensity transitions, but rather are subsequently defined by hand by the investigator in concordance with knowledge-based anatomic subdivisions (Filipek et al., 1994). In principle, the segmentation algorithms identify, classify, and create a continuous outline corresponding only to those voxel locations constituting the specified anatomic border. The software interface is tailored to enhance productivity of typical segmentation operations in order to maximize the number of scans processed per time unit, given the interactive nature of the process. This system makes an explicit tradeoff, utilizing a significant amount of user interaction, but permitting a comprehensive anatomic analysis based upon a single, relatively temporally efficient image acquisition. These operations have been described in greater detail elsewhere (Kennedy, Filipek, & Caviness, 1989; Filipek, Kennedy, Caviness, Spraggins, Rossnick, & Starewicz, 1989; Filipek, Richelme, Kennedy, & Caviness, 1994).

1. Positional Normalization

Spatial contiguity, especially in the presence of finite voxel resolution, exists between groups of tissue classes which require different anatomic labels. Therefore, definitions must be adopted. These definitions result in dependencies on brain orientation. Therefore, to optimize the criteria for delimiting anatomic structures across multiple scans, a technique for insuring standardized orientation and anatomic presentation, *positional normalization,* of the MRI scans has been developed (Filipek et al., 1994). This involves reformatting and reslicing the volumetric image data in accordance with the orientation described for the Talairach atlas (Talairach and Tournoux, 1988). The standard points of reference include the midpoints of the decussations of the anterior (AC) and posterior (PC) commissures, and the genu of the corpus callosum (to define the interhemispheric plane). By selection of these reference points and coordinate systems, we can define the image transformation (rotation and translation) necessary to create new, positionally normalized coronal images such that the AC–PC line segment is aligned along one axis, and the plane of the interhemispheric fissure is oriented in the sagittal plane. By using this postprocessing technique, the need for any special positional protocol during the image acquisition itself is essentially eliminated.

IV. Example Applications

We now review a number of example applications which characterize the use of volumetric analysis and span the range of spatial dimension and anatomic resolution. Our approach of anatomic segmentation and cortical localization analysis (parcellation) uses MRI to establish a hierarchy of anatomic description that spans from the *whole brain* to the *systems* level description, and to localize foci of activation or lesions within parcellation units that are defined by topographical landmarks of the particular brain under investigation.

A. Volume Measurement Hierarchy

Plate 5 shows a representation of some of the multiple spatial scales which are amenable to measurement using moderately high resolution MR image data. The spatial domains include: whole brain (Filipek et al., 1994), lobes [callosal-based subdivisions (Filipek et al., 1992)], and gyral-based topography [approximately systems-level (Rademacher, Galaburda, Kennedy, Filipek, & Caviness, 1992)]. The finer-grained analysis requires additional structural definitions. It is important to make these definitions relative to the information which is present in the image itself, as opposed to requiring inferences based upon unseen information.

B. Localization Using Cortical Parcellation

The topology of individual normal brains is constant, in so far as they each contain the same logical processing units (Mesulam, 1985). The topography, and hence the spatial deployment of processing areas of individual brains, is quite variable. However, these functionally distinct regions have been shown to bear a consistent relationship to the surface features of the brain. We have developed a method of cortical parcellation which subdivides the cortex into 48 topologically defined regions per hemisphere (Rademacher et al., 1992; Kennedy, Meyer, Filipek, & Caviness, 1994). These regions are identified by fissures and landmarks

readily identifiable in high resolution structural MR imaging. Our method of cortical parcellation is defined by a set of limiting nodes (planes and landmarks) and fissures. These features are identified in volumetric anatomic MR images (i.e., 3D Spoiled Grass (SPGR), Fast, Low-Angle Shot (FLASH) or Magnetization Prepared-Rapid Acquisition by Gradient Echo. (MP-RAGE)). Optimum visualization and identification of each of these features requires positional normalization and the ability to navigate and interact with the image data from all cardinal image orientations (coronal, sagittal, and axial). See Plate 6. We have developed a unique interactive user interface to interact with the volumetric MRI image data. The sequence of steps includes: segmentation of cortical ribbon, identification of nodes and sulci, subdivision of cortical ribbon relative to nodes and fissures, and anatomic labeling of parcellation units. Plate 7 demonstrates the cortical parcellation applied to a normal subject. The resulting segmented, parcellated, and colorized coronal images are shown. These cortical regions can be subsequently used for morphometric analysis and localization in functional studies.

C. Spatial Distribution of Cortical Parcellation Units

The gyral topography of the brain, and hence the parcellation units, is spatially complex. Significant effort is expended in understanding and visualizing the relationship between various brain structures. Hence, we have developed a number of visualization tools which use the results of cortical parcellation as the basis for visualizing the complex three-dimensional surface anatomy of the cortex in a two-dimensional format. One can represent the presence of each parcellation unit relative to the coronal (anterior–posterior) slice location (see Plate 8). With this class of presentation, the entire relative layout of the parcellation units, and hence the gyral topography, can be appreciated at a glance.

D. Generalized Cortical Parcellation Display

The form of the preceding presentation permits the next level of generalization for display purposes. A schematic representation of the cortical parcellation system can be created by giving each parcellation unit a standard (unit) size representation. The relative topology of the brain is *not* maintained in this representation, but it provides a *standard form* upon which to codify regional results, and facilitate intersubject comparison. In this example (see Plate 9), each parcellation unit is color-coded by its lobe.

E. Structural–Functional Correlation Using Cortical Parcellation

Functional task-activation studies are typically done in conjunction with anatomic imaging studies. The spatial correlation of these anatomic and functional data provides a basis for anatomic interpretation of the functional task-activation process. Examples of these classes of analysis will be shown to illustrate this concept in the specific case of functional MRI and cortical parcellation.

In a given fMRI session, the spatial registration between a task-activation study and an anatomic scan is, to first approximation, controlled by the scanning parameters, and is known. Methods have already been established to compensate for subject motion which may have occurred over the course of the experiment, and permits sub-voxel registration between functional and anatomic studies (Woods, Cherry, & Mazziotta, 1992; Jiang, Kennedy, Baker, Weisskoff, Tootell, Woods, et al., 1995). Once cortical parcellation is applied to the anatomic image data, the assessment of the fMRI signal change relative to the anatomically defined cortical areas is possible. The classes of measurement which can then be made include:

- localization of activation foci
- assessment of number of voxels and percentage of parcellation unit exceeding the activation threshold
- laterality measures per parcellation unit
- reproducibility of activation within and between paradigms
- intersubject comparisons within and between paradigms

Specifically, we can assess localization by observation of the intersection of local extrema with the parcellation units, or as a binary decision for each unit if any activated voxels intersect that unit. We can quantify the extent of activation as the total number of voxels, or as a percentage of parcellation unit which exceeds a given threshold. A number of graphical representations of these measures will be shown later.

For an explicit demonstration of this analysis technique, we applied fMRI and cortical parcellation to 3 subjects who underwent a passive word reading and verb generation task (visual presentation of written words, covert generation of related verbs). We specifically analyzed the 13 perisylvian cortical parcellation regions from the complete system which are considered to be involved in language processing in the dominant hemisphere (Caplan, Gow, & Makris, 1995). The selected regions were identified in high resolution anatomic MRI scans of the subjects, using the individuals' own sulci and landmarks as identified using the cross-referential display system. Plate 10 shows an example slice showing the correspondence between the functional statistical map and the anatomic image. The images include the results of sulcal identification, and permit interpretation in terms of the cortical parcellation system. For a number of the activation regions seen in this figure, the demarcation of regional activation corresponds well with observed gyral boundaries.

This same statistical map can now be summarized relative the generalized cortical parcellation display, and each parcellation unit can be given a grayscale intensity which is proportional to the percentage of the parcellation unit, which is activated above the $p<.0001$

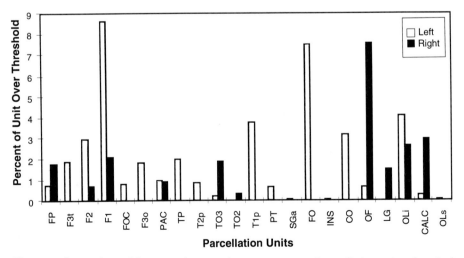

Figure 3 Comparison of the extent (expressed as a percentage of parcellation unit volume) of cortex involved in a passive word reading task between the left and right cerebral hemispheres. Only units which contained activation are shown.

level (Plate 11). This example can also be further extended to include the spatial distribution of significant activation. In Plate 12, the locations of the parcellation units, as well as the presence of activation, are indicated for the verb generation task in the 13 perisylvian language-related parcellation units.

F. Regional Analysis

In addition to identification of the spatial characteristics of parcellation units involved in a given paradigm, it is also desirable to quantify the extent to which the unit is involved. One example follows (Fig. 3), demonstrating the comparison of the extent (expressed as a percentage of the parcellation unit volume) of cortex involved in a passive word reading task between the left and right cerebral hemispheres. Only units which contained activation are shown, and they are grouped by lobar structure.

V. Discussion

Morphometric analysis is widely applied in many areas of study. Application of these methods to *in vivo* imaging of the brain is a logical extension of existing methodologies. These methods have been developed and refined concurrently with advances in image acquisition. The literature abounds with reports of morphometric measurement (predominantly size-based) used in the static population diagnostic characteristic domain of analysis. These include Alzheimer's disease (Ashtari, Zito, Gold, Lieberman, & Borenstein Herman, 1990; Jack, Sharbrough, Twomey, Cascino, Hirschorn, Marsh, et al., 1990; Scheltens, Leys, Barkhof, 1992; Seab, Huglo, Weinstein, & Vermersch, 1988), dyslexia (Duara, Jagust, Wong, Roos, Reed, & Budinger, Gross-Glen, Kushch, et al., 1991; Hynd, Semrud-Clikeman, Lorys, Novey, Eliopulos, 1990), attention deficit disorder (Hynd et al., 1990; Hynd, Semrud, Clikeman, Lorys, Novey, Eliopulos, & Lygtinen, 1991), schizophrenia (Shenton, Kikinis, Jolesz, Pollak, LeMay, & Wible, 1992), multiple sclerosis (Wicks, Tofts, Miller, du Bonlay, & Feinstein, 1992; Simon, Schiffer, Rudick, & Herndon, 1987), Huntington's disease (Harris, Pearlson, Peyser, Aylward, Roberts, & Berta, 1992), and obsessive-compulsive disorder (Breiter, Filipek, Kennedy, et al., 1992). As experience increases, and the methods become more standardized and available, the analysis of the time rate of change of the morphometric measurement will be used as a monitor of development and aging processes in both the normal and pathologic populations.

There are concurrent technical developments driving the imaging and computation analysis fields. In the areas of structural and functional imaging, the thrust is on maximizing spatial and temporal resolution. In the areas of computational analysis, the emphasis is to enhance the degree of automation which can be applied to image segmentation and morphometric analysis. This is critical in order to broaden the range of applicability of morphometric studies which can be carried out in the research and clinical settings. There is also a push to develop analysis methods which enable the finest-grained spatial resolution possible. In addition, it is not sufficient to have spatial anatomic resolution unless there is a concomitant functional validity to the analysis system. These areas will now be explored further.

A. Segmentation Is a Bottleneck

The preceding evidence shows that the morphometric assessment of many neurologically based disorders can benefit from an area or volumetric treatment. Thus, each morphometric study of this nature requires anatomic segmentation as the first step. Subsequent analysis after the initial segmentation can include fine-grained cerebral cortical subparcellation (Rademacher et al., 1992), volumetric analysis (Filipek et al., 1994), anatomic shape analysis (Kennedy et al., 1990), and localization analysis, in addition to the correlative studies of function and clinical symptoms. While nearly every neurologic and psychiatric disorder, as well as our knowledge of normal brain development, could potentially benefit from the quantitative analysis of brain structure, there cannot be a widespread proliferation of this methodology while the procedure remains highly time consuming and interactive. Invariably, the investigator is faced with the tradeoff of spending multiple days for the comprehensive analysis of each brain, or settle for a limited set of measures which can be made in a temporally efficient fashion in terms of human interaction and computational resources. The later option invariably results in a *limited* picture of the actual changes which have occurred and the results must be interpreted with extra caution.

In order to alleviate the bottleneck created by the segmentation step, we and others are actively pursuing the automation of these procedures. The advantages conferred through the automation of the segmentation are numerous:

- Increased accuracy, reproducibility, and reliability. Even semiautomated segmentation and anatomic labeling is a tedious, labor intensive task. A constant vigilance must be maintained in order to produce accurate results. Mechanically achieved results are less variable than human results when the algorithm and the data are deterministic. In addition, a computational system that performs the segmentation automatically is not only blind to subject identification, but also blind to the hypothesis which is being tested. Therefore, the automatic routines serve as a completely unbiased observer. It will, however, be inadvisable to completely remove the human expert from the loop. At some level, the resulting analysis must be reviewed and accepted as valid.

- Decreased cost. There are many sources of cost savings associated with automation. First, the computational resources which will be required cost less than full-time technicians performing the same task; computers also have less down time. In addition, the semiautomated methods require expert users and training to become proficient in both the conceptualization of the anatomic task and the operational requirements of the system. Third, costs are also reduced by the increased number of analyses per time unit which automation provides.
- New classes of questions can be asked. One of the most important benefits of increased efficiency is that the investigators will begin to formulate new types of questions, which would have been exorbitant in the amount of extra human time required over and above the time for segmentation.
- Increased availability. Finally, without automation, it is difficult to ". . . attract or convince physicians to use such technologies as a common tool in daily routine" (Stiehl, 1990). Automation will encourage more investigation at more widely dispersed sites to be able to address these classes of structural questions.

The elimination of this segmentation bottleneck through advances in automation will allow a more complete analysis to be performed and will provide benefits for clinical work as well as basic brain research. For example, in a study of the correlations between brain structure and a given pathology, a complete segmentation may not currently be performed because the researcher is interested in testing a hypothesis involving only certain brain regions. This decreases the amount of analysis and makes the study tractable. However, in advance, it may not be known where to find a correlation, or else the correlation may be in higher order statistics, (e.g. the ratios of measurements or a correlation in the variance of a group of measurements) (Filipek et al., 1994). A *complete* segmentation provided by automatic analysis may therefore provide information that would not otherwise be practical to obtain. Moreover, a complete analysis not only allows additional questions to be asked of the data, but also allows a rapid succession of questions and answers to lead to possibly unanticipated conclusions. As seen through the previously discussed applications, the precedence for such findings has already been established.

In addition to a more complete analysis for research, there are also potential clinical benefits. Automatic segmentation raises the possibility that every MRI brain scan taken can be run through a routine quantitative analysis. By comparing the results of such an analysis with "normal" measured shapes and sizes, a great deal of additional diagnostic information can be acquired. In applications to patients undergoing treatment, such routine use could provide increased feedback into the benefit of a specific treatment regimen, and potentially lead to the evolution of more efficacious treatment protocols.

B. Systems-Level Anatomic Description

The cortical parcellation system reviewed here is a comprehensive localization system for the cerebral cortex. It is defined relative to within-subject topographic reference and serves to provide additional localization information relative to the Talairach coordinate system (Talairach and Tournoux, 1988). This method can be used to summarize the results of a complete experimental paradigm from the entire cortex in a 1 or 2D plot of a suitably chosen measure per parcellation unit. While the time required for the anatomic analysis is long, it is not excessive given that the anatomic analysis need only be performed once per subject (assuming the ability to perform intrasubject registration between sessions). The correspondence between topographically defined anatomic regions and functional activation foci is an open empirical question; this methodology provides a means to assess the degree to which this correspondence exists. This method permits a more fine-grained approach to anatomic localization, since it is based solely upon the observed topology of the individual subject, not by reference to a typified anatomy as provided in an atlas-based system. The potential to identify further subdivisions of the parcellation units as defined by *functional* specialization will provide further insight into the functional architecture of the human brain.

In conclusion, it is clear that the quantitative analysis of both anatomic and functional structures will play a significant role as the field of developmental neuroimaging expands. Many developmental disorders have already been shown to have structural and functional correlates. Moreover, there are an untold number of disorders yet to be examined with these methodologies, each with a potential to shed new insight into the development and operation of the brain. Elucidation of the complete picture of the functional orchestration of the brain will require synergistic compilation of information from the microscopic, receptor, neural systems, and behavioral domains of information.

Acknowledgments

This work was supported in part by the following grants from the National Institute of Health: NS27950, NS34189, DA09467, and a grant from the Fairway Trust. The authors wish to thank Dr. Randall Benson for the functional MRI language task-activation data.

References

Amartur, S. C., Piraino, D., & Takefuji, Y. (1992). Optimization neural networks for the segmentation of magnetic resonance images. *IEEE Transactions on Medical Imaging, 11*(2), 215–220.

Ashtari, M., Zito, J. L., Gold, B. I., Lieberman, J. A., & Borenstein Herman, P. G. (1990). Computerized volume measurement of brain structure. *Investigative Radiology, 25*, 798–805.

Bear, D., Schiff, D., Saver, J., Greenberg, M., & Freeman, R. (1986). Quantitative analysis of cerebral asymmetries. *Archives of Neurology, 43*, 598–603.

Breiter, H. C., Filipek, P. A., Kennedy, D. N., Baer, L., Pitcher, D. A., Olivares, M. J., Renshaw, P. F. and Caviness, V. S., Jr. (1994). Retrocallosal white matter abnormalities in patients with obsessive–compulsive disorder, *Archives of General Psychiatry, 51*, 663–664.

Belliveau, J. W., Kennedy, D. N., McKinstry, R. C., Buchbinder, B. R., Weisskoff, R. M., Cohen, M. S., Vevea, J. M., Brady, T. J., & Rosen, B. R. (1991). Functional mapping of the human visual cortex by magnetic resonance imaging, *Science, 254*, 716–719.

Bhanu, B., & Holben, R. D. (1990). Model-based segmentation of FLIR images. *IEEE Aerospace Elect. Systems, 26*(1), 2–11.

Bister, M., Cornelis J., & Taeymans, Y. (1991). Towards automated analysis in 3D cardiac MR imaging. *Proc Information Processing in Medical Imaging, 12*, 205–221.

Bowmans, M. (1990). 3-D segmentation of MR images of the head for 3-D display. *IEEE Transactions on Medical Imaging, 9*(2), 177–183.

Brummer, M. E., Mersereau, R. M., Eisner, R. L., & Lewine, R. R. J. (1991). Automatic detection of brain contours in MRI data sets. *Proc. Information Processing in Medical Imaging, 12*, 188–204.

Caplan, D., Gow, D., & Makris, N. (1995). Analysis of lesions by MRI in stroke patients with acoustic-phonetic processing deficits, *Neurology, 45*, 293–298.

Caviness, V. S., Filipek, P. A., and Kennedy, D. N. (1989). MRI technology in human brain science: Blueprint for a program based upon morphometry. *Brain and Development, 11*, 1–13.

Churchland, P. S., and Sejnowski, T. J. (1988). Perspectives on cognitive neuroscience. *Science, 242*, 741–745.

Cohen, M. A., and Grossberg, S. (1984). Some global properties of binocular resonances: Disparity matching, filling-in, and figure-ground synthesis, In P. Dodwell, & T. Caelli, (Eds.), *Figural synthesis*, pp. 117–151, Hillsdale, NJ: Erlbaum.

Dawant, B. M., Zijdenbos, A. P., and Margolin, R. A. (1992). A surface fitting approach to the correction of spatial intensity variations in

MR images. *Proceedings of the SPIE. Biomedical Image Processing and Three-Dimensional Microscopy 1660*, 2–13.

de Lacoste, M.-C., Horvath D. S., & Woodward, D. J. (1990). Measures of gender differences in the human brain and their relationship to brain weight. *Biological Psychiatry, 28*, 931–242.

Duara, R., Kushch, A., Gross-Glen, K., et al. (1991). Neuroanatomic differences between dyslexic and normal readers on MRI scans, *Archives of Neurology, 48*, 410–416.

Edelman, G., and Mountcastle, V. (1978). *The mindful brain: Cortical organization and the group-selective theory of higher brain function.* Cambridge: MIT.

Ehrlich, R, and Weinberg, B. (1970). An exact method for characterization of grain shape, *Journal of Sedimentary Petrology, 40*(1), 205–212.

Filipek, P. A., Kennedy, D. N., Caviness, V. S., Jr., Spraggins, T. A., Russnick, S. L., & Starcwicz, P. M. (1989). MRI-based brain morphometry: Development and application to normal controls. *Annals of Neurology, 25*, 61–67.

Filipek, P. A., Kennedy, D. N., and Caviness, V. S., Jr. (1991) Morphometric analysis of central nervous system neoplasms, *Pediatrics Neurology 7*, 347–51.

Filipek, P. A., Kennedy, D. N., Caviness, V. S., Jr. (1992). Neuroimaging in child neuropsychology, In F. Boller & J. Grafman, (Eds.), *Handbook of neuropsychology*, Vol. 6, pp. 301–329, Elsevier, Amsterdam.

Filipek, P. A., Richelme, C., Kennedy, D. N., Caviness, V. S., Jr. (1994). The young adult human brain: An MRI-based morphometric analysis. *Cerebral Cortex, 4*, 344–360.

Fox, P. T., Mintun, M. A., Raichle, M. E., Miezin, F. M., Allman, J. M., & Van Essen, D. C. (1986). Mapping human visual cortex with positron emission tomography, *Nature (London), 323*, 806–809.

Fox, P. T., & Raichle, M. E. (1986). Focal physiological uncoupling of cerebral blood flow and oxidative metabolism during somatosensory stimulation in human subjects, *Proceedings of the National Academy of Sciences, U.S.A., 83*, 140–1144.

Fox, P. T., Raichle, M. E., Mintun, M. A., & Dence, C. (1988). Nonoxidative glucose consumption during focal physiologic neural activity, *Science, 241*, 462–464.

Galaburda, A., LeMay, M., Kemper, T. L., & Geschwind, N. (1978). Right-left asymmetries in the brain. *Science 199*, 852–856.

Geman, D., Geman, S., Graffigne, C., & Dong, P. (1990). Boundary detection by constrained optimization, *IEEE PAMI, 12*(7), 609–628.

Gerig, G., Martin, J., Kikinis, R., Kobler, O., & Jolesz, F. A. (1991). Automating segmentation of dual-echo MR head data. *Proc Information Processing in Medical Imaging, 12*, 175–187.

Geschwind, N, & Galaburda, A. (1987). *Cerebral lateralization.* Cambridge, MA: MIT.

Geschwind, N., & Levitsky, W. (1968). Human brain: Left–right asymmetries in temporal speech region. *Science, 161*, 186–187.

Goodglass, H., & Butters, N. (1988). *Psychobiology of Cognitive Processes. In Stevens Handbook of Experimental Psychology* (R. Atkinson, R Herrnstein, D. Luce & G. Lindsey, Eds.), New York: Wiley Interscience.

Grossberg, S, & Todorovic, D. (1988). Neural dynamics of 1-D and 2-D brightness perception: A unified model of classical and recent phenomena. *Perception and Psychophysics, 43*, 241–277.

Habib, M., Robichon, F., Levrier, O., Khalil, R., & Salanon, G. (1995). Diverging asymmetries of temporo-parietal cortical areas: A reappraisal of Geschwind/Galaburda theory. *Brain and Language, 48*, 238–258.

Hall, L. O., Bensaid, A. M., Clarke, L. P., Velthuizen, R. P., Silbiger, M. S., & Bezdek, J. C. (1992). A comparison of neural network and fuzzy clustering techniques in segmenting magnetic resonance images of the brain. *IEEE Transactions on Neural Networks, 3*(5), 672–682.

Haralick, R. M., & Shapiro, L. G. (1985). Survey: Image segmentation techniques, computer vision. *Graphics and Image Processing, 29,* 100–132.

Harris, G. J., Pearlson, G. D., Peyser, C. E., Aylward, E. H., Roberts, J., Barta, P. E., Chase, G. A., & Folstein, S. E. (1992). Putamen reduction on magnetic resonance imaging exceeds caudate changes in mild Huntington's disease, *Ann. Neurol., 31,* 69–75.

Hertz, J., Krogh, A., & Palmer, R. G. (1991). *Introduction to the theory of neural computation* (pp. 81–87). Redwood City, CA: Addison–Wesley.

Hynd, G. W., Semrud-Clikeman, M., Lorys, A. R., Novey, E. S., & Eliopulos, D. (1990). Brain morphology in developmental dyslexia and attention deficit/hyperactivity, disorder. *Archives of Neurology, 47,* 919–926.

Hynd, G. W., Semrud-Clikeman, M., Lorys, A. R., Novey, E. S., Eliopulos, D., & Lyytinen, H. (1991). Corpus callosum morphology in attention deficit disorder (ADHD): Morphometric analysis of MRI, *Journal of Learning Disabilities, 24,* 141–146.

Jack, C. R., Sharbrough, F. W., Twomey, C. K., Cascino, G. D., Hirschorn, K. A., Marsh, W. R., Zinsmeister, A. R., & Scheithaure, B. (1990). Temporal lobe seizures: Lateralization with MR volume measurements of the hippocampal formation. *Radiology, 999,* 423–429.

Jernigan, T. L., Press, G. A., & Hesselink, J. R. (1990). Methods for measuring brain morphologic features on magnetic resonance images: Validation and normal aging. *Archives of Neurology, 47,* 27–32.

Jiang, A. J., Kennedy, D. N., Baker, J. R., Weisskoff, R. M., Tootell, R. B. H., Woods, R. P., Benson, R. R., Kwong, K. K., Brady, T. J., Rosen, B. R., & Belliveau, J. W. (in press). Motion detection and correction in functional MR imaging, *Human Brain Mapping. 3,* 224–235.

Kennedy, D. N., Filipek, P. A., & Caviness, V. S., Jr. (1989). Anatomic segmentation and volumetric analysis in nuclear magnetic resonance imaging. *IEEE Transactions on Medical Imaging, 7,* 1–7.

Kennedy, D. N., Filipek, P. A., & Caviness, V. S., Jr. (1990). Fourier shape analysis of anatomic structures, In J. S. Byrnes & J. L. Byrnes (Eds.), *Recent advances in Fourier analysis and its applications.* Dordrecht, The Netherlands: Klewer Academic Press.

Kennedy, D. N., Meyer, J. W., Filipek, P. A., & Caviness, V. S., Jr. (1994). MRI based topographic segmentation. In R. Thatcher, M. Hallett, T. Zeffiro, R. John, & M. Huerta, (Eds.), *Functional neuroimaging: Technical foundations.* Orlando, FL: Academic Press.

Kimura, D. (1975). In Human communication and its disorders. D. B. Tower, (Ed.), *The nervous system,* (Vol. 3), pp. 365-372, New York: Raven.

Knox, C., & Kimura, D. (1970). Cerebral processing of non-verbal sounds in boys and girls. *Neuropsycologia, 8,* 227–37.

Mesulam, M. M. (1985). Patterns of behavioral neuroanatomy: Association areas, the limbic system, and hemispheric specialization. *Principles of behavioral neurology* (pp. 1–70). Philadelphia: Davis.

Minor, L. G., & Sklansky, J. (1981). The detection and segmentation of blobs in infrared images. *IEEE Transactions on Systems, Man, and Cybernetics, 11,* 194–201.Olhander, R., Price, K., & Reddy, D. R. (1978). Picture segmentation using a recursive region splitting method. *Computer Graphics and Image Processing, 8,* 313–333.

Ozkan, M., Sprenkels, H. G., & Dawant, B. M. (1990). Multi-spectral magnetic resonance image segmentation using neural networks. *Proceedings IJCNN, 1,* 429–434.

Perona, P., & Malik, J. (1990). Scale-space and edge detection using anisotropic diffusion. *IEEE Transactions on Pattern Analysis and Machine Intelligence, 12*(7), 629–639.

Pfefferbaum, A., Mathalon, D. H., Sullivan, S. V., Rawles, J. M., Zipyrsky, R. B., & Lim, K. O. (1994). A quantitative magnetic resonance imaging study of changes in brain morphology from infancy to late adulthood. *Archives of Neurology, 51,* 874–887.

Phelps, M. E., Kuhl, D. E., & Mazziotta, J. C. (1981). Metabolic mapping of the brain's response to visual stimulation: Studies in humans. *Science, 211,* 1445–1448.

Prichard, J., Rothman, D., Novotny, E., Petroff, O., Kuwabara, T., Avison, M., Howseman, A., Hanstock, C., & Shulman, R. (1991). Lactate rise detected by 1H NMR in human visual cortex during physiologic stimulation, *Proceedings of the National Academy of Science. U.S.A., 88,* 5829–5831.

Raya, S. P. (1990). Low-level segmentation of 3-D magnetic resonance brain images: A rule-based system, *IEEE TMI, 9*(3), 327–337.

Rademacher, J., Galaburda, A. M., Kennedy, D. N., Filipek, P. A., & Caviness, V. S., Jr. (1992). Human cerebral cortex: Localization, parcellation and morphometry with magnetic resonance imaging. *Journal of Cognitive Neuroscience, 4,* 352–374.

Rosenfeld, A., & Kak, A. C. (1982). *Digital picture processing.* Orlando, FL: Academic.

Sacks, J. A., Kennedy, D. N., Filipek, P. A., Caviness, V. S., Jr. (1990). MRI-based three-dimensional analysis of shape. *Proceedings of the Society of Magnetic Resonance in Medicine, 9,* 100.

Scheltens, P., Leys, D., Barkhof, F., Huglo, D., Weinstein, H. E., Vermersch, P., Kuiper, M., Steinling, M., Wolters, E. C., & Valk, J. (1992). Atrophy of the medial temporal lobes on MRI in "probable" Alzheimer's disease and normal aging: Diagnostic value and neuropsychological correlates. *Journal of Neurology, Neurosurgery, and Psychiatry, 55,* 967–972.

Seab, J. P., Jagust, W. J., Wong, S. T., Roos, M. S., Reed, B. R., & Budinger, T. F. (1988). Quantitative NMR measurements of hippocampal in Alzheimer's disease. *Magnetic Resonance in Medicine, 8,* 200–208.

Shenton, M. E., Kikinis, R., Jolesz, F. A., Pollak, S. D., LeMay, M., Wible, C. G., Hokcma, H., Martin, J., Metcalf, D., Coleman, M., & McCarley, R. W. (1992). Abnormalities of the left temporal lobe and thought disorder in schizophrenia: A quantitative MRI study. *New England Journal of Medicine, 327,* 604–612.

Simon, J. H., Schiffer, R. B., Rudick, R. A., & Herndon, R. M. (1987). Quantitative determination of MS-induced corpus callosum atrophy *in vivo* using MR imaging, *American Journal of Neuroradiology, 8,* 599–604.

Snyder, W., Logenthiran, A., Santago, P., Link, K., Bilbro, G., & Rajala, S. (1991). Segmentation of magnetic resonance images using mean field annealing. *Proceedings of the Information Processing in Medical Imaging, 12,* 218–226.

Sperry, R. (1985). Consciousness, Personal Identity, and the Divided Brain. In D. F. Benson & E. Zaidel (Eds.), *The dual brain: Hemispheric specialization in humans.* New York: The Guilford Press.

Stiehl, H. S. (1990). 3D image understanding in radiology. *IEEE Engineering in Medicine and Biology, 9*(4), 24–28.

Swaab, D. F., & Hofman, M. A. (1984). Sexual differentiation of the human brain: A historical perspective. *Progress in Brain Research, 61,* 361–373.Talairach, J., & Tournoux, P. (1988). *Co-planar stereotaxic atlas of the human brain.* New York: Thieme Medical.

Van Essen, D. C., & Anderson, C. H. (1990). In E. Schwartz (Ed.), *Computational neuroscience.* Cambridge, MA: MIT.

Wang, T., Zhuang, X., & Xing, X. (1992). Robust segmentation of noisy images using a neural network model. *Image and Vision Computing, 10*(4), 233–240.

Wicks, D. A., Tofts, P. S., Miller, D. H., du Boylay, G. H., Feinstein, A., Sacares, R. P., Harvey, I., Brenner, R., & McDonald, W. I. (1992). Volume measurement of multiple sclerosis lesions with magnetic resonance images: A preliminary study. *Neuroradiology, 34,* 475–479.

Woods, R. P., Cherry, S. R., & Mazziotta, J. C. (1992). *JCAT, 16*(4), 620–633.

Worth, A. J., Lehar, S., & Kennedy, D. N. (1992). A recurrent cooperative/competitive field for segmentation of magnetic resonance brain images. *IEEE Transactions Knowledge and Data Engineering 4*(2), 156–161.

Zatz, L. M., Jernigan, T. J., & Ahuada, A. J. (1982). Changes on computed cranial tomography with aging: Intracranial fluid volume. *American Journal of Neuroradiology, 3,* 1–11.

Zeki, S., Watson, J. D. G., Lueck, C. J., Friston, K. J., Kennard, C., and Frackowiak, R. S. J. (1991). A direct demonstration of functional specialization in human visual cortex. *Neuroscience (Oxford), 11,* 641–649.

Zilles, K. (1990). In G. Paxinos (Ed.), *The human nervous system.* Orlando, FL. Academic.

4

Measurement and Analysis Issues in Neurodevelopmental Magnetic Resonance Imaging

Eric Courchesne* and Elena Plante†

*Neurosciences Department, School of Medicine, University of California at San Diego, La Jolla, California 92093, and Autism and Brain Development Research Laboratory, La Jolla, California 92037; †Scottish Rite/University of Arizona Center for Childhood Language Disorders, Tucson, Arizona 85701, and Department of Speech and Hearing Sciences, University of Arizona, Tucson, Arizona 85721

I. Introduction

Magnetic resonance (MR) imaging is the most powerful technique yet invented for imaging the structure of the living human brain (Plate 13). Amazingly, it is simultaneously the most readily available and widely used imaging technique. It is possible for nearly anyone—from first quarter freshmen to radiology professors—to sit at an MR console and direct the acquisition of anatomical (or functional) images of the human brain. Given a modest amount of money and administrative permission, even those with virtually no prior training in MR imaging, neurosciences, experimental design, or statistical analysis can collect MR brain images with the help of a clinical medical technologist, (who may in turn also have relatively little detailed knowledge of human brain anatomy or training in scientific research procedures).

Once images have been obtained, anyone with a Macintosh computer can use free NIH software to measure MR images in any way he or she sees fit. Frequently, there is no convenient means available for one neuroscientist to objectively evaluate the image acquisition and analysis procedures reported by another researcher. Given this current state of affairs, the potential for erroneous measurements and effects to find their way into the literature is not insubstantial. In fact, historically this problem has accompanied the introduction of other powerful research technologies used

to image human brain structure or function (e.g., ERPs, PET). The process of winnowing methodological and interpretational grain from chaff in studies using these powerful tools has been and remains of paramount importance.

It is sometimes tempting to confer a "privileged" status to research that uses new and powerful techniques such as MR imaging. The enthusiasm concerning a technique's potential for scientific breakthrough can temper concerns for the limits of its application. However, the potential power of a technique in no way guarantees that the data it produces will be interpretable in all cases. In fact, MR imaging analyses are as capable of producing highly reliable but spurious results as any other research technique (Plante & Turkstra, 1991). Rather than being a methodologically privileged technique, the principles that are basic to good scientific design and statistical interpretation also apply to MR imaging research. Therefore, the degree to which MR imaging produces valid results relies on the investigator's sophistication in designing a study that considers and controls a variety of threats to research validity.

II. What Should Be Measured?

Scientific research is predicated upon the formulation of a hypothesis and the collection and analysis of data that empirically test that hypothesis. Given this,

DEVELOPMENTAL NEUROIMAGING

the validity of a study begins with the hypothesis and the translation of the ideas it contains into the specifics of a research design. Therefore, the ideas, or constructs, contained in a hypothesis provide a good starting point for the examination of validity. A strong hypothesis meets two basic requirements: (1) It is scientifically tenable, and (2) The specifics of the hypothesis are a good match to the capabilities of MR imaging as a research tool.

A scientifically tenable hypothesis is one that is specific and empirically or theoretically supported. The first of these components, specificity, is essential. To the extent that the constructs represented in the hypothesis are specific, specific approaches can be developed to target the hypothesized effects.

In contrast, hypotheses that are only vaguely defined can lead to the use of methods that are a poor match for the nature of the disorder. For example, the hypothesized construct of "atypical development" in a developmental disorder could be manifested in a variety of ways, including anomalous regions of subcortical gray matter, disturbed gyral patterns, disturbed asymmetries, or altered regional volumes (larger or smaller). However, not all of the neuroanatomic effects that reflect atypical development can reasonably be expected to occur in all developmental disorders. Specificity concerning which particular features are likely to be found in a disorder can promote the kinds of methodological approaches that are most likely to find those features.

The alternative to the development of specific techniques to match the specific ideas contained in a well-formulated hypothesis, is to develop a single protocol that is applied to the study of multiple disorders. This might be thought of as a "one-size-fits-all" approach. Although the protocols in these cases may produce highly reliable measures using recognizable anatomical divisions, the risk is that such protocols can be suboptimal for application to the specific characteristics of a particular disorder. For example, if a measurement protocol combines areas known to be altered with additional tissue that is typically spared, any effect may be substantially diluted. This problem occurs when the regions of interest in a standard protocol are large, or when the hypothesized effect occurs in a relatively restricted region. In these cases, a lack of specificity in either the hypothesis or in the match between the hypothesis and the measurement protocol can lead to erroneous interpretation of the resulting data.

In addition to being specific, a strong hypothesis is empirically or theoretically supported. A hypothesized neuroanatomic effect might be well-supported for one developmental disorder, but be unjustified or inappropriate for another. A good example of this is the examination of brain asymmetries in developmental disorders. Several investigators (e.g., Hynd, Semrud-Clikeman, Lorys, Novey, & Eliopulos, 1990, Leonard, Voeller, Lombardino, Morris, Hynd, Alexander, 1993, Plante , Swisher, Vance, Rapcsak, 1991, Plante and Turkstra, 1991) have hypothesized that patterns of asymmetry for structures in the region of the sylvian fissure would be disturbed in studies of developmental language and learning disabilities. For these disorders, this hypothesis is theoretically supported by the tie between the neuroanatomical structures involved in the asymmetry measures and the types of skill deficits (e.g. language) frequently exhibited in these disorders. It is empirically warranted, because the modal left-greater-than-right asymmetry in the general population (Chi, Dooling, & Gilles, 1977; Geschwind & Levitsky, 1968; Wada, Clarke, & Hamm, 1975, Witelson & Pallie, 1973) provides a relatively stable base from which to judge deviations. Furthermore, interpretation of altered asymmetries in these areas as evidence of altered brain development has construct validity, because the prenatal origin of this asymmetry (e.g., Chi et al., 1977; Wada et al., 1975, Witelson & Pallie, 1973) is a neuroanatomic trait that is consistent with the developmental nature of these disorders. Therefore, there is an empirical and theoretical base for predicting altered asymmetry of perisylvian structures in developmental language and learning disorders and interpreting altered asymmetries as evidence of a developmental effect.

In contrast, routine asymmetry calculations for perisylvian structures for other types of disorders lack theoretical support if there is no presumed tie between these neuroanatomic regions and the particular disorder. Furthermore, the not uncommon practice of calculating asymmetries for any and all interhemispheric measures lacks empirical support because not all brain regions have reliable standing asymmetries in the general population. Therefore, there is no theoretical or data-based reason to predict changes in asymmetry for every brain region measured in a study, or for every disordered population.

Once a specific and supported hypothesis is proposed, the links between the hypothesis and MR imaging capabilities can be systematically examined. This process necessitates careful consideration of both the hypothesized neuroanatomical effect, and how this effect should manifest within the parameters and limitations of the available MR imaging techniques. Neuroanatomic effects can be thought of as falling along a continuum from effects that occur at a microscopic level to those that affect large regions of the brain (see Fig. 1). In order for MR imaging to be considered an

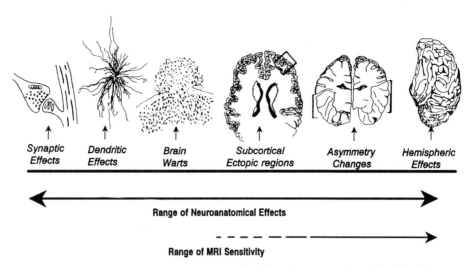

Figure 1. Neuroanatomic effects range from subcellular changes to effects that alter the gross anatomical structure of the full brain. The current resolution of MRI scans permits detection of effects only at the gross end of this continuum. Hypothesized effects must fall within the current resolving power of MRI in order for it to be used effectively as research tool.

appropriate research tool, the hypothesized neuroanatomical effect must be one that MR imaging techniques can detect. This is not a trivial issue. Although the resolution of MR imaging continues to improve, the most commonly used scan protocols are relatively *insensitive* to many types of developmental neuroanatomic effects.

For MR imaging to be an appropriate research tool, the hypothesized neuroanatomic effect must be of sufficient magnitude and imagibility to be detected through the investigator's scanning and quantification protocols. With some exceptions (e.g., Damasio et al., 1991, Clark, Courchesne, & Grafe, 1992), current scan protocols are limited to visualization of gross anatomy. Although a disorder, like dyslexia, may involve both micro- and macroscopic brain anomalies on autopsy, most imaging protocols will only reveal the latter. Therefore the specific hypotheses for an imaging study must lie within the relative sensitivity of MR imaging as a research tool. Even when this is the case, the methodological decisions that the investigator makes in employing MR imaging as a research tool will largely determine his or her ability to detect a hypothesized effect. The most well-formulated and well-supported hypothesis will not overcome the weaknesses of ill-considered decisions within the research design. The following section will address selected methodologic concerns that can greatly influence the viability of MR imaging-based investigations of developmental disorders.

III. How Well Can We Measure It?

In MR studies, three key steps are subject selection, anatomic visualization, and anatomic quantification. At each step, biases and error can reduce validity. Error consists of excess, random variation, the result of which is a decreased ability to detect true effects. Bias, on the other hand, is an unintended but systematic and directional effect that increases or decreases measured values. As such, "biases are irreversible, undetectable and potentially absolutely catastrophic" (Gundersen & Jensen, 1987), because they can both obscure some true effects and create effects that are spurious. Both bias and error in the research method lead to a loss of statistical power and the increased potential for false negative reports. The successful researcher naturally attempts to increase the chances of finding true effects (that speak to an a priori specific hypothesis), and to avoid false ones (that come from excessive error or biases). In other words, the researcher attempts to maximize the internal validity of the study.

Since there is no one single method for selecting subjects and optimizing the MR protocol for measurement of every possible neuroanatomic feature, the first and most important step in the optimization of procedures is to know what you are measuring and why it should be measured in a particular population. That is, one must have a specific a priori hypothesis. Put simply, those who know exactly what they must measure and why, will be able to take steps to guard against systematic measurement biases, and to maximize their chances of finding true effects and avoiding false ones, by carefully tailoring their sampling procedures to fit the specific needs for a test of an a priori hypothesis.

Conversely, those who do not, will not. That is, those who do not begin with specific theoretically-based hypotheses, and so do not know precisely what should be measured or why, cannot optimize their MR sampling procedures for every structure imaged. Such approaches will run the risk of unacceptably high error or "catastrophic" biases in their data sets. Such an approach is most diplomatically characterized as exploratory and runs the risk of missing true effects and reporting false ones. The results of such exploratory attempts to "measure everything" will be less accurate than and noncomparable (though possibly complementary) to results from studies that have successfully optimized subject selection and anatomic visualization and quantification.

The following sections examine selected principles that influence the internal validity of MR imaging studies of developmental disorders. We will provide examples of issues that concern all phases of the method: subject selection, decisions concerning scanning parameters, and anatomic segmentation. These include methodological components that are currently under investigator control, as well as some that are on the horizon as MR technology continues to improve.

A. Current Concerns

1. Subject Selection

a. Patients: Specificity versus Heterogeneity If the goal of a study is to find neuroanatomical common denominators associated with a developmental neurological disorder, it behooves the researcher to use specific, conservative, and narrow diagnostic criteria that best distinguish that disorder from others. Use of broadly inclusive patient selection criteria will introduce diagnostic heterogeneity into study samples. Patient heterogeneity is likely to mask true neuroanatomical differences from what is considered normal, since different disorders are usually associated with different underlying brain pathologies. For example, infantile autism, Asperger syndrome, and Rett syndrome, though distinctly diagnostically different from each other (DSM-IV), all fall within the same domain of pervasive developmental disorders. Quantitative MR studies of the vermis in these three diagnostic categories reveal anatomic differences between them. In autism, hypoplasia of the vermis is present from infancy onward (Hashimoto, Tayama, Murakawa, Yoshimoto, Miyazaki, Harada, et al., 1995; Courchesne, 1995

and 1995b; Saitoh, Yeung-Courchesne, Press, Lincoln, Hass, 1994); Asperger patients have normal vermis size (Lincoln, Courchesne, & colleagues, in preparation); and Rett patients have minimal vermian loss in early childhood, but substantial vermian atrophy by young adulthood (Murakami, Courchesne, Haas, Press, & Yeung-Courchesne, 1989). Use of broadly inclusive patient selection criteria that allowed autistic, Asperger and Rett patients to be combined into a single MR study sample of "autistic disorders" or "autistic-like disorders" would clearly produce muddled results.

For some disorders, like language or learning disabilities, it is not at all clear which behavioral features constitute a single phenotype, and when variation may signal multiple and biologically distinct disorder subtypes. For example, it is now widely recognized that early language development is predictive of later reading ability, and that many individuals identified as dyslexic show poor oral language skills during early development. Therefore, there is substantial overlap between the developmentally language-disordered and dyslexic populations. However, the degree of overlap, or whether these populations are identical, remains controversial.

Furthermore, when a disorder is behaviorally defined and identified through behavioral testing, the accuracy (statistical sensitivity and specificity) of the tests used to identify subject groups is frequently unreported or unknown; (see Plante & Vance, 1994 for a detailed illustration of this problem). A related problem arises when an identification scheme combines information from several tests, such as in discrepancy formulas for identifying learning disabilities (see Francis, Fletcher, Shaywitz, Shaywitz, & Rouke, 1996, for a review of these issues). This lack of documentation for validity and accuracy of the identification method can lead to significant error or bias in subject selection, including overidentification of normal individuals as disordered and misidentifications of individuals who have the disorder as "normal."

Developmental disorders are not unique in terms of their behavioral overlap. The same concern applies to disorders of aging such as dementia, which can be caused by more than 60 disorders with widely disparate underlying brain pathologies (Haase, 1977). If patients with different types of dementia were included as a single study group in a quantitative and statistical MR research design, the different underlying abnormalities would be averaged together and may well result in statistically insignificant, or "negative" findings; any positive findings from such a diverse group would be misleading, since no meaningful interpretation can be made to determine the actual variety of brain abnormalities underlying the different types of dementia.

So, whether due to a disorder of development or aging, neurobehavioral dysfunction may be caused by widely disparate underlying brain pathologies. At one time, children with infantile autism, phenylketonuria (PKU), Lesch–Nyhan syndrome, Rett syndrome, fragile-X, Asperger syndrome, and so on would all have been similarly classified as "social failures." Broad subject selection criteria that includes such a spectrum of developmental disorders does little to advance understanding of the specific and characteristic brain bases and etiologies of each separate disorder. As with dementia, if a research design included the broad spectrum of different patients with overlapping behavioral symptoms into a single study group, false negative or misleading MR findings would likely result. The best chance for obtaining valid quantitative and statistical information on the anatomical bases of a neurological disorder, whether it be autism or Alzheimer's disease, is to use diagnostically sensitive, specific, and conservative, rather than broadly inclusive, patient selection criteria.

b. Normal Controls: Normal Volunteers versus "Normal" Patients The only way to demonstrate an anatomical abnormality in a disorder is by reference to "normal." Unfortunately, all too often the high cost of MR imaging presents a strong incentive for the methodological shortcut of utilizing, as controls, clinical patients whose scans have been deemed "normal" by routine clinical radiological review. However, the use of MR imaging to investigate the neuroanatomy of neurological disorders has arrived at a stage where quantitative differences in brain structures between clinical and normal populations are being sought. Clinical patients seek clinical consultation because they do not feel healthy and normal; even if qualitative radiologic review returns with a "normal" diagnosis, meaning "disease has not been detected," the probability of true normality among these patients is, by definition, lower than that for normal volunteers.

This concern is magnified if "normative" developmental data are collected from pediatric patients with negative scans. A normal infant or child is seldom referred for MR brain imaging unless sufficient history or symptoms justify the procedure (for which sedation is usually advised to ensure motionlessness). Frequent reasons for MR referrals are developmental delay and seizure disorder with chronic therapy. These conditions carry a high probability that some brain structures would have subnormal sizes due to underdevelopment or atrophy. For example, analyses show that vermian measures in pediatric patients are signifi-

cantly smaller than those reported in studies using normal, healthy volunteers (Fig. 2).

Other characteristics of any non-normal (i.e., "normal" patient) control group may also impact outcome. To the extent that the non-normal control group and target patient group are truly independent with regard to the variables under study, statistical effects will be maximized. Conversely, if such a non-normal control group is "contaminated," the effect will be compromised. For example, when a disorder is familial (e.g., language and learning disabilities), the effect size for between-group comparisons will be reduced if the control group inadvertently includes subjects with a

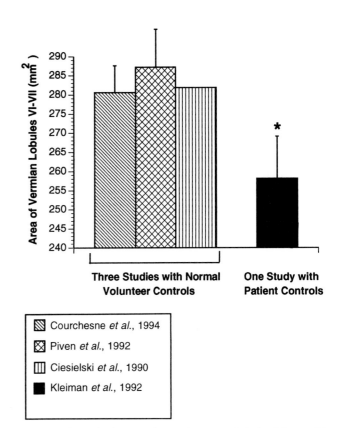

Figure 2 Example showing that patient controls judged "normal" by routine radiologic clinical criteria may not have normal neuroanatomy when quantitatively measured. Among four MR studies of vermian lobules VI–VII in infantile autism, three studies used control subjects who were normal, healthy volunteers (Ciesielski et al., 1990; Piven et al., 1992; Courchesne, Saitoh, et al., 1994), but one study used pediatric patients as controls (Kleiman et al., 1992). Although MR scans from these pediatric patients were judged to be normal at clinical radiologic examination, the areas of vermian lobules VI–VII in these "normal" pediatric patients were significantly smaller than the healthy, normal volunteer subjects in other studies (Ciesielski et al., 1990; Piven et al., 1992; Courchesne, Saitoh, et al., 1994a). * = Significantly different from normal, healthy volunteer subjects. [Note: In this figure, the mean from Courchesne, Saitoh, et al. (1994a) represents the mean of the 44 normal volunteers from that report (from Courchesne, Yeung-Courchesne, et al., 1994c).]

family history for the disorder under study (Leonard et al., 1993; Plante, 1991). This may be a particular problem when parents refer their children as control subjects because they have concerns about their child's developmental status.

Selection of a normal, healthy volunteer control group should be based on criteria that make good neurobiological sense such as normality of developmental milestones, normality of medical, psychiatric, family, and educational history, normality of current intellectual and physical functioning, absence of a history of exposure to environment risk factors, and so on. Nonbiological criteria such as native language background or social economic status (SES) are of questionable value. Brain growth may be affected by some factors that may be correlated with these types of criteria, (e.g., poor nutrition or exposure to environmental toxins with SES; ethnicity with native language background). However, if these associated factors are of concern, the strongest approach would be to identify the factors explicitly and control their occurrence in the subject group directly.

In the absence of such identifiable risk factors, the idea that brain growth is correlated with all manner of subject characteristics in the normal, healthy, risk-free fetus, infant, and child remains unproven. To illustrate the case with the example of SES, the authors suspect that brain growth is not strongly correlated with whether an individual's parents are poor poets who preferred working in a small town library after high school to attending a mediocre junior college or are rich pet rock inventors living on Fifth Avenue in New York after four years of pro forma enrollment in college! Moreover, over the last decade, we have noticed the remarkable ebb and flow of educational, social, and job opportunities that make the SES of any individual mutable. If you lose your job as an aeronautical design engineer and now wrap burgers and fries, will your children develop abnormal sulcal configurations? Ill-considered restriction on the selection of either normal or disordered subjects can lead to a sample that does not represent the population to whom we hope to generalize the research findings.

In sum, qualitative review of an MR scan is insufficient to ensure "normality"; so-called "normal" scans from patients are not a substitute for scans from normal, healthy volunteers; the neurodevelopmental and family history of volunteers should not intersect with that of the patient study groups; and subject selection criteria should be neurobiologically grounded.

c. Contrast Patient Groups   In MR neuroanatomy studies, biological theory should determine the choice of contrast patient groups. The common uses of normal volunteers and contrast patient groups stem from distinctly different purposes. Normal controls provide the opportunity to demonstrate abnormality. Contrast patient groups are often used for one of two purposes. In some studies, contrasted disorder groups are used to obtain neurobiological evidence that dissociates two disorders that frequently co-occur in the population (e.g., dyslexia and attention deficit/hyperactivity disorder (ADHD) in Hynd et al., 1990). In such studies, some overlap in the anomalous neuroanatomical traits are expected between the two disorders, but findings of one or more traits unique to each supports the interpretation of the disorders as biologically separable.

Other investigators use a contrast disorder group for a different purpose: to determine whether such abnormalities are "specific" to the primary disorder of interest. This particular use of contrasting disorder groups is problematic. For instance, a large set of distinctly different etiological, microscopic anatomical, and physiochemical abnormalities can potentially underlie any particular MR size abnormality. Therefore, and contrary to popular belief, similar anatomical MR size abnormalities in two contrasting patient groups does not say anything really interesting about specificity of underlying etiological, microscopical, or physiochemical abnormalities in the two disorders. Autism and PKU both involve cerebellar hypoplasia, but whereas autism involves Purkinje neuron loss, PKU involves retarded neuron growth. The superficial macroscopic similarities belie deeper and more important etiological, anatomical, and functional dissimilarities. Moreover, precisely the same etiological insult to the same developing structure can lead to distinctly different outcomes, depending on the precise timing and magnitude of the insult (e.g., Altman, 1982). Thus, the practice of contrasting two or more neuropsychiatric patient groups (e.g., autism and non-autistic retarded patients or language-impaired patients; or Williams and Down syndrome patients) can reflect a misconception of developmental biology and the phenomenon of developmental convergence, as well as a naivete about what level of anatomic abnormality and specificity is revealed by macroscopic MR anatomical measures. In sum, a potential contrast patient group must make good neurobiological sense vis-à-vis specific neurobiological hypotheses about the target patient disorder, or it should not be used at all.

2. Quantitative versus Qualitative Approaches to MR Image Analysis

During initial studies of a disorder whose neuroanatomical substrate is unknown, qualitative analyses of MR images can occasionally lead to the discovery of some abnormalities if they are rather obvious, and in doing so, can quickly orient further quantitative analyses. An example comes from infantile autism, in which the discovery of hypoplasia in cerebellar vermian lobules VI and VII was initially made by a qualitative radiologic examination of a single patient with autism (Courchesne, Hesselink, Jernigan, & Yeung-Courchesne, 1987), which had been prompted by an earlier theory linking neocerebellar structures to autism (Courchesne, 1985). Verification of this single case radiologic finding was then accomplished via detailed quantitative analyses of a large number of patient and normal subjects (Courchesne, Yeung-Courchesne, Press, Hesselink, & Jernigan, 1988, Courchesne, Saitoh, Yeung-Courchesne, Press, Lincoln, Haas, & Schreibman, 1994; Courchesne, Townsend, & Sartoh, 1994). Presently, anatomical abnormalities of the cerebellar vermis and hemispheres in autism have been reported in 16 quantitative MR and autopsy studies from nine laboratories involving more than 254 autistic (and 220 normal) patients (Table 1). An analogous story is emerging for the parietal lobes in autism (Courchesne, Press, & Yeung-Courchesne, 1993; Egaas, Courchesne, & Saitoh, 1995;

Townsend & Courchesne, 1994; Townsend, Courchesne, & Egaas, in press).

Although qualitative analyses may sometimes succeed in detecting abnormalities of a rather large magnitude, even the most practiced and sensitive radiologic eye may often be unable to discern significant abnormality. Rett syndrome provides an example. This disorder involves severe brain maldevelopment, readily identifiable neurologic manifestations, relatively little clinical heterogeneity, and high diagnostic confidence in typical cases. Brain maldevelopment is so severe in Rett syndrome that a simple tape measurement of head circumference is frequently sufficient to show microcephaly in affected children, adolescents, and adults, and autopsy examination reveals gross abnormalities in brain weight and neural growth. Moreover, in a recent MR study of Rett patients, quantitative and statistical analyses readily identified abnormality in the cerebellum, cerebrum, brainstem, and basal ganglia (Murakami et al., 1992). By contrast, qualitative MR radiologic examination did not detect any abnormality in the majority of these same patients (Murakami et al., 1992).

So, reports of no neuroanatomical abnormality in a patient sample based solely on qualitative MR radiologic impressions should be received with extreme caution if not frank skepticism, especially since real anatomical differences in many neurodevelopmental disorders may be relatively small. Qualitative analysis is much less sensitive to subtle abnormalities in size, as only size abnormalities of a rather large magnitude are discernable to even a practiced eye (Fig. 3). From a research standpoint, qualitative, radiologic analysis, being less sensitive, is therefore prone to "false negatives." At the same time, since only obvious abnormalities are likely to be judged "abnormal" by qualitative evaluation, it is also more conservative, and the probability of a "false positive" report is much lower. The strength of qualitative evaluation lies in identifying possible abnormalities. Verification, however, is better accomplished through quantitative measurement.

3. Anatomic MR Visualization and Quantification

When visualizing and quantifying anatomic MR data, mismeasurements can often be traced back to any one of several sources: the MR scan protocol, the analysis approach, segmentation algorithms, and accuracy in anatomic identification.

a. MR Scan Protocol Crucial steps in any MR project are decisions about the number, orientation, and in-plane spatial resolution of MR slice samples. Decisions are driven by theoretical, experimental, and practical considerations. Theoretical and experimental

Table 1 The Cerebellar Abnormalities in Infantile Autism: Quantitative MR Imaging and Autopsy Evidence

---

Studies finding abnormalities

Williams et al., 1980 (autopsy)

Bauman & Kemper, 1985 (autopsy)

Ritvo et al., 1986 (autopsy)

Bauman & Kemper, 1986 (autopsy)

Gaffney et al., 1987 (MR)

Courchesne et al., 1988 (MR)

Murakami et al., 1989 (MR)

Bauman & Kemper, 1990 (autopsy)

Ciesielski et al., 1990 (MR)

Arin et al., 1991 (autopsy)

Bauman, 1991 (autopsy)

Piven et al., 1992 (MR)[a]

Kleimen et al., 1992 (MR)[a]

Courchesne, Saitoh, et al., 1994 (MR)

Saitoh et al., 1995 (MR)

Hashimoto et al., 1995 (MR)

Studies finding no abnormalities

Garber and Ritvo, 1992 (MR)

Holttum et al., 1992 (MR)

---

[a]Evidence based on reanalyses of study data by Courchesne, Townsend, & Saitoh, 1994.

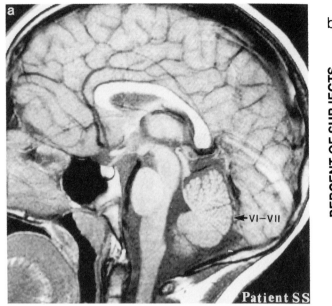

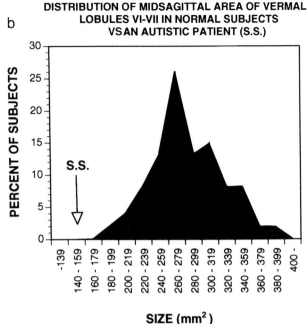

Figure 3 Appearances can be deceptive. (a) Midsagittal MR (T1-weighted, 600/12) of a 7-year-old autistic child (S.S.) was judged to be normal at clinical radiologic examination. (b) Quantitative analyses of anatomy in this patient showed substantial deviation from normal. For example, as compared to the distribution of size for vermian lobules VI–VII in normal, healthy volunteers (Courchesne, Saitoh, et al., 1994a), the size of this patient's vermian lobules VI–VII (arrow: subject S.S.) fell well below normal values (from Courchesne, Yeung-Courchesne, et al., 1994).

stereological studies have examined different methods for estimating volumes and cross-sectional areas of a variety of irregularly shaped biological objects (Gundersen & Jensen, 1987). They demonstrated mathematically and empirically that the most efficient and unbiased general method, (based on the Cavalieri principle), involves systematic sampling of an object using a series of sections, each composed of a regular x-y grid of sample points. This is directly analogous to the routine MR procedure of obtaining a series of MR slices, each composed of an x-y grid of voxel values.

Moreover, Gundersen & Jensen (1987) developed a method for predicting the number of sample slices and in-plane x-y sample points needed to obtain a given coefficient of error. For example, when estimating the volume of even very irregularly shaped biological structures, they showed that as few as 10 slices may be sufficient to obtain estimates having a coefficient of error of less than 5%, a value smaller than most group effect sizes. However, with even fewer slices (e.g., 3 or 4), volume estimates may be in substantial error. Slice orientation, thickness, and gaps between slices are less important parameters than the number of slices passing through a structure of interest when attempting to obtain volume estimates of that structure. Mayhew & Olsen (1991) showed that these sampling and estimation methods generalize to MR data samples. In esti-

mating the volume of the human brain by MR in postmortem and *in vivo* cases, they found that the coefficient of error of the volume estimate was 1.7% for 14 slices, <4% for 7 to 8 slices, and >10% for 3 slices.

The results of these studies have several important implications for the use of MR imaging to quantify neuroanatomical volumes in the normal and abnormal brain. First, to achieve low coefficients of error (<5%) in volume estimates, MR protocols must provide at least 7 slices through every anatomical structure whose volume is to be quantified. A common approach is to obtain an MR data set composed of 1.5- to 5-mm gapless slices in one or another direction (coronal, axial, or sagittal). In any one such data set, volume estimates of some structures, such as the entire cerebrum, will be based on a large number of slices and will have a very small coefficient of error (<1%), while volume estimates of other structures, such as a single gyrus, the head of the caudate, the thalamus, or the amygdala, will be based on a much smaller number of slices and will have a larger coefficient of error. Such differences are important when making statistical power calculations, choosing measurement and analysis approaches, and drawing inferences from results.

Second, an orientation that might allow a sufficient number of slices to pass through one set of structures (e.g., the cerebellum viewed sagittally), might preclude the possibility of collecting a sufficient number of slices through other structures (e.g., the hippocampus viewed sagittally). The investigator may need to trade off on the number of regions that can be theoretically measured for increased accuracy in certain regions, in order to keep the total scan time within the limits of patient tolerance. Therefore, the investigator may need to prioritize the potential regions of interest and select slice thickness and orientation to optimize volume estimates of those regions that are critical to the research hypothesis.

The dependence of volumetric accuracy on the number of slices used to obtain the volume estimate, even when the orientation of those slices may vary, has particular relevance for developmental research. It implies that longitudinal MR volumetric studies can be readily and reliably done by following the principles and methods derived by Gundersen & Jensen (1987), and has been demonstrated with MR brain imaging by Mayhew and Olsen (1991). Thus, the principal requirements for a longitudinal MR study of the brain are that on each sampling occasion, a sufficient number of slices and a suitable orientation of slices be obtained for each structure of interest. A "sufficient" number of slices can be determined by taking into account the minimum longitudinal effect size that one wants to be able to resolve for a given structure of interest, the coefficient of error for different numbers of slices through that structure, and the desired statistical power level in statistical analyses.

A "suitable" orientation is one that provides good visualization of the critical landmarks and boundaries defining the structure of interest and minimizes confounding partial voluming effects. These are important caveats that apply to the principle of volume estimation from serial slices. Even when a protocol provides a satisfactory number of slices through a structure of interest, for some neuroanatomical structures some orientations will provide better visualization of defining landmarks and boundaries than will other orientations. For example, sagittal MR slices cut orthogonally through the vermis reveal in complete detail all surface features known to define anatomically and functionally separate regions (Courchesne et al., 1989; Press & Courchesne, 1992a,b). In contrast, axial MR slices cut the vermis obliquely and provide poor visualization of its surface features, especially when such oblique orientations cause landmarks and structural boundaries to become blurred or lost through partial voluming with neighboring structures. So, in general, as compared to more optimal MR slice orientations, orientations that provide poor visualization will lead to an increased potential for inaccurate delineation of critical anatomical landmarks and struc-

tural boundaries during quantitative analyses, and to greater inaccuracy of volume estimates.

Precision and comparability of MR slice orientation is of paramount importance when anatomic quantification involves area measures obtained from a single slice or only a very few slices, rather than volume measures. Examples of such instances include measurements of the cross-sectional areas of the corpus callosum (Egaas et al., 1995), the vermis (Courchesne, Saitoh, et al., 1994), and the body of the hippocampus (Saitoh, Courchesne, Egaas, Lincoln, & Schreibman, 1995; see also Courchesne, Yeung-Courchesne, & Egaas, 1994) (Fig. 4). In these instances, the error inherent to minimal slice numbers can be offset by standardizing the structure's orientation for all subjects. In such situations, routine clinical positioning procedures are not acceptable. For example, in a benchmark paper published on hippocampal size in patients with amnesia, Press, Amaral, and Squire (1989) demonstrated the principle that, in quantitative studies of a single slice or only a very few slices, alignment of MR sections should be based on critical anatomic features that are intrinsic to the specific structure to be quantified, rather than on structures extrinsic to the structure of interest, as is commonly practiced.

When misalignment does occur, some may advocate reslicing the MR data set after the original acquisition step. Reslicing involves interpolating values between in-plane voxels to obtain an estimation of voxel values that should occur in an alternate plane of view. However, given comparable scan parameters, resliced images do not provide the same degree of high anatomical fidelity as images which are obtained with initially accurate alignment. Presently, MR protocols typically offer 3 to 4 times higher resolution in-plane than out-of-plane, and reslicing algorithms necessarily mix the two resolutions. The extent of error from measurement of resliced images will depend on a number of factors, including the magnitude of misalignment, slice thickness, in-plane resolution, and the algorithm used to calculate the resliced image from the original data set. When small group differences are at issue, analyses based on resliced images may be too coarse to resolve such differences due to the error inherent in the interpolated image data.

Of greater concern, however, is the danger of introducing bias through reslicing image data. When there is a systematic difference in the original slice angle obtained for two or more subject groups, the reslicing of image data could introduce a systematic effect of sufficient magnitude to produce a statistically significant between-group difference. Systematic differences in the default orientation for subject groups could occur for various reasons. For some developmental disorders, like Down syndrome, differences in the skull shape between the disordered and normal group will affect the tilt of the head as it lays naturally in the scanner. Similarly, the degree of rostral–caudal head tilt for a supine subject varies with the age of the subject. This age effect could result in significant bias in longitudinal studies, particularly for anatomical structures that are imaged over few slices. Likewise, this age effect on slice orientation could obscure the ability to detect cross-generational similarities in familial studies, by introducing a source of variance that is extraneous to the anatomical features under study. (See Fig. 5: Differences in a mother–daughter pair.)

b. Signal Intensity Inhomogeneities

In quantitative analyses, after suitable MR brain images have been obtained, the most important next step is the accurate classification of all pixels into gray matter, white matter, and cerebrospinal fluid (CSF). This can be a monumental task. For example, the 1160 cm^3 of a typical cerebrum corresponds to several million MR image pixels. The convoluted surface of the cerebral cortex makes the manual tracing of all tissue boundaries a tedious, difficult, and error-prone undertaking. To reduce the manual labor involved in this step, some have developed computer algorithms that simplify or speed experimenter decisions during manual tracing, while others have developed automatic algorithms that classify pixels.

Regardless of which path is chosen, a major problem is encountered. Signal intensity inhomogeneities are present in all MR brain scans as a result of the MR device itself. That is, because of properties inherent in the MR device, if one could take the identical sample of gray matter (or white matter or CSF), and image it in different locations within a head coil, it would have different signal intensities. As shown in Figure 6a, a pronounced dropoff occurs in the superior–inferior axis, and the signal may be reduced by as much as 30% in the inferior cerebellum relative to the cerebral lobes. Figure 6B shows a ring of reduced signal on an axial proton density-weighted image of a pure water phantom. Similar effects can be observed in axial brain images in the posterior pole.

Thus, it is clear that thresholding algorithms intended to aid tracing or pixel classification are potentially biased by MR device-based signal intensity inhomogeneities. They can lead to the overestimation of the number of gray matter pixels in some regions, and the underestimation of them in another. In this way, the mean total (global) volume of gray matter pixels may appear to approximate correct published data, while in fact local estimates may be in substantial error. It is therefore inadequate to use such total estimates as the only evidence validating the accuracy of

any pixel classification approach. This is a major problem because, as previously discussed, gray matter, white matter, and CSF do not produce signal values that uniquely and separately encode them. Signal differences between tissue types are relative and graded. Therefore, virtually all computer classification algo-

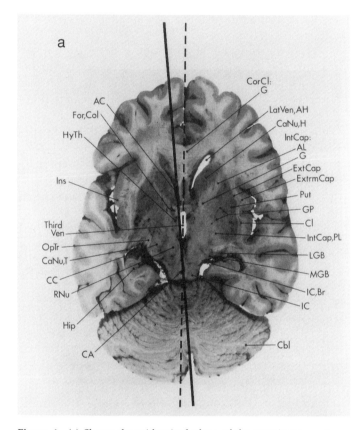

Figure 4 (a) Shows the midsagittal plane of the vermis may not necessarily be the same as the midsagittal plane for nonvermian structures such as the fornix, anterior commissure, third ventricle, or aqueduct of Sylvius. The midsagittal plane of the vermis (*solid line* in figure) is frequently not naturally aligned with the midsagittal plane of nonvermis structures (*dotted line* in figure). Nonetheless, several MR studies (Garber et al., 1989; Garber & Ritvo 1992; Holttum et al., 1992) of the vermis in autism have oriented MR sections based on one or more of these nonvermian structures. Alignment based on such nonvermian midsagittal planes can in many cases result in a misalignment relative to the midsagittal position of the vermis. Any MR study that uses such misalignments will report erroneous measures of the vermis. Since, in developmental disorders, the differences from normal in vermian structures may be small—many neural structures in disorders with severe maldevelopment such as Rett syndrome may differ from normal by 15% or less—such errors can mask real differences and cause negative findings to be reported. Transverse brain section reproduced from D. H. Haines, *Neuroanatomy: An Atlas of Structures, Sections and Systems*, Figure 4–20. *Dotted line:* midsagittal alignment based on noncerebellar structures including the columns of the fornix (For, Col), anterior commissure (AC), third ventricle (Third Ven), and aqueduct of Sylvius (CA). *Solid line:* midsagittal alignment based on vermian landmarks.

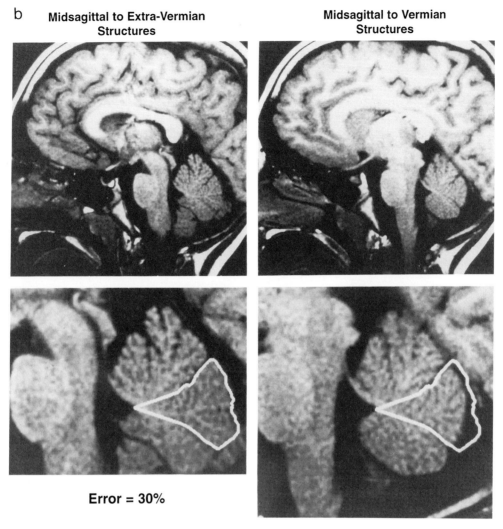

b   **Midsagittal to Extra-Vermian Structures**   **Midsagittal to Vermian Structures**

Error = 30%

Figure 4   (continued) (b) The principle of optimizing MR slice alignment based on the anatomy intrinsic to the structure to be quantified, rather than on other structures which may be merely convenient, applies generally. Example shows that alignment based on nonvermian midsagittal landmarks (left panels) can result in misalignment relative to the actual midsagittal position of the vermis (right panels), and an erroneous measure of the size of vermian lobules VI–VII. The area of vermian lobules VI–VII derived from the nonvermis-based alignment (traced area on left) is 30% larger than measure derived from vermis-based alignment. For comparison, the traced area on the left is superimposed on a properly aligned vermian image on the right, T1-weighted, 600/12 MR images (from Courchesne, Yeung-Courchesne, et al., 1994).

rithms, as well as the majority of those that aid manual tracing, must use some form of thresholding. So, the distinctions between algorithms fraught with much error and those that inject little error lie in the details of the thresholding approach taken by each. It is a serious matter that neither the algorithmic details necessary to evaluate thresholding approaches, nor the detailed evidence of actual performance, accompany the majority of quantitative MR studies of the brain.

Approaches that are able to directly account for the signal intensity inhomogeneities inherent in the MR device (Fig. 6) can provide more accurate results. While manual tracing does have its obvious draw-backs, its use by an expert anatomist is as good a method as any for circumventing device dependent signal intensity inhomogeneity. In part, this is because when deciding upon whether a set of pixels belongs to one or another tissue type (e.g., gray matter), the expert is able to take into account local contrast among pixels as well as global contrast. Automatic algorithms can be devised to perform an analogous process. In the Courchesne laboratory, Stuart Hinds and Brian Egaas have developed two such algorithms. One, fully automated algorithm, first models the device-dependent signal intensity inhomogeneity, and then takes the further step of refining final pixel classifications by using

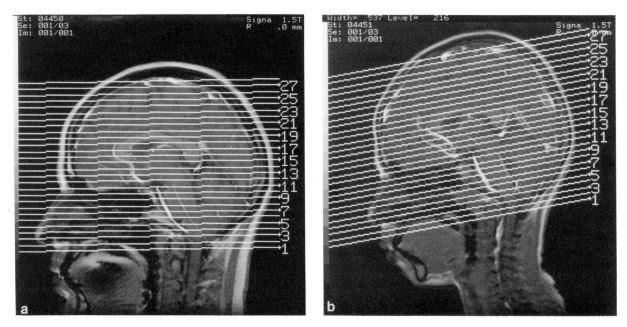

Figure 5 The developmental difference in the tilt of the head as it rests in the scanner is a potential source of bias when cross generational or longitudinal studies are planned. Figure shows an example from MR scans of a mother (a) and her daughter (b). Uncontrolled and systematic variation in the original tilt and in error inherent in slice reconstruction could produce spurious effects under some conditions.

local contrast information (Egaas, in manuscript). Resulting segmented images show excellent fidelity with the original MR images (Plates 13C, 13D, and 13E).

c. Anatomic Identification Even when protocols provide acquisition of a satisfactory number and orientation of slices, in-plane spatial resolution, tissue type differentiation, and so on, there still remains the

potential for large experimenter error during the next step of anatomic identification. The following is a vivid example: One of us was approached by a researcher in another lab about an apparent discrepancy in the midsagittal area of the vermis in patient and normal subjects. Two experimenters in that lab had traced the vermis on each midsagittal scan; each experimenter traced each midsagittal image twice. Re-

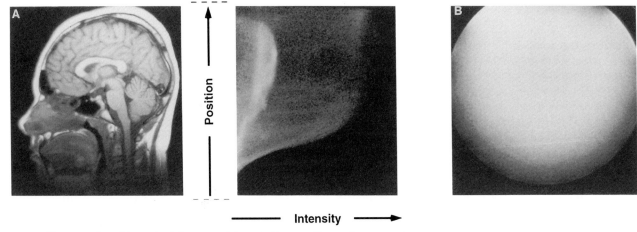

Figure 6 Signal intensity inhomogeneities in MR scans. These effects must be considered when using automatic algorithms to measure brain tissue. (a) A pronounced dropoff is apparent in the superior–inferior axis of this T1-weighted image. Signal may be reduced by 30% in the inferior cerebellum relative to the cerebral lobes. (b) Axial proton density-weighted image of a pure water phantom shows a ring of reduced signal. Similar effects are observed in axial brain images at the posterior pole. (Adapted from Egaas, in preparation.)

sults of this apparently very careful procedure showed high intraexperimenter reliability in tracing and high between-experimenter correlations. In other words, each experimenter traced each midsagittal scan in a very similar way. Unfortunately, each also frequently traced the *wrong* cerebellar anatomy! For instance, on some images, these experimenters included portions of the superior posterior cerebellar hemispheres and the cerebellar tonsil into their tracings of the midsagittal area of the vermis.[1] In one such instance shown to one of us, their erronoeous tracing resulted in a whopping 27% measurement error of the vermis!

Needless to say, large measurement error can just as easily be present in computer automated algorithms, which of course are merely implementations of human decisions about how to identify anatomy. While computer implementations do have the virtue of being consistent, sometimes they can also have the vice of being consistently in error. The problem of automating identification of classical neuroanatomic locations and boundaries is formidable. One well-known effort was undertaken by Talairach and colleagues (Talairach, Szikla, Tournoux, Prossalentis, Bordas-Ferrer, Covello, et al., 1967; Talairach & Tournoux, 1988). They developed a stereotactic proportional grid method for telencephalic localization. Across different individuals, even the most reliably present cerebral landmarks, such as the central sulcus, show large variation in their exact location within this proportional grid system (Steinmetz, Furst, & Freund, 1989). Exhaustive study of cerebral sulci shows great individual variation in the presence and patterning of sulci, even major sulci (Ono, Kubick, & Chad, 1990). In concluding their MR imaging study of localization of cerebral sulci using the Talairach grid method, Steinmetz et al. (1989) state, "As new developments in the field of MR provide decreasing slice thickness and volume measurements, and 3D rendering, the indirect grid method can be partly replaced by a more precise direct experimenter identification of . . . sulci between different cortical areas." Once again, the expert knowledge and accuracy of the experimenter is of central importance.

Whether measurement involves manual tracing, proportional grids, thresholding, or some other technique, the importance of having expert neuroanatomical knowledge when conducting MR neuroanatomical research cannot be overemphasized. Moreover, the importance of rigorous training of any nonexpert (whether technician, student, or physician) who is entrusted with measuring MR neuroanatomical images also cannot be overemphasized. Interexperimenter or intraexperimenter statistical reliability and computer automation do not by themselves ensure accuracy in anatomic identification and measurement.

B. Problems Calling for New Approaches in Quantitative MR Imaging

1. Myeloarchitectonics and MR Quantification of Cortical Volume and Thickness

The presence of neuron cell bodies and dendrites defines cerebral gray matter (cortex). Cerebral white matter does not have these neural elements, but instead has only axons, the majority of which are myelinated. There are significant signal intensity differences between brain parenchyma with and without myelin; that is, MR is intrinsically highly sensitive to the myelin content in brain parenchyma, and indeed, this has traditionally been the principal biologic feature used to classify brain pixels into gray matter and white matter.

However, the gray matter of the cerebral cortex also contains myelinated axons (Fig. 7) (Braak, 1980, 1984; Vogt & Vogt, 1919), the amount of which varies with cortical region and age (Braak, 1984; Smith 1907; Vogt & Vogt, 1919). Up to three horizontal stripes of myelin—the stripe of Kaes-Bechterew in layer III, the outer stripe of Baillarger in layer IV, and the inner stripe of Baillarger in layer Vb—may appear in different cortical lamina (Fig. 7) (Braak, 1980, 1984; Smith 1907; Vogt & Vogt, 1919). Different cerebral cortical regions have different amounts of intracortical myelin and different intracortical laminar patterns of myelination (Fig. 7). These topographic differences are the basis of myeloarchitectonic maps of the human cerebral cortex, such as the one in Figure 8 from Smith (1907). There appears to be a good correspondence between myeloarchitectonic and cytoarchitectonic maps (Economo, 1929, p. 7; Kemper & Galaburda, 1984). In 1955, maps were constructed by Sarkissov and Filimonoff that form the most comprehensive synthesis available today of the Vogt myeloarchitectonic and Brodmann cytoarchitectonic maps (Braak, 1980). In addition, some hold that myeloarchitecture provides even "finer differentiation within cerebral cortex" (Brodmann, 1909; Kemper & Galaburda, 1984).

Cytoarchitectural features cannot be imaged by current MR devices, and there is an imperfect match between different cytoarchitectonic regions and gyral and sulcal landmarks (Sarkissov, 1966; Stensaas, Ed-

---

[1] These two structures are part of the huge cerebellar hemispheres and appear on midsagittal images along with the inferior vermis in a large percentage of people.

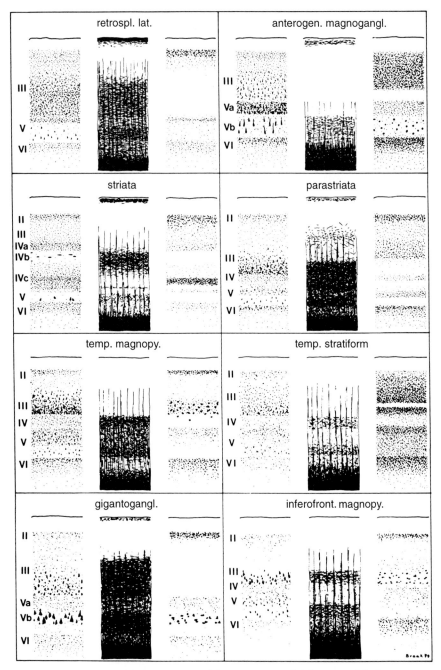

Figure 7. Diagrammatic representation of the appearance of eight areas of the human cerebral cortex in the Nissl, the myelin, and the pigment preparation (left, middle, and right sections of each panel). Abbreviations stand for cerebral cortical areas (left panel to right panel from top to bottom): retrosplenialis lateralis, anterogenualis magnaganglionaris, striata, parastriata, temporalis magnopyramidalis, temporalis stratiformis, gigantoganglionaris, and inferofrontalis magnopyramidalis centralis. (From Braak, 1980.)

dington, & Dobelle, 1974; Galaburda & Sanides, 1980; Murphy, 1985). However, it does appear that the best opportunity for obtaining *in vivo* architectural information about the human cerebral cortex is via MR imaging and analysis of intracortical myeloarchitectonic patterns.

The first MR study to successfully do this used MR to identify myeloarchitectonic regions of cerebral cortex directly by estimating the relative concentration of myelin within cortical lamina (Clark et al., 1992). In this study, we were able to identify striate Brodmann's area 17 and neighboring extrastriate cortex *in vivo* (Fig.

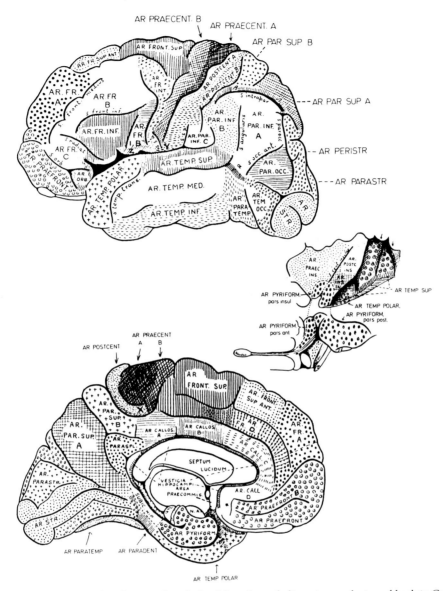

Figure 8   The beginnings of myeloarchitectural analysis of the telencephalic cortex can be traced back to Gennari (1782), Vicq d'Azyr (1786), and Baillarger (1840), who examined the whitish stripes of myelinated intracortical fibers in unstained preparations.

Such attempts to study the cortex macroscopically reached their peak in the work of the Australian Grafton Elliot Smith (1871–1937). He made use of the local variations of the two stripes of Baillarger, which can be recognized even with the un-aided eye. Smith finally arrived at a subdivision of the human cortex into about 50 areas. His map, which appeared in a short paper in 1907, is in many respects superior to that of Campbell. Although Smith was quite aware that he was apt to overlook real differences by limiting his investigations to only the gross appearance of cortical myelinated fibers, his work clearly illustrates the value of myeloarchitectonic studies. As a rule, even the unexperienced investigator is capable of de-lineating cortical areas with the aid of myelin preparations. Moreover, macroscopical or low-power microscopical examina-tion is actually an appropriate way of studying the architectonics of the brain, since it permits easy recognition of principal cortical variations. The resolution is not so great, however, that one necessarily sees the subtle and confusing differences ap-parent in Nissl preparations. Analysis is therefore much easier.

In Smith's map, the allocortex is much less pertinently parcellated than the isocortex. There is, for instance, no substan-tiation to unite as he did the basal parts of the frontal lobe with adjacent ones of the insula and the entorhinal region.

The main territories of the isocortex are clearly delineated. Smith has the merit of distinguishing a peristriate territory from a parastriate area which immediately surrounds the visual core. The extent of the acoustic core appears exaggerated, an error which is understandable since the areas which accompany the acoustic core are almost as heavily myelinated as the core itself. The cortex covering the superior temporal gyrus is sharply set off from that spreading over the subjacent gyri. The latter is described as an almost uniform territory showing only variations in the total thickness of the cortex. Smith points already to the fact that isocortical areas are for the most part bounded by relatively sharp borderlines. (Text from Braak, 1980; figure from Smith, 1907.)

9); this was confirmed with postmortem studies (Fig. 10) (Clark et al., 1992). In such myeloarchitectonic analyses of cortical lamina, the most important source of error is from the "Gibbs" artifact (Kelly, 1987); methods of assaying for its presence have been devised by Brian Egaas (Clark et al., 1992, pp. 421–422). As MR imaging technology improves, this noninvasive method has the potential to identify and discriminate among more than 46 cortical regions and subregions (Fig. 8) in the living human brain.

For the very same reason that the presence of myelin within cortical lamina provides an opportunity to test specific a priori hypotheses about cortical structure and function in normal and patient populations, it presents a serious and thorny problem for the accurate quantification of cortical gray matter volume and thickness. That is, the more intracortical myelin contained in a voxel, the greater the likelihood that that pixel will be erroneously classified as white matter. Every currently used approach—hand tracing and computer algorithm alike—makes this sort of quantification error. The error will be greatest in cortical regions with the greatest intracortical myelination, and least in those with the least myelination.

In studies of disorders that involve delay, deviation, or degeneration in intracortical myelination, the use of current imaging and analysis approaches could lead to erroneous results and conclusions. Imagine, for instance, a disorder that results in a loss of pyramidal cells in layers III and Va, which provide the myelinated axon collaterals that form the outer and inner stripes of Baillarger, respectively (Braak, 1984). Using current MR imaging and quantification methods, the loss of neurons should translate into obtaining fewer pixels classified as gray matter, but this could be offset by the loss of intracortical myelin, which should translate into obtaining more pixels classified as gray matter. The net result might well be thickness and volume estimates that erroneously appear to be similar to normals' (whose thicker cortices would also be embedded with more myelin). To obtain more accurate quantifications of cortical thickness and volume would require very high-resolution MR devices and new approaches to imaging and image analysis. Our MR study of cerebral cortical myeloarchitectonics represents a new starting point for such an effort (Clark et al., 1992).

2. Cerebral Cortical Sulci and MR Quantification of Cortical Surface Area

Two-thirds of the entire surface of cerebral cortex lies within sulci, and this is as true for newborns as for adults (Economo, 1929; Blinkov & Glezer, 1968, Table 186, p. 376). Unfortunately, this intrasulcal surface is most difficult to accurately image with MR in normal, healthy young children. In our experience with the healthy young cerebral cortex, accurate delineation of the opposing walls of sulci is difficult, because they are typically very narrow (indeed) and often tightly juxtaposed to each other. An even bigger concern, however, is the accurate determination of the depth of many sulci, because sulcal floors are difficult to locate, even for expert observers. This is true even in some postmortem protocols, which optimize spatial resolution and myelin vs gray matter resolution. (Compare the ambiguity and clarity of sulcal walls and floors on MR images and microtome slices in Figs. 2b and 2c from Clark et al., 1992.) Because of partial voluming

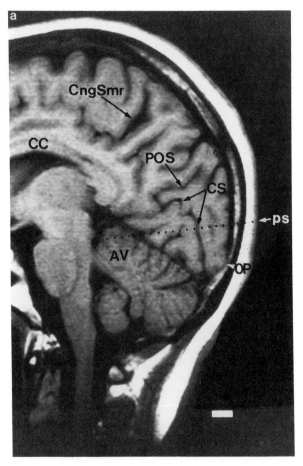

Figure 9 MR images of a living volunteer. (a) Shows plane of sectioning (ps) for (b). It is possible to identify the calcarine sulcus (CS) anterior to the occipital pole (OP), the parietooccipital sulcus (POS), and the marginal ramus of the cingulate sulcus (CngSmr). The corpus callosum (CC) and the anterior vermis of the cerebellum (AV) can also be identified.

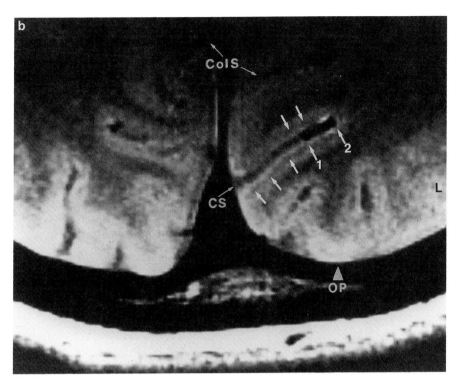

Figure 9. **(cont.) (B)** Shows the stria of Gennari *in vivo:* PD-weighted oblique SE image (TR = 3000 msec, TE = 23 msec, 4 NEX, FOV = 10 cm, matrix = 256 × 256, thickness = 3.0 mm) of the left hemisphere (L) using a 5″ surface coil. The collateral sulcus (ColS) is situated anterior to the calcarine sulcus. Arrows point to the stria of Gennari, which is seen as a layer of low signal intensity within middle cortical lamina in this region. Region of cortex between arrows marked 1 and 2 was used for statistical analysis and laminar intensity curves. Scale bars, 1 cm. (From Clark et al., 1992.)

effects, ambiguity and error will be worse with lower spatial resolution protocols (i.e., thicker slices and lower in-slice resolution). The difficulty is further aggravated by the fact that even in MR protocols using thin slices, sections will inevitably cut most sulci at oblique angles. Furthermore, the location of sulcal walls and floors (and therefore the depth of sulci), cannot be easily modelled because cortical thickness varies so greatly between and within cortical regions (Economo, 1929; Blinkov & Glezer, 1968). For example, cortical thickness varies from crown to sulcal floor by as much as 50%, and cortex at gyral crowns in some regions may be as much as 6 times thicker than cortical gyral crowns in other regions (Economo, 1929). Because two-thirds of all cortical surface is in sulci, even modest errors in attempts to model or manually trace the depth of sulci could result in a substantial measurement error.

The magnitude of such measurement errors can, unfortunately, vary with variables of special interest, including age and disorder. In our experience, sulcal width increases with age in normal, healthy controls from childhood through adulthood, so the accuracy of measuring sulcal surface and calculating total cerebral surface area also increases with age. Abnormalities resulting in cerebral volume loss can lead to excessive sulcal widening. Thus, when quantifying cortical surface area, substantial systematic measurement biases may exist between comparison groups (e.g., young vs old normal subjects; normal volunteers vs atrophy patients) due to large group differences in the clarity and certainty with which sulcal surfaces are visualized by current MR protocols. For instance, one can imagine the ironic situation where patients with less-than-normal surface area, but also with substantial cortical atrophy, are erroneously reported to have similar-to-normal surface area because their atrophy allows *visualization and measurement of the full extent and depth of their abnormally widened sulci.* Studies of cortical surface area therefore need to develop and provide evidence of bias-free measurement of sulcal surfaces.

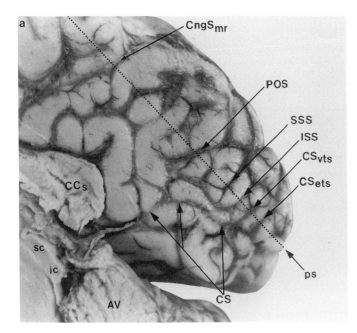
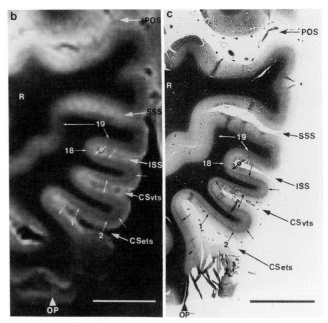

Figure 10 Photographic (a), MR (b), and myelin substance (c) images of the right hemisphere of a postmortem brain. (a) Photographic image of the right medial surface, showing the plane of sectioning (ps) for (b) and (c). It is possible to identify the calcarine sulcus (CS), and its external terminal segment (CS_{ets}) and vertical terminal segment (CS_{vts}), and also the inferior sagittal sulcus (ISS), the superior sagittal sulcus (SSS), the parieto-occipital sulcus (POS), and the marginal ramus of the cingulate sulcus ($CngS_{mr}$) (Ono et al., 1990). The splenium of the corpus callosum (CC_s), superior colliculus (sc), inferior colliculus (ic), and anterior vermis of the cerebellum (AV) can also be identified. (b) T1-weighted MR image (TR = 300 msec, TE = 25 msec, 14 NEX, FOV = 9 cm, matrix = 256 × 256, thickness = 3.0 mm) of the right (R) occipital lobe with 352 μm in-plane resolution. The occipital pole (OP) is at the bottom. T1 signal contrast is reversed in the fixed brain as compared to a living brain with this imaging sequence. (18) and (19) are Brodmann areas 18 and 19. (c) Microtome section, 40 μm thick, stained for myeloarchitecture, using eriochrome stain, cut on the same plane as (b). For (b) and (c), gray matter appears *white* and white matter is *gray* or *black*. *Small arrows* point to the stria of Gennari, which provides myeloarchitectonic verification of striate cortex. Arrow with naught indicates position of border between striate (area 17) and extrastriate (areas 18 and 19, indicated with arrows) cortical regions, which can be precisely located in the MR image to within a few millimeters. Extrastriate cortex extends to the anterior bank of the parieto-occipital sulcus. Region of striate cortex (between arrows marked 1 and 2 within CS_{ets}) were used for statistical analysis of laminar intensity. Scale bars (b) and (c), 1 cm. (From Clark et al., 1992).

IV. How Should We Analyze MR Measures?

A. Statistical Effects

The interpretation of scientific data typically relies on statistical analysis. However, ill-considered and inappropriate use of statistics can both mask true effects and identify spurious ones. In both cases, the statistical analyses compromise the validity of the study.

Central to any discussion of statistical validity is the concept of statistical power. Statistical power is defined as the probability of obtaining a statistically significant result in support of a hypothesis when the hypothesis is indeed true. Power reflects the relative contributions of various components. These include the magnitude of the hypothesized neuroanatomic re-

sult (i.e. effect size), *the amount of error variation,*[2] and the size of the subject sample. When error variation is held constant, smaller effect sizes require larger sample sizes to produce statistically significant results. When sample size is held constant, small effect sizes can still result in statistically significant differences if error variation is minimal. Therefore, the factors that influence effect size and error variation must be considered to determine appropriate sample sizes for an MR imaging study.

Effect sizes vary considerably in studies of developmental disorders. This variation is demonstrated in Table 2. The studies included in Table 2 are those that provided sufficient information to calculate an effect

---

[2]The term "error variation" is used in its statistical sense here.

Table 2 Effect Sizes Associated with Neuroanatomical Regions in Various Developmental Disorders

Authors	Subject group	General location	Range of effects
Neuroanatomic effects			
Courchesne et al. (1988)	Autism	Cerebellum	.02–.58
Duara et al. (1991)	Dyslexia	Anterior cerebral	.07–.11
Hynd et al. (1991)	ADD/H	Corpus callosum	.05–.36
Hynd et al. (1990)	ADD/H	Frontal cerebral	.00–.32
		Temporal/insular	.16–.38
		Posterior cerebral	.09–.17
	Dyslexia	Frontal cerebral	.05–.53
		Temporal/insular	.03–.48
		Posterior cerebral	.01–.11
Jernigan et al. (1991)	Language	Asymmetries	.05–.87
	Learning	Anterior cerebral	.13–.58
	Disabled	Posterior cerebral	.10–.73
		Basal ganglia	.51–.64
Kushch et al. (1993)	Dyslexia	Temporal lobe	.02–.29
Leonard et al. (1993)	Dyslexia	Temporal	.02–.37
		Parietal	.07–.33
Murakami et al. (1992)	Rett Syndrome	Brainstem	.40–.58
		Basal ganglia	.24–.50
		Cerebellum	.30–.66
		Corpus callosum	.61
Plante et al. (1991)	Language	Asymmetry	.45
	Impaired	Cerebral regoins	.27–.60
Schultz et al. (1994)	Dyslexia	Temporal lobe	.03–.70
Wang et al. (1992)	Down Syndrome	Cerebellum	.41
	Williams Syndrome	Cerebellum	.13
Weis (1991)	Down Syndrome	Brainstem	.38
		Cerebellum	.41
		Cerebral	.62–.67
		Subcortical	.00–.16
Selected measurement error effects			
Plante & Turkstra (1991)	Normal subjects	Hemispheres	.00–.11
		Cerebral regions	.00–.78

Note: Effect sizes are standardized to range between .00 (negligible effect) and 1.00 (maximal effect) in a comparison between disorder and control groups. NB: Smaller effects require a larger N to find statistically significant differences.

for a two-sample comparison for individual brain regions. These studies represent a variety of developmental disorders and include measurements from a variety of neuroanatomical regions. In these studies, the effects ranged from those that were marginal to those that were quite robust. Although larger effect sizes are much more likely to produce statistically significant effects, not all theoretically interesting effects are large. Therefore, it is worth considering the factors that serve to maximize the size of the predicted effects and minimize other sources of (error) variance, in order to detect true effects that may only be of a modest magnitude.

As discussed in the previous section, protocols that are effective (i.e., they represent the target structure reliably and accurately) tend to increase statistical power. Conversely, ineffective scan or measurement protocols can inflate error variance and reduce the chance of detecting true effects. To illustrate, Table 2 includes a range of effects that are associated with various sources of error that can affect measurement accuracy of selected neuroanatomic regions. It is not trivial that the effect sizes associated with error sources can exceed some of the effect sizes associated with developmental disorders. This demonstrates the ease with which extraneous sources of variability, left uncontrolled, can mathematically cancel smaller experimental effects. This extraneous variability can inflate the error variance component in a statistical analysis, with a resulting loss of power to detect any true effects.

B. Alpha Slippage

The converse to missing a true effect due to low power (Type II error) is the identification of an effect that occurred by chance (Type I error). Although it is a conventional standard to identify as statistically significant a difference that would rarely occur by chance (i.e., less than 5% or 1% of the time), these improbable chance events will sometimes occur. The likelihood of stumbling upon a chance finding increases as a direct function of the number of statistical analyses performed. Although a particular alpha level (e.g., $\alpha = .05$) may be chosen for an experiment, the actual probability of achieving statistical significance by chance on a single statistical comparison inflates with each additional comparison performed. This phenomenon is known as alpha slippage. The degree of slippage is quite easy to calculate through the formula $1 - (1 - \alpha)^c$, where c is equal to the number of comparisons performed. For example, whereas with one statistical comparison, the probability of a Type I error occurring is in fact .05, the performance of three comparisons inflates this probability to $1 - (1 - .05)^3$ or .14.

With MR imaging data, the number of possible comparisons can quickly escalate until it is virtually certain that one or more chance findings will occur. One article that we are acquainted with conducted 48 t-tests on various brain regions. With this many analyses, it is a virtual certainty that two or more of the comparisons would be significant by chance alone. This problem also occurs when a data set is reanalyzed for more than one publication. Unfortunately, when alpha slippage occurs, there is no way for the investigator to know which of the apparently significant findings are valid and which are chance.

There are several options available to the investigator to guard against the problem of alpha slippage. The first is to design studies that test well-founded hypotheses, and to distinguish between analyses that are direct tests of a limited number of hypotheses and those that "explore" the nature of the data beyond that point. When an effect is predicted from prior knowledge or theory, the plausibility of the effect occurring by chance alone is reduced. When a potential effect is identified through exploratory or post hoc analyses, the results must be considered more tenuous. These exploratory analyses require both protection against alpha slippage and replication of findings that were "unexpected," "unanticipated," or that were otherwise suggested only after the data had been examined.

Another option, if multiple areas are truly of theoretical interest, is to employ statistical techniques that provide protection against alpha slippage over multiple comparisons. Analysis of Variance (ANOVA) and regression techniques are familiar to most investigators. Other statistical techniques (e.g., confirmatory analyses of covariance structures, linear structural equation models) are available for testing specific hypothesized interrelations among multiple variables and can be employed to take a "system" approach to understanding the developmentally disordered brain (see Gonzales–Lima, this volume). Although these statistical techniques are capable of providing tests of complex interrelations among neuroanatomic measures, the cost to the investigator is that large groups of subjects are frequently needed to provide stable results. This may place these techniques beyond the capacity of many investigations of low-incidence populations. However, for investigators proposing a series of studies with multiple samples, a minimal amount of initial planning could produce an accumulated data set that would be appropriate for these types of analyses.

The final option available to avoid the problem of alpha slippage and the potential for chance findings is replication. This is widely recognized as the strongest test of an "unanticipated" finding. An investigator who has planned a series of studies may be in a position to integrate a replication phase into subsequent studies in the series. Replication can also be accomplished within a study. An investigator may be able to divide his or her sample in order to carry out exploratory analyses on one subset of the sample, reserving the remaining subjects for confirmatory analyses. This is an approach that is frequently used in studies that employ a discriminant analysis, but could be used with other statistical techniques as well. For an investigator to make use of this approach would require that the sample size within each subset be adequate for the planned statistical analyses.

The interpretation of statistical analyses relies on an understanding of the mathematical components that contribute to a statistical effect. The investigator can do much to enhance statistical power through design. Careful planning of design elements, including sample size and characteristics, MR imaging scan protocol sensitivity, and measurement accuracy, will enhance statistical power. The investigator must also assess, and should report, the probability that a true effect may have been missed or that a spurious effect may have occurred by chance, in order to make valid interpretations of the data.

V. Conclusions

In recent years, improvements in MR imaging capabilities have been striking and exciting. In general, researchers have been quick to take advantage of the new capacity for obtaining very high spatial resolution images (e.g., more than 100 gapless 256 × 256 matrix, 1–3 mm images) in relatively short scan times (10 to 20 min). There has been an emphasis on the need for thinner slices and gapless sampling, on measuring as many brain structures as possible on every protocol, and on using computer algorithms rather than manual tracing for image measurement.

While these are exciting technical improvements and are laudable methodological emphases, improvement in MR research depends as much on other factors. Accurate volume estimates are not solely a matter of absolute slice thickness (e.g., 1 mm or 5 mm), or absolute in-plane matrix (128 × 128 or 512 × 512), or whether the protocol was gapless, and so on. Rather, accurate volume estimates depend on having an adequate number of slices through every structure of interest, 100 to 200 in-plane sample points (voxels), and a slice orientation that provides the necessary visualization of landmarks and boundaries critical to delineating the structure of interest on each slice. This is true whether the structure of interest is the whole cerebrum or the left mammillary body. Thus, the importance of being able to obtain very high spatial resolution images really only comes into play when there is a need to image relatively small structures (such as a single cortical gyrus or a mammillary body) or some convoluted structure (such as cerebral sulci or cerebellar sulci and folia), whose landmarks and boundaries would be obscured by partial voluming in low resolution protocols, cortical myeloarchitectonic structure, and so on. Similarly, accurate 2D area measures (e.g., of the corpus callosum or vermis) depend on accurate slice orientation and positioning, and 100–200 in-plane sample points.

Accurate measurement is also not solely a matter of whether computer algorithms or manual tracing is employed. Any method that fails to account for signal intensity inhomogeneities will be fraught with error. Whether approaches use global thresholding computer algorithms, slice by slice experimenter-controlled thresholding procedures, or some other procedure, details and validation of the approach should be published information. Manual tracing can be an effective, though time consuming, method of circumventing MR device-dependent signal intensity inhomogeneities, but it does not guarantee accuracy in anatomical identification. Whether measurement involves manual tracing, computer algorithms, pro-portional grids, thresholding, or some other technique, the importance of having expert neuroanatomical knowledge when conducting MR neuroanatomical research cannot be overemphasized. Moreover, the importance of rigorous training of any nonexpert (whether technician, student, or physician) who is entrusted with measuring MR neuroanatomical images also cannot be overemphasized. Interexperimenter or intraexperimenter statistical reliability and computer automation do not by themselves ensure accuracy in anatomic identification and measurement.

Lastly, whether an MR study employs the latest in image analysis hardware and software or the expertise of a neuroanatomist, there remains no substitute for knowing why you are conducting an expensive MR analysis of the brain. To best match the MR protocol to a structure, it is necessary to begin with specific a priori hypotheses about which structures will be measured. To insure sufficient statistical power to detect true effects and avoid false positive and false negative reporting, it is necessary to begin with specific a priori hypotheses that allow one to calculate the number of subjects needed, the number of slices needed, and so on. To choose a useful contrast patient group, it is necessary to begin with a priori hypotheses that point to how such a contrast group specifically contributes to illuminating the neurobiological issues under study. In sum, as with any neurobehavioral field of study, good MR studies of the developing brain begin with good ideas.

Acknowledgments

Supported by National Institute of Neurological Diseases and Stroke grant 5-R01-NS-19855 and National Institute of Mental Health 1-R01-MH-36840 awarded to E. Courchesne, and National Institute on Deafness and Other Communication Disorders grant K08 DC-00077 awarded to E. Plante, and support by the Tucson Scottish Rite Charitable Foundation.

References

Altman, J. (1982). Morphological development of the rat cerebellum and some of its mechanisms. In S. L. Palay & V. Chan-Palay (Eds.), *The cerebellum: New vistas* (pp. 8–49). New York: Springer-Verlag.

Arin, D. M., Bauman, M. L., & Kemper, T. L. (1991). The distribution of Purkinje cell loss in the cerebellum in autism. *Neurology, 41*(Suppl 1), 307.

Baillarger, J.-G.-F. (1840). Recherches sur la structure de la couche corticale des circonvolutions du cerveau. *Memories des l'Academie Royale de Medicine, 8,* 149.

Bauman, M. L. (1991). Microscopic neuroanatomic abnormalities in autism. *Pediatrics, 87,* 791–796.

Bauman, M. L., & Kemper, T. (1985). Histoanatomic observations of the brain in early infantile autism. *Neurology, 35,* 866–874.

Bauman, M. L., & Kemper, T. L. (1986). Developmental cerebellar abnormalities: A consistent finding in early infantile autism. *Neurology, 36*(Suppl. 1), 190.

Bauman, M. L., & Kemper, T. L. (1990). Limbic and cerebellar abnormalities are also present in an autistic child of normal intelligence. *Neurology 40*(Suppl. 1), 359.

Blinkov, S. M., & Glezer, I. I. (1968). *The human brain in figures and tables: A quantitative handbook.* New York: Plenum.

Braak, H. (1980). *Architectonics of the human telencephalic cortex.* Berlin: Springer-Verlag.

Braak, H. (1984). Architectonics as seen by lipofuscin stains. In A. Peters & E. G. Jones, (Eds.), *Cerebral cortex* (pp. 59–104). New York: Plenum.

Brodman, K. (1909). *Vergleichende Lokalisationslehre der Grosshirnrinde in ihren Prinzipien dargestellt auf Grund des Zellenbaues.* Leipzig: Barth.

Ciesielski, K. T., Allen, P. S., Sinclair, B. D., Pabst, H. F., Yanossky, R., & Ludwig, R. (1990). Hypoplasia of cerebellar vermis in autism and childhood leukemia. In *Proceedings of the 5th International Child Neurology Congress; Tokyo, Japan; November.*

Chi, J. G., Dooling, E. C., & Gilles, F. H. (1977). Left–right asymmetries of the temporal speech areas of the human fetus. *Archives of Neurology, 34,* 346–348.

Clark, V. P., Courchesne, E., & Grafe, J. (1992). *In vivo* myeloarchitectonic analysis of human striate and extrastriate cortex using magnetic resonance imaging. *Cerebral Cortex, 2,* 417–424.

Courchesne, E. (1985). The missing ingredients in autism. Presented at *The conference on brain and behavioral development: Biosocial dimension, Elridge, MD., May 19–22.*

Courchesne, E. (1995a). New evidence of cerebellar and brainstem hypoplasia in autistic infants, children and adolescents: The MR study by Hashimoto and colleagues. *Journal of Autism and Developmental Disorders, 25,* 19–22.

Courchesne, E. (1995b). Infantile autism. Part I: MR imaging abnormalities and their behavioral correlates. *International Pediatrics, 10,* 50–63.

Courchesne, E., Hesselink, J. R., Jernigan, T. L., & Yeung-Courchesne, R. (1987). Abnormal neuroanatomy in a nonretarded person with autism: Unusual findings with magnetic resonance imaging. *Archives of Neurology, 44,* 335–334.

Courchesne, E., Press, G. A., Murakami, J., Berthody, D., Hesselink, J. R., & Wilen, C. A. (1989). The cerebellum in sagittal plane: Anatomical MR correlation. Part I: The Vermis. *American Journal of Neuroradiology, 10,* 659–665.

Courchesne, E., Press, G. A., & Yeung-Courchesne, R. (1993). Parietal lobe abnormalities detected on magnetic resonance images of patients with infantile autism. *American Journal of Roentgenology, 160,* 387–393.

Courchesne, E., Saitoh, O., Yeung-Courchesne, R., Press, G. A., Lincoln, A. J., Haas, R. H., & Schreibman, L. (1994). Abnormality of cerebellar vermian lobules VI and VII in patients with infantile autism: Identification of hypoplastic and hyperplastic subgroups by MR imaging. *American Journal of Roentgenology, 162,* 123–130.

Courchesne, E., Townsend, J., & Chase, C. (1994). Neurodevelopmental principles guide research on developmental psychopathology. In D. Cicchetti (Ed.), *A manual of developmental psychopathology,* pp. 195–226.

Courchesne, E., Townsend, J., & Saitoh, O. (1994). The brain in infantile autism: Posterior fossa structures are abnormal. *Neurology, 44,* 214–223.

Courchesne, E., Yeung-Courchesne, R., & Egaas, B. (1994). Methodology in neuroanatomic measurement. *Neurology, 44,* 203–208.

Courchesne, E., Yeung-Courchesne, R., Press, G. A., Hesselink, J. R., & Jernigan, T. L. (1988). Hypoplasia of cerebellar vermal lobules VI and VII in autism. *New England Journal of Medicine, 318,* 1349–1354.

Damasio, H., Kuljis, R. O., Yuh, W., Van Hoesen, G. W., & Ehrhardt, J. (1991). Magnetic resonance imaging of human intracortical structure *in vivo. Cerebral Cortex, 1,* 374–379.

Duara, R., Kushch, A., Gross-Glenn, K., Barker, W. W., Jallad, B., Pascal, S., Loewenstein, D. A., Sheldon, J., Rabin, M., Levin, B., & Lubs, H. (1991). Neuroanatomic differences between dyslexic and normal readers on magnetic resonance imaging scans. *Archives of Neurology, 48,* 410–416.

Economo, C. (1929). *The cytoarchitectonics of the human cerebral cortex.* London: Oxford.

Egaas, B., Courchesne, E., & Saitoh, O. (1995). Reduced size of corpus callosum in autism. *Archives of Neurology, 52,* 794–801.

Francis, D. J., Fletcher, J. M., Shaywitz, B. A., Shaywitz, S. E., & Rourke, B. P. (1996). Defining learning and language disabilities: Conceptual and psychometric issues with the use of IQ test. *Language, Speech and Hearing Services in Schools 27,* 132–143.

Gaffney, G. R., Tsai, L. Y., Kuperman, S., & Minchin, S. (1987). Cerebellar structure in autism. *American Journal of Diseases in Children, 141,* 1330–1332.

Galaburda, A. M., & Sanides, F. (1980). Cytoarchitectonic organization of the human auditory cortex. *Journal of Comparative Neurology, 190,* 597–610.

Garber, H. J., & Ritvo, E. R. (1992). Magnetic resonance imaging of the posterior fossa in autistic adults. *American Journal of Psychiatry, 149,* 245–247.

Gennari, F. (1782). *De Peculiari Structura Cerebri Nonnullisque Eius Morbus.* Parma, Italy: Ex Regio Typographeo.

Geschwind, N., & Levitsky, W. (1968). Human brain: Asymmetries in the temporal speech region. *Science, 161,* 186–187.

Gundersen, H. J. G., & Jensen, E. B. (1987). Stereological estimation of the volume-weighted mean volume of arbitrary particles observed on random sections. *Journal of Microscopy, 138,* 127–142.

Haase, G. R., (1977). Diseases presenting as dementia. In C. D. Wells, (Ed.), *Dementia* (2nd Ed., pp. 27–67). Philadelphia, PA: Davis.

Haines, D. E. (1987). *Neuroanatomy: An atlas of structures, sections, and systems.* (p. 61). Baltimore/Munich: Urban and Schwarzenberg.

Hashimoto, T., Tayama, M., Murakawa, K., Yoshimoto, T., Miyazaki, M., Harada, M., & Kuroda, Y. (1995). Development of the brainstem and cerebellum in autistic patients. *Journal of Autism and Developmental Disorders, 25,* 1–18.

Holttum, J. R., Minshew, N. J., Sanders, R. S., & Phillips, N. E. (1992). Magnetic resonance imaging of the posterior fossa in autism. *Biological Psychiatry, 32,* 1091–1101.

Hynd, G. W., Semrud-Clikeman, M., Lorys, A. R., Novey, E. S., & Eliopulos, D. (1990). Brain morphology in developmental dyslexia and attention deficit disorder/hyperactivity. *Archives of Neurology, 47,* 919–926.

Hynd, G. W., Semrud-Clikeman, M., Lorys, A. R., Novey, E. S., Eliopulos, D., and Lyytinen, H. (1991). Corpus callosum morphology in attention deficit-hyperactivity disorder: morphometric analysis of MRI. *Journal of Learning Disabilities, 24,* 141–146.

Jackson, T., & Plante, E. (in press). Gyral morphology in the posterior perisylvian region in families affected by developmental language disorder. *Neuropsychological Review.*

Jernigan, T. L., Hesselink, J. R., Sowell, E., & Tallal, P. A. (1991). Cerebral structure on magnetic resonance imaging in language-impaired and learning-impaired children. *Archives of Neurology, 48,* 539–545.

Kelly, W. (1987). Image artifacts and technical limitations. In M. Brant-Zawadzki & D. Norman (Eds.), *Magnetic resonance imaging of the central nervous system* (pp. 43–82). New York: Raven.

Kemper, T. L. B., & Galaburda, A. M. (1984). Principles of cytoarchitectonics. In A. Peters & E. G. Jones (Eds.), *Cerebral cortex* (pp. 35–57). New York: Plenum.

Kirk, R. E. (1982). *Experimental design: Procedures for the behavioral sciences* (2nd Ed.). Monterey, CA: Brooks–Cole.

Kleiman, M. D., Neff, S., & Rosman, N. P. (1992). The brain in infantile autism: Are posterior fossa structures abnormal? *Neurology, 42,* 753–760.

Kushch, A., Gross-Glenn, K., Jallad, G., Lubs, H., Rabin, M., Feldman, E., & Duara, R. (1993). Temporal lobe surface area measurements on MRI in normal and dyslexic readers. *Neuropsychologia, 31,* 811–821.

Leonard, C. M., Voeller, K. S., Lombardino, L. J., Morris, M. K., Hynd, G. W., Alexander, A. W., Anderson, H. G., Garofalakis, M., Honeyman, J. C., Mao, J., Agee, O. F., & Staab, E. V. (1993). Anomalous cerebral structure in dyslexia revealed with magnetic resonance imaging. *Archives of Neurology, 50,* 461–469.

Lyman, F. L. (1963). *Phenylketonuria.* Springfield, IL: Thomas.

Mayhew, T. M., & Olsen, D. R. (1991). Magnetic resonance imaging (MRI) and model-free estimates of brain volume determined using the Cavalieri principle. *Journal of Anatomy, 178,* 133–144.

Murakami, J. W., Courchesne, E., Press, G. A., Yeung-Courchesne, R., & Hesselink, J. R. (1989). Reduced cerebellar hemisphere size and its relationship to vermal hypoplasia in autism. *Archives of Neurology, 46,* 689–694.

Murakami, J. W., Courchesne, E., Haas, R. H., Press, G. A., & Yeung-Courchesne, R. (1992). Cerebellar and cerebral abnormalities in Rett syndrome: A quantitative MR analysis. *American Journal of Roentgenology, 159,* 177–183.

Murphy, G. M. (1985). Volumetric asymmetry in the human striate cortex. *Experimental Neurology, 88,* 288–302.

Ono, M., Kubick, S., & Chad, D. (1990). *Atlas of the Cerebral Sulci.* New York: Thieme.

Piven, J., Nehme, E., Simon, J., Barta, P., Pearlson, G., & Folstein, S. E. (1992). Magnetic resonance imaging in autism: measurement of the cerebellum, pons, and fourth ventricle. *Biological Psychiatry, 31,* 491–504.

Plante, E. (1991). MRI findings in the parents and siblings of specifically language-impaired boys. *Brain and Language, 40,* 67–80.

Plante, E., Swisher, L., Vance, R., & Rapcsak, S. (1991). MRI findings in boys with specific language impairment. *Brain and Language, 40,* 52–66.

Plante, E., & Turkstra, L. (1991). Sources of error in the quantitative analysis of MRI scans. *Magnetic Resonance Imaging, 9,* 589–595.

Plante, E., & Vance, R. (1994). Selection of preschool language tests: A data-based approach. *Language, Speech, & Hearing Services in Schools, 25,* 5–24.

Press, G. A., Amaral, D. G., & Squire, L. R. (1989). Hippocampal abnormalities in amnesic patients revealed by high-resolution magnetic resonance imaging. *Nature (London), 341,* 54–57.

Press, G. A., & Courchesne, E. (1992a). Atlas of the cerebellum and vermis. In L. A. Hyman & V. C. Hinck (Eds.), *Clinical brain imaging: Normal structure and functional anatomy* (pp. 251–279). St. Louis, MO: Mosby Yearbook.

Press, G. A., & Courchesne, E. (1992b). Cerebellar hemispheres and vermis. In L. A. Hyman and V. C. Hinck (Eds.), *Clinical brain imaging: Normal structure and functional anatomy* (pp. 281–286). St. Louis, MO: Mosby Yearbook.

Ritvo, E. R., Freeman, B. J., Scheibel, A. B., Duong, T., Robinson, H., Guthrie, A., & Ritvo, A. (1986). Lower Purkinje cell counts in the cerebella of four autistic subjects: Initial findings of the UCLA–NSAC autopsy research report. *American Journal of Psychiatry, 143,* 862–866.

Saitoh, O., Courchesne, E., Egaas, B., Lincoln, A. J., & Schreibman, L. (1995). Cross-sectional area of the posterior hippocampus in autistic patients with cerebellar and corpus callosum abnormalities. *Neurology, 45,* 317–324.

Sarkissov, S. A. (1966). *The structure and functions of the brain.* Bloomington, IN: Indiana Univ. Press.

Schultz, R. T. (1994). Brain morphology in normal and dyslexic children: The influence of gender and age. *Annals of Neurology, 35,* 732–742.

Smith, G. E. (1907). A new topographical survey of the human cerebral cortex, being an account of the distribution of the anatomically distinct cortical areas and their relationship to the cerebral sulci. *Journal of Anatomy, 41,* 237–254.

Steinmetz, H., Furst, G., & Freund, H.-J. (1989). Cerebral cortical localization: Application and validation of the proportional grid system in MR imaging. *Journal of Computer Assisted Tomography, 13,* 10–19.

Stensaas, S. S., Eddington, D. K., & Dobelle, W. H. (1974). The topography and variability of the primary visual cortex in man. *Journal of Neurosurgery, 40,* 747–755.

Talairach, J., Szikla, G., Tournoux, P., Prossalentis, A., Bordas-Ferrer, M., Covello, L., Jacob, M., Mempel, A., Buser, P., & Bacaund, J. (1967). *Atlas d'Anatomie Stereotaxique du Telencephale.* Paris: Masson.

Talairach, J., & Tournoux, P. (1988). *Co-planar stereotaxic atlas of the human brain: A 3-dimensional proportional system: An approach to cerebral imaging.* New York: Thieme.

Townsend, J., & Courchesne, E. (1994). Parietal damage and narrow "spotlight" spatial attention. *Journal of Cognitive Neuroscience, 6,* 218–230.

Townsend, J., Courchesne, E., & Egaas, B. (in press). Slowed orienting of covert visual-spatial attention in autism: Specific deficits associated with cerebellar and parietal abnormality. *Development and Psychopathology.*

Vicq d'Azyr, F. (1786). *Traite d'Anatomie et de Physiologie.* Paris: Didot.

Vogt, C., & Vogt, O. (1919). Allgemeinere Ergebnisse unserer Hirnforschung. *Journal of Psychology and Neurology, 25,* 279–461.

Wada, J. A., Clarke, R., & Hamm, A. (1975). Cerebral hemisphere asymmetry in humans. *Archives of Neurology, 32,* 239–246.

Wang, P. P., Hesselink, J. R., Jernigan, T. L., Doherty, S., & Bellugi, U. (1992). Specific neurobehavioral profile of Williams' syndrome is associated with neocerebellar hemispheric preservation. *Neurology, 42,* 1999–2002.

Weis, S. (1991). Morphometry and magnetic resonance imaging of the human brain in normal controls and down's syndrome. *The Anatomical Record, 231,* 593–598.

Williams, R. S., Hauser, S. L., Purpura, D. P., DeLong, R., & Swisher, C. N. (1980). Autism and mental retardation: Neuropathological studies performed in four retarded persons with autistic behavior. *Archives of Neurology, 37,* 749–753.

Witelson, S. F., & Pallie, W. (1973). Left hemisphere specialization for language in the newborn. *Brain, 96,* 641–646.

II

NEUROIMAGING OF PERCEPTUAL AND COGNITIVE DEVELOPMENT

5

Spatio-Temporal Modeling of Brain Waves

Peter C. M. Molenaar, Hilde M. Huizenga, and Han L. J. van der Maas

Faculty of Psychology, University of Amsterdam, 1018 WB Amsterdam, The Netherlands

I. Introduction

The appearance of the Nunez (1981) treatise on electric fields of the brain constituted an important hallmark in the analysis of space–time characteristics of electrocortical activity. Part of that treatise is devoted to equivalent dipole modeling of the spatial layout of brain potential fields, while another part discusses brain wave modeling of spatio-temporal electroencephalogram (EEG) organization. Presently, over a decade later, equivalent dipole models belong to the standard equipment of applied brain topography. Moreover, the dipole models themselves have been increasingly refined, especially from a biophysical point of view. In contrast, the present status of Nunez's brain wave model seems to be less well-established in that it has been applied in only a limited number of brain topographic studies. It is our intention, among other things, to show that the brain wave model can provide us with a unique set of mathematical–statistical tools to uncover the spatio-temporal organization of potential fields in a valid and reliable way.

The next two sections can be read as comments on Nunez's work. In section II we will address the mathematical dipole model from an application-oriented point of view. That is, we will discuss whether the source is modeled as an infinitesimal dipole or as an extended dipole layer, and, regardless of the way in which inhomogeneities in the medium are accounted for, whether or not the fit of an equivalent dipole model boils down to an instance of nonlinear regression analysis. We will scrutinize currently fashionable approaches to the fit of dipole models and propose a more principled way of fitting and evaluating these models. In section III, the focus is on applied brain wave modeling. It will be shown that there is an important weakness in the way empirical orthogonal wave functions appear to be determined in Nunez (1981, chap. 7), making the results thus obtained possibly uninterpretable. A special unitary rotation technique which removes this weakness will be introduced. In addition, we mention an extension of the orthogonal wave function approach which can accommodate nonstationary potential fields.

Both an equivalent dipole model with time-varying moments and the applied brain wave model belong to the class of linear dynamic models of potential field fluctuations in the microsecond domain. At the level of modeling the evolution of potential field organization across the life span of individuals, however, one enters the realm of nonlinear dynamics which flourishes in developmental biology (e.g., Murray, 1988). In section IV we will consider recent attempts at modeling such age-dependent reorganizations of spatio-temporal brain fields, note the resemblance of some of these models to a particular class of artificial neural networks, and discuss their implications for applied brain topography. In the closing section, section V, we speculate about some new extensions of the techniques presented in the preceding sections.

Evidently, we will only be able to scratch the surface of many of the issues raised within the limited confines of this chapter. The discussion mainly will proceed at a general level in which empirical evidence will only be presented in summarized form (for further details the reader is referred to the original sources). On request, listings of the source codes of the computational techniques used in sections II–IV will be made available.

II. Nonlinear Regression Analysis of the Dipole Model

Consider the registration of the scalp potential field using an n-lead montage. Let y denote the $(n \times 1)$ column vector of potential values at the n scalp locations, and let X denote the $(n \times 2)$ matrix of coordinates of the latter scalp locations. (Vector-valued variables always will be represented by italicized lowercase letters and matrix-valued variables by italicized uppercase letters.) A schematic representation of the mathematical dipole model is given by

$$E[y] = m[X,a; b], \tag{1}$$

where $E[.]$ is the expectation operator, a is the vector of dipole parameters, and b is a vector of nuisance parameters. The model function $m[.]$ is nonlinear in the parameter vector a, and depends upon assumptions about the source and the head geometry. The vector b consists of nuisance parameters like the boundaries of, and conductivities in, piecewise homogeneous regions.

Many successful efforts have been made to study the effects of deviations of the real source and/or head geometry from the restrictive assumptions underlying $m[.]$. For instance De Munck (1989) carried out a beautiful series of simulation studies in which the effects of neglecting the source extension and erroneous conductivity parameters were determined. Presently, however, much less attention has been paid to the statistical aspects of fitting $m[.]$ to the data. An ordinary least squares (OLS) technique is almost always employed, in which the measurements are represented as

$$y = m[X,a; b] + e, \tag{2}$$

where the components of e are assumed to be identically and independently distributed. The OLS estimate a^* is then obtained by minimizing $S(a)$ with respect to a:

$$a^* : \min_a S(a) = \min_a \{y - m[X,a; b]\}^t \{y - m[X,a; b]\}, \tag{3}$$

where the superscript t denotes transposition. Often the goodness-of-fit of the model is evaluated on the basis of a criterion like $D = S(a^*)/\{y^t y\}$.

In order to compare the statistical properties of this popular approach to equivalent dipole fitting, it was considered to be an instance of nonlinear regression analysis and, within this standard statistical paradigm, subjected to an intensive simulation study. Such an integral reconceptualization of dipole fitting not only enables the derivation of a more principled measure of goodness-of-fit, which has much better statistical properties than (variants of) D, but also provides an encompassing differential geometrical characterization of the biasing effects of nonlinearities on the sampling distribution of a^* (cf. Seber & Wild, 1990). These biasing effects in particular, with regard to their dependence on the number (n) of leads, were further substantiated in the simulation study. It was found that with a 19-lead montage, positioned according to the 10–20 system, both a^* and its estimated standard error may be substantially biased. In contrast, the sampling distribution of a^* approached normality, and the bias in a^* and its standard error were small, if a 41-lead montage (which can be obtained by coupling two 21-channel machines) was employed. For a detailed presentation of the nonlinear regression framework and results of the simulation study, the reader is referred to Huizenga & Molenaar (1994).

Within the same nonlinear regression analytic framework, we undertook another large scale simulation study of various methods to accommodate spatial autocorrelation of the components of e. This can be accomplished if the OLS approach based on Eq. (3) is replaced by the generalized least squares (GLS) criterion:

$$a\# : \min_a \{y - m[X,a; b]\}^t V_e^{-1} \{y - m[X,a; b]\}, \tag{4}$$

where V_e denotes the $(n \times n)$ covariance matrix of e. In fact, the elements of V_e can be regarded as a set of nuisance parameters like b, but in contradistinction to b, one rarely has available a priori information about V_e. In each application to real data, V_e will therefore have to be estimated together with $a\#$ in a multistage optimization of Eq. (4). Notice that for typical values of the number n of leads, V_e consists of many free elements. Consequently, it may be difficult to obtain stable estimates in a straightforward approach. A less direct approach, for instance, first modeling the spatial structure of V_e in terms of a spatial autoregression involving a limited number of free parameters, will often yield better-conditioned estimates.

In Huizenga & Molenaar (1995) four alternative multistage GLS methods were applied to spatially correlated potential field data. The results of this simulation study clearly show that the GLS methods outperform the OLS estimator in that both $a\#$ and the associated standard errors are less biased. For instance, a consistent finding with data obeying a simple distance-dependent spatial correlation structure was that OLS-estimated standard errors are too small. Occasionally, the OLS standard error was more than five times smaller than the true standard error. Evidently, such substantial biases will give rise to unwarranted confidence in the reliability of results thus obtained.

Together, these simulation studies emphasize the importance of taking due recognition of the statistical characteristics of equivalent dipole modeling. Specifically, it appears that the fashionable OLS approach can yield overly optimistic assessments of the reliability of a source model, while the parameter estimates and their standard errors are considerably off the mark. Nonlinear regression analysis has much to offer to improve the fidelity of model fitting in these respects. In fact, it can be expected that along this line additional gains in the validity and reliability of equivalent dipole modeling can be obtained. This can be done, for instance, by employing generalized models accounting for uncertainties in X, the scalp locations of the leads. Another possibility to improve the statistical performance of equivalent dipole modeling involves the fit of a source model to a time-series of consecutive n-channel potential values. In general, this will increase the power of the analysis, but one then has to deal with the presence of both spatial and time-lagged autocorrelation. A flexible way in which this could be accomplished is by using a recursive multistage GLS estimator (cf. Molenaar, 1994). Several other promising extensions of statistical methods for the fit of equivalent dipole models can be envisaged, but have still remained largely unexplored.

III. Applied Brain Wave Modeling

The linear wave equation constitutes a basic tool in the analysis of spatio-temporal electromagnetic fluctuations. For instance, retarded potentials associated with an elemental time-varying dipole field obey a nonhomogeneous linear wave equation (cf. Robinson & Silvia, 1981). Nunez (1981) has shown that even a simple homogeneous 1D linear wave model can already be of considerable help in understanding the spatio-temporal organization of potential fields. His theoretical developments along these lines, culminating in a coupled set of brain wave equations, will not however, be considered in what follows. Instead, we will focus on the determination of the empirical eigenfunctions associated with a 2D wave model.

Consider again an n-lead montage in which the electrodes are positioned on a finite 2D manifold. Let $y(t, r_n)$, $t = 1, \ldots, T$ and $n = 1, \ldots, N$, represent a multidimensional series of potential values, where t denotes time and r_n is the vector of orthogonal coordinates of the nth electrode. The temporal Fourier Transform of this series is $y(f, r_n)$, $f = k/T$, $k = 0, 1, \ldots, T - 1$. Now let $y(f) = [y(f, r_1), \ldots, y(f, r_n)]^t$ and consider the model

$$E[y(f)] = H(f)x(f), \qquad (5)$$

where $x(f)$ is an ($m \times 1$) source vector (m is usually much smaller than n) and $H(f)$ is an ($n \times m$) matrix. This model corresponds to Nunez's expansion of the electroencephalogram (EEG) in terms of empirical spatial eigenfunctions (Nunez, 1981, p. 269). That is, each column in $H(f)$ is taken to be analogous to a normal mode function associated with the 2D manifold.

The expansion of the EEG in terms of empirical spatial eigenfunctions defined by Eq. (5) is especially useful for applied brain wave modeling. In view of this, one would like to have available a stringent formal specification of its relationship to 2D wave models. The suggested relationship between empirical spatial eigenfunctions and normal mode functions certainly is a plausible one, but needs a definite mathematical proof. Such a proof perhaps might be given if the solution of a wave equation is represented by a convolution of the 2D Green's Function (cf. Robinson & Silvia, 1981) with a general source function.

In the remainder of this section we will concentrate on some important issues with the way in which the empirical spatial EEG eigenfunctions have been determined in applied research. As Eq. (5) defines a frequency-dependent orthogonal expansion, it follows that $H(f)$ can be determined by means of complex-valued principal component analysis in the frequency domain. That is, the solution of Eq. (5) is obtained from the eigenvalue decomposition of the spectral density matrix $S(f) = E[y(f), y(f)^\$]$, where the superscript $\$$ denotes transposition of the complex conjugate. Principal component analysis in the frequency domain is an established technique in time series analysis, especially due to the important work by Brillinger (1975). Yet there has been a persistent problem with this type of analysis. In contrast to the eigenvalue decomposition of a real-valued covariance matrix, which is unique (the so-called rotation problem here is a phantom), the analogous decomposition of a complex-valued covariance matrix like $S(f)$ is, in a special sense, not unique. To elaborate, we will denote the first column vector in $H(f)$ as $h_1(f)$, the standardized eigenvector associated with the first eigenvalue of $S(f)$. Then $\exp[-ia]h_1(f)$, where i is the imaginary unit and a is an arbitrary real variable, is also a standardized eigenvector associated with this first eigenvalue. Consequently, each column vector in $H(f)$ is only unique up to unitary rotation.

The special type of nonuniqueness of complex-valued eigenvectors complicates the interpretation of Eq. (5) (cf. Brillinger, 1975, p. 354; Priestley, Subba Rao, & Tong, 1973). It implies that the phase angles of these eigenvectors are not completely identifiable. To illustrate, we write the *kth* element of the first column in $H(f)$ in polar form:

$$h_{k1}(f) = |h_{k1}(f)| \exp[-ip_{k1}(f)], \qquad (6)$$

where $|x|$ denotes the absolute value of x and $p_{k1}(f)$ is the phase angle. It then is immediately apparent that unitary rotation will change the phase angle, but leave the absolute value invariant. Notice that phase angles are of eminent importance in applied wave modeling. For instance, if a wave model is postulated then it follows that there exists a definite, so-called dispersion relation between temporal and spatial frequencies, which can be expected to provide the principle link between theory and experiment (cf. Nunez, 1981, p. 325). Hence the nonuniqueness of phase angles in $H(f)$ is a quite unfortunate result.

One way to try to circumvent the unitary rotation problem is to constrain the value of the phase angle at one location at zero. For instance $p_{11}(f) = 0$ for all f. This implies that only phase differences with respect to the first lead are considered. Another way to deal with this problem is to take the output of the principal component analysis routine at face value. This appears to be the way in which Nunez approached the issue. (If this supposition is correct, then his plots of the real and imaginary parts and the amplitude–phase diagrams of $H(f)$ are uninterpretable.) There is, however, a more definite, principled way to solve the special unitary rotation problem. This solution has been detailed in Molenaar (1987). The key observation is to conceive of Eq. (5) as an input–output system, where $x(f)$ is the input, $y(f)$ is the output, and $H(f)$ is the system's transfer function. Such a conception of wave propagation has been elaborated upon by Robinson & Silvia (1981, section 1.3), implying that $H(f)$ represents the relationships between a brain wave at different lead locations on the 2D manifold. Now, take the inverse Fourier Transform of Eq. (5), yielding the time domain representation:

$$y(t) = \sum_{u=-T}^{T} H(u)x(t-u). \qquad (7)$$

Notice that according to Eq. (7) the output $y(t)$ is determined by past (u positive), instantaneous (u zero), and future (u negative) input values $x(t-u)$. Of course, the latter dependence of $y(t)$ on future inputs

cannot be obtained with real brain waves, and $H(u)$ in Eq. (7) is therefore called a physically unrealizable filter. However, it can be shown (Robinson & Silvia, 1981, Section 1.6) that if a strictly causal, physically realizable filter exists, then its phase angle in Eq. (6) has minimum value. It follows immediately that the physically realizable spatial eigenfunctions in $H(f)$, if they exist, have minimum phase angle.

The unique solution to the unitary rotation problem is obtained by rotation of each complex-valued eigenvector in $H(f)$ to the minimum phase angle. In Molenaar (1987), a mathematical proof and illustrative outcome of a simulation study are presented, showing that this rotation is necessary to obtain faithful and sensible results in any application of principal component analysis in the spectral domain. An application to real EEG data obtained with a single subject is discussed in Molenaar (1994). In the latter study, exactly the same procedures were followed as described by Nunez (1981, Chap. 7), save for two exceptions. The first exception concerned the additional application of the special unitary rotation described above. The second exception involved the interpretation of the (minimum) phase angles of complex-valued eigenvectors. It is only possible to obtain a complete view of these phase angles, and therefore of the lead–lag pattern across leads in the time domain, if the entire multidimensional phase spectrum at all frequencies is considered. One way to display this multidimensional phase information is to construct spectra of phase differences between all pairwise combinations of leads. It is then possible to detect linear trends which are indicative of systematic lead–lag patterns.

The results of the application to the single-subject EEG data show that unitary rotation to the minimum phase angle indeed has a large effect on the multidimensional phase spectra. Only after carrying out this rotation did a remarkably clear lead–lag pattern emerge, which could be interpreted as being caused by a time-varying source located in a deeper layer at the temporal region. Also noteworthy is that the spectral power was not very large at $T4$ in comparison with the other channels. (In accordance with the procedures followed by Nunez, recordings were only made at the right side of the head.) This nicely corresponds to the observation made by Nunez (1981, p. 337) that the location of maximum amplitude does not necessarily coincide with a source.

We expect that principal component analysis in the spectral domain, in combination with unitary rotation to the minimum phase angle and scrutiny of the complete multidimensional phase spectrum, will become an important tool in applied brain wave modeling. Its solid mathematical and statistical qualities have been thoroughly documented by Brillinger (1975), while Nunez (1981) indicated its close relationship with theoretical brain wave models. Also, this technique can be readily generalized in several interesting ways. To mention one such generalization, a confirmative factor analysis in the spectral domain can be formulated along the same lines. In this so-called dynamic factor model (Molenaar, 1985; Molenaar, de Gooijer, & Schmitz, 1992), it then is possible to define $x(f)$ as a linear combination of a transient and random part. This generalization would seem to be especially appealing for application to event-related potential (ERP) data, which almost by definition are transient phenomena; (for further details, cf. Molenaar, 1989, 1995).

IV. Nonlinear Ontogenesis of Brain Potential Fields

In this section we leave the millisecond domain and enter the realm of life span development. That is, we focus on age-dependent evolution of the structure of brain potential fields. Following the seminal work by Courchesne (e.g., 1978) on developmental relationships between cognitive information processing and ERPs, and by the Thatcher group (e.g., Thatcher, Krause, & Hrybyk, 1986) on cognitive development and EEG, there has been an increasing interest in age-dependent changes in brain topography. Some of our own empirical studies have been reviewed in van der Molen and Molenaar (1993). Here we will be mainly concerned with a concise discussion of mathematical models that might be helpful in explaining particular aspects of these developmental data.

One can distinguish two general types of ontogenetic models of brain topography: finite– and infinite–dimensional models. The finite–dimensional type involves models in which spatial characteristics are represented by a finite set of dependent variables, the evolution of which can be described by a system of ordinary differential or difference equations. For instance, Thatcher's (1991) developmental model of mean EEG coherence belongs to this type. Also, models pertaining to age-dependent evolution of the parameters in an equivalent dipole model, or the parameters in a brain wave model, would belong to this type. In contrast, infinite–dimensional models are represented by partial differential equations describing the evolution of brain maps along the temporal as well as spatial coordinates. Many interesting examples of this type of model can be found in the study of pattern formations in developmental biology (cf. Murray, 1988). In what follows, we will first discuss at some length finite–dimensional models and

then outline a few promising instances of the second type.

The finite–dimensional evolution models of brain topography we have in mind are nonlinear and will be referred to as nonlinear dynamical systems. The main reason for bypassing the ubiquitous linear dynamical models is that these linear models cannot explain several important characteristics of developmental processes. For instance, developmental processes can have emergent properties, undergo sudden transitions to qualitatively new ways of functioning, display symmetry breaking in their spatio-temporal organization, give rise to stable limit cycles, and yield chaotic growth patterns. Typical developmental characteristics like these can only be generated by nonlinear dynamical models. In particular, the occurrence of sudden transitions to qualitatively new ways of functioning, which constitutes the landmark of stagewise development, requires for its proper analysis the use of sophisticated nonlinear dynamical modeling techniques. In the developmental sciences, such stage transitions are conceived of as the outcome of so-called epigenetic processes (cf. Edelman, 1987), where the eipigenetic processes concerned are considered to be inherently nonlinear and capable of dynamic self-organization. It then follows (Molenaar, 1986a,b) that many theoretical questions about stage transitions can be resolved in a mathematical bifurcation analysis (see below) of these self-organizing epigenetic processes.

The empirical results obtained by Courchesne, (1978), Thatcher, and in our laboratory suggest that periods involving major reorganization of brain potential fields coincide with the time table of stage transitions in cognitive development. It would therefore seem plausible to try to represent the ontogenesis of brain potential fields by a nonlinear epigenetic process model. The self-organizing stage transitions in such a process model could then be studied in a bifurcation analysis. This approach will be illustrated by a concise discussion of Thatcher's conjecture that a nonlinear population dynamic model can simulate some of the critical features of the development of EEG coherence (e.g., Thatcher, 1992). Please notice that our discussion will proceed on the general level of mathematical modeling, and does not present new empirical results.

Thatcher's conjecture pertains to a predator–prey population model. The traditional predator–prey model is a special instance of the following bivariate Lotka–Volterra system:

$$dx/dt = x(a + bx + cy); \qquad (8)$$
$$dy/dt = y(d + ex + fy),$$

where d/dt denotes differentiation with respect to time. If c and d are smaller than zero and $b = f = 0$, then one obtains the well known predator–prey equations in which x denotes the density of prey and y that of predators. In their textbook on the theory of evolution and dynamical systems, Hofbauer and Sigmund (1988, section 18.2) prove that Eq. (8) has at least one particular shortcoming in that it cannot generate structurally stable periodic oscillations. Moreover, they state that "... even the slightest intraspecific competition destroys the periodicity altogether" (Hofbauer & Sigmund, 1988, p. 152). Consequently, the typical behavior of Eq. (8) does not appear to be stable, and to get a more robust model one has to generalize it. As to this, consider the schematic representation:

$$dx/dt = ax + xP_x(x,y); \qquad (9)$$
$$dy/dt = by + yP_y(x,y),$$

where $P_x(x,y)$ and $P_y(x,y)$ denote interaction terms. Notice that the interaction terms are linear in Eq. (8). Hofbauer and Sigmund prove (1988, section 18.4) that structurally stable behavior can be obtained under general conditions if these interaction terms are allowed to be nonlinear (as is the case in Thatcher's model; R. W. Thatcher, 1994). Accordingly, this allowance will be made in what follows.

Now the occurrence of sudden transitions to qualitatively new ways of behavior of Eq. (9) could be made explicit in a bifurcation analysis. In such a bifurcation analysis the equilibria of Eq. (9), which are defined by setting dx/dt and dy/dt at zero, are charted as functions of the model parameters (a, b, and the parameters entering the interaction terms). That is, if each model parameter is varied continuously, then in general, the equilibrium set of Eq. (9) will also vary continuously. But, at distinct values of a model parameter, the equilibria may suddenly change in a qualitative way: existing equilibria may disappear and/or new types may emerge. For instance, an existing stable focus may give way to an unstable focus together with a stable limit cycle (so-called supercritical Hopf bifurcation). For simple nonlinear dynamical systems, a bifurcation analysis can be carried out mathematically, but usually one has to take recourse to a numerical approach. A sophisticated set of computational procedures for carrying this out can be found in Kubicek and Marek (1983).

What can be said about a bifurcation analysis of a system like Eq. (9)? Before we try to answer this question, we first present an interesting relationship between Lotka–Volterra systems and a particular class of artificial neural networks. Consider the case in which $P_x(x,y)$ and $P_y(x,y)$ involve modulation of the interacting x and y variables by a sigmoid function $S(z) = 1/(1$ $+ \exp[-z])$, $z = x,y$. If a and b in Eq. (9) are also smaller than zero, then one obtains one of Grossberg's basic forms of an artificial neural network, in which x and y denote mean excitatory and inhibitory network activities, respectively (e.g., Grossberg, 1988). This formal relationship is fortunate for at least the following reasons. First, it may help in reinterpreting a predator–prey system in terms which are more familiar to neurophysiologists, namely excitatory and inhibitory neural activity. Second, the large body of mathematical results concerning the stability of Lotka–Volterra systems (cf. Hofbauer & Sigmund, 1988) can thus be brought to bear on artificial neural network systems, and in reverse, recent analytic results concerning the storage capacity of artificial neural networks (cf. Amit, 1989, chap. 6) might be applied to Lotka–Volterra systems. Third and finally, this relationship is also helpful for our present purposes. Schuster and Wagner (1990, Fig. 2) published the results of a bifurcation analysis of a neural network that in a formal sense resemble Eq. (9). More specifically, their neural network scheme (which simulates the 40–60 Hz synchronized oscillations over large distances across the visual cortex, as reported by Gray, Konig, Engel, & Singer, 1989) is obtained by modulating the interacting x and y variables by the sigmoid function already alluded to, and adding an input term I_x to the excitatory part of the model. Continuous variation of the input I_x then induces a number of bifurcations of the equilibrium set of their model, including a Hopf bifurcation to limit cycle oscillations. In our own reconstruction of this bifurcation diagram, it was also found that the basin of attraction of an equilibrium (that is, the range of initial x values which are attracted to it) may shrink substantially as function of I_x. In conclusion, the (numerical) bifurcation analysis of this artificial neural network nicely illustrates the detailed information about stage transitions which can thus be obtained. Of course, the Schuster and Wagner model pertains to brain activity in the millisecond domain, and therefore specific conclusions about its bifurcation diagram cannot be directly generalized to life span models like the Lotka–Volterra systems. But it can be expected that a bifurcation analysis of a predator–prey system will yield similar results, given its formal resemblance to such artificial neural networks.

It would seem that bifurcation analysis provides a royal road to the construction of nonlinear dynamical models explaining the ontogenesis of brain potential fields. Unfortunately, however, this is not entirely the case. In contrast to linear dynamical models, only a limited number of which have to be considered in any application to real data, the number of conceivable nonlinear variants seems to be unbounded. Typical characteristics of developmental processes like the occurrence of stage transitions or limit cycles can be the result of a large variety of nonlinear dynamical systems. The identification of a unique nonlinear dynamical model from empirical data (in contrast to a deductive bifurcation analysis of an already given model) is still an unresolved problem, if no further a priori information is available. It is, in general, not sufficient to show that a postulated nonlinear model fits the data well, because there will be an unknown number of alternative models that fit the data equally well or even better. What is called for is a kind of abstract bifurcation analysis which covers all conceivable nonlinear dynamical models without depending on their detailed mathematical specifications. Such an abstract bifurcation indeed exists, and is called "catastrophe theory" (Gilmore, 1981). As has been argued elsewhere (van der Maas & Molenaar, 1992), catastrophe theory allows for the detection of stage transitions, even if no mathematical model of the developmental process is available. It suffices to test for the presence of a set of seven so-called catastrophe flags like sudden jumps, hysteresis, and anomalous variance (for a mathematical derivation of these flags, cf. Gilmore, 1981, chap. 9). All that is required for an application to brain potential field data is to choose a suitable operationalization for each of the catastrophe flags, and then carry out the tests (cf. van der Maas & Molenaar, 1992, for an application to cognitive development).

In closing this section, we will briefly discuss infinite-dimensional developmental models of brain topography (although, to the best of our knowledge, no such models have yet been considered in the neurophysiological literature). Remember that these models describe developmental processes along the temporal as well as spatial coordinates, such as age-dependent changes in topographic amplitude maps of the EEG. Strong arguments can be given that so-called reaction–diffusion models with finite interaction velocity will prove to be especially useful (cf. Vasiliev, Romanovskii, Chernavskii, & Yakhno, 1987, chap. 2). For ease of presentation we will only consider one spatial coordinate x. A schematic representation of such a reaction–diffusion is:

$$u_t = u_{xx} + f(u, u_x, x, t), \qquad (10)$$

where partial derivatives are denoted by subscripts. In Eq. (10) u_{xx} denotes the diffusion part and $f(.)$ the reaction part. Of course, a reaction–diffusion model for age-dependent changes in EEG amplitude maps would require two spatial coordinates. For the same reasons as given above, $f(.)$ has to be nonlinear in order to capture the characteristic features of developmental processes.

Reaction–diffusion models have been successfully applied in developmental biology after much of the groundwork has been laid by Nicolis and Prigogine (1977). In particular, the monograph by Meinhardt (1982) presents many detailed simulations of biological pattern formation (as well as a listing of the source code of the simulation program). More recently, Feistel and Ebeling (1989, section 9.4) considerably extended the range of applications, including a consideration of a Lotka–Volterra reaction–diffusion model. All this work contains many Ansatzes for the construction of plausible reaction–diffusion models of the ontogenesis of brain potential fields.

V. Discussion

In the foregoing sections we presented a bird's eye view of several aspects of the mathematical modeling of brain potential fields. The models in question either are already regularly employed in studies of brain topography, or else appear to be on the verge of being applied in this way. In this closing section, we will leave this reference point behind and speculate about some possibly interesting innovative developments. One of these pertains to the substantial biological effects of imposed, extremely low-frequency (ELF), electric fields (Adey & Lawrence, 1984). Imposed ELF fields also appear to affect the membranes of neurons and therefore could have psychophysiological side effects. This raises the question of whether there are also detectable effects of these ELF fields on properly filtered brain potential fields. If this is indeed the case, one could consider the possibility of employing the latter effects in inverse modeling techniques (e.g., based inverse scattering theory) of neural sources.

Another speculation also involves the possibility to improve neural source modeling techniques. Computerized tomography is based on the Radon Transform, which reconstructs a 2D distribution from corresponding line–integral projections. Recently, a new application of the Radon Transform has been proposed to reconstruct the distribution of radar backscatter intensity as a function of range delay and Doppler Shift (cf. Bernfeld, 1990). Perhaps other new applications can be worked out along this line. In so far as dynamical systems like the working brain generate regular manifolds in phase space, and if suitable carrier signals can be found which are attenuated by these manifolds, one could in principle use the Radon Transform to reconstruct them. This would provide a truly dynamic computerized tomography (CT) scan of ongoing brain activity.

Of course the speculations given above (and one could think of various other ones) are just that: purely speculative. In contrast, the discussion in the preceding sections focussed on more definite modeling techniques in applied brain topography. All sections taken together, however, are intended to provide a global map of the many exciting possibilities of further progress in the applied mathematical modeling of brain potential fields. We hope that our map will be of some help in this continuing search.

References

Adey, W. R., & Lawrence, A. F. (eds.) (1984). *Nonlinear electrodynamics in biological systems.* New York: Plenum.

Amit, D. J. (1989). *Modeling brain function: The world of attractor neural networks.* Cambridge: Cambridge Univ. Press.

Bernfeld, M. (1990). Tomography in radar. In L. Auslander, T. Kailath, & S. Mitter (Eds.), *Signal processing, Part I: Signal processing theory.* Berlin: Springer-Verlag.

Brillinger, D. R. (1975). *Time series: Data analysis and theory.* New York: Holt, Rinehart, & Winston.

Courchesne, E. (1978). Neurophysiological correlates of cognitive development: Changes in long-latency event-related potentials from childhood to adulthood. *Electroencephalography and Clinical Neurophysiology, 45,* 468–482.

De Munck, J. C. (1989). *A mathematical and physical interpretation of the electromagnetic field of the brain.* Unpublished Ph.D. Thesis, University of Amsterdam, Amsterdam.

Edelman, G. M. (1987). *Neural Darwinism: The theory of neuronal group selection.* New York: Basic Books.

Feistel, R., & Ebeling, W. (1989). *Evolution of complex systems: Selforganization, entropy and development.* Dordrecht, The Netherlands: Reidel.

Gilmore, R. (1981). *Catastrophe Theory for Scientists and Engineers.* New York: Wiley.

Gray, C. M., Konig, P., Engel, A. K., & Singer, W. (1989). Oscillatory responses in cat visual cortex exhibit inter-columnar synchronization which reflects global stimulus properties. *Nature (London), 338,* 334–337.

Grossberg, S. (1988). *Neural networks and natural intelligence.* Cambridge, MA: MIT Press.

Hofbauer, J., & Sigmund, K. (1988). *The theory of evolution and dynamical systems.* Cambridge: Cambridge Univ. Press.

Huizenga, H. M., & Molenaar, P. C. M. (1994). Estimating and testing the sources of evoked potentials in the brain. *Multivariate Behavioral Research, 29,* 237–262.

Huizenga, H. M., & Molenaar, P. C. M. (1995). Equivalent source estimation of scalp potential fields contaminated by heteroscedastic and correlated noise. *Brain Topography, 8,* 13–33.

Kubicek, M., & Marek, M. (1983). *Computational methods in bifurcation theory and dissipative structures.* New York: Springer-Verlag.

Meinhardt, H. (1982). *Models of biological pattern formation.* London: Academic Press.

Molenaar, P. C. M. (1985). A dynamic factor model for the analysis of multivariate time series. *Psychometrika, 50,* 181–202.

Molenaar, P. C. M. (1986a). Issues with a rule-sampling theory of conservation learning from a structuralist point of view. *Human Development, 29,* 137–144.

Molenaar, P. C. M. (1986b). On the impossibility of acquiring more powerful structures: A neglected alternative. *Human Development, 29,* 245–251.

Molenaar, P. C. M. (1987). Dynamic factor analysis in the frequency domain: Causal modeling of multivariate psychophysiological time series. *Multivariate Behavioral Research, 22,* 329–353.

Molenaar, P. C. M. (1989). Aspects of dynamic factor analysis. In *Analysis of statistical information.* Tokyo: The Institute of Statistical Mathematics.

Molenaar, P. C. M. (1994). Dynamic factor analysis of psychophysiological signals. In J. R. Jennings, P. Ackles, & M. G. H. Coles (Eds.), *Advances in psychophysiology,* Vol. 5, pp. 229–302. London: Jessica Kingsley Publishers.

Molenaar, P. C. M. (1995). Dynamic latent variable models in developmental psychology. In A. von Eye & C. C. Clogg (Eds.), *Analysis of latent variable in developmental research,* pp. 155–180. Newbury Park, CA: Sage.

Molenaar, P. C. M., de Gooijer, J. G., & Schmitz, B. (1992). Dynamic factor analysis of nonstationary multivariate time series. *Psychometrika, 57,* 333–349.

Murray, J. D. (1988). *Mathematical biology.* Berlin: Springer-Verlag.

Nicolis, G., & Prigogine, I. (1977). *Selforganization in nonequilibrium systems: From dissipative structures to order through fluctuations.* New York: Wiley.

Nunez, P. L. (1981). *Electric fields of the brain: The neurophysics of EEG.* New York: Oxford Univ. Press.

Priestley, M. B., Subba Rao, T., & Tong, H. (1973). Identification of the structure of multivariate stochastic systems. In P. R. Krishnaiah (Ed.), *Multivariate analysis III.* New York: Academic Press.

Robinson, E. A., & Silvia, M. T. (1981). *Digital foundations of time series analysis, Volume 2: Wave-equation space-time processing.* San Francisco: Holden-Day.

Schuster, H. G., & Wagner, P. (1990). A model for neuronal oscillations in the visual cortex: Mean-field theory and derivation of the phase equations. *Biological Cybernetics, 64,* 77–82.

Seber, G. A. F., & Wild, C. J. (1990). *Nonlinear regression.* New York: Wiley.

Thatcher, R. W. (1992). Cyclic cortical reorganization during early childhood. *Brain and Cognition, 20,* 24–50.

Thatcher, R. W. (1991). Maturation of the human frontal lobes: Physiological evidence for staging. *Developmental Neuropsychology, 7,* 397–419.

Thatcher, R. W., Krause, P., & Hrybyk, M. (1986). Cortico-cortical association fibers and EEG coherence: A two compartmental model. *Electroencephalography and Clinical Neurophysiology, 64,* 123–143.

van der Maas, H. L. J., & Molenaar, P. C. M. (1992). Stagewise cognitive development: An application of catastrophe theory. *Psychological Review, 99,* 395–417.

van der Molen, M. W., & Molenaar, P. C. M. (1993). Cognitive psychophysiology: A window to cognitive development and brain maturation. In G. Dawson & K. W. Fischer (Eds.), *Human behavior and the developing brain,* pp. 456–490. New York: Guilford Publications.

Vasiliev, V. A., Romanovskii, Yu.M., Chernavskii, D. S., & Yakhno, V. G. (1987). *Autowave processes in kinetic systems: Spatial and temporal selforganization in physics, chemistry, biology and medicine.* Dordrecht, The Netherlands, Reidel.

6

PET and fMRI in the Detection of Task-Related Brain Activity: Implications for the Study of Brain Development

Guinevere F. Eden* and Thomas A. Zeffiro†

Section on Functional Brain Imaging, National Institute of Mental Health, National Institutes of Health, Bethesda, Maryland 20892; and †Laboratory of Diagnostic Radiology Research, National Institutes of Health, Building 13, Room 3W13, 9000 Rockville Pike, Bethesda, Maryland 20892

I. Introduction

Functional neuroimaging has become an increasingly popular research tool over the last decade. The ability to make measurements of *in vivo* physiologic information such as regional cerebral metabolism or blood flow have allowed previously impossible studies of human brain function in health and disease. These studies have contributed important new information concerning the neurophysiological mechanisms of sensation, cognition, and movement. In this chapter we examine the use of two neuroimaging techniques, positron emission tomography (PET) and functional magnetic resonance imaging (fMRI), and discuss the possibilities for future applications of functional neuroimaging in aiding our understanding of human brain development. For technical and ethical reasons, imaging studies with children have been few in number, compared to those with adults. The introduction of functional neuroimaging techniques better suited to studies involving children or adolescents will allow larger numbers of developmental studies in the future. We will examine how these new brain imaging methods, such as fMRI, may allow new approaches to the study of development.

II. Functional Neuroimaging Techniques

A. Positron Emission Tomography

Neural information processing in humans has been indirectly measured using behavioral, electrophysiological, and neuroimaging techniques. Of these three approaches, functional neuroimaging has appeared most recently, and potentially holds the most promise for precisely mapping the processes underlying human perception, movement, and cognition. PET is considered by many to be the "gold standard" among the available functional neuroimaging techniques, as it allows the measurement of changes in neural activity by monitoring changes in regional cerebral blood flow (rCBF). PET can be used to measure blood flow and blood volume, which change in relation to neuronal activity changes in the neocortex (Roy & Sherrington, 1890). PET radiotracer techniques also allow the study of glucose and oxygen metabolism, as well as other physiological variables (for a review of techniques, see Herscovitch, 1994). Many studies employing PET have revealed precise mapping of various neuronal functions related to vision (Zeki, Watson, Lueck, Friston, Kennard, & Frackowiak, 1991), audition (Price, Wise, Ramsay, Friston, Howard, Patterson, et al., 1992), movement (Colebatch, Deiber, Passingham, Friston, & Frackowiak, 1991; Sadato, Zeffiro, Campbell, Konishi, Shibasaki, & Hallett, 1995), language (Wise, Chollet,

Hadar, Friston, Hoffner, & Frackowiak, 1991; Petersen, Fox, Posner, Mintun, & Raichle, 1988), working memory (Jonides, Smith, Koeppe, Awh, Minoshima, & Mintun, 1993), and attention (Pardo, Fox, & Raichle, 1991; Corbetta, Miezin, Dobmeyer, Shulman, & Petersen, 1990).

As predicted by Roy and Sherrington in 1890, activity in a particular region of the brain results in a corresponding change in local cerebral blood flow. In subsequent animal studies it has been shown that there is an interrelationship between local flow, glucose metabolism, and functional activity (Sokoloff, 1981). The details of the complicated relationship among these physiological variables is not yet clear. Nevertheless, human behavioral studies utilizing PET have capitalized on this relationship: PET measurements, mainly using bolus injections of 30–80 mCi of H_2 ^{15}O for the assessment of rCBF, or 5–10 mCi of [^{18}F] deoxyglucose (FDG) for glucose metabolism, have been used to assess brain function in health (Phelps & Mazziotta, 1985), development (Chugani, Phelps, & Mazziotta, 1987), aging (Hoffman, Guze, Baxter, Mazziotta, & Phelps, 1989), and disease (Mazziotta, Phelps, Pahl, Huang, Baxter, Riege, et al., 1987). For rCBF, the relatively short 2 minute half-life of ^{15}O (compared to a 110 minute half-life for FDG), allows multiple scans to be performed in each subject. Since the relationship between rCBF and tissue count is almost linear (Fox & Mintun, 1989), changes in rCBF can be estimated from observed tissue counts following injection of this freely diffusible tracer. Instead of having to use arterial blood sampling and perform a calculation based on a model of the tracer's diffusion, images of tissue counts normalized for total brain radioactivity can be reconstructed and subjected to statistical analysis. While this technique has been extremely useful, the spatial resolution obtained from conventional PET is low, limited by the distance a positron may travel before colliding with an electron and emitting the coincident photons that are detected by the gamma camera in the PET scanner (see section I.C. for improved 3D PET techniques). Moreover, it is necessary to wait at least 5 tracer half-lives between scans to allow the tracer to decay to a level allowing a new measurement with acceptably low background noise. In the case of H_2 ^{15}O this results in a minimum interscan interval of 10 minutes, limiting the number of scans that can be obtained from any individual in a 2 hour experiment to a practical maximum of 12. Experimental designs requiring a larger number of scans either need extremely compliant subjects or repeat scanning on another day, with attendant problems of spatial registration of the images from the 2 separate scan sessions. Therefore, functional imaging techniques based on magnetic resonance technology, offering the promise of higher spatial resolution and shorter data acquisition times, have generated particular excitement in the community of researchers interested in brain and cognitive development.

B. Functional Magnetic Resonance Imaging

Belliveau and colleagues first demonstrated that high resolution magnetic resonance imaging with bolus injections of contrast material could be used to study visual processing in humans (Belliveau, Kennedy, McKinstry, Buchbinder, Weisskoff, Cohen, et al., 1991). These results generated immediate and sustained interest in the functional neuroimaging community and rapid technical development followed. Very soon, a completely noninvasive method for measuring blood oxygenation change using magnetic resonance functional neuroimaging was reported by Kwong and his collaborators, using an effect reported by Ogawa (Ogawa, Lee, Nayak, & Glynn, 1990). They clearly demonstrated changes in cortical activation in the calcarine fissure of the visual cortex during photic stimulation (Kwong, Belliveau, Chesler, Goldberg, Weisskoff, Poncelet, et al., 1992). Since then, functional magnetic resonance imaging has been used in numerous laboratories at both 1.5 and 4 tesla to investigate the processes underlying human movement and perception (Turner, Jezzard, Wen, Kwong, Le Bihan, Zeffiro, et al., 1993; Bandettini, Wong, Hinks, Tikofsky, & Hyde, 1992; Ogawa, Tank, Menon, Ellermann, Kim, Merkle, et al., 1992; Frahm, Bruhn, Merbold, & Hanicke, 1992; Blamire, McCarthy, Gruetter, Rottman, Rattner, Hyder, et al., 1992).

Functional MRI is based on the principle that the recorded MRI signal may change in response to changes in the magnetic character of the intravascular contents. These changes may result from injection of contrast material or from changes in the magnetic properties of the contents of red blood cells. Since deoxygenated hemoglobin is more paramagnetic than oxygenated hemoglobin (Thulborn, Waterton, Matthews, & Radda, 1982), it acts as an endogenous intravascular paramagnetic contrast agent (Ogawa, et al., 1990; Turner, Le Bihan, Moonen, & Frank, 1991). Animal studies first demonstrated that variations in blood oxygenation affect the MR image intensity, hence the term blood oxygenation level dependent contrast (BOLD) (Ogawa et al., 1990). It is this phenomenon on which fMRI is based; specific tasks thought to be associated with increased regional brain activity have been shown to have concomitant local increases in signal intensity. During increased neural activity, there is an elevation of cerebral blood flow, which is greater than that required to support local oxygen consumption. As a result of this discrepancy, the relative local concentration of deoxyhemoglobin is decreased. On a magnetic susceptibility $T2^*$ weighted image, this results in increased signal intensity, which as in PET, allows estimation of neural activation when compared to a baseline image.

C. Comparison of Characteristics of PET and fMRI

Both PET and fMRI have their unique advantages. Data acquisition with fMRI can be accomplished rapidly. Some fMRI methods, such as echo-planar imaging (EPI), are extremely fast (Mansfield, 1977; Cohen & Weisskoff, 1991), allowing single plane imaging times of 40 msec. The obvious advantage is that rapid changes of brain activity, which may well be less than some tens of milliseconds in duration, may be tracked with greater accuracy than is possible with PET ^{15}O studies, with their minimum 40 sec sampling time. The brief single frame data acquisition period possible with EPI is somewhat misleading though, as the changes in fMRI signal lag the neuronal changes by some 4–10 sec, resulting in a distortion of the neuronal "signal" by the effect of the hemodynamic response function (Bandettini, 1993; Friston, Jezzard, & Turner, 1994). It is the latency of the hemodynamic response time, which may or may not be the same for all areas of the brain, that sets the ultimate limit on temporal resolution.

Fast imaging techniques such as EPI do avoid some of the problems of brain or subject motion artifact. Rapid image acquisition reduces the chances of including motion; only interscan subject motion remains and can be corrected (Woods, Cherry, & Mazziotta, 1992). As a further benefit, faster acquisition times allow more scans per session. Increasing the number of samples in an experimental session results in increased statistical power and therefore sensitivity to signals of lesser amplitude. Hence, single subject analysis can be carried out, or several different tasks can be employed in the same session, in the context of more complex experimental designs.

Another advantage of fMRI is the possibility of obtaining high spatial resolution. This higher spatial resolution reduces signal inaccuracies due to partial volume effects (Mazziotta, Phelps, Plummer, & Kuhl, 1981). However, it should be pointed out that there has been improvement in PET technology, allowing 4–6 mm in-plane spatial resolution.

Data acquisition using PET also has some advantages. PET allows 3D acquisition of parallel slices of the entire brain in cameras with a 15 cm field of view. Most of the fMRI experiments conducted so far make use of only a few slices in a particular area of interest in the brain. It is possible to acquire whole-head volumes with fMRI using a whole-head coil, but since the images are nevertheless acquired slice by slice, as the number of slices is increased, the acquisition time increases. As a result, there is a time delay between the acquisition of the first slice and the last slice, raising some uncertainty about the timing of the physiological changes and the usual possible problems associated with intrascan head motion. Three dimensional fMRI methods are being developed (van Gelderen, Ramsey, Liu, Duyn, Frank, Weinberger, et al., 1995), which circumvent these problems and have their own advantages such as no inflow effects.

As with all new techniques, there have been some attempts to use fMRI in areas previously not explored with functional neuroimaging techniques. This is inviting because fMRI is suited to studies in which the use of other techniques, such as PET, are limited or impossible. The obvious advantage with fMRI is that it allows study of subjects where radiation dosimetry limits the use of the technology, such as PET scans of healthy children. It also allows studies involving repeated scanning over many days or weeks; this may be the case for longitudinal studies over several sessions, or in order to perform numerous tasks in the same session. Also, fMRI lends itself to single subject analysis, which not only allows for the study of smaller sample sizes, but gives information concerning between-subject variation. However, single subject studies can now also be carried out using PET. As demonstrated by Watson and colleagues (Watson, Myers, Frackowiak, Hajnal, Woods, Mazziotta et al., 1993), using a 3D PET scanner, the activation maps generated from data of a single subject can be mapped onto the subject's own MRI, allowing superior neuroanatomical localization. In fact, the advent of fMRI has occurred in parallel with improvements in PET technology, so that many of the advantages of fMRI are not always as exclusive as may be first assumed.

One very substantial difference between the two techniques is that currently fMRI approaches relying on the BOLD contrast phenomenon do not provide direct measures of physiological parameters. PET can measure absolute blood flow, but BOLD contrast detects only signal change between control and activation conditions, using the signal intensity of $T2^*$ weighted images. (There are ways to calculate blood flow and blood volume measurements with MRI using a contrast agent, but these are of course, invasive.) It should be noted that numerous PET studies are also done qualitatively rather than quantitatively, by omitting arterial blood lines and instead capitalizing on the fact that tissue counts in reconstructed PET images closely correspond to CBF, at least at low blood flow rates (Fox & Mintun, 1989). PET, however, does have the advantage of offering quantitative measures, and PET offers numerous other methods for assessing physiological mechanisms, such as neuroreceptor and transmitter systems and blood–brain barrier permeability.

A practical consideration when choosing between these two techniques is the maturity of data processing software available; image software analysis is much more developed with respect to statistical analysis of PET data, since this is a well-established technique. While there is broad consensus concerning methods for PET data analysis and display (Friston's Statistical Parametric Mapping system is a notable example; Friston, Frith, Liddle, & Frackowiak, 1991), similar consensus concerning analysis strategies for fMRI data has not yet occurred.

With regard to financial considerations, MRI is a much more affordable technique. While many investigators use scanners equipped for EPI to allow for the advantages of rapid image acquisitions, it is possible to perform fMRI experiments with conventional scanners (Connelly, Jackson, Frackowiak, Belliveau, Vargha-Khadem, & Gadian, 1993; Cohen, Forman, Braver, Casey, Servant-Schreiber, & Noll, 1994; Cuenod, Bookheimer, Hertz-Pannier, Zeffiro, Theodore, & Le Bihan, 1995). In addition, ^{15}O PET studies require a cyclotron on site for isotope generation, which is one of the reasons making this the more costly technique.

The advantages of fMRI over PET, in summary, are absence of radiation exposure, direct mapping of functional and anatomical data within a single imaging modality, improved temporal resolution, and the ability to perform longitudinal studies. PET, like fMRI, does offer the possibility of single subject studies. It also offers fairly good resolution, and while fMRI is even better in this regard, it is always at the expense of increased signal averaging to achieve statistical significance. The problems encountered with fMRI may appear quite numerous now, but this is largely due to the infancy of this technique. With the large amount of interest in the development of fMRI among a range of scientific communities who see potential for their field with this method, many of these problems are likely to be solved in the very near future.

D. Direct Comparison of PET and fMRI: A Study of PET and fMRI Using a Visual Stimulus in Adults

Although the two techniques are based on different methods, one would predict good agreement between the outcome of PET and fMRI studies. Several fMRI studies have reported findings that confirm previous PET experiments performed utilizing similar tasks. For example, the study by McCarthy and others (McCarthy, Blamire, Rothman, Gruetter, & Shulman, 1993) used fMRI to show activation during a word generation task, and the results are in agreement with Petersen's PET study (Petersen et al., 1988). Studies on the motor system with PET (Colebatch et al., 1991) and fMRI (Bandettini, 1993) have shown corresponding task-related signal changes in the primary motor cortex in relation to hand movements. Belliveau and colleagues (Belliveau, Kwong, Kennedy, Baker, Stern, Benson, et al., 1992) have shown the existence of a clear overlap of their fMRI data with data on CBF percentage change obtained from another laboratory's PET study (Fox & Raichle, 1985), when subjects were visually stimulated across a range of temporal frequencies in both studies. While these suggest good agreement between these two techniques, they do not represent a direct comparison. Our group carried out an fMRI validation using PET data acquired under similar experimental conditions (Eden, Maisog, Jezzard, VanMeter, Herscovitch, Giedd, et al., 1994). We assessed to what extent the results were in agreement with one another, given that all other conditions were comparable. We examined the suggestions that some of the reported task-related fMRI signal changes may be artifactual (Hajnal, Myers, Oatridge, Schwieso, Young, & Bydder, 1994).

To carry out a study in which the identical task is being performed and analyzed in a comparable way, the relevant advantages and disadvantages of PET and fMRI had to be considered. For example, although fMRI has the potential of resolving millimeter details in the region of interest in a single subject, this is at the expense of increased number of scans and longer acquisition times for larger volumes. The number of scans that can be acquired in this time period will influence the contrast–to–noise ratio. In this comparison study we used relatively large volumes rather than just a few slices. For both PET and fMRI we used similar voxel sizes, to allow for a true comparison. The fMRI data was acquired using isometric voxels, therefore working with a cubic volume of equal subdivisions in all three directions.

For both the PET and MRI studies, the subjects consisted of healthy, normal volunteers, selected using the same selection criteria. (For PET scanning procedures see Eden et al., 1994.) In brief, the subjects' head motion was reduced with thermoplastic masks as they lay supine in the PET scanner. RCBF changes were assessed, using images obtained by summing the activity over 60 sec following the first detection of cerebral radioactivity, after the intravenous bolus injection of

33 mCi of ^{15}O–water. For the control scans, the subjects were instructed to maintain fixation on a central cross hair. For the visual stimulation scans, the subjects maintained fixation on the cross hair, centered on a reversing checkerboard. The scans (four in total) were individually corrected for interscan motion (Woods et al., 1992).

Multislice fMRI data were acquired using EPI on a 1.5 tesla system with a 5″ surface coil positioned in a coronal orientation at the back of the head. Twenty contiguous 5mm slices (field of view (FOV) 32 cm, matrix 64 × 64, echo time (TE) 40 msec) were collected in 2 seconds. This procedure made it possible to acquire volumes consisting of 5mm cubic voxels that spanned the occipital and posterior parietal cortex. One volume was obtained each minute, as in the PET study, but a total of 72 acquisitions were made for each subject. The stimuli were the same as those used in the PET study. FMRI data were also corrected for interscan head motion with the same realignment procedure utilized for the PET data (Woods et al., 1992).

Larger numbers of observations obtained with fMRI allowed for statistical analysis of single subjects. Detection of regional task-related signal change was performed by computing t-statistic maps contrasting task and control states. These maps were transformed to the standard normal distribution (z-scores) for comparison with the results of the rCBF measurements, using $z = 4.5$ as the minimum critical threshold. Time series at locations corresponding to local maxima were examined for verification that the signal changes were task-related. Neuroanatomical localization was determined by comparison of the echo-planar images with co-planar spin echo images.

Plate 14 is an example of the fMRI results in one subject, and Figure 1 depicts a corresponding time series. Local maxima are shown in calcarine sulcus and lingual gyrus. The individual z-scores for these maxima were 8.3 and 6.9, respectively (this corresponds to 1.5% and 1.1% increase above the baseline).

Task minus control subtractions in the same single subjects are shown for the PET data in Plate 15, displaying a signal increase above 20% (the small number of observations prevented single subject statistical analysis). This examples illustrates agreement between these two techniques on the neuroanatomical localization of the task-related responses. The large area of signal increase for the PET scans reflects the lower resolution of this technique. Similarly, a group data comparison in a sample of 8 subjects (Eden, VanMeter, Maisog, Jezzard, Herscovitch, Rapoport, et al., 1995) demonstrated that the fMRI single subject analysis was able to delineate spatially discrete foci in striate and extrastriate cortex

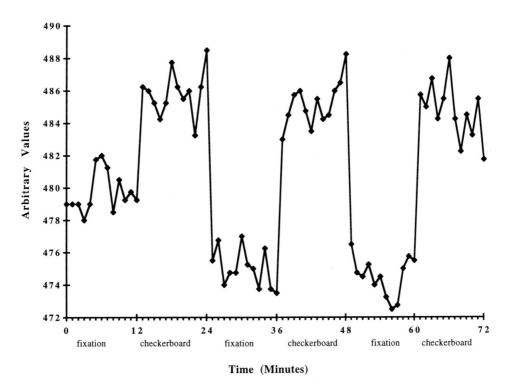

Figure 1. An example of an fMRI time series (mean signal intensity change averaged from 4 voxels) from the calcarine sulcus.

that appeared to be merged when using PET group analysis Statistical Parametric Mapping (SPM). fMRI gave more information on the spatial extent and response variability between the subjects in the extrastriate areas. Steps were taken to reduce interscan head motion, and the resulting pattern of signal changes recorded did not differ from that observed in the PET experiment. A more accurate PET/fMRI comparison will now be feasible with the use of gamma cameras operating in 3D mode (Watson et al., 1993; Cherry, Dahlbom, & Hoffman, 1992).

III. Imaging and the Study of Brain Development

A. Processes Underlying Brain Maturation

Brain development and maturation occur as a result of morphological, biochemical and physiological changes in the central nervous system. In agreement with animal studies (O'Kusky & Colonnier, 1982), human postmortem histological examination has revealed that developmental changes are most dramatic in neonates and during the first few postnatal years (Conel, 1939–1963; Huttenlocher & de Courten, 1987). The reason for this initial explosive growth is a large overproduction of neurons in early development, followed by selective elimination, leaving only functionally specific and efficient neuronal populations (Changeux & Danchin, 1976). While neuronal loss decreases in the later phase of maturation, synapse elimination occurs up until the later years of childhood (e.g., in human striate cortex, 40% of synapses are lost between ages 8 months and 11 years, Huttenlocher & de Courten, 1987). Even though these changes are most dramatic in the newborn brain, some dendritic growth occurs in adult brains and this may be related to learning, memory, and recovery of function following brain damage (Reinis & Goldman, 1980).

Early maturational changes have been monitored electrophysiologically (ERP and EEG) and behaviorally (for a review, see Holmes, 1986), and have been characterized to be age-dependent. Numerous complex events are thought to occur simultaneously, such as changes in the abundance of dendrites, axons, and synapses, myelination of axons, and other biochemical maturation. Imaging provides a method of relating behavioral developmental changes to some of the processes underlying brain maturation. Conventional MRI has been used to measure some of these changes in early infancy and throughout childhood, by making morphometric assessments (Pfefferbaum, Mathalon,

Sullivan, Rawles, Zipursky, & Lim, 1994), and measuring myelination (Jernigan & Tallal, 1990; Jernigan, Trauner, Hesselink, & Tallal, 1991; Holland, Haas, Norman, Brant-Zawadzki, & Newton, 1986; McArdle, Richardson, Nicholas, Mirfakhraee, Hayden, & Amparo, 1987). Myelination is known from autopsy studies to continue into late childhood (Yakovlev & Lecours, 1967) and can be assessed in a limited fashion by white matter/gray matter segmentation of the MRI image. These anatomical findings are accompanied by functional changes. PET has been used to demonstrate changes in measures of local cerebral glucose metabolic rates from early to late childhood (Chugani et al., 1987).

There appears to be regional variation in developmental processes across the brain, which has been detected in most of the assessment techniques used. Different areas mature at different rates. In humans for example, synaptic density changes, measured with tissue staining techniques, are completed in occipital areas before frontal areas (Huttenlocher & de Courten, 1987; Huttenlocher & Raichelson, 1989). MRI studies have found reductions of gray matter volume mainly in the superior, compared to the inferior cortical areas of the cortex (Jernigan et al., 1991). Functionally, cortical and subcortical structures show different patterns of metabolic activity changes throughout development (Chugani et al., 1987). Some time courses of anatomical development can be related to physiological changes; however, not all studies corroborate one another. In fact, some research supports concurrent synaptogenesis in different cortical regions rather than regional variation for this process (Rakic, Bourgeois, Eckenhoff, Zecevic, & Goldman-Rakic, 1986).

There is now increasing opportunity to use functional brain imaging as a measure of brain development and relate it to cognitive skills. This approach assumes that there is agreement as to what cognitive functions rely on what types of brain organization and the development needed to make them efficient. In this way, certain brain regions are specialized to perform specific types of information processing. While the measure of structure–function relationship in the normal developing brain may be explored using functional brain imaging, it is not clear what to expect in the case of brain dysfunction or delayed maturation. In the case of developmental abnormalities, areas may consist of networks that behave like immature neurons; alternatively, abnormal development could result in poorly myelinated axons that would have poor conduction and be responsible for reduced spread of electrical activity. How these would differentially affect fMRI signal intensities is an area that requires further research.

B. Practical Considerations in Studying Children

Artifacts produced by head movement are among the most serious obstacles to successful collection of data in functional neuroimaging experiments. This problem is likely to be especially severe in fMRI studies of children. In general, due to the small task-related signal expected in fMRI experiments, a large number of scans needs to be carried out to achieve statistical significance. The exact number of repetitions depends on the efficacy of the stimulus in producing a neuronal response. These artifacts, a problem also with PET, are a greater problem in fMRI studies in which a smaller voxel size is likely to be used (Green, Seidel, Stein, Tedder, Kempner, Kertzman, et al., 1994). It is extremely important to have no head movement between scans to avoid head motion artifact. The ability to carry out naturalistic tasks with padding or other head restraint devices is quite difficult in the physically limiting environment of the MR scanner. Young children are not likely to be easily amenable to lying motionless in the confined environment of an MR scanner. Claustrophobic reactions are made more probable with the use of a whole-head coil. Foam padding is comfortable and may decrease some head motion, but more rigid stabilization mechanisms, such as a bite bar, are difficult to use with children. While some motion during the scan can be corrected by using available re-registration algorithms (Woods et al., 1992), children tend to be less disciplined about minimizing motion and the excitement of performing a "game" in the scanner will accentuate this difficulty. Particularly restless subjects, such as children with attention deficit/hyperactivity disorder (ADHD), are likely to be particularly problematic in this respect. However, new technical approaches are being developed to eliminate gross head motion. One promising approach utilizes head motion monitoring devices, the information from which may used to correct interscan head motion artifacts (Jezzard & Goldstein, 1994).

Movement of the entire head is not the only problem. The brain itself has intrinsic pulsation motion, which will contribute to the problem of motion artifact. These displacements are small, particularly at the cortical surface. Brain parenchyma motion has been found to be most prominent in the proximity of the foramen magnum in the caudal direction, and around the thalami in the lateral direction. The largest displacement measured is 0.5 mm (Poncelet, Wedeen, Weisskoff, & Cohen, 1992). Investigators with an interest in the thalami and surrounding areas will have to design analysis strategies to minimize the effects of this class of artifacts.

Monitoring task performance will be of key importance in many developmental studies, where task accuracy will be correlated with signal intensity changes to identify areas of task-related activity. Given the limited space around the subject in the MR scanner, it is often not possible to observe the subject as easily as it is in a PET scanner. This situation may be improved with monitoring devices that can function in high magnetic fields, but for now, control of task performance requires careful experimental design and proper preparation of the subject. Complex verbal or motor responses induce motion and therefore investigators have sometimes asked their subjects to respond with a simple button push or by "saying" words in their mind. A lack of a direct response can be to some extent compensated for by having a set of questions to be answered when the subject comes out of the scanner, which may be used to assess the subject's performance. Whatever the strategy used for the activation condition, there remains the problem of determining or controlling mental activity during the resting state condition. There is no direct way to assess what is going through the child's mind or if he or she is awake and attentive. Particularly for children, it may be advisable to dismiss the usual "rest" scan, in which the subject is fixating on a spot or keeping his or her eyes closed. Instead, an active control condition that requires compliance would be used, and this would differ from the other activation condition by the cognitive or perceptual component that is the object of study (for example, see Binder, Rao, Hammcke, Yetkin, Jesmanowicz, Bandettini, 1994).

Another practical obstacle arises from technical difficulties caused by small field inhomogeneities. These field inhomogeneities result from field gradients established at the boundaries of regions of the sample which have different magnetic susceptibility properties. Prominent examples of this are the air–tissue interface of the sinuses around the frontal lobes, and the bone–tissue interface around the petrous bone. A procedure known as "shimming" alleviates some of these problems. Also, methods are available to correct geometric distortion in echo-planar images at the data processing stage, using information gathered on field inhomogeneities at the time of scanning (Jezzard & Balaban, 1995). However, this is time consuming and can take varying lengths of time in different individuals. It may not resolve the problem entirely. Some areas of interest, such as the frontal lobes, are more difficult to image due to the proximity of air sinuses. This could be an obstacle for investigators interested in the study of psychiatric frontal lobe disorders (David, Blamire, & Breiter, 1994).

Most fMRI studies gather data on a small number of selected slices. Preliminary studies suggest different patterns in task-related activity related to language in children compared to adults, as the distribution of information processing appears to be more diffuse (Hertz–Pannier, Gaillard, Mott, Cuenod, Bookheimer, Weinstein, et al., 1994). If a task activates a greater spatial extent in a child's brain, there may be a need to gather data on larger brain volumes. This would increase scanning time and make the study more prone to head motion related artifacts.

Duration of a study depends on the type of protocol employed. In general, it is possible to complete a study in about one hour, which is a time period tolerated by most children. It is reasonable to carry out an fMRI experiment in this time, even if psychiatric disorders or phobias are present. Shorter scans have another obvious benefit, as they require less time and therefore cost less. Depending on the specifics of the experimental setup, large amounts of time may be consumed correcting for field inhomogeneities and the other sources of artifact discussed above.

Nevertheless, there are numerous reasons to pursue the possibility of utilizing fMRI to study development in children. There is opportunity for this technique to be applied much more widely than other neuroimaging techniques, since most MRI scanners in clinical use have the potential to be used for fMRI. Much has improved in fMRI data collection techniques. The rapid advances promise to overcome the types of problems described above. One of these advantages is that fMRI employing measurements of BOLD contrast is noninvasive; there are no concerns about radiation. Second, this method allows repeat studies for monitoring of cognitive development in the same child over days, weeks, or years. The magnetic field strengths used in fMRI pose no biological dangers (Balaban, 1992). Higher field strengths offer advantages (Turner et al., 1993) such as increased signal intensity, therefore affecting sensitivity and spatial resolution. On the other hand, certain artifacts are magnified at higher field strengths, such as geometric distortion. The potential advantages a high magnetic field may have to offer a developmental study could possibly be counterbalanced by other problems. Since high field magnets (e.g., 4 tesla) are relatively rare compared to 1.5 tesla magnets, which are found abundantly in clinical settings, the expectation is that the majority of studies in the near future may be performed on these instruments, perhaps using conventional imaging. While there have been reports of adverse effects when echoplanar imaging (EPI) is used in combination with very short gradient switching times (therefore creating very rapidly alternating magnetic fields), these effects are known and can be avoided in adults and children (Cohen, Weisskoff, Rzedzian, & Kantor, 1990).

C. Functional Imaging in Normal Development and Developmental Disorders

Wide availability of fMRI research facilities will allow more emphasis on the study of the neural processes associated with normal perceptual, cognitive, and motor development. The inclusion of healthy children has been very rare in neuroimaging studies for ethical reasons. (Some examples of studies with children and adolescents are Lou, Henriksen, & Bruhn, 1984, for xenon 133; and DeVolder, Bol, Michel, Congneau, & Goffinet, 1987; Zametkin, Liebenauer, Fitzgerald, King, Minkunas, Herscovitch, et al., 1993; Chugani et al., 1987, for PET using FDG.) Unfortunately, many of the children that have been included in PET studies come from populations that encompass a wide range of medical or developmental histories. Usually, these subjects are normal for the purpose of the question addressed in a study, but potential doubts introduced by the clinical problems may limit the interpretive generality of the results. For example, patients may be drawn from populations with complex partial seizures (CPS). Also, PET studies carried out in children so far have made use of FDG, the only apparent example of an H_2 ^{15}O in a youth with CPS, participating in a study assessing hemispheric dominance for language (Pardo & Fox, 1993). While the data from these FDG studies has been useful in studying metabolism in children and adolescents, they do not give measures of rCBF changes between different activation states. Measuring activation changes during functional brain mapping of different cognitive states in a short time duration is bound to be very popular for developmental studies.

Concern about the possible biological effects of tracer doses of radiation has made it difficult to justify the study of healthy children with PET. For this reason, much of what has been learned from neuroimaging studies concerning the spatial distribution of cognitive processes has come from adult experiments. The degree to which these results generalize to younger, developing populations is a matter of debate. FMRI now allows the observation of brain activity at the time when the disorder first presents itself. This may eventually allow early functional discrimination between individuals with developmental disorders and healthy controls. Studying children during the early course of a disease will eliminate the problem of retrospective diagnosis and the unknown effects of the developmental disorder on brain activation patterns over many years (Zametkin et al., 1993). Whether or not early identification and initiation of treatment of developmental disorders will be possible with imaging remains to be seen.

Normal development may be studied by precise mapping of maturational changes in brain activity. Experimental approaches to the study of human brain maturation using fMRI can make good use of information available from the study of anatomical, functional, and organizational changes observed in animal studies, as well as human postmortem data. Much is already known about the anatomical distribution of substrate utilization (glucose) during brain maturation in humans. It was discovered almost 40 years ago that cerebral blood flow in healthy children was about 1.8 times that of young adults (Kennedy & Sokoloff, 1957). Chugani and colleagues have shown how human cerebral glucose metabolism changes dramatically during the first decade of life (Chugani et al., 1987). Individual differences can be measured between cortical and subcortical structures in their glucose utilization, and these are reflected in the behavioral patterns thought to be associated with these structures. Glucose metabolic landscapes look similar at the age of 1 year to those of adults, but adult metabolic rates are not reached until about the second year. However, it is the next decade and a half that will be of interest, since glucose metabolism values appear to be double those of adults by the age of 3 to 4 years, remain at this level until approximately 9 years of age, and from there on steadily decline until the age of 18, to reach and maintain adult levels. These changes have been explained in terms of high energy demand during development associated with the excess production of neurons and synapses. As previously discussed, there appears to be regional variation in the rate of brain development. The exact timing of regional synaptogenesis or synapse elimination may play a crucial role in cortical reorganization or plasticity of different areas of the brain.

Along with the morphological changes observed during normal development using conventional MRI, functional information can now provide insight into structure–function correlations. Pfefferbaum and colleagues (Pfefferbaum et al., 1994) have demonstrated that cortical gray matter volume increases until the age of 4 years, after which a decrease is observed, while cortical white matter volume continues steady volumetric increase until the age of 20. It is possible that these changes in brain composition are reflected in activation changes measured by fMRI, as suggested by metabolic studies (Chugani et al., 1987).

fMRI has the ability to precisely integrate an individual's structural information with functional patterns, as both are acquired in the same experiment. Neuroimaging (CT and MRI) in populations with developmental disorders has shown that there are differences in cerebral morphology when compared to controls. In the developmental reading disorder dyslexia, for example, some of the brain structures identified to be morphologically different compared to normals (Hier, LeMay, Rosenberg, & Perlo, 1978; Hynd & Semrud-Clikeman, 1989; Hynd, Hall, Novey, Eliopulus, Black, Gonzalez, et al., 1995) are thought to reflect deviations from normal *in utero* development (Geschwind & Galaburda, 1985). Anomalies in the cortical morphology of the left temporoparietal and frontal regions seen with MRI (Hynd, Semrud–Clikeman, Lorys, Novey, & Eliopulos, 1990), and in postmortem studies (Galaburda, Sherman, Rosen, Aboitiz, & Geschwind, 1985), may be associated with the abnormal performance observed during phonological tasks, as PET studies in adults with dyslexia seem to suggest (Gross–Glenn, Duara, Barker, Loewenstein, Chang, Yoshii, et al., 1991; Rumsey, Andreason, Zametkin, Aquino, King, Hamburger, et al., 1992).

Unfortunately, not all morphometric findings have been consistent. First, there is great variation in the morphological data. It has been suggested (Galaburda et al., 1985) that there is a lack of the normal left-greater-than-right asymmetry of the planum temporale in dyslexics (about 75% of the normal population had L>R asymmetry in a postmortem study; Geschwind & Galaburda, 1987). The hypothesis is that the dyslexic brains are more symmetric due to an increased right temporal planum. Galaburda and colleagues (1985) have argued that, as seen in animal studies (Goldman–Rakic & Galkin, 1978), these observations may be the result of early lesions, affecting architectonic and connectional organization of immediate and distal areas in the brain. There are great inconsistencies in the human neuroimaging results, where some studies have been able to confirm this loss of asymmetry in dyslexics (Hier et al., 1978; Hynd & Semrud-Clikeman, 1989; Hynd et al., 1990; Larsen, Hoien, Lundberg, & Odegaard, 1990; Rosenberger & Hier, 1980; Rumsey, Dorwart, Vermess, Denkla, Kruesi, & Rapoport, 1986), but others have not (Haslam, Dalby, Johns, & Rademaker, 1981; Leonard, Voeller, Lombardino, Morris, Hynd, Alexander, et al., 1993; Levin & Pinker, 1991; Schultz, Cho, Staib, Kier, Fletcher, Shaywitz, et al., 1994). These studies are riddled with problems of definition criteria, handedness, age, and sex, all of which can change the outcome of morphometric analysis (Jancke, Schlaug, Huang, & Steinmetz, 1994; Schultz et al., 1994). There are variations in the method used to acquire and analyze the data as well as defining anatomical regions. Gender plays an important role. Anatomical and behavioral differences that have been observed between genders may well be reflected in the activation patterns studied in these groups. In fact, fMRI studies in adults have shown such differences in lateralization of a phonological task (Shaywitz, Shaywitz, Pugh, Constable, Skudlarski, Fulbright, et al., 1995).

The principal goal of many of these studies has been to link brain abnormalities to behavioral differences, and this has not been uniformly successful. For example, even if the findings for dyslexia were more consistent, since about 25% of the normal population have brains with symmetrical plana, loss of the asymmetry is not enough to cause dyslexia. This raises the question of whether or not any morphometric findings are truly causally related to dyslexia. Even in normal subjects without developmental disorders, it is not clear precisely how morphometric measures relate to language skills or language lateralization (for example, Jancke & Steinmetz, 1994). In the case of dyslexia, where in addition to their reading problems individuals demonstrate deficits in language abilities such as phonological awareness (Liberman, Shankweiler, Fischer, & Carter, 1974; Stanovich, 1988), there have been reports of non-language related behavioral differences. The specific nature of these deficits, for example slower visual temporal processing, abnormal eye movements, and other visually related deficits (Lovegrove, Martin, & Slaghuis, 1986; Lovegrove, Heddle, & Slaghuis, 1980; Eden, Stein, Wood, & Wood, 1994; Eden, Stein, Wood, & Wood, 1995) and their role in dyslexia will need to be clarified, in order to establish clear behavioral–functional relationships. The use of fMRI in the study of visual processing has provided evidence for differences in the regional functional organization of the cortical visual system in dyslexics (Eden, VanMeter, Rumsey, Maisog, Woods, & Zeffiro, in press).

Much of our knowledge about normal language development has been obtained by observation of patients with acquired focal lesions. It has been suggested that some developmental disorders result from a brain lesion early in life (Galaburda et al., 1985). The structural change resulting from an early lesion may be difficult or impossible to detect later in life. As such, it is not clear how well the principally affected area in dyslexia will be detected using neuroimaging techniques, in the same way that acquired lesions are. The data collected so far suggests a diffuse or symmetrical reduction of particular volumes of brain structures in developmental disorders. Focal lesions have not been seen. In addition, the early lesion may not be focal in the spatial sense, but may be focal in the functional sense, perhaps limited to a particular neurochemical system.

An *in utero* lesion, as has been speculated, might give rise to an unusual spatial distribution of neuronal processing associated with a particular cognitive or motor process. This difference in the spatial distribution of processing could well be detected in the population under study. The observation of such a functional abnormality may be complicated by the process of adaptive plasticity or the fact that children with developmental disorders may employ different strategies (therefore different neuronal circuits) to carry out a particular task compared to normals. Nevertheless, with fMRI, a change in the spatial distribution of brain processes or differences in signal change within a functional area associated with developmental disorders is an observation we are hopeful to make.

D. Examples of fMRI Studies in Children

Although there have been no developmental reports using fMRI, a number of fMRI studies have been performed studying children and will be briefly described here. Just as with conventional MRI, with fMRI children under sedation can be scanned easily and the information is valuable, particularly in disease. For example, fMRI has been used to monitor focal seizures in a 4-year-old boy (Jackson, Connelly, Cross, Gordon, & Gadian, 1994). Language and the cortical changes that occur as a child acquires complex linguistic abilities and written language is likely to be one of the most interesting areas to be studied with fMRI in development. Language lateralization has been successfully studied in healthy adults using fMRI (McCarthy et al., 1993; Cuenod et al., 1995; Rueckert, Appollonio, Grafman, Jezzard, Johnson, Le Bihan, et al., 1993). Similar studies are possible in children. Using a silent word generation task, Herz–Pannier and colleagues (Hertz–Pannier et al., 1994) have studied seven children with CPS (age range 9.1 to 17.5 years). The fMRI study, using EPI, demonstrated that language lateralization can be observed, thereby offering a suitable method for preoperative assessment. A number of areas of activation were observed (anterior frontal cortex and posterior inferior frontal gyri), all of which were included to determine language lateralization. This study has now been extended to include 11 children (L. Hertz-Pannier, personal communication February, 1995), and Wada testing was carried out in 6 of these, confirming language lateralization as assessed with fMRI. These results establish the feasibility of using fMRI to determine language localization in children. All children complied with the task and remained in the magnet for 75 minutes. However, 4 of the children were scanned a second time, since motion artifact resulted in invalid data the first time. Nevertheless, even if it requires several scans, this form of noninvasive, low risk assessment is an advance in the field of epilepsy surgical planning. An additional finding in this study was the observation of a more diffuse activation pattern than that seen in adults (Hertz-Pannier et al., 1994). This finding is in concordance with observations on regional maturation patterns (Huttenlocher & de Courten, 1987) and metabolic imaging studies (Chugani et al., 1987) in the developing brain, which are thought to be a reflection of ongoing maturation.

FMRI has been used to examine changes in the spatial distribution of neuronal processing following focal injury. Cao and colleagues (Cao, Vikingstad, Huttenlocher, & Towle, 1994) have used fMRI to demonstrate changes of the functional organization in the developing brain. Functional maps in adolescents and young adults with unilateral neonatal brain injury showed how sensorimotor cortex contralateral to the lesion had undergone reorganization. The patients in this study had unilateral brain damage since birth and were asked to perform a simple motor task. For example, in one subject during finger opposition of the nonparetic hand, contralateral activation was demonstrated in the intact hemisphere, as seen in normal subjects. However, movement of the paretic hand activated the ipsilateral as well as the contralateral hemisphere. Activation (measured in volumes of activated brain tissue) was seen around the area of the lesion on the contralateral hemisphere, and in the non-Rolandic zone (mainly posterior to the central sulcus) in the intact, ipsilateral hemisphere. This study with fMRI in adolescents and young adults has demonstrated the same type of functional reorganization as previously seen with PET (Weiller, Chollet, Friston, Wise, & Frackowiak, 1992), and is in agreement with patterns of reorganization seen in animal lesion studies (Huttenlocher & Raichelson, 1989). It is therefore possible to demonstrate and characterize plasticity of the developing brain using fMRI, even in children. The amount of plasticity and resulting reorganization depends on the type of lesion that has occurred, the site of the lesion, and at what age the lesion occurred, with earlier damage in life predicting better functional reorganization.

In summary, there have been few studies utilizing fMRI in children, but there are current efforts underway and their results are awaited eagerly. The findings from these studies predict successful mapping of functional organization or reorganization in the developing brain. Their small number is a reflection of the novelty of this technique, difficulties validating this method, and the problems that are still being worked out even for studies involving healthy adults.

IV. Conclusions and Implications for the Study of Brain Development

With the recent advances in noninvasive imaging with fMRI it is tempting to apply this technique to unexplored areas, such as noninvasive monitoring of brain development. While the future looks promising, there are still a number of practical problems that need to be addressed. One of the arguments for not choosing fMRI may be the fact that there is still much about this technique that is not fully understood. There are a number of factors that can affect the MR signal (e.g., oxygen extraction rate, blood velocity, and hematocrit), and the exact relationship between the rate of $T2^*$ relaxation rate and CBF is not yet clarified. This relationship is also affected by field strength, diffusion distance, and pulse sequences. Less is known about the effect of decreased CBF on fMRI signal. The use of MRI for the acquisition of functional information in humans is a novel development and requires further validation and improvement, in order to understand the signal physiology obtained with this technique.

As this technique is further developed and improved, it should be possible to establish correlations between the neurobehavioral findings observed during development with normal anatomy, as well as in developmental disorders, with their hypothesized alterations in brain morphology findings. This will guide the identification of brain regions as potential candidates for functional neuroimaging studies. Advances in reliable morphometry, mapping of physiologic phenomena in normals, and linking these findings to architectonic localization may bring us closer to diagnosis and treatment of developmental disorders. In this way, neuroimaging could constitute a significant part of the large body of research examining the etiology and treatment of developmental disorders.

Acknowledgments

The authors thank Peter Herscovitch, John vanMeter, Peter Jezzard, and Joe Maisog for their contributions to the work presented here and Lucie Pannier for valuable discussions. We are grateful to the *in vivo* NMR Center for the use of the NMR facilities. Thanks to Michelle Williams for her kind assistance in acquiring the MRI data. Also, we would like to express our appreciation to the staff at the NIH cyclotron facility.

References

Balaban, R. (1992). Magnetic resonance imaging and spectroscopy at high magnetic fields *in vivo*. NHLBI Conference, NIH.

Bandettini, P. A. (1993). MRI studies of brain activation: temporal characteristics. *Functional MRI of the brain* (pp. 143–151). Berkley, CA: Society of Magnetic Resonance in Medicine.

Bandettini, P. A., Wong, E. C., Hinks, R. S., Tikofsky, R. S., & Hyde, J. S. (1992). Time course EPI of human brain function during task activation. *Magnetic Resonance in Medicine, 25,* 390–397.

Belliveau, J. W., Kennedy, D. N., McKinstry, R. C., Buchbinder, B., Weisskoff, R. M., Cohen, M. S., Vevea, J. M., Brady, T. J., & Rosen, B. R. (1991). Functional mapping of the human visual cortex by magnetic resonance imaging. *Science, 254,* 716–710.

Belliveau, J. W., Kwong, K. K., Kennedy, D. N., Baker, J. R., Stern, C. E., Benson, R., Chesler, D. A., Weisskoff, R. M., Cohen, M. S., Tootell, R. B. H., Fox, P. T., Brady, T. J., & Rosen, B. R. (1992). Magnetic resonance imaging mapping of brain function: Human visual cortex. *Investigative Radiology, 27,* S59–S65.

Binder, R. J., Rao, S. M., Hammeke, T. A., Yetkin, F. Z., Jesmanowicz, A., Bandettini, P. A., Wong, E. C., Estkowski, L. D., Goldstein, M. D., Haughton, V. M., & Hyde, J. S. (1994). Functional magnetic resonance imaging of the human auditory cortex, *Annals of Neurology, 35* (6), 662–672.

Blamire, A. M., McCarthy, G., Gruetter, R., Rottman, D. L., Rattner, Z., Hyder, F., & Shulman, R. G. (1992). Echo planar imaging of the left inferior frontal lobe during word generation. *Proceedings of the Eleventh Annual Meeting of the Society of Magnetic Resonance in Medicine,* 1834.

Cao, Y., Vikingstad, E. M., Huttenlocher, P. R., & Towle, V. L. (1994). Functional magnetic resonance studies of the reorganization of the human hand sensory motor area after unilateral brain injury in the perinatal period. *Proceedings of the National Academy of Sciences, USA, 91,* 9612–9616.

Changeux, J.-P., & Danchin, A. (1976). Selective stabilization of developing synapses as a mechanism for the specification of neural networks. *Nature (London) 264,* 705–712.

Cherry, S. R., Dahlbom, M., & Hoffman, E. J. (1992). Evaluation of a 3-D reconstruction algorithm for multi-slice PET scanners. *Physics, Medicine and Biology, 37,* 779–790.

Chugani, H. T., Phelps, M. E., & Mazziotta, J. C. (1987). Positron emission tomography study of human brain functional development. *Annals of Neurology, 22,* 487–497.

Cohen, J. D., Forman, S. D., Braver, T. S., Casey, B. J., Servant-Schreiber, D., & Noll, D. C. (1994). Activation of the prefrontal cortex in nonspatial working memory task with functional MRI. *Human Brain Mapping, 1,* 293–304.

Cohen, M. S., & Weisskoff, R. M. (1991). Ultra-fast imaging. *Magnetic Resonance Imaging, 9,* 1–37.

Cohen, M., Weisskoff, R., Rzedzian, R., & Kantor, H. (1990). Sensory stimulation by time-varying magnetic fields. *Magnetic Resonance in Medicine, 14,* 409–414.

Colebatch, J., Deiber, M.-P., Passingham, R., Friston, K., & Frackowiak, R. (1991). Regional cerebral blood flow during voluntary arm and hand movements in human subjects. *Journal of Neurophysiology, 65*(6), 1392–1401.

Conel, J. L. (1939–1963). *The postnatal development of the human cerebral cortex.* Cambridge, MA: Harvard Univ. Press.

Connelly, A., Jackson, G. D., Frackowiak, R. S. J., Belliveau, J. W., Vargha-Khadem, F., & Gadian, D. G. (1993). Functional mapping of activated human primary cortex with a clinical MR imaging system. *Radiology, 188,* 125–130.

Corbetta, M., Miezin, F., Dobmeyer, S., Shulman, G., & Petersen, S. (1990). Attentional modulation of neural processing of shape, color and velocity in humans. *Science, 248,* 1556–1559.

Cuenod, C. A., Bookheimer, S. Y., Hertz-Pannier, L., Zeffiro, T. A., Theodore, W., & Le Bihan, D. (1995). FMRI during a word generation game using conventional equipment: A potential tool for language localization in the clinical environment. *Neurology, 45*(10), 1821–1827.

David, A., Blamire, A., & Breiter, H. (1994). Functional magnetic resonance imaging. *British Journal of Psychology, 164,* 2–7.

DeVolder, A., Bol, A., Michel, C., Congneau, M., & Goffinet, A. M. (1987). Brain glucose metabolism in children with the autistic syndrome: Positron tomography analysis. *Brain Development, 9,* 581–587.

Eden, G. F., Maisog, J. M., Jezzard, P., VanMeter, J. W., Herscovitch, P., Giedd, J., Rapoport, J. L., & Zeffiro, T. A. (1994). A comparison of PET and MRFN in the neuroanatomical localization of visual processing. *Proceedings of the Second Annual Meeting of the Society of Magnetic Resonance, 2,* 691.

Eden, G. F., VanMeter, J. W., Maisog, J. M., Jezzard, P., Herscovitch, P., Rapoport, J. L., & Zeffiro, T. A. (1995). A comparison of PET and MRFN techniques using a visual stimulus. *Human Brain Mapping,* S39.

Eden, G. F., Stein, J. F., Wood, H. M., & Wood, F. B. (1994). Differences in eye movements and reading problems in dyslexic and normal children. *Vision Research, 34*(10), 1345–1358.

Eden, G. F., Stein, J. F., Wood, H. M., & Wood, F. B. (1995). Verbal and visual problems in reading disabled and normal children. *Journal of Learning Disabilities, 28*(5), 272–290.

Eden, G. F., VanMeter, J. W., Rumsey, J. M., Maisog, J. M., Woods, R. P., & Zeffiro, T. A. (1996). Functional MRI differences in visual motion processing in dyslexia. *Nature,* in press.

Fox, P. T., & Mintun, M. A. (1989). Noninvasive functional brain mapping by change-distribution analysis of averaged PET images of $H^{2\ 15}O$ tissue activity. *Journal of Nuclear Medicine, 30,* 141–149.

Fox, P. T., & Raichle, M. E. (1985). Stimulus rate determines regional brain blood flow in striate cortex. *Annals of Neurology, 17,* 303–305.

Frahm, J., Bruhn, H., Merbold, T. K.-D., & Hanicke, W. (1992). Dynamic MRI of human brain oxygenation during rest and photic stimulation. *Magnetic Resonance Imaging, 2,* 501–505.

Friston, K. J., Frith, C., D., Liddle, P. F., & Frackowiak, R. S. J. (1991). Comparing functional (PET) images: The assessment of significant change. *Journal of Cerebral Blood Flow Metabolism, 11,* 690–699.

Friston, K. J., Jezzard, P., & Turner, R. (1994). Analysis of functional MRI time-series. *Human Brain Mapping, 1,* 153–171.

Galaburda, A. M., Sherman, G., Rosen, G. D., Aboitiz, F., & Geschwind, N. (1985). Developmental dyslexia: Four consecutive cases with cortical anomalies. *Annals of Neurology, 18,* 222–233.

Geschwind, N., & Galaburda, A. M. (1985). Cerebral lateralization biological mechanisms, associations, and pathology: A hypothesis and program for research. *Archives of Neurology, 42,* 428–459.

Geschwind, N., & Galaburda, A. (1987). Ultimate origins of asymmetry. *Cerebral Lateralization biological mechanisms, associations, and pathology* (pp. 223–239). Cambridge, MA: Bradford.

Goldman-Rakic, P. S., & Galkin, T. W. (1978). Prenatal removal of frontal association cortex in the fetal rhesus monkey: Anatomical and functional consequences in the postnatal life. *Brain Research, 152,* 451–485.

Green, M. V., Seidel, J., Stein, S. D., Tedder, T. E., Kempner, K. M., Kertzman, C., & Zeffiro, T. A. (1994). Head movement in normal subjects during simulated PET brain imaging with and without head restraint. *Journal of Nuclear Medicine, 35*(9), 1538–1546.

Gross-Glenn, K., Duara, R., Barker, W. W., Loewenstein, D., Chang, J.-Y., Yoshii, F., Apicella, A. M., Pascal, S., Boothe, T., Sevush, S., Jallad, B. J., Novoa, L., & Lubs, H. (1991). Positron emission tomographic studies during serial word-reading by normal and dyslexic adults. *Journal of Clinical and Experimental Neuropsychology, 13*(4), 531–544.

in functional imaging of the brain. *Magnetic Resonance in Medicine, 31,* 283–291.

Haslam, R., Dalby, J., Johns, R., & Rademaker, A. (1981). Cerebral asymmetry in developmental dyslexia. *Archives of Neurology, 38,* 679–682.

Herscovitch, P. (1994). Radiotracer techniques for functional neuroimaging with positron emission tomography. In R. W. Thatcher, M. Hallett, T. Zeffiro, E. Roy John, & M. Huerta (Eds.), *Functional neuroimaging: Technical foundations* (pp. 29–46). San Diego: Academic Press.

Hertz-Pannier, L., Gaillard, W. D., Mott, S., Cuenod, C. A., Bookheimer, S. Y., Weinstein, S., Conry, J., Theodore, W., & Le Bihan, D. (1994). Pre-operative assessment of language by FMRI in children with complex partial seizures: Preliminary study. *Proceedings of the Second Annual Meeting of the Society of Magnetic Resonance, 1,* 326.

Hier, D. B., LeMay, M., Rosenberg, P. B., & Perlo, V. B. (1978). Developmental dyslexia: Evidence for a subgroup with reversal of cerebral asymmetry. *Archives of Neurology, 35,* 90–92.

Hoffman, J., Guze, B., Baxter, L., Mazziotta, J., & Phelps, M. (1989). [18F]-fluorodeoxyglucose (FDG) and positron emission tomography (PET) in aging and dementia. *European Neurology, 29(3),* 16–24.

Holland, B. A., Haas, D. K., Norman, D., Brant-Zawadzki, M., & Newton, T. H. (1986). MRI of normal brain maturation. *American Journal of Neuroradiology, 7,* 201–208.

Holmes, G. L. (1986). Morphological and physiological maturation of the brain in the neonate and young child. *Journal of Clinical Neurophysiology, 3(3),* 209–238.

Huttenlocher, P. R., & de Courten, C. (1987). The development of synapses in striate cortex in man. *Human Neurobiology, 6(1),* 1–9.

Huttenlocher, P. R., & Raichelson, R. (1989). Effects of neonatal hemispherectomy on location and number of corticospinal neurons in the rat. *Developmental Brain Research, 47,* 59–69.

Hynd, G. W., Hall, J., Novey, E. S., Eliopulus, D., Black, K., Gonzalez, J. J., Edmonds, J. E., Riccio, C., & Cohen, M. (1995). Dyslexia and corpus callosum morphology. *Archives of Neurology, 52,* 32–38.

Hynd, G., & Semrud-Clikeman, M. (1989). Dyslexia and brain morphology. *Psychological Bulletin, 106(3),* 447–482.

Hynd, G., Semrud-Clikeman, M., Lorys, A., Novey, E., & Eliopulos, D. (1990). Brain morphology in developmental dyslexia and attention deficit disorder/hyperactivity. *Archives of Neurology, 47,* 919–926.

Jackson, G. G., Connelly, A., Cross, J. H., Gordon, I., & Gadian, D. G. (1994). Functional Magnetic resonance imaging in focal seizures. *Neurology, 44,* 850–856.

Jancke, L., Schlaug, G., Huang, Y., & Steinmetz, H. (1994). Asymmetry of the planum temporale. *Neuroreport, 5(9),* 1161–3.

Jancke, L., & Steinmetz, H. (1994). Auditory lateralization and planum temporale asymmetry. *Neuroreport, 5(2),* 169–72.

Jernigan, T., & Tallal, P. A. (1990). Late childhood changes in brain morphology observable with MRI. *Developmental Medicine and Child Neurology, 32,* 379–385.

Jernigan, T., Trauner, D. A., Hesselink, J. R., & Tallal, P. A. (1991). Maturation of human cerebrum observed *in vivo* during adolescence. *Brain, 114,* 2037–2049.

Jezzard, P., & Balaban, R. S. (1995). Correction for geometric distortion in echo planar images from B0 field variations. *Magnetic Resonance in Medicine, 34(1),* 65–73.

Jezzard, P., & Goldstein, S. R. (1994). A head position monitoring device for use in functional MRI studies. *Proceedings of the Second Annual Meeting of the Society of Magnetic Resonance, 2,* 684.

Jonides, J., Smith, E., Koeppe, R., Awh, E., Minoshima, S., & Mintun, M. (1993). Spatial working memory in humans revealed by PET. *Nature (London), 363,* 623–625.

Kennedy, C., & Sokoloff, L. (1957). An adaptation of the nitrous oxide method for the study of cerebral circulation in children; normal values for cerebral blood flow and cerebral metabolic rate in childhood. *Journal of Clinical Investigation, 36,* 1130–1137.

Kwong, K. K., Belliveau, J. W., Chesler, D. A., Goldberg, I. E., Weisskoff, R. M., Poncelet, B. P., Kennedy, D. N., Hoppel, B. E., Cohen, M. S., Turner, R., Cheng, H.-M., Brady, T. J., & Rosen, B. R. (1992). Dynamic magnetic resonance imaging of human brain activity during primary sensory stimulation. *Proceedings of the National Academy of Sciences, USA, 80,* 5675–5679.

Larsen, J., Hoien, T., Lundberg, I., & Odegaard, H. (1990). MRI evaluation of the size and symmetry of the planum temporale in adolescents with developmental dyslexia. *Brain and Language, 39,* 289–301.

Leonard, C. M., Voeller, K. K. S., Lombardino, L. J., Morris, M. K., Hynd, G. W., Alexander, A. W., Andersen, H. G., Garofalakis, M., Honeyman, J. C., Mao, J., Agee, O. F. & Staab, E. V. (1993). Anomalous cerebral structure in dyslexia revealed with MRI. *Archives of Neurology, 50(5),* 461–569.

Levin, B., & Pinker, S. (1991). Introduction to special issue of *Cognition* on lexical and conceptual semantics. *Cognition, 41,* 1–7.

Liberman, I. Y., Shankweiler, D., Fischer, F. W., & Carter, B. (1974). Explicit syllable and phoneme segmentation in the young child. *Journal of Experimental Child Psychology, 18,* 201–212.

Lou, H. C., Henriksen, L., & Bruhn, P. (1984). Focal cerebral hypoperfusion in children with dysphasia and/or attention deficit disorder. *Archives of Neurology, 41,* 825–829.

Lovegrove, W. J., Heddle, M., & Slaghuis, W. (1980). Reading disability: Spatial frequency specific deficits in visual information store. *Neuropsychologia, 18,* 111–115.

Lovegrove, W. J., Martin, F., & Slaghuis, W. (1986). A theoretical and experimental case for visual deficit in specific reading difficulty. *Cognitive Neuropsychology, 3,* 225–267.

Mansfield, P. (1977). Multi-planar image formation using NMR spin echoes. *Journal of Physics C, 10,* L55–L58.

Mazziotta, J. C., Phelps, M. E., Pahl, J. J., Huang, S.-C., Baxter, L. R., Riege, W. H., Hoffman, J. M., Kuhl, D. E., Lanto, A. B., Wapenski, J. A., & Markham, C. H. (1987). Reduced cerebral glucose metabolism in asymptomatic subjects at risk for Huntington's disease. *New England Journal of Medicine, 316(7),* 357–362.

Mazziotta, J. C., Phelps, M. E., Plummer, D., & Kuhl, D. E. (1981). Quantititation in positron computed tomography. 5. Physical-anatomical effects. *Journal of Computer Assisted Tomography, 5,* 734–743.

McArdle, C. B., Richardson, C. J., Nicholas, D. A., Mirfakhraee, M., Hayden, C. K., & Amparo, E. G. (1987). Developmental features of the neonatal brain: MRI imaging: Part I. Gray–white matter differentiation and myelination. *Radiology, 162,* 230–234.

McCarthy, G., Blamire, A., Rothman, D., Gruetter, R., & Shulman, R. (1993). Echoplanar magnetic resonance imaging studies of frontal cortex activation during word generation in humans. *Proceedings of the National Academy of Sciences, U.S.A., 90,* 4952–4956.

Ogawa, S., Lee, T. M., Nayak, A. S., & Glynn, P. (1990). Oxygenation-sensitive contrast in magnetic resonance image of rodent brain at high magnetic fields. *Magnetic Resonance in Medicine, 14,* 68–78.

Ogawa, S., Tank, D. W., Menon, R., Ellermann, J. M., Kim, S.-G., Merkle, H., & Urgubil, K. (1992). Intrinsic signal changes accompanying sensory stimulation: Functional brain mapping using MRI. *Proceedings of the National Academy of Sciences, U.S.A., 89,* 5951–5955.

O'Kusky, J., & Colonnier, M. (1982). Postnatal changes in the number of neurons and synapses in the visual cortex (A17) of the macaque monkey. *Journal of Comparative Neurology, 210,* 291–306.

O'Kusky, J., & Colonnier, M. (1982). Postnatal changes in the number of neurons and synapses in the visual cortex (A17) of the macaque monkey. *Journal of Comparative Neurology, 210,* 291–306.

Pardo, J. V., & Fox, P. T. (1993). Preoperative assessment of the cerebral hemispheric dominance for language with PET. *Human Brain Mapping, 1,* 57–68.

Pardo, J. V., Fox, P. T., & Raichle, M. E. (1991). Localization of human system of sustained attention by positron emission tomography. *Nature (London), 349,* 61–64.

Petersen, S. E., Fox, P. T., Posner, M. I., Mintun, M., & Raichle, M. E. (1988). Positron emission tomographic studies of the cortical anatomy of single word processing. *Nature (London) 331,* 385–389.

Pfefferbaum, A., Mathalon, D. H., Sullivan, E. V., Rawles, J. M., Zipursky, R. B., & Lim, K. O. (1994). Aquantative magnetic resonance imaging study of changes in brain morphology from infancy to late adulthood. *Archives of Neurology, 51,* 874–887.

Phelps, M., & Mazziotta, J. (1985). Positron emission tomography: Human brain function and chemistry. *Science, 228,* 799–809.

Poncelet, B. P., Wedeen, V. J., Weisskoff, R. M., & Cohen, M. S. (1992). Brain parenchyma motion: Measurement with cine-echo-planar MR imaging. *Radiology, 185*(3), 645–51.

Price, C., Wise, R., Ramsay, S., Friston, K., Howard, D., Patterson, K., & Frackowiak, R. (1992). Regional response differences within the human auditory cortex when listening to words. *Neuroscience Letters, 146,* 179–182.

Rakic, P., Bourgeois, J.-P., Eckenhoff, M. F., Zecevic, N., & Goldman-Rakic, P. S. (1986). Concurrent overproduction of synapses in diverse regions of primate cerebral cortex. *Science, 232,* 232–234.

Reinis, S., & Goldman, J. (1980). *The development of the brain.* Springfield, IL: Thomas.

Rosenberger, P., & Hier, D. (1980). Cerebral asymmetry and verbal intellectual deficits. *Annals of Neurology, 8,* 300–304.

Roy, C. S., & Sherrington, C. S. (1890). On the regulation of the blood-supply of the brain. *Journal of Physiology, 11,* 85–108.

Rueckert, L., Appollonio, I., Grafman, J., Jezzard, P., Johnson, R., Le Bihan, D., & Turner, R. (1993). MRI functional activation of left frontal cortex during covert word production. *Journal of Neuroimaging, 4,* 67–70.

Rumsey, J., Andreason, P., Zametkin, A., Aquino, T., King, A., Hamburger, S., Pikus, A., Rapoport, J., & Cohen, R. (1992). Failure to activate the left temporoparietal cortex in dyslexia. *Archives of Neurology, 49*(5), 527–534.

Rumsey, J., Dorwart, R., Vermess, R., Denkla, M. B., Kruesi, M. J. P., & Rapoport, J. (1986). Magnetic resonance imaging of brain anatomy in severe developmental dyslexia. *Archives of Neurology, 43,* 1045–1046.

Sadato, S., Zeffiro, T., Campbell, G., Konishi, J., Shibasaki, H., & Hallett, M. (1995). Regional cerebral blood flow changes in motor control areas after transient anesthesia of the forearm. *Annals of Neurology, 37,* 74–81.

Schultz, R. T., Cho, N. K., Staib, L. H., Kier, L. E., Fletcher, J. M., Shaywitz, S. E., Shankweiler, D. P., Katz, L., Gore, J. C., Duncan, J. S., & Shaywitz, B. A. (1994). Brain morphology in normal and dyslexic children: the influence of sex and age. *Annals of Neurology, 35,* 732–742.

Shaywitz, B. A., Shaywitz, S. E., Pugh, K. R., Constable, R. T., Skudlarski, P., Fulbright, R. K., Bronen, R. A., Fletcher, J. M., & Shankweiler, D. P. (1995). Sex differences in the functional organization of the brain for language. *Nature (London), 373,* 607–609.

Sokoloff, L. (1981). Relationships amongst local functional activity, energy metabolism and blood flow in the central nervous system. *Federation Proceedings, 40,* 2311–2316.

Stanovich, K. E. (1988). Explaining the differences between the dyslexic and the garden-variety poor reader: The phonological-core variable-difference model. *Journal of Learning Disabilities, 21,* 590–612.

Thulborn, K. R., Waterton, J. C., Matthews, P. M., & Radda, G. K. (1982). Oxygenation dependence of the transverse relaxation time of water protons in whole blood at high field. *Biochimica et Biophysica Acta, 714,* 265–270.

Turner, R., Jezzard, P., Wen, H., Kwong, K. K., Le Bihan, D., Zeffiro, T., & Balaban, R. S. (1993). Functional mapping of the human visual cortex at 4 and 1.5 Tesla using deoxygenated contrast EPI. *Magnetic Resonance in Medicine, 29,* 281–283.

Turner, R., Le Bihan, D., Moonen, C. T. W., & Frank, J. (1991). Echoplanar imaging of deoxygenation episodes in cat brain at 2T. *Journal of Magnetic Resonance Imaging, 1*(2), 227.

van Gelderen, P., Ramsey, N., Liu, G., Duyn, J., Frank, J., Weinberger, D. R., & Moonen, C. T. (1995). Three dimensional functional MRI of human brain on a clinical 1.5T scanner. *Proceedings of the National Academy of Sciences, USA, 92*(15), 6906–6910.

Watson, J. D. G., Myers, R., Frackowiak, R. S. J. Hajnal, J. V., Woods, R. P., Mazziotta, J. C., Shipp, S., & Zeki, S. (1993). Area V5 of the human brain: Evidence from a combined study using positron emission tomography and magnetic resonance imaging. *Cerebral Cortex, 3,* 79–94.

Weiller, C., Chollet, F., Friston, K., Wise, R., & Frackowiak, R. (1992). Functional reorganization of the brain in recovery from striatocapsular infarction in man. *Annals of Neurology, 31*(5), 463–72.

Wise, R., Chollet, F., Hadar, U., Friston, K., Hoffner, E., & Frackowiak, R. S. J. (1991). Distribution of cortical neural networks involved in word comprehension and word retrieval. *Brain, 114,* 1803–1817.

Woods, R. P., Cherry, S. R., & Mazziotta, J. C. (1992). Rapid automated algorithm for aligning and reslicing PET images. *Journal of Computer Assisted Tomography, 16,* 620–633.

Yakovlev, P., & Lecours, A. (1967). The myelogenetic cycles of regional maturation of the brain. In A. Minkowski (Ed.), *Regional development of the brain in early life* (pp. 3–70). Philadelphia, PA: Davis.

Zametkin, A. J., Liebenauer, L. L., Fitzgerald, G. A., King, A. C., Minkunas, D. V., Herscovitch, P., Yamada, E. M., & Cohen, R. M. (1993). Brain metabolism in teenager with attention-deficit hyperactivity disorder. *Archives of General Psychiatry, 50,* 333–340.

Zeki, S., Watson, J. D. G., Lueck, C. F., Friston, K. J., Kennard, C., & Frackowiak, R. S. J. (1991). A direct demonstration of functional specialization in human visual cortex. *Journal of Neuroscience, 11*(3), 641–649.

7

Neuroimaging of Cyclic Cortical Reorganization during Human Development

Robert W. Thatcher

*Medical Research Services, VA Medical Center, Bay Pines, Florida 33504; and Departments of Neurology and
Radiology, University of South Florida College of Medicine, Tampa, Florida 33612*

I. Introduction

A. Functional Organization of the Human Cortex

A new view of the functional organization of the cerebral cortex is emerging from the spatial integration of electrophysiological and magnetoencephalographic studies. Whereas earlier studies tended to emphasize the functions of individual neurons in isolated cortical regions, current views of the functional organization of the cortex are focusing on the spatio-temporal dynamics of distributed network processing in which the allocation of resources occurs through the self-organization of coherent regions of neural activity (Gray, Konig, Engel, & Singer, 1989; Eckhorn, Bauer, Jordan, Brosch, Kruse, Munk, et al., 1988; Murthy & Fetz, 1992; Singer, 1995; Toro, Wang, Zeffiro, Thatcher, & Hallett, 1994; Thatcher, Toro, Pflieger, & Hallett, 1994c). Recent studies have indicated that the rules that govern the self-organizational properties of the cortex involve traveling waves of coherent neural activity. For example, Linas and Ribary (1992) have shown a cyclic rostral–caudal traveling wave of coherent 40Hz activity which is in continuous motion in the human cerebral cortex. Other examples of traveling waves of coherent neural activity have been noted in a wide number of studies (Lilly and Cherry, 1954, 1955; Gorbach, Tsicalov, Kuznetsova, Shevelev, Budko, & Sharaev, 1989; Verzeano and Negishi, 1960; 1961;

Nunez, 1981; Thatcher and John, 1977). One of the notable aspects of these studies are that the electromagnetic traveling waves behave in an orderly fashion and exhibit specific spatial directions and velocities. The most commonly observed spatial directions are along the lateral-to-medial and the rostral-to-caudal anatomical axes of the cerebral cortex.

B. Spatial Coordinates for Developmental Neuroimaging

Recent embryological and developmental studies suggest a common anatomical dynamic that organizes coherent neural activity in the lateral-to-medial and rostral-to-caudal planes. These data suggest a spatial temporal nesting of spiral processes which may constitute a generalized recapitulation of a lateral-to-medial anatomical rotation that operates in human evolution, ontogenesis, and learning. For example, the evolution of the lateral cortical system predates the evolution of the medial cortical system by several million years (Lohman and Smeets, 1990; Shimizu and Karten, 1990). A similar spatial–temporal sequence, involving a three-dimensional spiral of growth, was observed during mouse (Smart, 1983) and rat (Bayer and Altman, 1991) prenatal neurogenesis. Medio-lateral and anterior–posterior spatial gradients have also been observed during human postnatal cortical development (Thatcher, 1992b, 1994a, 1994b). In the latter studies, a wave-like growth began in the rostral–

lateral cortical regions and spread to the caudal–medial systems. Finally, magnetoencephalographic studies have demonstrated a spiral spatial movement of dipole generators of the P300 electrocortical potential during the performance of cognitive tasks (Rogers, Baumann, Papanicolaou, Bourbon, Alagarsamy, & Eisenberg, 1991). The successively activated P300 dipole sources followed an orderly course from deep thalamic structures to the outer lateral cortical regions at a velocity of approximately 1 mm every 5 msec (or 1 cm every 50 msec). The Rogers et al. (1991) findings of a millisecond range spiraling sequence of dipoles involved in learning and memory also follows a lateral–medial anatomical path, which may recapitulate similar anatomical paths followed in ontogeny and phylogeny.

The purpose of the present chapter is to focus attention on some of the spatio-temporal dynamics that may be operative during postnatal human cerebral development and, thus, lend themselves to quantitative neuroimaging analysis. Special emphasis will be placed on computerized electroencephalogram (EEG) analyses obtained from the scalp of children ranging in age from birth to 16 years. These analyses have revealed spatio-temporal patterns of EEG coherence that are present throughout the postnatal period, and reflect specific spatial gradients in which a cyclic lateral–medial and rostral–caudal reorganization process was observed.

II. Lifespan Human Cortical Development Using EEG Coherence

Nineteen channel analyses of the development of EEG coherence were conducted on a subset of 577 normal children ranging in age from 2 months to 26.4 years (Thatcher, Walker, & Giudice, 1987). The children had a mean full scale I.Q. of 106.4, and they had no history of neurological disorders or abnormalities in the prenatal, perinatal, and postnatal developmental period. There were many examples of rapid and significant increments in EEG coherence which could be characterized as "growth spurts." In previous studies (Thatcher et al., 1987), 2- to 4-year oscillations in the lifespan development of EEG coherence were commonly evident using 1-year means. In order to increase the frequency resolution of the rhythms of coherence, sliding averages were computed using 1-year epochs and .25-year increments, from a mean of .513 years to a mean of 15.98 years of age (Thatcher, 1991). This provided a total of 64 means, or four means per year in a limited sample of children (i.e., $N = 436$). This limited sample of 436 subjects was selected be-

cause of an adequately large sample size (Ns ranged from 15 to 53 per group) at each age period, and the stability of the data set (e.g., relatively equal variances and constant coefficients of variation across age), (Thatcher et al., 1987; Thatcher, 1991). The demographics of the data were 242 males, 174 females, and handedness of children over the age of 3 (i.e., when handedness could be measured) was approximately 88% right handed, 9% left handed, and 3% ambidextrous. Varimax factor analyses of the 64 point sliding average time series of EEG coherence from all intrahemispheric interelectrode combinations revealed that from 9 to 11 factors accounted for at least 90% of the variance within each frequency band (i.e., delta, theta, alpha, and beta). Furthermore, the factors for the different frequency bands were consistently periodic and showed consistent anatomical patterns (Thatcher, 1991).[1]

A. Growth Spurts as Periods of "In-Phase" Activity

Growth spurts were defined by peaks of velocity or those postnatal ages where there was a maximum increase in mean coherence as measured by the first derivative. The point of maximum increase in EEG coherence (i.e., peak velocity) was considered to reflect either an increase in the number and/or strength of connections between two or more intracortical systems. The criterion for defining a peak in velocity as a growth spurt was that only "in-phase" EEG coherence trajectories that loaded >0.80 on a factor were evaluated. The criteria of "in-phase" developmental trajectories was generally satisfied by a significant loading on a given factor (Thatcher, 1991). That is, each factor represented the commonality between developmental trajectories of EEG coherence and therefore, by definition, reflected "in-phase" activity. In-phase trajectories were considered important since they reflect shared activity between specific intracortical connection systems and not localized or spurious changes, and, the first derivative must exhibit a positive peak. The velocity, or first derivative, was selected rather than the

---

[1]Replicated and stable factor structures were observed in the delta, theta, alpha, and beta frequency bands (Thatcher, 1991). Because of space limitations, only the analyses of the theta frequency band are presented. The critical features of this study, such as cyclic recurrence of growth spurts and the spatial dimensions of rostral–caudal, ventral–dorsal, and left-versus-right hemisphere were present in all frequency bands. The most conspicuous differences between frequency bands were between beta and delta, with the former exhibiting strong oscillatory and localized trajectories and the latter exhibiting slightly less pronounced oscillatory behavior and less anatomical specificity.

second derivative (acceleration), or peaks in mean co-herence, because velocity reflects the point in time when growth or change in coherence is at a maximum. The second derivative reflects the time of onset of a growth spurt, as well as points of inflection. However, the second derivative is more susceptible to noise and may or may not eventually lead to a positive first de-rivative peak, or to a significant increase in mean co-herence. Mean coherence values represent the target or end point of the growth spurt as measured by the first derivative. However, the end point is when growth or change is at zero; therefore, maximum mean coherence values were not used to define a growth spurt. A four-point least-squares procedure was used to compute the first derivative (i.e., velocity) or instantaneous rate of change in EEG coherence means from the 436 children in each developmental time series (Savitzky and Golay, 1964). The first four points (mean ages of .513 to 1.292 years) were used to estimate the derivatives, and these points were set at zero. Therefore, no estimates of growth spurts prior to 1.495 years of age were made. Figure 1 shows the ve-locity curves from the subgroupings of electrode pairs that had the highest loadings (e.g., >.80) on the first five factors in the theta frequency band. These factors accounted for a total of 65.7% of the variance. Factor 1 accounted for 22.3% of the variance, factor 2 ac-counted for 12.9% of the variance, factor 3 accounted for 10.4% of the variance, factor 4 accounted for 10.8% of the variance, and factor 5 accounted for 9.3% of the variance (Thatcher, 1991). Left temporal–frontal and left parietal–frontal developmental trajectories loaded on factor 1, right temporal–frontal developmental tra-jectories loaded on factor 2, bilateral local frontal tra-jectories loaded on factor 3, left occipital frontal trajec-tories loaded on factor 4, and bilateral posterior cortical trajectories loaded on factor 5. Periodic "in-phase" activity was present at different ages for each of the 5 factors. The fact that multiple electrode com-binations were often involved indicated that the "growth spurts" or "in-phase" activity reflected the in-volvement of relatively large numbers of neuronal systems over relatively short periods of time (e.g., 6 months to 1 year).

B. Cyclic Micro-Cycles of Development

Figure 2 is a summary of the ages and durations of "in-phase" activity for the five factor groupings shown in Figure 1.[2] An iterative and sequential anatomical pattern of growth spurts was evident. For example, at age 1.5 years, growth spurts were relatively localized (e.g., 6 cm interelectrode distances) and confined to the left parietal and left central to left lateral–temporal re-gions. At age 2.5 years, there was a lengthening along the rostral–caudal dimension (e.g., 12 cm interelec-trode distances) with a lateral-to-medial rotation of parietal–frontal relations to include left parietal to left dorsal medial–frontal regions (i.e., P3–F3 and T3–F1). At age 3 years, there was a further lengthening of in-tracortical relations along the rostral–caudal dimen-sion (e.g., 18 to 24 cm interelectrode distances) with continued involvement of dorsal medial–frontal to posterior cortex. This sequence of lengthening along the rostral–caudal dimension and rotation along the lateral-to-medial dimension between 1.5 and 3 years was repeated again between ages 5.5 to 6.5 years and finally again between 14.5 to 15.5 years and is referred to as a "microcycle" of cortical development. The label of a pattern as a micro–cycle or a subcycle is used to emphasize the presence of a cyclical pattern. The im-portant point, whether a sequence is labeled as a mi-crocycle or a subcycle, or as a stage or substage, is that sequential developmental processes are nested within cyclic anatomical patterns.

C. Expansion of Left Intracortical Connections

Figure 3A shows the sequential lengthening of left hemisphere intracortical growth spurts in EEG coher-ence at ages of approximately 1.5 to 3.0 years. For ex-ample, a peak in the first derivative of EEG coherence occurred in short-distance parietal-to-ventral temporal leads around age 1.6 years (e.g., P3–T3, approx. 6 cm). This was followed by a peak in the first derivative around 2.5 years in the parietal-to-lateral frontal (e.g., P3–F7, approx. 12 cm), and this was followed by a peak in the first derivative around 3.1 years in a longer distance connection system (e.g., F7–O1, approxi-mately 21 cm).

Figure 3B shows a similar sequential lengthening of left hemisphere intracortical growth spurts during the period from 5.5 years to 6.5 years. The short distance connection system of the parietal-to-lateral temporal regions (e.g., approx. 6 cm) exhibited a growth spurt at approximately 5.5 years and was followed by growth spurts at 18 cm (e.g., F7–01), followed by a growth spurt at 6.5 years at approximately 24 cm (e.g., F1–O1). It should be noted that a 180-degree phase reversal be-tween long distance versus short distance connection systems was observed in both figures 3A and 3B.

---

[2] Although most of the first derivative peaks were single points, several peaks were broad, involving more than one point. Therefore, for clarity, only approximate ages of first derivative peaks are repre-sented in the text and figures. Since Julian ages were used (Thatcher et al., 1987), the designation of the age of a first derivative peak was the six month period it was nearest to.

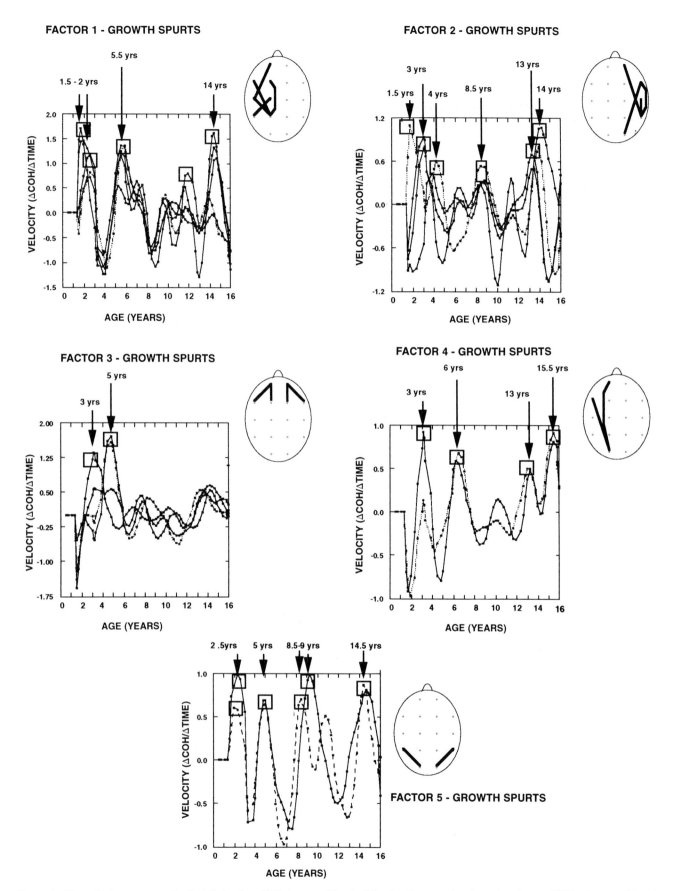

Figure 1 The velocity curves or the first derivatives (Δ Coherence/Time) of the developmental trajectories of mean EEG coherence from the sub-groupings of electrode pairs that had the highest factor loadings (e.g., >.80) (Thatcher, 1991). Growth spurts were defined by a positive

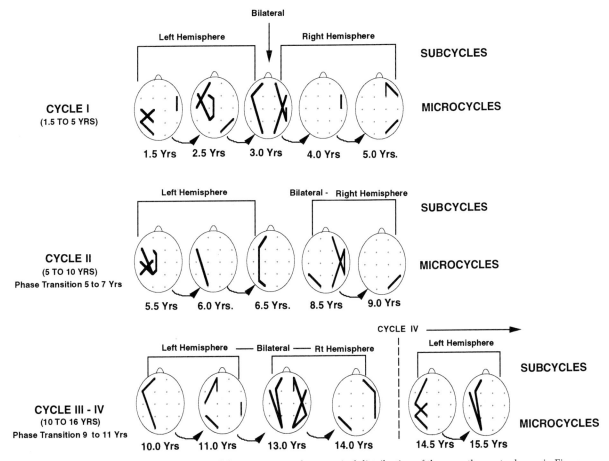

Figure 2 Diagrammatic representation of the sequence and anatomical distribution of the growth spurts shown in Figure 1. Lines connecting two electrode locations correspond to the electrode locations in Figure 1 for the various developmental trajectories that loaded (>.80) on the first five factors (Thatcher, 1991). Microcycles were defined by a developmental sequence involving a rostral–caudal lengthening of interelectrode distances and a lateral–medial rotation that cycles from the left hemisphere to bilateral to right hemisphere in approximately 4-year periods. The microcycles were grouped into subcycles and the subcycles were grouped into cycles as defined by the age 5–7 and age 9–11 bifurcations (from Thatcher, 1994a).

D. Contraction of Right Intracortical Connections

The right hemisphere pattern of contraction appeared to be the reverse of the left hemisphere pattern of expansion. For example, in cycle 2 between 8.5 and 9 years, and between 13 and 14 years in cycle 3, (and possibly between 3 and 4 years in cycle 1), the right hemisphere exhibited a sequence of contraction or consolidation of long distance rostral–caudal intracortical relations (e.g., 18 cm) to shorter distance right caudal cortex (i.e., 6 cm, right occipital–temporal). Figures 4A and 4B support the notion that this may be a functional sequence by the larger first derivative values in the short distance connections, in comparison to the preceding growth spurt in long distance connections, and the tendency toward inverse phase relationships. A similar sequence of contraction was also observed in right hemisphere connections between ages 3 and 4 (see Fig. 2).

Figure 1 (cont.) peak in the first derivative (i.e., a postnatal time of maximum growth) in multiple interelectrode combinations. Since each of the trajectories loaded heavily on a factor (i.e., >.80), this was considered sufficient evidence that a trajectory represented "in-phase" or anatomical synchrony of growth. See Figure 2 to determine more precisely which intracortical connections exhibited growth spurts at the different postnatal ages (from Thatcher, 1994a).

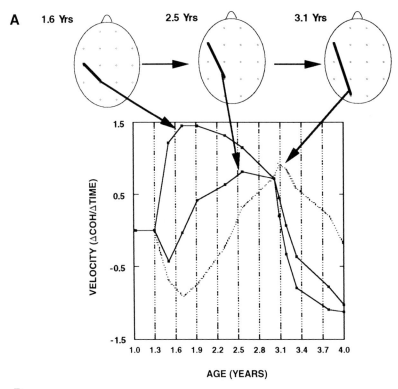

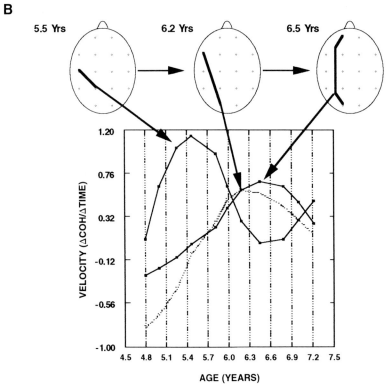

Figure 3 (A and B) Examples of left hemisphere expansion sequences from short distance intracortical connection systems to longer distance systems (see Fig. 2). (A) Sequence of expansive growth spurts in mean EEG coherence trajectories during the 1.5 to 3 year period. A peaks in velocity occurred first in the short distance intracortical connection system (e.g., 6 cm interelectrode distance) in the left parietal lateral–temporal region at age 1.6 years, and was followed by a peak in the intermediate distance intracortical system of the left parietal–lateral frontal region at 2.5 years (e.g., 12 cm interelectrode distance), and then, finally, followed by a peak in velocity in the longer distance lateral frontal–occipital region at 3 years postnatal.

E. Age 3 as the Intermediate Point in a Lateral-to-Medial Anatomical Rotation

Figure 5A shows the full sequence of left and right hemisphere growth spurts between the ages of approximately 1.5 and 3.5 years. A sequential left hemisphere expansion of intracortical growth spurts was followed by a right hemisphere sequence of intracortical contractions. This process can be visualized as a left-to-right, lateral-medial rotational vector in which the "north pole" is reached at approximately age 3. Figure 5B shows the left and right dorsal frontal growth spurts which are present at approximately age 3 years. Note that near age 3, there is an approximately 2- to 3-month phase lag between left and right hemisphere growth spurts, with the left hemisphere leading the right.

F. Rostral–Caudal Expansion of Intracortical Connections

A rostral–caudal pole of development was evident by: 1. a frontal-to-caudal dominance of cortico-cortical EEG coherence changes in both the left and right hemispheres (Thatcher et al., 1987; Thatcher, 1991), and 2. a developmental sequence from short distance rostral–caudal interelectrode combinations (e.g., P3–T3 or T5–C3), to longer distance rostral–caudal electrode combinations (e.g., P3–F7 or P3–F1), to even longer rostral–caudal electrode combinations (e.g., O1–F1). Figure 6A shows a sequential caudal-to-rostral expansion in the length of intracortical growth spurts. The expansion begins around the age of 4.7 years with a growth spurt between short distance intracortical connections (i.e., O1–P3, approx. 6 cm), followed by a growth spurt in longer distance connections (i.e., O1–C3, approx. 12 cm), followed by a growth spurt in a longer distance connection system (i.e., O1–F3, approx. 18 cm) followed, finally, by a longer distance growth spurt at approximately age 6.7 years (i.e., O1 F1, approx. 24 cm). This entire process is completed in approximately 2 years and represents a sequence of growth spurts in intracortical connections that lengthens from 6 cm to 24 cm, and exhibits

a velocity of approximately 2 cm/2 years or 1 cm/month.

As shown in Figure 6B, a similar sequential lengthening of intracortical connections was observed in the rostral-to-caudal direction. This growth process occurred during the same postnatal interval of approximately 4.7 to 6.7 years as observed for the growth process in the caudal-to-rostral direction. However, the timing of growth spurts for a given interelectrode distance was somewhat different for the two directions of growth. For example, the growth spurt in the 12 cm distance in the caudal-to-rostral direction (e.g., O1–C3) occurred at approximately age 5.8 years, whereas the same distance in the rostral-to-caudal direction (e.g., F1–C3) exhibited a growth spurt at approximately 5.4 years.

A prominent feature of the rostral–caudal directional growth spurts was a 180° phase reversal between short distance versus long distance connections. As discussed elsewhere (Thatcher, Krause, & Hrybyk, 1986; Thatcher, 1991, 1992a, 1992b) 180° phase reversals often reflect a competitive relationship, especially in dynamical nonlinear systems (Thom, 1975; Thompson and Stewart, 1986).

G. An Age 5.0 Right Frontal Pole Growth Spurt

Figure 7A shows a spatial gradient in the magnitude of a right frontal pole growth spurt around the age of 4.75 to 5.0 years. A maximum first derivative is in the short distance right frontal pole interelectrodes of F2–F8 and F2–F4 (i.e., approx. 6 cm); a smaller growth spurt is simultaneously present in the longer distance frontal pole interelectrodes of F2–T4 and F2–C4 (i.e., approx. 12 cm), and no growth is present in the frontal pole to occipital electrode pairs (i.e., approx. 28 cm). A comparison to the same electrode pairs in the homologous left hemisphere is shown in Figure 7B. Only very small first derivatives were present with no spatial gradient evident.

These data suggest that a uniquely localized right frontal lobe growth spurt was present around the age of 4.5 to 5.0 years.

Figure 3   (cont.) (B) Sequence of expansive growth spurts in mean EEG coherence trajectories during the 5.5 to 6.5 year period. A peaks in velocity again occurred first in the short distance intracortical left parietal lateral–temporal region at age 5.5 years (e.g., 6 cm interelectrode distance), and was followed by a velocity peak in the intermediate distance intracortical systems in the left lateral fronto–occipital region at 6.2 years (e.g., 12 cm), and finally, followed by a peak in velocity in the longer distance medial–frontal–occipital region (e.g., 24 cm interelectrode distance). A third left hemisphere expansion was noted between 14.5 and 15.5 years (see Fig. 2) (from Thatcher, 1992b).

RIGHT HEMISPHERE CONTRACTION   (18 cm ➝ 6 cm)

A

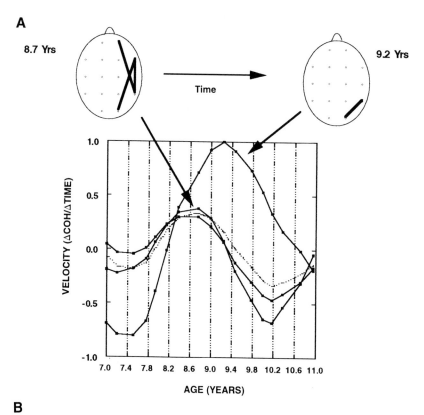

B

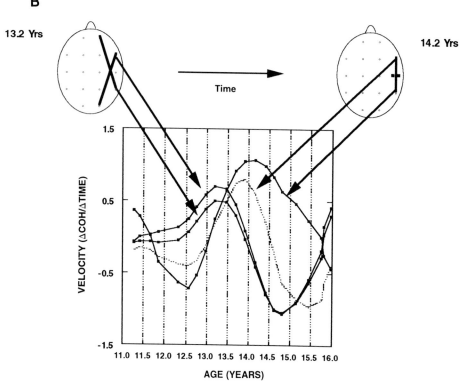

III. Summary

A. The Issue of Cycles versus Stages

In general, the dynamics of intracortical development reviewed in this chapter support modern neo-Piagetian models of cognitive development (Fischer, 1980, 1983; Fischer and Pipp, 1984; Fischer and Farrar, 1987; Case, 1985, 1987; Pascual-Leon, 1976; van Geert, 1991). Specifically, children's thought processes proceed through time-bound cycles between birth and 16 years of age, with each cycle divided into a number of subcycles, and the structure of one cycle or subcycle hierarchically emerges from those of the previous cycle or subcycle (Case, 1985, 1987). While Fischer and Case differ in the exact timing of cycles and in their emphasis on the relative importance and meaning of different cycles, these two workers have done a commendable job of formulating cyclical theories of behavioral development. The data from the present study strongly supports Fischer's and Cases's theories by pointing out some of the physiological processes that may underlie the emergence of "stages" of child development. One of the most important contributions by the neo-Piagetian's, especially Fischer and Case, is their perception of "cycles" as opposed to simply "stages" of child behavioral development. A "cycle" is defined by events that repeat themselves in the same order and over approximately the same interval of time. In contrast, a "stage" is a discrete process or step. There are many examples in biology whereby cycles of growth give rise to an outward manifestation of stages. For example, organisms that construct nests or hives on a seasonal basis, often produce step-like structures. It is argued in the present paper that the presence of stages in cognitive development is merely the outward manifestation of underlying cycles of brain growth, and that the underlying neurophysiological gradients and cycles are the engines that drive cognitive development. Thus, human cognitive development contains both continuous and discontinuous processes. One possible source of the stages in cognitive development is the fact that different regions of the brain develop at different ages. Although a cyclic process drives differential anatomical development, the outward manifestation of qualitatively different behaviors is due, in part, to the growth of different neural structures at different ages. In order to emphasize this point, the nomenclature of "subcycles" and "microcycles" was chosen to distinguish different spatial extents of the cyclic process. It should be kept in mind that the label of an anatomical organization of growth spurts as a subcycle or a microcycle is somewhat arbitrary. The particular divisions are to emphasize the presence of cyclical patterns of predominantly left, bilateral, and right hemispheric development. The important point, whatever divisions of age one chooses, is that sequential developmental processes are nested within cyclic anatomical patterns.

B. Left versus Right Hemispheric Development

It would appear that a specific cognitive function, mediated by a particular hemisphere, does not simply develop at a specific age and then cease in its development. Rather, a cyclic reorganization and reintegration seems to operate at each cycle or subcycle of development.

It is not surprising that the left and right hemispheres develop at different rates, since this is consistent with the neuropsychological literature. However, a new finding is that there are anatomical poles and gradients of postnatal cortical development and phase transitions which operate differently for the two hemispheres. Further, the findings of qualitatively different phase transitions between left and right hemispheres (Thatcher, 1994a, 1996a), and different directions of change (left lengthening in intracortical connections and right contracting, Figs. 3 and 4), suggests that these developmental processes reflect the precursors of differential hemispheric functioning in the adult. For example, it is consistent with the notion that the function of the adult left hemisphere is differential, an-

Figure 4 (A and B) Examples of right hemisphere contraction sequence from long distance intracortical connection systems to shorter distance systems (see Fig. 2). (A) Growth spurts in mean EEG coherence trajectories during the 7 to 11 year period. Peaks in the first derivative occurred first in long distance intracortical connection systems (e.g., 12 to 18 cm interelectrode distances) in the right fronto–temporal and right fronto–occipital areas at age 8.5 years, and were followed by a larger amplitude peak in the short distance intracortical systems (e.g., 6 cm interelectrode distance) in the right parietal–occipital regions at 9 years postnatal.

(B) Growth spurts in mean EEG coherence trajectories during the 11 to 16 year period. Peaks in the first derivative again occurred first in the long distance intracortical right fronto–temporal regions at age 13.2 years, and were followed by a larger amplitude peak in the short distance intracortical systems in the right temporal and fronto–temporal regions at 14.2 years. A third right hemisphere contraction sequence was present between 3 and 4 years (see Fig. 2) (from Thatcher, 1994a).

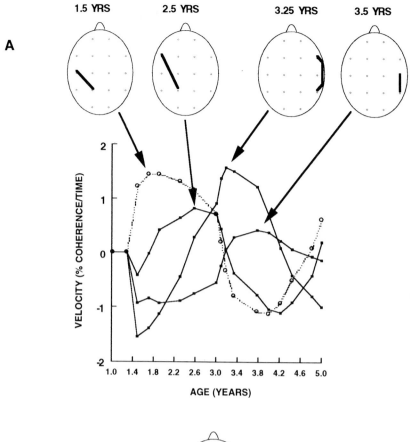

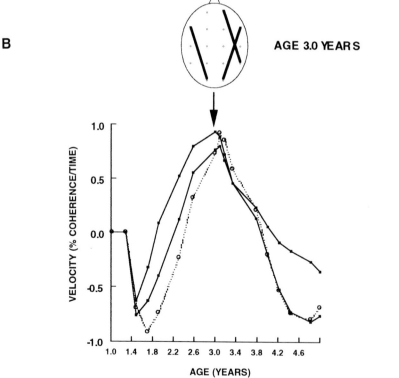

Figure 5   (A) shows a sequence of expanding and contracting growth spurts that reflect a clockwise anatomical rotation. The process begins at age approximately 1.5 years in the left temporal–parietal region, rotates and extends at approximately age 2.5 years to the left lateral frontal–parietal region, then rotates at approximately age 3.2 years to the right lateral frontal–posterior temporal region and finally, rotates and contracts to the right lateral temporal–posterior temporal region at age 3.5 to 4 years.

(B) shows the long distance cortico-cortical growth spurts which are present near the dorsal medial cortex around the age of 3.0 years. Age 3.0 represents the "12 o'clock" or "north pole" of the lateral-to-medial rotational vector, and is characterized by a phase lag of about .25 years between long distance left hemisphere frontal connections and the long distance right hemisphere frontal connections (from Thatcher, 1992b).

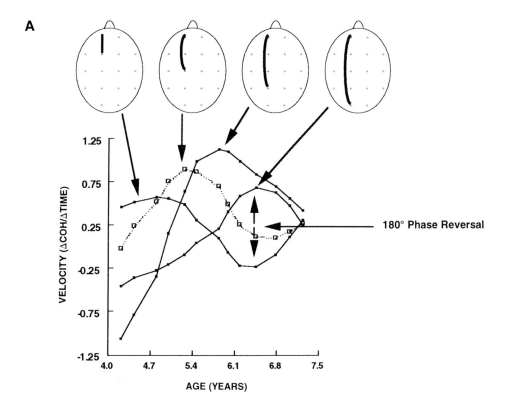

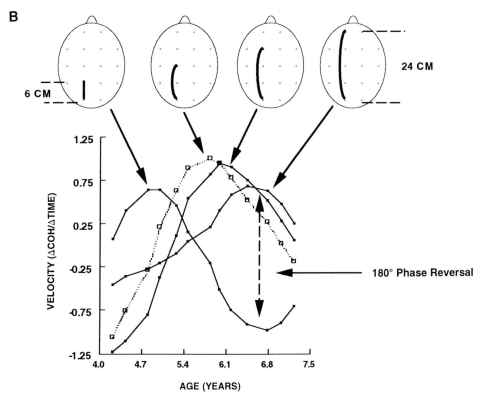

Figure 6 Legend on next page.

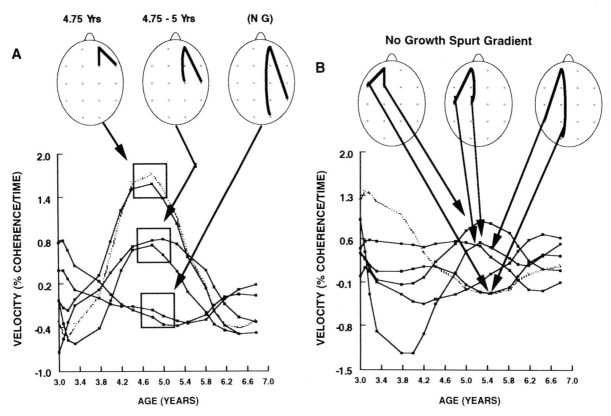

AGE 4.5 TO 5 YEARS

Figure 7   (A) shows a right frontal pole growth spurt around the age of 4.5 to 5.0 years. Right frontal pole localization of the growth spurt is demonstrated by the spatial gradient in the decline of the first derivative from right frontal pole electrode pairs at approximately 6 cm (i.e., F2–F4/F8), to longer distance frontal pole electrode pairs at approximately 12 cm (i.e., F2–C4/T4), to no growth (N G) at approximately 18 to 24 cm (i.e., F2–O2/T6).

(B) shows first derivative values from the homologous left frontal pole as those shown in (A). No spatial gradient was evident and only minor first derivative values were observed (from Thatcher, 1992b).

alytical, and sequential while the function of the right hemisphere is spatial, holistic, and integrative (Kinsbourne, 1974). The developmental sequence of the left hemisphere, from short distance differentiated subsystems to long distance integration of the subsystems, mirrors the functional differences between the two hemispheres. Left hemisphere development can be likened to a process that functionally integrates differentiated subsystems. In contrast, the development of the right hemisphere, from long distance connections to short distance subsystems, can be likened to a process of functional differentiation of a previously in-

Figure 6   (A) shows an expanding sequence of rostral-to-caudal growth spurts which occur in the medial–dorsal plane. This process begins at approximately age 4.5 years in the left frontal pole–dorsal frontal region, then expands at approximately age 5.3 to the left frontal pole–central region, then expands at age approximately 6.0 to the left frontal pole–parietal region and finally, expands at approximately 6.5 years to the left frontal pole–occipital region. A 180° phase reversal between the short distance intracortical electrode pair (i.e., F1–F3) and the long distance intracortical electrode pair (i.e., F1–O1) is evident around age 6.5 years.

(B) shows a complementary and nearly simultaneous expanding sequence to that observed in (A), but in the caudal-to-rostral direction. This process begins at approximately age 4.5 in the left occipital–central region, then expands to the left occipital–dorsal frontal at approximately 6.0 years and finally, expands to the left occipital–frontal pole at approximately age 6.5 years. A 180° phase reversal between the short distance intracortical electrode pair (i.e., O1–P3) and the long distance intracortical electrode pair (i.e., O1–F1) is again evident around age 6.5 years (adapted from Thatcher, 1992b).

tegrated system. These observations suggest that the complementary functions of the left and right hemispheres are established early in human development through complementary developmental sequences. For example, the adult left hemisphere is specialized for analytical and sequential processing which involves a high degree of local differentiation (Kinsbourne, 1974). However, differentiated subsystems require coordination and integration to operate efficiently. The developmental sequence of the left

hemisphere is from differentiation to integration, and this order may play an important role in the eventual maturation of left hemisphere analytical and sequential processing observed in the adult. In contrast, the specialized functions of the right hemisphere involve holistic and integrative information processing (Kinsbourne, 1974). Accordingly, the developmental order of the right hemisphere begins from an integration of distributed subsystems and then converges to a differentiated or specialized subsystem. Presumably, this it-

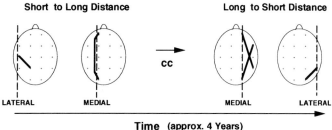

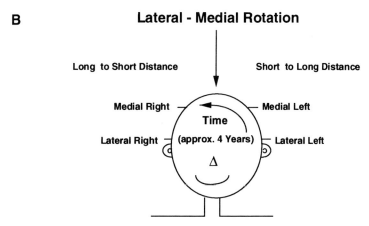

Figure 8 (A) A diagrammatic representation to illustrate the rostral–caudal sequence of development in the left and right hemispheres. The left hemisphere exhibited a sequential lengthening of intracortical connection systems, described as a developmental process of integrating differentiation. The right hemisphere exhibited a sequential shortening of the intracortical connection systems, described as a developmental process of differentiating integration (see Figs. 2, 3, & 4).

(B) A diagrammatic representation to illustrate the lateral–medial sequence of development. The sequence begins at left lateral cortex, then intrahemispherically expands to left dorsal medial cortex, then projects through the corpus callosum to the right dorsal medial cortex, and then intrahemispherically contracts in the right lateral cortex (see Figs. 1, 2, & 4) (adapted from Thatcher, 1994a).

erative sequence reflects a consolidation of the holistic functioning of the right hemisphere to relatively localized regions of the right parietal and right frontal and temporal lobes. Figure 8 is a summary of the specialized integration–differentiation distinctions of the two hemispheres.

C. Cyclic Convergence as a Schemata Formation Process That Narrows the "Gap" between Structure and Function

The data from this and previous studies (Thatcher et al., 1987; Thatcher, 1991, 1992b) indicate that various intracortical connection systems iteratively exhibit growth spurts on an approximately 2- to 4-year cycle. The dominant patterns of the developmental trajectories of EEG coherence over the period from 1.5 years to age 16 indicate "poles" of development from which there are spatial gradients of organizational structure. The left–right, rostral–caudal, and lateral–medial poles of development reflect the three major anatomical axes of the cerebral cortex. That is, the major dimensions of anatomical differentiation, as manifested in differences in neocortical cytoarchitecture and intracortical connections, are along these three axes. Furthermore, gross anatomical differentiation along the three major axes is largely established prenatally (Rakic, 1985) and, as evidenced by longitudinal MRI analyses, is essentially complete by the second year of life (Salamon, Raynaud, Regis, & Rumeau, 1990). However, at age 2 there is a large disparity between structure and function in that adult anatomical differentiation is established early, while adult behavioral development only slowly emerges during the postnatal period (Piaget, 1952, 1971, 1975; Fischer and Pipp, 1984; Fischer, 1980; Fischer and Farrar, 1987; Case, 1985, 1987). Thus, the iterative growth spurts and patterns of development during the postnatal period may reflect a convergence process which narrows the disparity between structure and function by slowly sculpting and shaping the brain's micro-anatomy to eventually meet the demands and requirements of an adult world. According to this notion, an individual's gross anatomical structure is established early in development, and the postnatal iterative sculpting process is used to fine tune anatomical structure to meet the needs of diverse and unpredictable environments. The sculpting process unlocks or tailors the functional potential of the stable gross anatomy according to individual needs and environmental demands. The mechanisms by which this may occur, whether by changes in the number of synapses or changes in the coupling strength of existing synapses, is unknown (Singer, 1995).

D. Neural Plasticity and Sensitive Periods

A cyclic reorganization model of human brain development explicitly integrates neural plasticity with sensitive periods. That is, each cycle of synaptic surplus followed by pruning represents a "sensitive period" in anatomically localized and interconnected brain regions. Thus, sensitive periods are continuously occurring since they are driven by a diffusion wave of anatomically circulating nerve growth factor. A staging or discontinuous aspect of this process arises because of inherent nonlinearities in both space and time. Spatially, the nonlinearities arise because of the segregation of differentiated functions in distributed ensembles of neurons. The functionally differentiated anatomy of the brain guarantees spatial nonlinearities as the wave of growth hormone sweeps across domains of cells. Thus, stages or "sensitive periods" are present because functionally differentiated regions of the brain develop at different ages. A stage-plateau sequence in cognitive development is an outward manifestation of both the continuous and discontinuous aspects of the process. Each stage or period represents rapid synaptic growth within functionally differentiated neural systems and, as a consequence, neural plasticity involves the genetically driven over-production of synapses and the environmentally driven maintenance and pruning of synaptic connections. An important point of the theory, whatever divisions of age one chooses, is that sequential developmental processes are nested within cyclic anatomical patterns, and the synaptic drives mediated through frontal cortico-cortical connections play a crucial role in human development, especially in the process of synaptic pruning and synaptic selection (Thatcher, 1996a, 1996b).

E. Implications for Developmental Neuroimaging

The oscillations and significant velocity peaks shown in Figure 1 represent only approximately a 5 to 20% variation around the trajectory of mean EEG coherence at different ages. Thus, the variation in number or strength of synaptic connections as indicated by quantitative EEG is relatively small and may be difficult to detect using fMRI or optical imaging techniques in general. This is especially likely since the signal strength of blood flow change using a 1.5 tesla magnet is only approximately 2 to 5%. Even with echo-planar imaging techniques or higher magnetic fields, it is unlikely that eyes closed conditions will significantly deviate on the order of a few months as shown in this chapter. A more promising technique is nuclear magnetic resonance spectroscopy, or MRS, as described in

Drs. Minshew's and Pettigrew's chapter in this volume. One would expect, for example, that periodic growth spurts involve periodic and anatomically localized changes in phosphate concentrations and membrane phospholipid metabolism. The naturally occurring P^{31} phosphorous nucleus uniquely provides a method to assay developmental changes in membrane and synaptosomal structure, which can be noninvasively measured *in vivo* (Minshew and Pettigrew, this book). Changes in phosphomonoester levels can be quantified by MRS and, if a sufficiently large data sample per age is used, then subtle changes in phosphomonoesters related to synaptogenesis may be detected. The unfulfilled promise of MRS may someday be realized if there is increased funding and increased recognition of the value of this technique.

References

Bayer, S. A., & Altman, J. (1991). *Neocortical development*. New York: Raven.

Case, R. (1985). *Intellectual development: Birth to adulthood*. New York: Academic Press.

Case, R. (1987). The structure and process of intellectual development. Internat. *Journal of Psychology, 22*, 571–607.

Eckhorn, R., Bauer, R., Jordan, W., Brosch, M., Kruse, W., Munk, M., & Reitboek, H. J. (1988). Coherent oscillations: A mechanism of feature linking in the visual cortex? *Biological Cybernetics, 60*, 121–130.

Fischer, K. W. (1980). A theory of cognitive development: The control and construction of hierarchies of skills. *Psychological Review, 87*, 477–531.

Fischer, K. W. (1983). Developmental levels as periods of discontinuity. In K. W. Fischer (Ed.), *Levels and transitions in children's development*. San Francisco: Jossey-Bass.

Fischer, K. W., & Farrar, M. J. (1987). Generalizations about generalization: How a theory of skill development explains both generality and specificity. *International Journal of Psychology, 22*, 643–677.

Fischer, K. W., & Pipp, S. L. (1984). Processes of cognitive development: Optimal level and skill acquisition. In R. J. Sternberg (Ed.), *Mechanisms of cognitive development* (pp. 45–80). New York: Freeman.

Gorbach, A. M., Tsicalov, E. N., Kuznetsova, G. D., Shevelev, I. A., Budko, K. P., & Sharaev, G. A. (1989). Infrared mapping of the cerebral cortex, *Thermology, 3*, 108–112.

Gray, C. M., Konig, P., Engel, A. K., & Singer, W. (1989). Oscillatory responses in cat visual cortex exhibit inter-columnar synchronization which reflects global stimulus properties. *Nature (London), 338*, 334–337.

Kinsbourne, M. (1974). Mechanisms of hemisphere interaction in man. In M. Kinsbourne & L. Smith (Eds.), *Hemispheric disconnection and cerebral function*. (pp. 71–86). Springfield, IL: Thomas.

Lilly, J. C., & Cherry, R. (1954). Surface movements of click responses from the acoustic cerebral cortex of the cat: The leading and the trailing edges of a response figure. *Journal of Neurophysiology, 17*, 521–532.

Lilly, J. C., & Cherry, R. (1955). Surface movements of figures in the spontaneous activity of anesthetized cerebral cortex: The leading and trailing edges, *Journal of Neurophysiology, 18*, 18–32.

Linas, R. R., & Ribary, U. (1992). Rostrocaudal scan in human brain: A global characteristic of the 40-Hz response during sensory input. In E. Basar and T. H. Bullock (Eds.), *Induced rhythms in the brain* (pp. 147–154). Boston: Birkhauser.

Lohman, A. H. M., & Smeets, W. J. A. J. (1990). The dorsal ventricular ridge and cortex of reptiles in historical and phylogenetic perspective. In B. L. Finlay, G. Innocenti, H. Scheich (Eds.), *The neocortex*. New York: Plenum.

Murthy V. N. & Fetz, E. E. (1992). Coherent 25 to 35 Hz oscillations in the sensory motor cortex of awake behaving monkeys. *Proceedings of the National Academy of Science U.S.A. 89*, 5670–5674.

Nunez, P. (1981). *Electric fields of the brain*. Boston: Oxford Univ. Press.

Pascual-Leone, J. (1976). A view of cognition from a formalist's perspective. In K. F. Riegel & J. Meacham (Eds.), *The developing individual in a changing world*. The Hague: Mouton.

Piaget, J. (1952). *The origins of intelligence*. New York: International Univ. Press.

Piaget, J. (1971). *Psychology of intelligence*. Littlefield, Adams & Co., NJ.

Piaget, J. (1975). *Biology and knowledge*. (2nd ed.). Chicago: Univ. of Chicago Press.

Rakic, P. (1985). Limits of neurogenesis in primates. *Science, 227*, 1054–1056.

Rogers, R. L., Baumann, S. B., Papanicolaou, A. C., Bourbon, T. W., Alagarsamy, S., & Eisenberg, H. M. (1993). Localization of the P3 sources using magnetoencephalography and magnetic resonance imaging. *EEG and Clinical Neurophysiology, 79*, 308–321.

Salamon, G., Raynaud, C., Regis, J., and Rumeau, C. (1990). *Magnetic resonance imaging of the pediatric brain*. New York: Raven.

Savitzky, A., & Golay, M. J. E. (1964). Smoothing and differentiation of data by simplified least squares procedures. *Analytical Chemistry, 36*, 1627–1639.

Shimizu, T., & Karten, H. J. (1990). Multiple origins of neocortex: Contributions of the dorsal ventricular ridge. In B. L. Finlay, G. Innocenti, & H. Scheich (Eds.), *The Neocortex*. New York: Plenum.

Singer, W. (1995). Development and plasticity of cortical processing architectures. *Science, 270*, 758–764.

Smart, I. H. M. (1983). Three dimensional growth of the mouse isocortex. *Journal of Anatomy, 137*, 683–694.

Thatcher, R. W. (1991). Maturation of the human frontal lobes: Physiological evidence for staging. *Developmental Neuropsychology, 7*(3), 397–419.

Thatcher, R. W. (1992a). Are rhythms of human cerebral development "traveling waves"? *Behavior and Brain Sciences, 14*(4), 575.

Thatcher, R. W. (1992b). Cyclic cortical reorganization during early childhood development. *Brain and Cognition, 20*, 24–50.

Thatcher, R. W. (1994a). Cyclic cortical reorganization: Origins of human cognition. In G. Dawson & K. Fischer (Eds.), *Human behavior and brain development*. New York: Guilford.

Thatcher, R. W. (1994b). Psychopathology of early frontal lobe damage: Dependence on cycles of development. *Development and Psychopathology, 6*, 565–596.

Thatcher, R. W., Toro, C., Pflieger, M. E., & Hallett, M. (1994c). Human neural network dynamics using multimodel registration of EEG, PET, and MRI. In R. W. Thatcher, M. Hallett, T. Zeffiro, E. R. John, & M. Huerta (Eds.), pp. 269–278. *Functional Neuroimage Technical Foundations*. Orlando, FL: Academic Press.

Thatcher, R. W. (1996a). A predator/prey model of human cerebral development. In K. Newell & P. Molennar (Eds.), *Dynamical systems and development*. Hillsdale, NJ: Erlbaum.

Thatcher, R. W. (1996b). Human Frontal Lobe Development: A Theory of Cyclic Cortical Reorganization. In N. Krasnegor; R. Lyon, & P. Goldman-Rakic, (Eds.), *Prefrontal cortex: Evolution, neurobiology and behavior.* Baltimore: Brooks.

Thatcher, R. W., & John, E. R. (1977). *Functional neuroscience: Foundations of cognitive processing,* Hillsdale, NJ: Erlbaum.

Thatcher, R. W., Krause, P., & Hrybyk, M. (1986). Corticocortical association fibers and EEG coherence: A two compartmental model. *Electroencephalography and Clinical Neurophysiology, 64,* 123–143, 1986.

Thatcher, R. W., Walker, R. A., & Giudice, S. (1987). Human cerebral hemispheres develop at different rates and ages. *Science, 236,* 1110–1113.

Thom, R. (1975). *Structural stability and morphogenesis.* Reading, MA: Benjamin.

Thompson, J., & Stewart, H. (1986). *Nonlinear dynamics and Chaos.* New York: Wiley.

Toro, C., Wang, B., Zeffiro, T. A., Thatcher, R. W., & Hallett, M. (1994). Movement related cortical potentials. Source analysis and PET/MRI correlation. In R. W. Thatcher, M. Hallet, T. Zeffiro, E. R. John, & M. Huerta, (Eds.). (pp. 259–267. *Functional Neuroimaging.* San Diego: Academic Press.

van Geert, P. (1991). A dynamic systems model of cognitive and language growth. *Psychological Review, 98,* 3–53.

Verzeano, M., (1972). Pacemakers, synchronization, and epilepsy. In H. Petsche & M. A. B. Brazier (Eds.), *Synchronization of EEG activities in epilepsies* (pp. 154–188). New York: Springer-Verlag.

Verzeano, M., & Negishi, K. (1960). Neuronal activity in cortical and thalamic networks. *Journal of General Physiology (Suppl.), 43,* 177.

Verzeano, M., & Negishi, K. (1961). Neuronal activity in wakefulness and in sleep. In G. E. W. Wolstenholme & M. O'Connor (Eds.), *The nature of sleep* (pp. 108–126). London: Churchill.

8

Nuclear Magnetic Resonance Spectroscopic Studies of Cortical Development

Nancy J. Minshew* and Jay W. Pettegrew[†]

*University of Pittsburgh School of Medicine Departments of Psychiatry and Neurology, Pittsburgh, Pennsylvania 15213; and [†]Health Services Administration, Pittsburgh, Pennsylvania 15213

I. Introduction

Magnetic resonance spectroscopy (MRS) is an emerging technology in neuroscience, with the capacity for investigating the molecular and metabolic underpinnings of normal brain development and aging, and the various disease states throughout life that disrupt these processes. MRS is particularly suited to the study of neuronal organization and its disorders, because of its capacity for directly assaying high energy phosphate and membrane phospholipid metabolism. In addition, *in vivo* MRS is noninvasive and relies on the naturally occurring isotope of the atomic nucleus under consideration (^{31}P, ^{1}H), making repeated studies and the study of children both possible and safe.

Although spectroscopy was the original scientific application of the now familiar nuclear magnetic resonance (NMR) phenomenon, its initial application in medical science was in the form of imaging. Magnetic resonance spectroscopy has lagged significantly behind magnetic resonance imaging (MRI) in achieving recognition for its unique capabilities for contributing to the delineation of pathophysiologic mechanisms underlying neurologic disorders. Insights into these mechanisms may provide a link between basic neuroscience observations and neuroanatomic abnormalities revealed by other brain imaging techniques.

From a neuroscience perspective, MRS of the naturally occurring phosphorus nucleus (^{31}P) is particularly suited to the study of the brain, since among current research imaging techniques it uniquely provides an assay of both brain energy and membrane metabolism. Since neural membrane, and especially synaptosomal structure, dynamics, and function are of vital importance to normal neurochemical, neurophysiological, and neuropharmacological function, ^{31}P MRS has the potential for providing important information related to brain function. With ^{31}P MRS, the chemistry of the living brain can be studied *in vivo* and, in greater detail, *in vitro*, using brain slices and brain tissue extracts. These investigations can also be extended to animal models, and to the analysis of solutions and solids, to address questions about physical chemical relationships important to *in vivo* molecular metabolic dynamics. Collectively, these various avenues provide a sophisticated and powerful approach to the study of brain physiology and pathophysiology.

Over the past 15 years, we have applied ^{31}P MRS to the *in vitro* study of brain maturation and aging in rats from the newborn period to senescence (Pettegrew, Panchalingam, Wither, et al., 1990), and the *in vivo* study of brain maturation and aging in normal individuals (Panchalingam, Pettegrew, Strychor, et al., 1990), including the study of synaptic pruning during adolescence (Minshew, Panchalingam, Dombrowski, Pettegrew, et al., 1992), Alzheimer's disease (Pettegrew, 1989a; Pettegrew, Klunk, Panchalingam, et al., 1993; Pettegrew, Panchalingam, Klunk, et al., 1994), schizophrenia (Pettegrew, Keshavan, Panchalingam, et al.,

1991), and autism (Minshew, Goldstein, Dombrowski, et al., 1993). These studies have demonstrated the capacity of ^{31}P MRS for monitoring *in vivo* neuronal membrane organizational events during development and normal aging in humans (Minshew, Goldstein, Dombrowski, Panchalingam, Pettegrew, et al., 1993; Panchalingam et al., 1990; Pettegrew, Keshavan, & Minshew, 1993), and the capacity for detecting pathologic states involving the synthesis (Minshew et al., 1993) or deterioration of brain membranes in humans (Pettegrew, 1989a, 1989b; Pettegrew et al., 1991; Pettegrew, Klunk, McClure, et al., 1991; Pettegrew, Klunk, et al., 1993). These MRS findings in Alzheimer's disease and schizophrenia have been replicated by other groups in the United States, Canada, and France, using both surface coil and localization techniques for MRS (Brown, Levins, Gorell, et al., 1989; Cuenod, Kaplan, Michot, et al., 1995; Nasrallah & Pettegrew, 1995; Smith, Gallenstein, Layton, et al., 1993; Stanley, Williamson, Drost, et al., 1993, 1994). Although MRS is still in its infancy as a developing clinical neuroscience research tool, these initial studies have demonstrated the significant contributions to the molecular and metabolic pathophysiology in the brain possible with this methodology.

II. Introduction to NMR

A. Historical Perspective and Effect of Sample State on Resonance Line Widths

The first NMR experiments were conducted in 1946 with the detection of proton nuclear magnetic resonance in solid paraffin and liquid water (Bloch, Hansen, & Packard, 1946; Purcell, Torrey, & Pound, 1946). Until about 1952, NMR research was dominated by the study of protons in solids which gave rise to broad resonance peaks, reflecting the relative immobility of protons in this state. However, in 1950 reports of chemical shifts in several compounds in solution and gaseous ions led to the development of high resolution NMR of liquids (Dickinson, 1950; Proctor & Yu, 1950). Since the rapid molecular motions in liquids result in very narrow lines compared to those in solids, much smaller chemical shifts could be detected. The technical development of sharp resonance lines in the early 1950s gave rise to a powerful technique for assaying the quantity and structure of organic molecules in solution. This resulted in the domination of high resolution NMR of liquids for the ensuing 30 years.

B. Expansion of Analytic Capabilities

Additional NMR technical advances resulted in: (1) High resolution MRS for identifying and quantitating molecules in complex mixtures and tissue extracts, (2) *in vivo* MRS techniques for noninvasively monitoring metabolites in intact animals and humans, (3) methods for structure determination of moderate size proteins, and (4) improved methods for structural characterization of solids and liquid crystals such as the detection of phase changes in membranes. The potential applications of MRS to neuroscience research are therefore numerous and broad. The present chapter focuses on (1) *in vitro* studies of brain development in an animal model and (2) *in vivo* studies of normal brain maturation in adolescence, brain aging in adults, and a developmental disorder of neuronal organization.

III. NMR Principles

The following is a basic description of the terms and principles pertinent to MRS research. A more detailed discussion of MRS is provided in several recent reviews (McClure, Panchalingam, Klunk, et al., 1996; Pettegrew, 1991; Pettegrew, Klunk, et al., 1993; Silverstein, Bassler, & Morrill, 1991).

A. Nuclear Dipole Moment

Atomic nuclei are composed of protons and neutrons, both of which have intrinsic spin. If a nucleus has an uneven number of protons and neutrons, it will have a magnetic moment. If the nuclear distribution of charge is asymmetrical, that is, nonspherical, then a polarized distribution of charge or a nuclear magnetic quadrupole exists. In the absence of a magnetic field, the orientations of nuclear magnetic dipoles and quadrupoles are degenerate, or random.

B. Nuclear Dipole Quantum Numbers

Atomic nuclei with nuclear dipole moments have nuclear spin angular momentum quantum numbers (m_I), which indicate the allowed number of excited states or excited state orientations of the dipole in a magnetic field (H_0). For atomic nuclei with biologic relevance, the number of allowed orientations or excited spin states ranges from two to six, with two being the number for both ^{31}P and ^{1}H. The number of allowed excited spin states, in conjunction with rotational correlation time and magnetic field strength, are important determinants of the linewidth of NMR resonance peaks.

C. Effect of Applied Static Magnetic Field

In the presence of an applied static magnetic field designated by convention as the main magnetic field

H_0, the nuclear magnetic dipoles precess or rotate around the axis of H_0, which by convention is chosen to project along the z-axis of the NMR coordinate system. This precession is called resonance. The precessional frequency of a nuclear magnetic dipole is called its Larmor frequency (ω_o), and is characteristic of the specific atomic nucleus and magnetic field strength. For example, the Larmor frequency for phosphorus at 1.5 T is about 26 MHz, and at 11.7 T is about 202 MHz. The Larmor frequencies for biologically relevant nuclei are in the radio frequency (rf) range (3–64 MHz at 1.5 Tesla (T)).

D. Effect of Pulsed Radio Frequency (RF) Field

In order to obtain a signal from precessing nuclear dipoles in a static magnetic field, a second magnetic field (H_1) at the Larmor frequency range of the nuclei under study is applied transiently as a pulse which is repeated over time (number of repetitions) to achieve a satisfactory signal to noise ratio. Under the resonance condition, the nuclear dipoles absorb energy at their Larmor frequency from this rf pulse, causing them to move from a ground state oriented along the z-axis to an excited state. The rf field pulse is applied along an axis orthogonal to the main magnetic field in such a way as to displace the nuclear magnetic dipole 90° from the z-axis to lie along the y-axis. The degree of displacement of the nuclear dipole is determined by the length and field strength of the rf pulse. The parameters that result in the desired 90° displacement of the dipoles are referred to as a 90° pulse.

E. Chemical Shift

When atomic nuclei are covalently bonded in molecules, the electron cloud distribution surrounding each nucleus is altered as a result of interactions with the electron clouds of neighboring nuclei in the molecule. Hence, the electron cloud around a phosphorus nucleus in glucose 6-phosphate is different from the electron cloud surrounding the phosphorus in inorganic orthophosphate, and each of the three phosphorus nuclei in adenosine 5'-triphosphate (ATP) are exposed to a different electron cloud distribution. In the presence of an applied magnetic field H_0, the electron cloud of a nucleus produces a magnetic field opposed to the main magnetic field, thus decreasing the actual magnetic field experienced by the nucleus and, in turn, its resonance frequency. (Fig. 1. *In vitro* ^{31}P NMR spectrum at 11.7 T of a brain extract.) The reduction in magnetic field by the electron cloud is referred to as diamagnetic shielding, and the resulting alteration in the resonance frequency of the nucleus is referred to as

chemical shift. Chemical shift is the basis of the analytic capabilities of MRS. The strength of the secondary magnetic field induced by diamagnetic shielding and, in turn, the magnitude of the chemical shift are proportional to H_0 field strength. Chemical shift dispersion, or the separation between resonance peaks, therefore increases with H_0 field strength.

Chemical shifts are usually reported in accordance with the International Union of Pure and Applied Chemistry convention in units of parts per million or ppm (δ), which are independent of field strength. Parts per million values are derived by dividing the resonance frequency by the applied frequency and multiplying by 10^6. Chemical shifts may also be reported in terms of frequency (Hz), but then applied field strength must also be specified, since chemical shift varies with field strength. Chemical shifts are defined relative to a standard reference resonance. For ^{1}H NMR, a typical reference standard is 3-(trimethylsilyl)propionic-2,2,3,3-d₄ acid, sodium salt (TMSP), at 0.0 ppm, and for ^{31}P NMR of the brain the signal of glycerol-3-phosphorylcholine is set at -0.13 ppm. Resonances upfield from the designated 0 ppm are positive numbers and resonances downfield have negative chemical shift numbers.

F. Resonance Splitting Pattern: Spin Coupling

Another chemical structure-dependent spectral characteristic is the splitting pattern of the resonance peak. This splitting is caused by the indirect coupling of nuclear spins through bonding electrons. This coupling is caused by the tendency of a bonding electron to pair its spin with the spin of the nearest nuclei, thus altering the spin of adjacent bonding electrons, which in turn affects the electron clouds of the next nuclei. These influences do not usually extend beyond three covalent bonds. Thus, the resonance peak from the β phosphorus of ATP exhibits triplet splitting as a result of spin coupling with the neighboring α and γ phosphoruses. The resonance peaks for the α and γ phosphoruses of ATP are characterized by doublet splitting, as are the α and β phosphorus peaks of adenosine 5'-diphosphate (ADP) (see Fig. 1). The magnitude and pattern of this splitting are characteristic of molecule structure and thus are an additional aide in peak identification.

G. MRS Signal and Fourier Transformation

When a nucleus in a main magnetic field (H_0) has been excited to one of its higher quantum spin states by an applied rf field pulse (H_1), it will begin losing its excited state energy and return to ground state and its

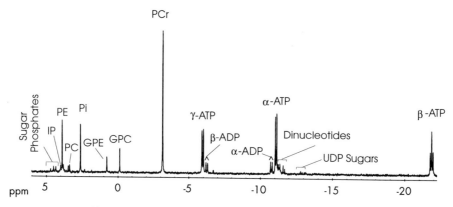

Figure 1 *In vitro* ^{31}P NMR spectrum of rat brain PCA extract at 11.7 T (for abbreviations, see p. 112).

original orientation precessing around H_0, once the applied field pulse is terminated. The excited state energy is emitted as an rf signal at the Larmor frequency of that nucleus. The receiving coil of the spectrometer records this signal in the time domain as a continuous wave, which is referred to as the free induction decay or FID (Fig. 2). The mathematical conversion of the FID to the frequency domain by Fourier transformation produces the conventional MRS spectrum seen in Fig. 1. Under the proper NMR experimental conditions, the integrated area under each resonance peak corresponds to the number of atoms of that particular moiety in the sample.

The signal emitted by the relaxing dipoles is maximally positive when the dipoles have been displaced 90° to lie along the y-axis, since the rf receiver coil is oriented to detect signals along the y-axis. A maximum negative signal is elicited if the dipoles are rotated 270° to be along the y-axis. Displacements of 0° and 180° will give no signal and are thus referred to as null points. For accurate quantitation, the rf pulse must

therefore produce a 90° displacement. There must also be sufficient time between pulses to allow complete relaxation, and this time is shorter after a 90° than a 270° pulse. If the nuclei are not given sufficient time to return to ground state before the next rf pulse, then the displacement of the dipoles will progressively increase with each succeeding pulse and the signal intensity will decrease, reaching a null point when the nuclei are displaced 180° or 360°. This problem is called saturation of the nuclear magnetization, and is avoided by providing a long enough time interval between successive pulses (time to repetition, TR) to prevent saturation effects. Only fully relaxed spectra provide accurate quantitation.

Since the relaxation process is time dependent, the earliest MRS signals in the FID are generated by the most rapidly relaxing components of the sample. Because molecular motion retards relaxation, the signals on the first part of the FID originate from the most immobile constituents of the sample detectable under the conditions of the study. In the brain, the earliest signals in the FID are from relatively immobile sources such as synaptic vesicles, which have long rotational correlation times. The later components of the MRS signal are from slowly relaxing, highly mobile, small molecules in solution, such as ATP, which are referred to as the short correlation time components of the spectra.

H. Relaxation Processes

The relaxation processes underlying energy dissipation include spin–lattice relaxation, which gives rise to the time constant T_1, and spin–spin relaxation, which gives rise to the time constant T_2. T_1 relaxation is produced by rapidly fluctuating magnetic fields directed along the x- and y-axes of the NMR coordinate system; it is a measure of how fast the z-component of the nuclear magnetic moment returns to its equilibrium state.

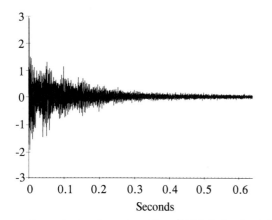

Figure 2 Free inducion decay signal from ^{31}P MRS of rat brain PCA extract at 11.7 T.

T_1 relaxation results from the transfer of energy between the nuclear magnetic spin system and the kinetic energy of the thermal motions of nuclei in adjacent molecules. T_1 is most sensitive to the environment, molecular mobility, and solvent. T_2 relaxation is produced by both rapidly and slowly fluctuating magnetic fields along the x-, y-, and z-axes (Farrar, 1989; Woessner, 1989), and is a measure of how fast the magnetic moments in the x–y plane lose their phase coherence and return to equilibrium state. T_2 relaxation is the result of the intramolecular interaction of nuclear spins.

Two molecule-dependent parameters are important determinants of the rate of relaxation. The first is the magnitude of the particular interaction contributing to relaxation, and the second is the rotational correlation time of the molecule. Molecular motion tends to retard the process of relaxation, therefore increasing T_1 and T_2, since more rapidly moving molecules experience fewer energy depleting events. The molecular motions found in liquids result in long T_2 relaxation times (and narrow linewidths). Molecules whose movements are more constrained have shorter T_2 relaxation times (and broader linewidths). The range of molecular motions detectable in an MRS study is dependent on rotational correlation time and Larmor frequency, and in particular, the rotational correlation time relative to Larmor frequency; both of these parameters are in turn affected by H_0 field strength. Phosphorus nuclei in molecules with extremely long rotational correlation times, such as the phosphorus atoms contained in the hypoxy–apatite crystals of bone, have a resonance which is so broad it is undetectable under the usual MRS experimental conditions.

The detectability of resonance signals can be altered by experimental conditions. For example, the longest rotational correlation time components detectable at 1.5 T may not be detectable at higher field strengths as a result of a change in the relationship between the Larmor frequency and rotational correlation time. Thus, the narrowing of linewidth of long correlation time components with increasing field strength may reflect a loss of signal, along with actual improvement in resolution due to increased chemical shift dispersion. Alternatively, the pulse–acquire time delay may be too long and result in failure to record the early signals from long correlation time components. This was a complication of some of the initial complex pulse sequences designed for signal localization, which delayed the onset of signal acquisition.

I. Resonance Linewidth

A number of factors contribute to resonance linewidth and therefore resolution. As mentioned ear-

lier, diamagnetic nuclei have from two to six excited state quantum levels or spin orientations, with two being the number for ^{31}P and ^1H. Relaxation from these two different spin states yields slightly different resonance frequencies. In slowly moving molecules, these slightly different signals are separably detected and merge in the spectrum to produce a broad resonance line. In rapidly moving molecules, these transitions are not detectable as separate signals and the linewidth is narrow. Complexation of molecules with cations such as Ca^{2+} and Mg^{2+} is also a source of line broadening, referred to as chemical exchange line broadening.

However, the biggest contributor to line broadening is H_0 inhomogeneity. If homogeneity varies across the magnetic field, identical spins in different locations will have slightly different Larmor frequencies. These different frequencies will result in a distribution of unresolved spectral lines which will appear as one broad resonance line. Field inhomogeneities are problematic in large bore magnets and in studies of intact tissue, either whole brain or brain slices. The small bore, high resolution magnets typically have good field homogeneity, and samples are frequently homogeneous solutions or tissue extracts.

J. Sensitivity of MRS

The major limitation of MRS is its sensitivity, reflecting the very low proportion of nuclear dipoles in the excited state. The MRS signal strength of a particular nucleus is a function of its intrinsic gyromagnetic ratio, the applied field strength, and the natural abundance of that nucleus. At 1.5 T and room temperature, the difference between the number of ground state and excited state proton dipoles relative to the total population of dipoles is 2.6×10^{-6}. In terms of sample concentration, the sensitivity of MRS is 10 nmol/ml for hydrogen containing molecules and approximately 1 μmol/ml for phosphorus-containing molecules. Signal strength can be increased by increasing field strength. For example, signal strength for phosphorus containing molecules is increased 3-fold by increasing field strength from 1.5 *T to 3.0 T and 17-fold between 1.5 T and 10 T.*

IV. ^{31}P NMR Spectrum of Mammalian Brain

A. *In Vitro* ^{31}P MRS Spectrum at 11.7 T

In vitro MRS provides chemical conditions more favorable to MRS analysis than occur in the living brain, and therefore greater sensitivity and resolution is achieved as compared to *in vivo* analytic approaches. Freeze clamping with liquid nitrogen preserves the high energy phosphate components, and perchloric acid tissue extraction removes cations and some lipids that contribute to line broadening. Field strength *in vitro* is also several times higher than *in vivo*, and the small bore magnets used for *in vitro* studies generally have good field homogeneity. In addition, a number of chemical procedures can be employed *in vitro* to improve resolution and facilitate peak identification. Sample pH can be titrated to identify the optimal pH for peak separation in complex mixtures, and can aid in identifying resonances from molecules containing acidic or basic functional groups. The characteristic splitting of signals due to spin coupling contributes to peak identification, and through decoupling experiments can identify signals originating from the same molecule. Finally, the identity of a resonance peak can be confirmed by adding a relatively small amount of a known compound to the mixture. Thus, *in vitro* NMR studies play a large and important research role in addressing many issues that cannot be fully defined or investigated *in vivo*.

1. Composition of the *in Vitro* Spectrum

The identities of the major peaks in the *in vitro* ^{31}P MRS spectrum of perchloric acid (PCA) extracts of freeze-clamped mammalian brain are well documented (Glonek, Kopp, Kot, Pettegrew, et al., 1982; Klunk, Xu, Panchalingam, et al., 1994) and are provided in Fig. 1. The *in vitro* ^{31}P spectrum at 11.7 T provides levels of:

(1) Phosphomonoesters (PME): α-glycerol phosphate (GP) (sugar phosphate), phosphocholine (PC), phosphoethanolamine (PE), and inositol-1-PIP
(2) Inorganic orthophosphate (Pi)
(3) The phosphodiesters (PDE): glycerophosphocholine (GPC) and glycerophosphoethanolamine (GPE)
(4) The high energy phosphates: phosphocreatine (PCr) and the polyphosphate regions of the spectrum, which in mammalian brain are primarily the contributions from ATP and ADP. Because there are multiple contributions to the polyphosphate resonances, these regions of the spectrum are more precisely referred to as the ionized ends region or resonance (−5 to −8ppm), the esterified ends resonance (−8 to −14ppm), and the middles resonance (−18 to −23ppm).

2. Quantitation of the *in Vitro* Spectrum

The quantitation of metabolites in brain tissue extracts can be accomplished by the addition of a known amount of an appropriate internal standard to the weighed tissue at the time of extraction. The results are then reported in absolute units of μmol/g. Alternatively, the tissue metabolites can be used as their own internal reference, in which case the results are expressed in relative units of mol%. The mol% method has the advantage of being independent of tissue volume, which is particularly important for *in vivo* work. A recent study comparing these two quantitation methods demonstrated essentially identical results for the μmol/g and mol% methods (Klunk et al., 1994). One objection proposed to the mol% method has been that a reduction in the concentration of a major component in the mixture might result in a false increase in other components. Although intuitively reasonable, the results of this empiric experiment have demonstrated that this does not occur (Klunk et al., 1994).

B. *In Vivo* ^{31}P MRS Spectrum

The *in vivo* ^{31}P MRS spectrum of the human brain at 1.5 T is considerably less well resolved than the *in vitro* spectrum, but provides excellent measures of the high energy phosphates and Pi, and of total phosphomonoester and phosphodiester levels. Despite loss of detail, the pioneering work of Ackerman, Grove, Wong, et al. (1980) established that *in vivo* MRS yields meaningful data that are both reliable and valid.

The lower resolution of the *in vivo* spectrum is partly due to the lower magnetic field strength used for *in vivo* studies (1.5 T versus 11.7 T). The absorption of radiofrequency power by the brain increases with field strength, thus limiting the highest practical field strength for *in vivo* MRS in humans to approximately 4 T. *In vivo* MRS resonance peaks are also broadened by the effect of the living tissue environment on the T_2 relaxation of molecules, in comparison to the relaxation of the same molecules in solution (Bolinger & Lenkinski 1992). Field inhomogeneity within the brain sample is yet another important contributor to line broadening *in vivo*. Thus, increased field strength of *in vivo* studies will improve spectral resolution to some extent, but will not yield the well-resolved spectra of *in vitro* MRS, because of the contributions of tissue and field inhomogeneity, long correlation time components, and chemical exchange broadening to the *in vivo* linewidths.

1. Composition of the *in Vivo* Spectrum

In vivo ^{31}P MRS of the human brain at 1.5 T provides spectral peaks for phosphomonoesters (PME), inorganic orthophosphates (Pi), phosphodiesters (PDE), phosphocreatine (PCr), and three polyphosphate peaks, representing the levels of the α, β, and γ phosphates of nucleotide triphosphates and the α and β phosphates of nucleotide diphosphates. The identification of the spectral peaks of the *in vivo* [31]P spectrum are based on the chemical shifts of the *in vitro* ^{31}P MRS spectrum (see Fig. 3, for identification of *in vivo* ^{31}P MRS resonances based on comparison with the *in vitro* spectrum).

2. Quantitation of the *in Vivo* Spectrum

Since the peaks in the *in vivo* spectrum overlap at the baseline, the areas of these resonances are quantified by a nonlinear curve fitting of Lorentzian peaks to the experimental data (Fig. 4). These methods produce values which have high reliability and validity. Test retest and intra- and interrater reliability have been demonstrated to be ≥.95 for these quantitation procedures in our laboratory, and *in vivo* values have been demonstrated to be highly comparable to previously published *in vitro* MRS data, and to determinations

with other classical analytic methods (Glonek et al., 1982; Klunk et al., 1994; Pettegrew, Minshew, Cohen, et al., 1984; Pettegrew et al., 1994).

3. Spatial Localization for *in Vivo* MRS

In contrast to *in vitro* MRS of solutions where the entire sample is analyzed, *in vivo* MRS requires the use of spatial localization methods, since only a portion of the neural tissue is of interest. In the *in vivo* studies described later, the depth pulse localization technique using a rf field gradient produced by a surface coil was employed. This technique uses a straightforward pulse–acquire sequence which minimizes the loss of spectral information at the beginning of the signal. This technique is governed by two basic principles: the size and shape of the surface coil, and the width of the rf pulse. The surface coil consists of two concentric coils, a larger outer transmitter coil and a smaller inner receiver coil. This arrangement ensures that the signal

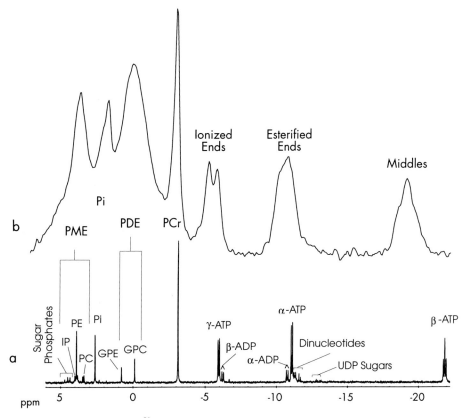

Figure 3 Comparison of (a) ^{31}P MRS *in vitro* spectrum of perchloric acid extract of freeze-clamped rat brain tissue at a magnetic field strength of 11.7 T, and (b) ^{31}P MRS *in vivo* spectrum of human brain (dorsal prefrontal cortex) at a magnetic field strength of 1.5 T. In the *in vivo* spectrum, ionized ends are γ-ATP and β-ADP, esterified ends are α-ATP and α-ADP, and middles are β-ATP. PME, phosphomonoesters; P_i, orthophosphate; PDE, phosphodiesters; PCr, phosphocreatine; IP, phosphoinositol; PE, phosphoethanolamine; PC, phosphocholine; GPE, glycerophosphoethanolamine; GPC, glycerophosphocholine; ATP, adenine triphosphate; ADP, adenine diphosphate; UDP, uridine diphosphate.

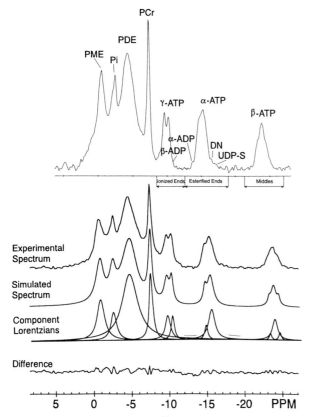

Figure 4 Quantitation of *in vivo* ³¹P NMR spectrum: unprocessed spectrum with deconvolution into component Lorentzian peaks.

recorded by the receiver coil is from within the region excited by the transmitter coil which, can be defined anatomically by an image produced with this coil. The rf field generated by the transmitter coil is conical in shape with its base at the surface of the skull and a depth equal to the radius of the coil. The rf pulse applied to a living animal dissipates as it penetrates tissue. Thus, pulse width can be adjusted so that the surface of the brain receives a 90° pulse, while skin and muscle on the surface of the skull receive a 180° or null pulse, essentially eliminating their contribution to the FID. The skull contributes no detectable signal to the *in vivo* spectrum because of the extremely long correlation times of the phosphates immobilized in bone. Thus, in the depth pulse localization technique, variation in rf flip angle, depth of tissue penetration, and size of the surface coil are used to localize the volume of brain tissue of interest (VOI).

Alternatively, complex spin–echo pulse sequences have been developed which provide simultaneous acquisition of spectra from several brain regions within a single 35 mm thick brain slice. The earliest of these methods tended to lose signal from the long correlation time phospholipid components of the spectrum,

because of the time required for the localizing gradients to be turned on and off before the receiver coil could be turned on. Recently developed short TE methods have eliminated this difficulty, as well as providing additional improvements in this methodology (Lim, Pauly, Webb, et al., 1994).

C. Chemical and Metabolic Information from the *in Vitro* and *in Vivo* ³¹P MRS Spectrum

The resonances related to bioenergetics (Pi, PCr, and the nucleoside phosphate resonances) are derived from small molecules. The simplest cases are Pi, which is solely derived from inorganic phosphate (mainly $H_2PO_4^{-1}$ and HPO_4^{-2} at physiologic pH), and PCr, which is derived solely from phosphocreatine. The nucleoside phosphates include contributions from adenosine, cytosine, guanosine, and uridine mono-, di-, and triphosphates (NMP, NDP, and NTP respectively), but the adenosine compounds are the predominant species. The ionized ends resonance (−5 to −8 ppm) is made up of the terminal, beta-phosphates of NDPs and the terminal, gamma-phosphates of NTPs, thus mainly representing ADP and ATP. The esterified ends resonance (−8 to −14 ppm) is made up of the nucleoside-coupled alpha-phosphates of NDPs and NTPs, again mainly representing ADP and ATP, but also including a minor contribution from dinucleotides such as nicotinamide adenine dinucleotide phosphate (NADP and NADPH) and uridine 5′-diphosphate (UDP) sugars. The middles resonance (−18 to −23 ppm) is the simplest of the nucleoside resonances, being composed only of the middle, beta-phosphate of NTPs, mainly ATP. The linewidth of these nucleoside resonances is increased by increased intracellular levels of free Ca^{2+} or Mg^{2+}, which form complexes with the nucleoside phosphates, producing chemical exchange line broadening (Pettegrew, Withers, Panchalingam, et al., 1988).

The resonances related to phospholipid membrane metabolism are no less complex. The PME resonance represents both small, rapidly tumbling molecules which give narrow linewidths and large, slowly moving macromolecules which give broad linewidths. The small molecules include PE, PC, IP, small amounts of phosphoserine (PS), NMP phosphates such as denosine 5′-monophosphate (AMP), sugar phosphates such as glucose-6-phosphate, and α-glycerol-phosphate (α-GP). The macromolecules are mainly composed of relatively mobile proteins containing phosphorylated serine and threonine residues. The macromolecular component appears to be relatively small, as at least 2/3 of the total *in vivo* PME concentration, reported to be approximately 3 μmol/g (Bottomley, Cousins, Pendrey, et al., 1992, Klausner, Sweeney, Deck, et al., 1992), is accounted for by the small water soluble metabolites. Phosphoethanolamine alone contributes about 1 µmol/g.

The PDE also have small and large molecular components. The small molecules are mainly GPC and GPE, which give relatively narrow linewidths. The large molecules are choline, ethanolamine, and serine phospholipids in small, mobile structures such as synaptic vesicles, and phospholipid vesicles such as those in the endoplasmic reticulum and Golgi (Kilby, Bolas, & Radda, 1991; Murphy, Bottomley, Salerno, et al., 1992; Pettegrew et al., 1994), which give the broad linewidth components. In practice, the broadest components originate from membrane bilayers and are typically not observed using typical spectral acquisition parameters, or are removed by processing the spectral baseline. Phospholipids in myelin, or even external cell membranes, or large organelle membranes, are also too immobile to be recorded with *in vivo* ^{31}P MRS (Kilby et al., 1991). Thus, as typically applied, the PDE peak of the *in vivo* ^{31}P MRS measures GPE, GPC, and mobile vesicular phospholipids. The mobile vesicular phospholipid contribution appears to predominate as the concentration of GPE plus GPC approaches 3 µmol/g brain in water soluble extracts, and the total PDE peak has been estimated to be on the order of 15 µmol/g *in vivo* (Bottomley et al., 1992; Klausner et al., 1992).

In vivo ^{31}P MRS also provides a direct assessment of intracellular pH, which is determined from the difference between the chemical shifts of PCr and Pi (Petroff, Prichard, Behar, et al., 1985). The *in vivo* measurement of brain pH is important as it provides information on physiochemical buffering capacity, consumption and production of metabolic acids such as lactic acid, and transmembrane fluxes of H^+ and HCO_3^-. Intracellular brain pH is also important because of its influence on enzymes and metabolic processes, such as creatine kinase, phosphofructokinase, redox ratios, and oxyhemoglobin dissociation (Siesjo, 1978).

In summary, *in vivo* ^{31}P MRS gives the following neurochemical information: The PME peak predominantly indicates levels of small, water soluble precursors of phospholipid membrane synthesis such as α-GP, IP, PE, and PC. The PDE peak gives information on both small, water soluble phospholipid membrane breakdown products (GPE and GPC), and mobile phospholipid vesicles such as synaptic vesicles. The Pi peak constitutes the final end-product of all of the phosphorus metabolites. The PCr peak specifically measures the level of this one high energy metabolite. PCr is the most metabolically labile of the high energy compounds, falling prior to ATP in situations of rapid energy consumption. The nucleoside phosphate reso-

nances (ionized ends, esterified ends, and middles) mainly represent levels of ATP and ADP. Changes in the ionized ends and/or esterified ends without a similar change in the middles resonance, suggest a change in ADP more than ATP. Changes in the middles resonance are mainly indicative of changes in ATP levels.

From a metabolic perspective, the PCr, ATP, ADP, Pi, and brain pH values provide information about the energy status of the brain. The phosphomonoesters (α-GP, IP, PE, and PC) are the building blocks of membrane phospholipids, and the relative concentrations of these metabolites are a measure of the active synthesis of membranes (Vance, 1991). Sources of PME include phosphorylation of their respective bases by kinases, phospholipase C cleavage of their respective phospholipids, phosphodiesterase cleavage of their respective PDE. The phosphodiesters (GPE, GPC) are the major catabolic products of membrane phospholipid degradation (Carlsson, 1988; Vance, 1991). They are the products of phospholipase A1 and A2 activity toward their phospholipids, and are converted to their respective PME by PDE phosphodiesterase activity.

D. MRS Data Compared to PET and SPECT Data

In contrast to bioenergetics data generated with positron emission tomography (PET) and single photon emission computed tomography (SPECT), ^{31}P MRS directly measures brain levels of ADP, ATP, PCr, and Pi, and also provides a measure of intracellular brain pH. Bioenergetics determinations with PET and SPECT are inferred from glucose uptake or blood flow. A second important difference between these methodologies is that MRS measures steady state metabolite levels, whereas PET and SPECT measure rate of consumption. These two measurements yield fundamentally different information about bioenergetics that are not equivalent. Alterations in bioenergetics determined with these different methods may therefore be in the same direction but may also be divergent. For example, a disorder characterized by an increased rate of energy utilization without alterations in steady state levels of energy metabolites could result in augmentation of cerebral blood flow and manifest PET and SPECT, but not ^{31}P MRS abnormalities. Conversely, a disorder characterized by normal cerebral blood flow and altered steady state levels of PCr and ATP would produce ^{31}P MRS alterations, but not PET or SPECT abnormalities. ^{31}P MRS is also distinguished from PET and SPECT methodologies by providing measurements of brain membrane phospholipid metabolism and by reliance on the naturally occurring isotope of the atomic nucleus.

V. ^{31}P MRS Studies of Normal Brain Development and Maturation

A. *In Vitro* Studies of Brain Development and Aging in an Animal Model

The sensitivity of ^{31}P MRS to changes in brain membranes and bioenergetics occurring with brain development and aging was initially investigated in an animal model. This was accomplished by studying perchloric acid extracts of the brain from Fisher 344 rats ranging in age from newborn (12 hours) through senescence, which in the rat corresponds to 12 to 24 months of age (Pettegrew et al., 1990). The brains were freeze-clamped to preserve the high energy metabolites, subjected to perchloric acid extraction, and analyzed with ^{31}P MRS at 4.7 T to obtain mole percent values for PCr, Pi, ATP, α-GP, PC, PS, PE, GPC, and GPE.

Brain development and maturation in the rat have been divided arbitrarily into five periods (McIlwain & Bachelard, 1985) (Table 1). Period I is the period of cellular division and extends up to birth, at which point the rat brain has no recordable electrical activity and has attained 15% of its adult weight. From birth to 10 days of age (Period II), there is growth in the size of individual cells, rapid outgrowth of axons, and rapid development of dendritic connections. These changes are

associated with a rapid increase in brain lipid content, which peaks at about 10 days of age. Naturally occurring cell death also begins during Period II, and continues through Period III (Clarke, 1985; Cowan, Fawcett, O'Leary, et al., 1984; Oppenheim, 1985; Pittman & Oppenheim, 1979). From 10–20 days of age (Period III), neuronal cell volume, synaptic density, and the number of nerve terminals rapidly increase. Simultaneously, intracellular K^+ space increases and the extracellular Na^+ and Cl^- space decreases. These changes are associated with the appearance of electrical activity on the electroencephalogram. Neurochemical correlates of the structural and neurophysiologic developments in Periods II and III are manifested in a steady increase after birth in adenosine triphosphatase activity, including $Na^+–K^+$ ATPase, and increases in the rate of glucose uptake, glycolysis, and oxidative phosphorylation, which reach adults levels during Period III. Periods II and III, or birth to approximately one month of age in the rat, are therefore a time of active neuronal growth, synaptogenesis, and neuronal organization. As in humans, naturally occurring cell death is also an integral part of the developmental process in the rat. Period IV in rat brain development begins at approximately 20 days of age, and is associated with active myelination but little further growth in brain size. During this phase, creatine phosphokinase activ-

Table 1 ^{31}P Magnetic Resonance Spectroscopy of Rat Brain Development and Aging

Period	Age	Anatomic event	MRS findings Phospholipid metabolism	PCr[a]
II	Birth–10 days	Neuronal organization • Rapid increase in brain lipid content • Synaptogenesis • Programmed cell death starts	PME levels high PDE levels low PME/PDE > 150	• PCr levels low • P_i levels high • PCr/P_i ratio low
III	10–20 Days	Neuronal organization • Synaptogenesis • EEG activity appears • Programmed cell death continues	PME levels decreasing PDE levels increasing	• Rapid increase in PCr and PCR/P_i ratio • Rapid decrease in P_i level, which correlates with development of glycolytic and oxidative pathways • Increase in Na^+-K^+ATPase and EEG activity
IV	20 Days–12 months	Myelination	PME/PDE $\approx$ 1–2	• Slight increase in PCr and P_i • PCr/P_i: no change
V	>12 months	Aging and senescence	PME/PDE < 1	• Slight increase in PCr and P_i • Slight increase in PCr/P_i suggesting decrease in PCr utilization

[a]There were no changes in adenosine triphosphate with age.

Note: PCr, phosphocreatine; PME, phosphomonoester; PDE, phosphodiester; P_i, inorganic orthophosphate; ATPase, adenosine triphosphatase; and EEG, electroencephalogram.

ity reaches maximum levels. Senescence in the rat (Period V) is thought to develop after 12 months of age, and certainly by 24 months of age.

High resolution ^{31}P MRS analysis of perchloric acid extracts of rat brain across this age spectrum demonstrated marked alterations in the measured levels of the membrane phospholipid and cellular high energy phosphate metabolites with brain development and more subtle effects with aging. (Figs. 5–7, Table 1). The phosphomonoesters, PC, PS, PE, and α-GP, were at very high levels at birth (Fig. 5). Between birth and 3 months of age, these levels dropped substantially ($p = .0001$), with the majority of this decline occurring in the first month of life. Between 3 and 12 months of life, the PC and α-GP levels remained stable, whereas there was a modest rise in PE and PS levels ($.01<p<.05$). Between 12 and 24 months of age, there was a slight decline in PME levels ($p<.001$). In contrast, the PDE levels, GPE and GPC, were low or undetectable in the newborn period and were substantially increased by 3 months of age ($p= .0001$), after which the levels rose at a slower rate up until 24 months of age (Fig. 6).

The PME/PDE ratio is an index of membrane phospholipid turnover, with values above 1 indicative of net anabolic activity and values below 1 indicating net catabolic activity. In the newborn period, the PME/PDE ratio in the rat brain was very high (>150), indicative of intense membrane synthetic activity and coinciding with the period of intense dendritic growth and synaptogenesis in the rat brain. After 10 days of age, the PME/PDE ratio was 10, declining to 2 by 3 months of age and remaining relatively stable until 12 months of age. During the period of brain senescence, the PME/PDE ratio fell below 1, signifying net membrane catabolic activity and net membrane loss during the aging process.

These MRS findings are indicative of very high phospholipid anabolic activity without appreciable

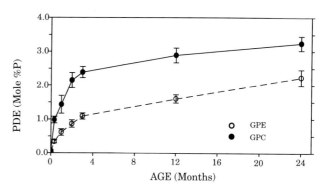

Figure 6 Effect of brain development and aging on PDE levels in rat brain.

catabolic activity between 12 hours and 10 days of age (Period II). This anabolic activity coincides with the increase in neuronal cell size, rapid outgrowth of axons, and rapid development of dendritic connections occurring during this phase of brain development in the rat. After 10 days of age (Period III), PME levels started to fall and there was a substantial increase in PDE levels, but the PME/PDE ratio remained high (<10). The increase in the PDE from 10–30 days of age is indicative of rising membrane catabolism, which may reflect the programmed cell death and synaptic remodeling that are integral parts of neuronal organization. From 1 to 3 months of age, the PME levels continued to decrease and the PDE to increase, but not as rapidly as before, and the PME/PDE ratio was 2. This metabolic activity could reflect ongoing low level remodeling of neuronal dendritic architecture, or perhaps myelination. Between 3 and 12 months, these metabolic dynamics continued, suggesting ongoing remodeling until the onset of aging. During aging, the PME levels fell, the PDE levels rose, and the PME/PDE ratio dropped below 1, suggesting that membrane catabolism was proceeding slightly faster than membrane anabolism, which corresponds to the slight loss of dendritic branching that occurs with aging.

The energy status of the brain also underwent dramatic changes with brain development and aging in the rat (Fig. 7). In the newborn rat brain, the levels of PCr were quite low and appeared to decrease further until 5 days of age. After day 5, the PCr levels increased rapidly up to 1 month of age, and less rapidly between 1 and 3 months of age. Thereafter, PCr levels underwent less dramatic, but steady, increases up to 24 months of age. Pi levels were relatively high at birth, decreased until 5 days of age, and then increased until 10 days of age. Thereafter, Pi levels fell rapidly until 3 months of age. Between 3 and 12 months of age the Pi levels remained essentially stable, and then declined between 12 and 24 months of age.

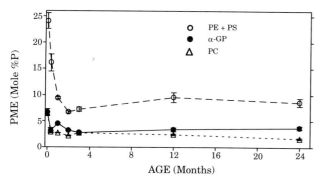

Figure 5 Effect of brain development and aging on PME levels in rat brain.

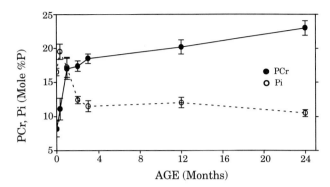

Figure 7   Effect of brain development and aging on bioenergetics in rat brain.

The PCr/Pi ratio provides a convenient measure of the energy status of the brain because it is the ratio of the most labile form of high energy phosphate (PCr) to the ultimate breakdown product of all high energy phosphate compounds (Pi). The PCr/Pi ratio was quite low in the newborn period until 5 days of age, after which time it rapidly increased until 3 months of age. After 3 months of age, the PCr/Pi ratio remained relatively constant up to 12 months of age, and then increased slightly between 12 and 24 months. The rapid increase in the PCr/Pi ratio in the first month of life in the rat coincides with the development of the glycolytic and oxidative pathways, increased Na^+-K^+ ATPase activity, and the onset of electroencephalographic activity. The increase in the PCr/Pi ratio between 12 and 24 months suggests declining utilization of PCr, and may be a reflection of the loss of dendritic spines and synapses that occurs with the aging process. Brain ATP levels in the rat did not change from birth to 24 months of age, which is consistent with the reliance on PCr to maintain stable ATP levels in brain.

This study of brain development and aging in the rat provides evidence of the sensitivity of MRS to the changes in membrane metabolism and cellular bioenergetics associated with neuronal organizational events. Marked developmental and smaller aging–related changes were documented in the precursors and degradation products of phospholipid membranes and in brain bioenergetics. These biochemical changes correspond to known histological and electrophysiological changes of neuronal organization in the brain during development and the loss of dendritic processes during aging.

B. *In Vivo* Studies of Brain Maturation and Aging in Normal Humans

Thus far, *in vivo* ^{31}P MRS data have been accumulated on approximately 150 normal adolescents and adults ranging in age from 10 to 80 years. These data

were collected from normal control subjects participating in several studies of neuropsychiatric disorders. Data are therefore confined to developmental events during adolescence, maturity, and aging.

1. Developmentally Regulated Changes in Brain Membrane Metabolism in Adolescence

During adolescence and young adulthood, phosphomonoester levels declined throughout adolescence and then remained stable during adulthood. PCr levels rose in adolescence to also remain stable during adulthood. The metabolic changes during adolescence may reflect the developmentally regulated processes in neuronal organization occurring during this time period, in particular those of programmed synaptic pruning.

2. Changes in Phospholipid and Energy Metabolism Related to Aging

With normal brain aging in humans, PME levels were observed to decline slightly and PCr levels to rise slightly. These small changes in phospholipid metabolism with normal aging are suggestive of decreased synthesis and increased breakdown of brain membranes, and are consistent with neuropathologic observations of a reduction in dendritic spines with normal aging. The slight rise in PCr levels with aging suggests a slight decrease in utilization of PCr, possibly due to loss of synapses which are the sites of highest utilization of high energy phosphates.

VI. ^{31}P MRS Studies in a Disorder of Neuronal Organization

A. *In Vivo* MRS in Adolescents and Young Adults with Autism

Autism is a developmental neurobiologic disorder of particular interest to neuroscience, as it involves deficits in complex cognitive abilities that provide the basis for adaptation and function in society and the development of the neural substrate subserving those abilities. Autism is now widely viewed as a disorder of neuronal organization, and is thought to involve both dendritic tree development and the development of brain organization at the neural systems level. Although abnormalities have been defined in the cerebral cortex, limbic system and cerebellum, a variety of evidence points to the association cortex and neocortical systems as the primary site of dysfunction in autism (reviewed in: Minshew, 1996; Minshew & Goldstein, 1993; Minshew, Goldstein, & Siegel, 1995).

The empiric support for a primary neocortex–neocortical systems abnormality in autism began accruing in 1979 with neurophysiology studies. The neurophysiology of autism has since been characterized with both evoked potential and oculomotor methodologies. Evoked potential studies in autism over the past 10 to 15 years have uniformly implicated late information processing, providing evidence of bilaterally symmetric neurophysiologic abnormalities referable to the parietal and frontal cortex. Early and midlatency potentials, including the N100 and N200 potentials, have been normal. This neuropsychologic profile has been replicated recently with oculomotor physiology. Cortically controlled eye movement tasks, analogous to those employed by Goldman–Rakic to investigate neocortical circuitry in nonhuman primates, have identified major alterations in the localized circuitry of the dorsal prefrontal cortex and parietal cortex in autism (Minshew, Sweeney, Furman, 1995). As with evoked potentials, studies of basic ocular motor and oculovestibular function in autism have provided evidence of intact function of subcortical pathways. Neuropsychologic studies in autism have demonstrated a similar pattern of function, providing evidence of the integrity of basic information acquisition abilities and generalized abnormalities in complex or higher order cognitive abilities. Specifically, deficits have been identified in complex reasoning and problem solving abilities, complex memory abilities including delayed recall, logical memory, and working memory, complex or higher order language abilities, complex motor abilities or praxis, and complex or higher cortical sensory abilities. The auditory and visual domains were equally affected. Deficits were best characterized across age and autism severity in terms of high information processing load relative to general intellectual level, and task dependence on association cortex. This pattern of generalized deficits in complex abilities is not that of a general deficit syndrome or mental retardation, since autistic subjects performed at average or above average levels in more basic abilities in these same functional domains, and deficits were either substantially below expectations based on age and IQ or abnormal at any IQ. This pattern of deficits is not readily explainable in terms of a common clinical deficit, but rather suggests that the deficits are unified at the neurobiologic level by a dependence on a common type of dendritic architecture specialized for the analysis of the most complex information. Functional methods have therefore been consistent in autism, both within and across methodologies, demonstrating a central abnormality in late or complex information processing by association cortex and its neural systems.

From a structural perspective, volumetric brain morphometry with MRI has provided evidence of an increase in the supratentorial size of the brain as a result of an increase in cortical grey and white matter, suggesting an increase in cerebral cortex and its projections. Neuropathologic studies have reported an increase in brain weight on the one hand, and on the other hand, a truncation in dendritic tree development in limbic system neurons, and reduced Purkinje and granule cell populations in the cerebellum.

The pathophysiologic bridge between the structural and functional alterations in the neocortex and its projections, and the histologic abnormalities in the limbic system and cerebellum, is suggested by the increase in white matter projections on MRI and the PET findings of a widespread decrease in the functional metabolic connections of frontal and parietal cortex, both intracortically as well as intrahemispherically, with limbic and subcortical structures. This constellation of neuroanatomic findings suggests a block in brain development at a stage of overgrowth of neocortex and its projections, with failure to attain normal connectivity of cortex with limbic and cerebellar structures, resulting in truncation of dendritic tree development in the limbic system and cell loss in cerebellum. Thus, it appears that the development and remodeling in neocortex is insufficient to adequately support the emergence of brain organization at the neural systems level.

1. *In Vivo* ^{31}P MRS of Frontal Cortex in Autism

The first and only ^{31}P MRS study published on autism to date was undertaken to investigate *in vivo* brain membrane phospholipid and energy metabolism in autism and its relationship to the pathophysiology of autism (Minshew et al., 1993). Phospholipid metabolism was of obvious interest because of the histologic evidence of alterations in dendritic tree development and in the development of cortical projections. Brain bioenergetics have received little attention in autism because of the lack of evidence to suggest a primary energy failure. However, recent PET and evoked potential mapping studies in normal individuals have provided evidence that brain activation and bioenergetics may also reflect neurophysiologic function. Specifically, mapping studies with cognitive evoked potentials and positron emission tomography in normal individuals have demonstrated less efficient brain function, that is, activation of more neural circuits, with incorrect answers, decreasing IQ, and new task learning (Gevins, Schaffer, Doyle, et al., 1983; Gevins, Morgan, Bressler, et al., 1987; Gevins, Cutillo, Bressler, et al., 1989; Haier, Siegel, MacLachlan, et al., 1992; Squire, Ojemann, Miezin, et al., 1992), suggesting a relationship between brain bioenergetics and neurophysiologic function. Such a relationship was actually suggested in autism in the first P300 studies, which had concluded that the neurophysiologic alterations in autism reflected the reliance by the brain on less efficient, alternative neural pathways for the processing of information (Novick, Kurtzberg, & Vaughn, 1979; Novick, Kurtzberg, Vaughn, et al., 1980).

In the present study, ^{31}P MRS of the dorsal prefrontal cortex was completed in 11 rigorously diagnosed high functioning autistic adolescents and young adults, and 11 normal control subjects individually matched on age, IQ, gender, and race, and group matched for family socioeconomic level (SES). MRS was performed using the well-described depth pulse localization method (Minshew et al., 1993; Pettegrew, Keshavan, et al., 1991; Pettegrew, Klunk, et al., 1991; Pettegrew et al., 1994 for review). The MRS phospholipid and energy metabolite levels were then compared with indices of the severity and deficits in autism. Specifically, full-scale IQ (FSIQ) and verbal IQ (VIQ) scores and language (composite score, Test of Language Competence) ability were used as overall indicators of relative autism severity (Venter, Lord, & Schopler, 1992). The perseverative error scores from the Wisconsin Card Sorting Test, delayed recall scores from the California Verbal Learning Test, Making Inferences subtest scores from the Test of Language Competence, and Token Test scores were used as indicators of the reasoning, complex memory, and higher order language deficits in autism.

Analysis of these data revealed intergroup differences for two metabolites and a consistent pattern of metabolic correlations with PME, PDE, and PCr across test scores in the autistic subjects, but not the controls. Decreased levels of PCr and esterified ends (α-ATP + α-ADP + dinucleotides + cytidine diphosphocholine and cytidine diphospho-ethanolamine + uridine diphosphosugars) were found for the autistic group. PCr is the most metabolically labile of the high energy phosphate sources. In the absence of alterations in brain pH that would alter the kinetics of the creatine kinase enzyme, this decrease in PCr levels suggests increased utilization of PCr to maintain ATP levels, or a hypermetabolic state. The esterified ends resonance region contains contributions related to bioenergetics, lipid and protein glycosylation, and membrane biosynthesis. In the absence of alterations in the other resonances to which ATP and ADP contribute, the reduction in the esterified ends resonance is more likely to be related to alterations in membrane biosynthesis rather than to bioenergetics.

The most significant findings of the study from a neurobiologic perspective were the pattern of clinical–metabolic correlations. In the autistic group, there was a consistent pattern of significant correlations between PME (membrane building blocks), PDE (membrane degradation products), and PCr levels across all clinical parameters. Specifically, as performance on these instruments declined in the autistic subjects, PCr and PME levels fell and PDE levels rose (see Table 2 and Figs. 8a–e). This pattern of correlations was not present in the age, IQ, gender, race, and SES matched control group. In addition, no significant clinical–metabolic

Table 2 ^{31}P MRS Study of Frontal Cortex in Autism: Metabolic Correlations with Clinical Measures of Severity

		PCr		PME		PDE	
		Aut	Ctrl	Aut	Ctrl	Aut	Ctrl
Full Scale IQ	r	0.92	−0.31	0.44	0.22	−0.76	−0.11
	p	0.0001	NS	NS	NS	0.01	NS
Verbal IQ	r	0.81	−0.26	0.70	0.40	−0.82	−0.14
	p	0.002	NS	0.02	NS	0.002	NS
TOLC	r	0.35	−0.09	−0.65	0.27	0.57	0.00
Composite	p	NS	NS	0.03	NS	NS	NS
Wisc. Card Sort. Test	r	−0.83	−0.18	−0.24	0.14	0.81	0.13
Perservative errors	p	0.01	NS	NS	NS	0.01	NS
CVLT	r	0.79	−0.33	0.33	0.02	−0.65	−0.04
Delayed recall	p	0.004	NS	NS	NS	0.03	NS
Test of Lang. Comp.	r	0.35	−0.09	−0.65	0.27	0.57	0.00
Making Inferences	p	NS	NS	0.03	NS	NS	NS
TOKEN Test	r	0.49	0.31	0.79	0.33	0.75	−0.58
Total score	p	NS	NS	0.003	NS	0.008	NS

Note: Data from 11 individually matched pairs of autistic and normal control subjects.

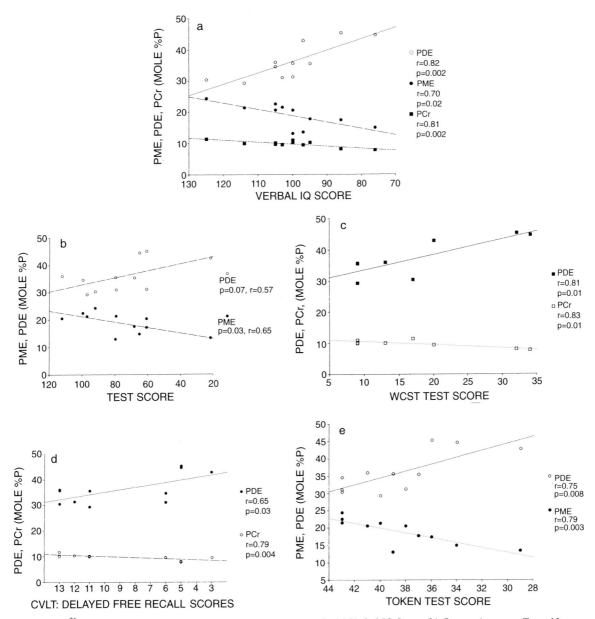

Figure 8 ^{31}P MRS metabolite correlations in autistic subjects with: (a) Verbal IQ Score; (b) Composite score, Test of Language Competence; (c) Perseverative error score, Wisconsin Card Sorting Test; (d) Delayed free recall score, California Verbal Learning Test; and (e) Token Test score.

correlations were found with age in either subject group or with IQ in the control group, suggesting that these findings were not the consequence of age or IQ effects. The positive correlation between falling PCr levels and declining test performance in autism is consistent with a hypermetabolic state. It is noteworthy that the cognitive evoked potential abnormalities in autism have been most prominent in the frontal cortex in autis-

tic subjects with comparable age, IQ, and gender to the declining subjects in this study. In view of the PET and cognitive evoked potential mapping data in normal individuals, suggesting increasing activation of neural circuitry with declining performance, it is possible that the hypermetabolic state demonstrated in this study is a reflection of the neurophysiologic abnormalities documented in autism.

The phospholipid correlations (↑PME–P↓PDE) in the autistic subjects with declining test performance is consistent with undersynthesis and enhanced degradation of brain membranes. This clinical–metabolic pattern in the frontal cortex of these high functioning autistic subjects is furthermore consistent with the predominance of neuropsychologic findings related to frontal lobe dysfunction in these individuals, the truncation in dendritic tree development in limbic structures with extensive frontal connections, and the anterior–posterior maturation of cortex during development, which would presumably leave frontal lobe and higher order processing systems most vulnerable to developmental pathology. The presence of evidence for enhanced degradation or turnover of brain membranes in autism has additional clinical significance, in that approximately ⅓ of autistic children present with regression and loss of previously acquired milestones, and a minority of older autistic children, experience a significant regression in later life. Consistent with MRS evidence of increased brain membrane turnover, Svennerholm and colleagues (Ahlsen, Rosengren, Belfrage, et al., 1993) have reported increased CSF ganglioside levels in autistic and autistic-like (pervasive developmental disorder, not otherwise specified) children. As gangliosides are considered synaptic markers, an increase in their levels suggests increased turnover of synaptic membranes in autism. Svennerholm and colleagues also found a three-fold increase in glial fibrillary acidic protein (GAP) in the cerebrospinal fluid (CSF) in autism. In the absence of gliosis (Bauman & Kemper, 1985; Bauman, 1991), the increase in GAP levels may also reflect increased turnover of synaptic membranes, since all synapses are insulated with astrocytic processes.

In summary, this pilot study provides preliminary evidence of alterations in brain energy and phospholipid metabolism that correlate with clinical deficits. These findings are consistent with a hypermetabolic energy state and undersynthesis and enhanced degradation of brain membranes, and may relate to the neurophysiologic and neuropathologic abnormalities in autism.

2. Metabolic Correlations in Autism as a Function of Information Processing Load

In a recent analysis of data from 8 additional autistic subjects, we investigated the dissociation between high and low information processing load tasks on a neuropsychologic battery in comparison to MRS phospholipid metabolites. As previously mentioned, neuropsychologic data in 85 high functioning autistic and 65 matched normal control subjects has revealed a dissociation between complex and simple tasks, with a generalized pattern of deficits in complex cognitive abilities across domains and sensory modalities, and intact or superior performance on simpler tasks in the same domains. To further explore the significance of this neuropsychologic dissociation in relation to the pathophysiology of autism, we defined two sets of variables—one set reflecting high information processing demand and the second, low information processing demand relative to general level of intellectual function. High information processing load variables included: the perseverative error score from the Wisconsin Card Sorting Test, the total number of moves and total number of problems solved from the Tower of Hanoi, the Logical Memory score from the Weschler Memory Scale, the delayed recall score for the Rey–Osterreith Figure, and the Making Inferences subtest score from the Test of Language Competence. Low information processing load variables from comparable areas of neuropsychologic function were chosen to reflect simpler more automatic skills in these same functional domains. These variables included: the Trails A score, the total error score from the Letter Cancellation test, and the reading decoding and spelling scores from the Kaufman Test of Educational Achievement. The correlations between scores on these instruments and PME and PDE levels in the frontal lobes of these subjects are provided in Table 3.

The preliminary analyses of these clinical–metabolic correlations revealed significant and consistent correlations with PME and PDE for the high information processing load variables, but also equal and opposite correlations with the low information processing variables. In this slightly younger group of autistic subjects, PME and PDE levels increased with increasing severity of the deficits, suggesting increasing production and turnover of brain membranes. This pattern is consistent with the increases in head circumference, gray and white matter on MRI, brain weight at autopsy, and the CSF evidence of increased turnover of synaptic membranes. The relationship between performance on low information processing load variables and the PME–PDE levels is in the opposite direction of the PME–PDE correlations with the high information processing load variables. This inverse relationship of high and low information processing variables to PME–PDE levels is precisely what is observed clinically, which is a tradeoff with developmental progress between the loss of excellence in their savant type simple skills, such as hyperlexia or incidental memory for details, and small gains in language comprehension and reasoning. We have speculated that this tradeoff reflects a neurobiologic relationship during information processing in which a "figure–ground transformation" of incoming environmental stimuli normally results in the emer-

Table 3 Neuropsychologic Correlations with PME and PDE Levels

	Neuropsych. Test Score Format[a]	PME[b]	PDE[c]
High Information Processing Load Variables			
Wisconsin Card Sorting Test: perseverative errors	↓	.69	.47
Tower of Hanoi: total number of moves	↓	.81	.49
Tower of Hanoi: total number solved	↑	−.87	−.45
Test of Language Competence: making inferences	↑	−.41	−.40
WMS–R, Logical Memory [story recall]	↑	−.42	−.06
Rey–Osterrieth Figure: delayed recall	↑	−.42	.12
Low Information Processing Load Variables			
Trails A: seconds	↓	−.03	.10
Letter Cancellation: errors	↓	−.02	−.16
K–TEA: reading decoding	↑	.53	−.26
K–TEA: spelling	↑	.49	.06
WMS–R: visual reproduction	↑	.44	−.28

[a] A ↓ indicates that higher scores are associated with poorer performance; a ↑ indicates higher scores reflect better performance.

[b] PME (phosphomonoesters) are the synthetic building blocks for brain membranes.

[c] PDE (phosphodiesters) are the membrane degradation products.

gence of a concept by suppressing some details. In autism, we suggest that abnormal information processing disturbs the "figure–ground" process, leaving these individuals with both an unusual clarity of memory for details and at the same time a poverty of concepts.

VII. Summary

In summary, the initial studies presented in this chapter demonstrate the potential of ^{31}P MRS for monitoring *in vivo* neuronal membrane organization events during normal brain development and aging, and for detecting pathologic states involving alterations in the synthesis and degradation of brain membranes, and possibly also the metabolic consequences of neurophysiologic alterations involving neural circuitry.

Acknowledgments

The careful and dedicated technical assistance of Evelyn J. Herbert is acknowledged and appreciated. This work was supported by NINDS grant NS33355 to Nancy J. Minshew.

References

Ackerman, J. J., Grove, T. H., Wong, G. G. et al. (1980). Mapping of metabolites in whole animals by 31P NMR using surface coils. *Nature (London), 283,* 167–170.

Ahlsen, G., Rosengren, L., Belfrage, M. et al. (1993). Glial fibrillary acidic protein in the cerebrospinal fluid of children with autism and other neuropsychiatric disorders. *Biological Psychiatry, 33,* 734–743.

Bauman, M. L. (1991). Microscopic neuroanatomic abnormalities in autism. Supplement to *Pediatrics, 87*(5), 791–796.

Bauman, M. L., & Kemper, T. L. (1985). Histoanatomic observations of the brain in early infantile autism. *Neurology, 35,* 866–874.

Bloch, F., Hansen, W. W., & Packard, M. E. (1946). Nuclear induction. *Physics Review 69,* 127.

Bolinger, L., & Lenkinski, R. E. (1992). Localization in clinical NMR spectroscopy. In L. J. Berliner and J. Reuben (Eds.), *Biological magnetic resonance 11 In Vivo spectroscopy* (pp. 1–53). New York: Plenum.

Bottomley, P. A., Cousins, J. P., Pendrey, D. L., et al. (1992). Alzheimer dementia: Quantification of energy metabolism and mobile phosphoesters with P-31 NMR spectroscopy. *Radiology, 183,* 695–699.

Brown, G. G., Levins, S. R., Gorell, J. M., et al (1989). In vivo ^{31}P NMR profiles of Alzheimer's disease and multiple subcortical infarct dementia. *Neurology, 39,* 1423–1427.

Carlsson A. (1988). The current status of the dopamine hypothesis of schizophrenia. *Neuropsychopharmacology, 1,* 179–186.

Clarke, P. G. (1985). Neuronal death in the development of the vertebrate nervous system. *Trends in Neurosciences 8,* 345–349.

Cowan, W. M., Fawcett, J. W., O'Leary, D. D., et al. (1984). Regressive events in neurogenesis. *Science, 225,* 1258–1265.

Cuenod, C., Kaplan, D. B., Michot, J., et al. (1995). Phospholipid abnormalities in early Alzheimer's disease. *Archives of Neurology 52,* 89–94.

Dickinson, W. C. (1950). Collisions of the second order and their effect on the field of the positive column of a glow discharge and mixture of the rare gases. *Physics Review 77,* 736.

Farrar, T. C. (1989). Principles of pulse NMR spectroscopy. In J. W. Pettegrew (Ed.), *NMR: Principles and applications to biomedical research* (pp. 1–36). New York: Springer-Verlag.

Gevins, A. S., Schaffer, R. E., Doyle, J. C., Cutillo, B. A., Tannehill, R. F., & Bressler, S. (1983). Shadows of thought: Shifting lateralization of human brain electrical patterns during brief visuomotor task. *Science, 220,* 97–99.

Gevins, A. S., Morgan, N. H., Bressler, S. L., Cutillo, B. R., White, R. M., Illes, J., Greer, D. S., Doyle, J. C., & Zeitlin, G. M. (1987). Human neuroelectric patterns predict performance accuracy. *Science, 235,* 580–585.

Gevins, A. S., Cutillo, B. A., Bressler, S. L., et al. (1989). Event-related covariances during a bimanual visuomotor task. II. Preparation and feedback. *Electroencephalogram Clinical Neurophysiology, 74,* 147–160.

Glonek, T., Kopp, S. J., Kot, E., Pettegrew, J. W., et al. (1982). P-31 nuclear magnetic resonance analysis of brain: The perchloric acid extract spectrum. *Journal of Neurochemistry, 39,* 1210–19.

Haier, R. J., Siegel, B. V., MacLachlan, A., et al. (1992). Regional glucose metabolic changes after learning a complex visuospatial/motor task: A positron emission tomographic study. *Brain Research, 570,* 134–143.

Kilby, P. M., Bolas, N. M., & Radda, G. K. (1991). 31P-NMR study of brain phospholipid structures *in vivo. Biochimica Biophysica Acta, 1085,* 257–264.

Klausner, J. D., Sweeney, J. P., Deck, M. D., et al. (1992). Clinical correlates of cerebral ventricular enlargement in schizophrenia. *Journal of Nervous and Mental Diseases, 180,* 407.

Klunk, W. E., Xu, C. J., Panchalingam, K., et al. (1994). Analysis of magnetic resonance spectra by mole percent: Comparison to absolute units. *Neurobiology of Aging, 15,* 133–140.

Lim, K. O., Pauly, J., Webb, P., et al. (1994). Short TE phosphorus spectroscopy using a spin-echo pulse. *Magnetic Resonance in Medicine 32,* 98–103.

McClure, R. J., Panchalingam, K., Klunk, W. E., et al. (1996). Magnetic resonance spectroscopy of neural tissue. *Methods in Neuroscience, 30,* 178–208.

McIlwain, H., & Bachelard, H. S. (1985). *Biochemistry and the central nervous system,* (5th ed., pp. 41–43). New York: Churchill Livingstone.

Minshew, N. J. (1996). Autism. In R. D. Adams and M. Victor (Eds.), *Principles of child neurology.* pp. 1713–1730. New York: McGraw-Hill.

Minshew, N. J., & Goldstein, G. (1993). Is autism an amnesic disorder?: Evidence from the California Verbal Learning Test. *Neuropsychology, 7,* 1–8.

Minshew, N. J., Goldstein, G., Dombrowski, S. M., Panchalingam, K., & Pettegrew, J. W. (1993). A preliminary ³¹P MRS study of autism: Evidence for undersynthesis and increased degradation of brain membranes. *Biological Psychiatry, 33,* 762–773.

Minshew, N. J., Goldstein, G., & Siegel, D. J. (1995). Speech and language in high functioning autistic individuals. *Neuropsychology, 9*(2), 255–261.

Minshew, N. J., Panchalingam, L., Dombrowski, S. M., & Pettegrew, J. W. (1992). Developmentally regulated changes in brain membrane metabolism. *Biological Psychiatry, 31*(5A Suppl.), 62A.

Minshew, N. J., Sweeney, J. A., & Furman, J. M. (1995). Evidence for a primary neocortical system's abnormality in autism (abstract). *Society for Neuroscience Abstracts, 21,* 735.

Murphy, D. G. M., Bottomley, P. A., Salerno, J., et al. (1992). *In vivo* brain glucose and phosphorus metabolism in Alzheimer's disease (abstract). *Society for Neuroscience, 18,* 567.

Nasrallah, H. A., & Pettegrew, J. W. (Eds.) (1995). *NMR spectroscopy in psychiatric brain disorders* Washington, D. C.: American Psychiatric Press.

Novick, B., Kurtzberg, D., & Vaughn, H. G., Jr. (1979). An electrophysiologic indication of defective information storage in childhood autism. *Psychiatry Research, 1,* 101–108.

Novick, B., Kurtzberg, D., Vaughn, H. G., Jr., et al. (1980). An electrophysiologic indication of auditory processing defects in autism. *Psychiatry Research, 3,* 107–114.

Oppenheim, R. W. (1985). Naturally occurring cell death during neural development. *Trends in Neurosciences, 8,* 487–493.

Panchalingham, K., Pettegrew, J. W., Strychor, S., et al. (1990). Effect of normal aging on membrane phospholipid metabolism by 31P *in vivo* NMR spectroscopy. *Society for Neuroscience Abstracts, 16,* 843.

Petroff, O. A. C., Prichard, J. W., Behar, K. L., et al. (1985). Cerebral intracellular pH by ³¹P nuclear magnetic resonance spectroscopy. *Neurology, 35,* 781–788.

Pettegrew, J. W. (1989a). Molecular insights into Alzheimer's disease. *Calcium Membranes, Aging, and Alzheimer's Disease Annals of the New York Academy of Sciences, 568,* 5–28.

Pettegrew, J. W. (Ed.) (1989b). *Nuclear magnetic resonance: The principles and applications of NMR spectroscopy and imaging to biomedical research.* New York: Springer-Verlag.

Pettegrew, J. W. (1991). Nuclear magnetic resonance: Principles and applications to neuroscience research. In F. Boller & J. Grafman (Eds.), *Handbook of neuropsychology* (Vol. 5, pp. 39–56). Amsterdam: Elsevier.

Pettegrew, J. W., Keshavan, M. S., Panchalingam, K., et al. (1991). Alterations in brain high-energy phosphate and membrane phospholipid metabolism in first-episode, drug-naive schizophrenics. *Archives of General Psychiatry, 48,* 563–568.

Pettegrew, J. W., Keshavan, M. S., & Minshew, N. J. (1993). 31P nuclear magnetic resonance spectroscopy: Neurodevelopment and schizophrenia. *Schizophrenia Bulletin, 19*(1), 35–53.

Pettegrew, J. W., Klunk, W. E., McClure, K., et al. (1991). Phosphomonoesters, phospholipids and high-energy phosphates in Alzheimer's disease: Alterations and physiological significance. In Z. S. Khachaturian & J. P. Blass (Eds.), *Alzheimer's disease: New treatment strategies* (pp. 193–212). New York: Dekker.

Pettegrew, J. W., Klunk, W. E., Panchalingam, K., et al. (1993). The diagnosis and prevention of Alzheimer's disease: The role of 31P NMR. In M. Nicolini, P. F. Zatta, & B. Corain (Eds.) *Advances in the Biosciences Alzheimer's Disease and Related Disorders* (Vol. 87, pp. 375–381). London: Pergamon.

Pettegrew, J. W., Minshew, N. J., Cohen, M. M., et al. (1984). P-31 NMR changes in Alzheimer's and Huntington's disease brain (abstract). *Neurology, 34*(Suppl. 1), 281.

Pettegrew, J. W., Panchalingam, K., Klunk, W. E., et al. (1994). Alterations of cerebral metabolism in probable Alzheimer's disease; A preliminary study. *Neurobiology of Aging, 15,* 117–132.

Pettegrew, J. W., Panchalingam, K., Wither, G., et al. (1990). Changes in brain energy and phospholipid metabolism during development and aging in the Fischer 344 rat. *Journal of Neuropathology and Experimental Neurology, 49,* 237–249.

Pettegrew, J. W., Withers, G., Panchalingam, K., et al. (1988). Considerations for brain pH assessment by ³¹P NMR. *Magnetic Resonance Imaging, 6,* 135–142.

Pittman, R., & Oppenheim, R. W. (1979). Cell death of motoneurons in the chick embryo spinal cord. IV. Evidence that a functional neuromuscular interaction is involved in the regulation of naturally occurring cell death and the stabilization of synapses. *Journal of Computer Neurology, 187,* 425–446.

Proctor, W. G., & Yu, F. C. (1950). The disorder of NMR frequency in chemical compounds. *Physics Review, 77,* 717.

Purcell, E. M., Torrey, H. C., & Pound, R. V. (1946). Resonance absorption by nuclear magnetic moments in solids. *Physics Review, 69,* 37.

Siesjo, B. (1978). Brain energy metabolism. In B. Siesjo (Ed.), *Brain energy metabolism* (Chap. 1 and 2). New York: Wiley.

Silverstein, R. M., Bassler, G. C., & Morrill, T. C. (1991). *Spectrometric identification of organic compounds.* New York: Wiley.

Smith, C. D., Gallenstein, L. G., Layton, W. J., et al. (1993). ^{31}P magnetic resonance spectroscopy in Alzheimer's and Pick's disease. *Neurobiology of Aging, 14,* 85–92.

Squire, L. R., Ojemann, J. G., Miezin, F. M., et al. (1992). Activation of the hippocampus in normal humans: A functional anatomical study of memory. *Proceedings of the National Academy of Sciences. 89,* 1837–1841.

Stanley, J. A., Williamson, P. C., Drost, D. J., et al. (1993). *In vivo* 31P MRS of schizophrenics: A reliability study. *Schizophrenia Research, 9,* 210.

Stanley, J. A., Williamson, P. C., Drost, D. J., et al. (1994). Membrane phospholipid metabolism and schizophrenia: An *in vivo* 31P-MR spectroscopy study. *Schizophrenia Research, 13,* 209–215.

Vance, D. E. (1991). Phospholipid metabolism and cell signalling in eucaryotes. In D. E. Vance and J. Vance (Eds.), *Biochemistry of lipids, lipoproteins and membranes* (Vol. 20, pp. 205–240). New York: Elsevier.

Venter, A., Lord, C., & Schopler, E. (1992). A follow-up study of high-functioning autistic children. *Journal on Child Psychology and Psychiatry 3,* 489–507.

Woessner, D. E. (1989). Relaxation theory with applications to biological studies. In J. W. Pettegrew (Ed.), *NMR: Principles and applications to biomedical research.* New York: Springer-Verlag.

9

Multimodal Assessments of Developing Neural Networks Integrating fMRI, PET, MRI, and EEG/MEG

Robert W. Thatcher

Medical Research Services, VA Medical Center, Bay Pines, Florida 33504, and Departments of Neurology and Radiology, University of South Florida College of Medicine, Tampa, Florida 33612

I. Introduction

Medical neuroimaging has rapidly evolved in the last few years. High resolution, three-dimensional (3D) tomographic information can now be obtained in a routine manner with magnetic resonance imaging (MRI) and computerized tomography (CT). Four-dimensional tomographic imaging of blood flow and metabolic information (i.e., space and time) can be obtained from the registration of position emission tomography (PET), single photon computed emission tomography (SPECT) and functional MRI (fMRI) images to conventional MRI images (Thatcher, Hallett, Zeffiro, John, & Huerta, 1994). However, the latter techniques have relatively poor temporal resolutions on the order of seconds and minutes and thus are unable to resolve the millisecond interactions of neuronal function. It is important for the field of developmental neuroimaging that methods be developed to visualize and quantify the fine temporal details involved in dynamic neural network development. For example, through the application of noninvasive high spatial and temporal resolution imaging methods, some of the most critical issues in human brain development may be brought under the scrutiny of the scientist. Issues concerned with linear versus nonlinear synaptogensis, changes in the strength and number of brain connections at different ages, or the presence or absence of cyclic reorganization processes may be ad-

dressed through the use of these new technologies. The purpose of this chapter is to discuss some of the methods involved in the development and application of multimodal registration of electroencephalography (EEG) and magnetoencephalography (MEG) with fMRI and conventional MRI. It is only by improving the temporal resolution of measures of neural network dynamics that the greatest benefits of neuroimaging can be realized.

II. Tomographic EEG/MEG and Multimodal Registration

The MRI and fMRI provide spatial resolutions on the order of 1mm. However, the MRI provides no temporal information, while the fMRI provides temporal information limited by hemodynamics, which is on the order of several seconds. An important goal for future developmental neuroimaging technologies is to create a marriage of different imaging modalities, whereby the strengths and weaknesses can combine and cancel to provided both high temporal and high spatial resolutions. Estimates of the spatial and temporal resolution of various imaging technologies are shown in Table 1. It can be seen that the noninvasive but rate-limited fMRI has a time resolution on the order of ten seconds with a spatial resolution of about 1 mm. In contrast, the EEG/MEG has a time resolution

Table 1

	Time Resolution	Spatial Resolution	Extent of Brain	Suitability for Humans	Network Dynamics
RCBF					
Xenon	10^1sec	1 cm	Cortex	Yes	No
Optical	10^0sec	1 cm	Surface	No	No
MRI	10^1sec	.1 cm	All	Yes	No
PET					
0^{15}	10^1sec	.5 cm	All	Limited	No
2DG	10^3sec	.5 cm	All	Limited	No
Single Unit	10^{-5}sec	10^{-3}cm	All	No	Yes
Multiple Unit	10^{-5}sec	10^{-2}cm	All	Very Limited	Yes
ERP Invasive	10^{-4}sec	10^{-2}cm	All	Very Limited	Yes
ERP Noninvasive	10^{-4}sec	5 cm	Cortex	Yes	Yes
EEG/MEG	10^{-4}sec	5 cm	Cortex	Yes	Yes

of about 1 millisecond and a spatial resolution of about 5 cm (assuming the proper density of scalp electrodes, see Nunez, 1981 and Gevins, Cutillo, DuRousseau, Le, Leong, & Smith, 1994 for details). Thus, the marriage of the fMRI (and conventional MRI) technology with EEG/MEG will maximize each modality's strengths while minimizing each modality's weaknesses. However, creating such a marriage is not a simple and straightforward process. There are a number of technical problems involved in identifying the sources of EEG/MEG events. Two recent solutions to these problems are: (1) The multimodal registration of the sources of EEG/MEG and evoked potentials which, by themselves, are not tomographic and, (2) low resolution electromagnetic tomography in which blurred EEG source locations are registered to a 3D brain coordinate system. For both of these solutions, when the sources of the EEG/MEG are properly registered to conventional tomographic imaging methods such as MRI, CT, PET and fMRI (Thatcher, Toro, Pflieger & Hallett 1994; Toro, Wang, Zeffiro, Thatcher, & Hallett, 1994; Wang, Toro, Wasserman, Zeffiro, Thatcher, & Hallett, 1994; Simpson, Bellevue, Foxe, Baker, & Vaughan, 1993; Simpson, Foxe, Vaughan, Mehta, & Schroeder, 1996), then the possibilities for tomographic EEG/MEG imaging immediately arise. For example, the root concept of "tomography" is "tomo" which is a "plane," "cut" or "section." Three dimensions are achieved when sections are placed in volumetric registration. It is in this manner that the two solutions mentioned above provide information about the 3D address of structures, events, and physiological

processes. While EEG/MEG may not be 3D in the same way that PET and MRI are, nonetheless, EEG/MEG can satisfy the dictionary definitions of tomo and tomography by providing a 3D address of physiological events. It is in this sense that the term "tomographic EEG/MEG" is used. One purpose of the present chapter is to explore the application of time domain analyses to the study of the development of human neural networks by presenting an example of the "tomographic" or 3D aspect of EEG sources whose spatial coordinates are corroborated by independent imaging techniques as well as by experimental design. It will be shown that the coregistration of these techniques may provide for spatial tomographic resolutions of the sources of EEG on the order of 1 cm, and time resolutions of interactions between EEG sources on the order of milliseconds. Once the uncertainty about the sources of EEG are minimized through independent registration with PET and/or fMRI, then the possibility of real-time analyses of the development of neural network switching during movement, perception, and cognition is available.

This chapter is not intended as a review of multimodal registration techniques such as are provided in other publications (Thatcher, Hallett, et al., 1994), nor is it a review of dipole source localization methods or model building. Instead, the purpose of this chapter is to discuss recent advances in "tomographic EEG/MEG" and their potential application to studies of human brain development, by reviewing examples and advancements in the multimodal registration of EEG, PET, and MRI, with special emphasis on the time domain analyses of the human brain. I refer to this new advancement as "tomographic EEG/MEG" since it involves a volumetric and sectional analysis of the location of the sources of the surface EEG which can be coregistered and strongly corroborated with structural imaging techniques such as the MRI and CT, as well as functional imaging techniques such as PET, SPECT, and fMRI.

Because our primary goal is the exploitation of the time domain, the initial conservative criteria for defining "Tomographic EEG/MEG" are: (1) Dipole sources involving primary sensory and/or motor systems must be involved; (2) The spatial coordinates of the dipole source analyses must be constrained by experimental design, established knowledge of functional neuroanatomy, and/or coregistration with PET or fMRI; and (3) the functional imaging technologies (i.e., fMRI, PET, SPECT, etc.) must be coregistered with conventional tomographic methods such as MRI and/or CT. I currently must limit dipole sources to the primary sensory and motor cortical regions because it is only in these areas that the source generators are sufficiently understood so that a priori constraints can be meaningfully used. For the moment I will restrict myself to the above conservative criteria and instead focus on some of the benefits to be derived through time series analyses of 4D or tomographic EEG/MEG. I expect that in the future, additional imaging and analytical advances will broaden the scope and range of tomographic EEG/MEG so that sources other than the primary sensory and motor systems can be included.

As mentioned previously, this is a rapidly developing field and specific techniques are changing almost weekly; thus, it is beyond the scope of this chapter to discuss in detail all of the methodologies for dipole source localization or all of the techniques for multimodal registration of EEG, PET, and MRI. In order to provide a practical perspective of the exploitation of the time domain in developing neuroimaging, a specific example will be presented using the coregistration of EEG, PET, and MRI in a study of voluntary finger movements. In this way, the reader can gain an understanding of some of the steps involved in the process of tomographic EEG/MEG using the noninvasive fMRI.

III. Summary of Concepts, Issues, and Procedures

A. EEG/MEG Recordings

The laws of electrodynamics elucidate the relations between electricity and magnetism and establish the equivalence and differences between EEG and MEG

(Nunez, 1981). Electric potentials and magnetic fields are precisely linked, as described by Maxwell's equations, and provide complementary information when recorded from the cranium. In general, all ionic current flow is accompanied by a magnetic flux that surrounds the current at a direction perpendicular to the current flow, with the flow of the current determined by the electrical potential and resistance of the tissues surrounding the sources and sinks. EEG electrical currents are conducted through the various tissues of the brain and are greatly influenced by the different conductivities of the tissue boundaries of scalp, skull, cerebral fluids, and parenchyma. In contrast, MEG offers the advantage of not being influenced by volume conduction and different tissue conductivities because the magnetic fields form a circle around the local sources from which they are generated. However, there are several negative aspects of MEG. One is the expense, a second is susceptibility to noise, and the third is MEG's insensitivity to radially oriented dipoles (i.e., a significant proportion of the cortical dipoles are oriented at right angles to the scalp surface, while MEG is primarily sensitive to tangentially oriented dipoles). In spite of the volume conductive nature of EEG, recent advances in digital signal processing have demonstrated the value of EEG dipole analyses and indicate a bright future for computerized EEG in general. It remains to be seen whether MEG will have a similar bright future when used alone, although the combination of EEG and MEG provides an important complimentary analysis. Therefore, in this chapter, primary emphasis will be placed on the EEG, while keeping in mind that much of what is discussed in this chapter pertains to both EEG and MEG.

The crucial factor in 4D tomographic EEG is the use of a sufficiently dense array of recording channels in a properly designed experiment using the appropriate dipole localization model. The relationship between the density of recording electrodes and the spatial resolution of dipole sources is discussed in several studies (Nunez, 1981; Gevins et al., 1994).

B. Skull and Scalp Measurements

A critical step in 4D EEG is coregistering the scalp location of the EEG electrodes to the scalp MRI. The most commonly used method is 3D digitization of the scalp electrodes and 3D digitization of a few skull landmarks (e.g., inion, nasion, auricles, canthus, etc.). A more recent and less expensive method involves photogrammatic analyses of the scalp and EEG electrodes in three dimensions. Another and simpler method is to carefully measure skull landmarks during the EEG electrode setup procedure using the 10–20 system of electrode placement (e.g., inion–nasion, auricle–to–auricle distance, canthus–meatal distance, canthus–auricle distance, etc.). These landmarks are then identified in the same subject's MRI, and the EEG electrode locations are registered to the MRI assuming an accurate and proportional 10–20 electrode placement. Once the 3D scalp location of the electrodes is determined, then one can coregister the EEG addresses to the scalp image in the MRI, using standard least squares fitting routines (Wang, Toro, Wasserman, Zeffiro, Thatcher, & Hallett, 1994; Pelizzari, Chen, Spelbring, Weichselbaum, & Chen, 1989). This step places the scalp EEG electrodes in registration with the underlying cerebral cortex. The magnitude of acceptable error for these different techniques has not yet been determined. Several studies indicate that coherent functional neural activity from a given brain region is seldom less than 1 cm in diameter (Thatcher, Toro, et al., 1994; Gray, Konig, Engal, & Singer, 1989; Eckhorn, Bauer, Jordan, Brosch, Kruse, Munk et al., 1988). Thus, accumulative errors of 1 cm $\pm$ 5 mm is close to acceptable.

C. Dipole Source Localization

The field of dipole source localization (DSL) is rapidly evolving with the recent emergence of many new and accurate techniques. Briefly, all of the DSL techniques require a surface and volume model by which the inverse and forward dipole solutions can be computed. DSL methods rely upon an equivalent dipole model, which assumes the presence of current flows between positive and negative poles in a large population of synchronous and similarly oriented pyramidal cells. The equivalent dipole source is determined using a least squares iteration method, in which a mathematical dipole model is moved around until the best possible solution to the distribution of scalp surface potentials is obtained. The inverse fields are then correlated with the forward solution to provide an estimate of the reliability of the fit of the scalp surface potentials to the model. The earliest DSL techniques involved a single sphere model, while later DSL techniques used a two and three sphere model to account for scalp, skull, and dura surfaces. More recently, realistic head models have been used in which the actual brain contours, rather than an idealistic geometric model, are used to compute the DSL (Roth, Balish, Gorbach, & Sato, 1993; Gevins & Bressler, 1988). In addition to the geometric models, DSL can be computed using a single dipole assumption or multiple dipole assumptions, a fixed point in time or a covariance of time points, and so on (Scherg and Berg, 1991). Finally, new and improved computational techniques such as the minimum norm technique (Scherg, 1992;

Wang, Williamson, & Kaufman, 1992; Wang, Kaufman, & Williamson, 1993) and regional analyses have been tested (Scherg, 1992). While progress has been made in improved accuracy and computational efficiency, DSL techniques are still quite tricky and require very careful applications of models, experimental designs, and procedures. For example, a spherical model fits the crown or crest of the cortex fairly well, but is a poor fit of the orbital frontal and basal temporal regions (Roth et al., 1993). Therefore, when one uses spherical models, an experimental design is recommended to optimize on the geometric fit of the model, such as a motor movement experiment or self-initiated mental practice that involves activation of the crown or crest of the cortex (Toro et al., 1994).

The DSL step is another critical step in the 4D tomographic EEG analysis because it provides a 3D or tomographic address for the sources of the surface EEG. The 3D addresses of the EEG sources can be registered to the MRI using the same least squares fitting techniques mentioned in the previous section (see reference Wang et al., 1994 for technical details).

D. Spatial Constraints and Independent Validation

With proper DSL modeling and experimental designs, it is possible to derive accurate and realistic dipole sources. For example, a spherical model consistently produces dipoles in the hand region of the motor cortex when subjects perform a hand movement (Toro, Matsumoto, Deuschl, Roth, & Hallett, 1993; Toro et al., 1994). This is prima facie validation of the location of the EEG dipole sources based solely on experimental design. However, in this new age of multimodal neural imaging, we can provide additional confidence about the location and orientation of the EEG dipole sources by independently validating the sources using PET or fMRI.

E. Psuedoinverse Calculations of Tomographic EEG

Once the location and orientation of the dipole sources of the EEG or MEG have been identified using DSL methods and corroborated by experimental designs, PET, or fMRI, then a simple mathematical technique can be applied to create a new time series from the corroborated dipole sources themselves (Thatcher, Toro, & Hallett, 1993a; 1993b; Thatcher, Toro, et al., 1994). This is a noninvasive equivalent to recording EEG from an implanted macroelectrode. The technique to accomplish this is called the "pseudoinverse" technique, which is one of a family of matrix manipulations to find the values of an unknown variable (Penrose, 1955). For example, if we know the 3D location and orientation of the dipole sources, then we can mathematically solve for the only unknown, that is, the amplitude at each instant in time. This procedure creates a new time series, which is a dipole EEG source that accounts for a significant amount of the variance of the surface EEG (e.g., > 95%).

Once a new dipole time series is created for each of the corroborated dipoles, then standard electrophysiological analyses can be performed on the dipole EEG, much as is done for the surface EEG. For example, coherence and phase analyses of the dipole EEG can be conducted to reveal the temporal dynamics of neural network coupling and decoupling processes that underlie human motor movements (Thatcher et al., 1993a; 1993b; Thatcher, Toro, et al., 1994).

Plate 16 is a diagrammatic chart of these summary concepts. Figure 1 shows estimates of error expected using different modeling (A) and registration (B) techniques.

IV. Instantaneous Coherence and Phase

Measurements of dynamic changes in the magnitude of neural network coupling require high temporal resolution. The discrete Wigner–Ville spectral distribution is one method that has been used to obtain high temporal resolution of changes in EEG covariance and phase (Gevins, Cutillo, Bressler, Morgan, White, Illes, et al., 1989a, 1989b; Gevin et al., 1994). This method, however, is computationally demanding and often difficult to interpret. In this chapter, we present a simple and easily implemented method to compute high temporal resolution EEG coherence and phase using the method of complex demodulation. We refer to this method as "instantaneous coherence and phase" or "event-related coherence and phase," since coherence and phase are explicitly evaluated in the time domain. This technique is distinctly different from frequency domain analyses associated with the Fourier transform, which is defined by an infinite inte-

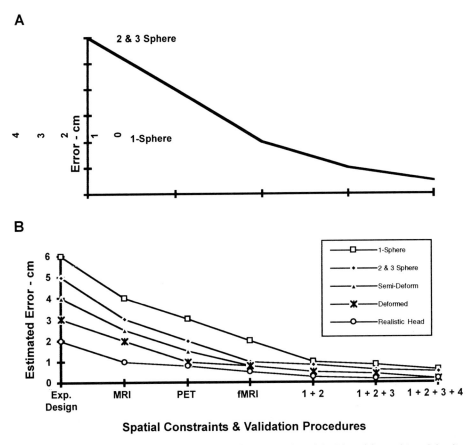

Figure 1 Estimates of error in centimeters for different head models (A) and for multimodal validation procedures (B), in which different images and EEG dipoles are placed into registration. These are only gross estimates of error based upon a survey of the literature.

gral over the time domain. In the latter analyses, integration precludes the ability to evaluate a signal at a specific instant in time.

It is also important to distinguish between the concept of "event-related coherence and phase" (ERCP) and the concept of "event-related average potential" (ERP). The latter involves the computation of an average or time invariant "signal" that is embedded in the background EEG which is usually treated as "noise." The background EEG, which is not time locked to the initiating stimulus, tends to cancel over repeated trials, while the time locked signal tends to emerge in the ERP. The trial by trial covariance of electrophysiological activity recorded in different channels is explicitly ignored by the ERP technique. In contrast, the computation of "event related coherence and phase" involves the use of a complex cross-correlation coefficient which explicitly computes the trial by trial covariance between channels while ignoring the "event related average potential." Thus, the ERCP and ERP are complementary analyses in which the averaged potential within and between channels could approach zero, while the coherence between channels could be high, and vice versa. The mathematical details of the computation of complex demodulation and instantaneous coherence and phase are given elsewhere (Otnes and Enochson, 1988; Thatcher, Toro, et al., 1994).

V. Neural Network Switching during Motor Movements

Instantaneous coherence and phase were computed from 32 channels of EEG obtained during a self-paced voluntary finger movement task (Thatcher et al., 1993b; Thatcher, Toro, et al., 1994; Toro et al., 1994). The computation was over 10 msec samples of EEG, from −600 msec premovement to +500 msec postmovement (i.e., 60 premovement samples + 50 postmovement samples) across 134 movement-related epochs. The DC (direct current) offset was removed from each trial by computing a mean value for the first 200 sample points and then subtracting the mean from each sample point. The complex demodulation filter was initialized at the beginning of each trial, then the sample points between −3000 msec and −600 msec were used as an extended warmup period for the filter.

Figure 2 shows some of the waveforms elicited during the self-paced voluntary finger movement task. The Bereitschaftpotential (BP), the negative slope (NS′), the peak of the NS′ (pNS′), and the frontal peak of the motor potential (fpMP) are indicated. Plate 17 shows the dipole source moments for the three equiva-

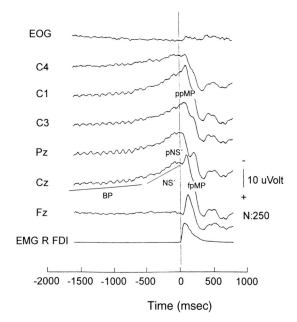

Figure 2 Waveform morphology of the movement response cortical potential (MRCP) elicited by self-paced voluntary finger abductions in the subject of this study ($N = 250$). The BP (Bereitschaftpotential), the negative slope (NS′), the peak of the NS′ (i.e., pNS′), the parietal peak of the motor potential (ppMP), the frontal peak of the motor potential (fpMP), and the FDI first dorsal interosis electromyogram EMG are shown. (Adapted from Thatcher et al., 1994.)

lent sources, which accounted for approximately 96% of the variance of the scalp measured waveforms elicited during the task. The arrows show the latency interval over which the dipole source localizations were computed. Figure 3 consists of head diagrams showing the locations of the three sources.

A. Multimodal Registration Procedures

The subject's head surface was used as a common framework to integrate the three types of data (i.e., EEG, MRI, and PET). The multimodal registration procedure was a four step process. First, the scalp surface and the location of each of the 29 electrodes were determined with a 3D magnetic digitizer. Second, the digitized scalp surface was registered with the scalp contour obtained from the same subject's MRI. Third, the three equivalent dipole sources determined by the BESA (Brain Electrical Source Analysis) program were mapped into the MRI coordinate system defined by the registered MRI and digitized scalp. Fourth, PET images obtained from the same subject undergoing the same motor movements were then superimposed on mapped MRIs by registering the brain contours ob-

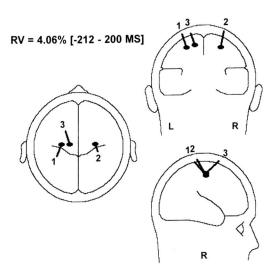

RV = 4.06% [-212 - 200 MS]

Figure 3 Dipole source analyses of the movement related cortical potentials (MRCPs) shown in Plate 16. The three dipole solutions over the latencies between −212 msec and +200 msec were calculated with two sources located on each side of the best fitting sphere (D1 = contralateral and D2 = ipsilateral) and one source (D3) located near to the SMA. These three sources accounted for approximately 96% of the variance of the MRCP.

tained from both the MRI and PET (see reference Wang et al., 1994 for further details).

B. Multimodal Registration of Equivalent Dipoles, PET, and MRI

Plate 18 shows the multimodal registration of PET, MRI and EEG dipoles. (A) shows the location of the ipsilateral motor cortex dipole two (D2) with respect to the registered MRI and PET. This equivalent dipole source registered within approximately 10 mm of the center of the active PET region located in the anterior bank of the ipsilateral central sulcus, near to the hand region. (B) shows the location of the contralateral motor cortex dipole one (D1). This equivalent dipole source registered within less than 3 mm of the center of the active PET region located in the anterior bank of the contralateral central sulcus, near to the hand region. (C) shows the location of the contralateral supplemental motor area (SMA) dipole three (D3). This equivalent dipole source registered within approximately 6 mm of the center of the active PET region located in the contralateral supplemental motor area.

These analyses show that there was relatively good coregistration between the location of the three equivalent dipoles and the independently obtained PET activation regions. In this way, the 3D or tomographic location of the EEG dipoles were corroborated by both experimental design (i.e., located in the hand region of the motor cortex, etc.) and by the PET scan.

C. Instantaneous Coherence between the Pseudoinverse Derived Dipole Time Series

Figure 4 shows the results of the instantaneous coherence analyses among the time series computed for the various combinations of the three dipoles (i.e., using the pseudoinverse procedure, see Section II.E). Although changes in coherence as a function of time were noted in the center frequency range from 3 to 25 Hz, the strongest effects were seen in the theta frequency band (i.e., 4 to 7 Hz). As seen in Figure 4(A), for dipoles 1 and 2, there was a bimodal change in theta coherence between −600 msec and −300 msec involving first a decline, then an increase, in the magnitude of coherence. This was followed by a relatively steady state level of coherence from −300 msec to 0 msec, after which there was an abrupt decrease in coherence between 0 msec and +50 msec postmovement. A slow recovery or increase in coherence was noted between +50 msec and 500 msec postmovement. In Figure 4(B), the coherence analyses for dipoles 1 and 3 were different than the analyses for dipoles 1 and 2. For example, there was a slow increase in coherence beginning at approximately −600 msec and reaching a peak at approximately −50 msec, after which there was a sudden drop in coherence just prior to movement (i.e., approximately −25 msec). During the postmovement period, coherence between dipoles 1 and 3 showed a marked increase, reaching a peak at approximately +200 msec and then declining sharply.

An inverse relationship was evident between the coherence trajectories from dipoles 1 and 3 and those from dipoles 2 and 3, as shown in Figure 4(C). That is, dipoles 2 and 3 exhibited a decrease in coherence between approximately −300 msec and −50 msec, after which there was a sudden increase in coherence just prior to movement (i.e., approximately −25 msec). During the postmovement period, coherence between dipoles 2 and 3 exhibited a decline, followed by a marked increase at approximately +200 msec.

D. Instantaneous Phase between the Pseudoinverse Derived Dipole Time Series

Figures 5(A) and (B) show a 180° phase reversal between the pseudoinverse derived time series from dipoles 1 and 2, and that from dipoles 1 and 3 during the premovement period. A rapid shift in phase from 180° to approximately 90° between dipoles 1 and 2 occurred at approximately +50 msec postmovement.

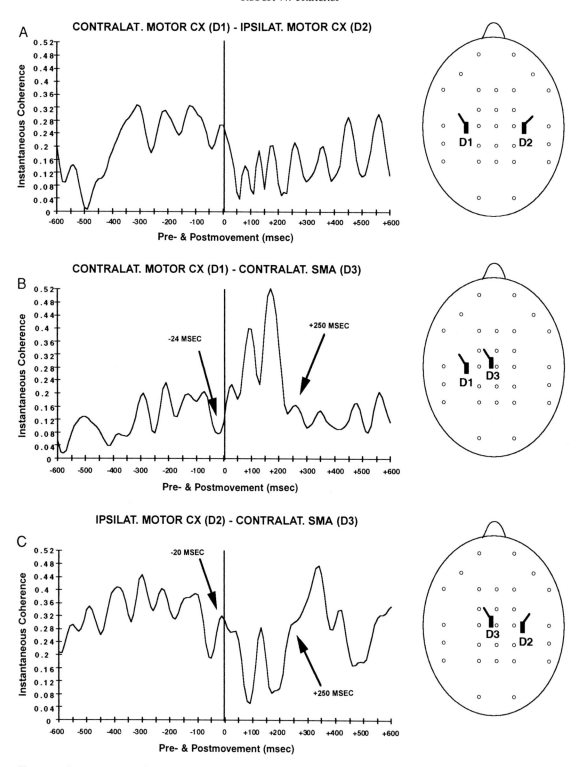

Figure 4 Instantaneous coherence (10 msec resolution) between the pseudoinverse derived dipole time series using a center frequency of 4.25 Hz and a bandwidth of 3.5 Hz. Instantaneous coherence on the y-axis is plotted against pre- and postmovement time (msec) on the x-axis. On the right side of the figure are diagrammatic representations of the location of the dipoles. (A) Instantaneous coherence between the ipsilateral motor cortex (D2) and the contralateral motor cortex (D1). (B) Instantaneous coherence between the ipsilateral motor cortex (D2) and the contralateral supplemental motor area or SMA (D3). (C) Instantaneous coherence between the contralateral motor cortex (D2) and the contralateral supplemental motor area or SMA (D3). (Adapted from Thatcher et al., 1994.)

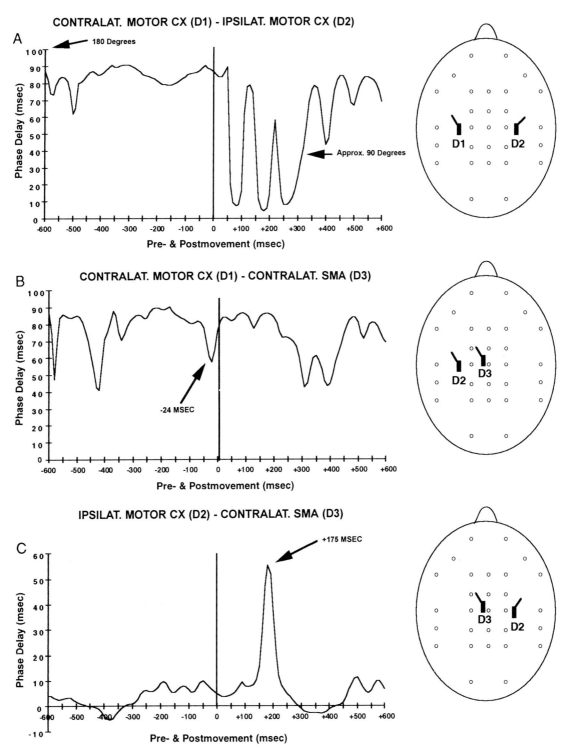

Figure 5 Instantaneous phase delay between the pseudoinverse derived dipole time series using a center frequency of 4.25 Hz and a bandwidth of 3.5 Hz. Phase delay (msec) on the y-axis is plotted against pre- and postmovement time (msec) on the x-axis. On the right side of the figure are diagrammatic representations of the location of the dipoles. (A) Instantaneous phase delay between the ipsilateral motor cortex (D2) and the contralateral motor cortex (D1). (B) Instantaneous phase delay between the ipsilateral motor cortex (D2) and the contralateral supplemental motor area or SMA (D3). (C) Instantaneous phase delay between the contralateral motor cortex (D1) and the contralateral supplemental motor area or SMA (D3). (Adapted from Thatcher et al., 1994.)

Rapid shifts in phase between dipoles 1 and 3 were noted in the premovement period as well as during the postmovement period. As seen in figure 5(C), a distinctly different phase trajectory was observed between dipoles 2 and 3. For example, the phase relationship was near to 0° during the entire premovement period, with a rapid increase in phase at approximately +150 msec postmovement.

VI. Discussion

A. Developmental Neuroimaging Application

In this technique, the original dipole locations and orientations are determined using averaged time domain data. The averaging procedure in effect throws away the "background EEG" activity that is not synchronized with the motor movement. The coherence analysis, on the other hand, is a frequency domain analysis of precisely this background EEG activity (i.e., with the average removed). Thus, the two forms of analysis are complementary approaches to the same data. Because the coherence analysis is not sensitive to the time-locked average activity used to estimate the set of dipole sources, the results of this analysis are of potential physiological interest because they are not dependent upon a signal–to–noise averaging process. Instead, the analysis focuses on the magnitude and timing of "coupling" relations that precede and follow the timing of evoked potential peaks. To this extent, the "dipole coherence" analysis may be of value in the study of the subsecond neural network dynamics involved in the mediation of perception and cognition, and in the development of neural networks. A further advantage of the pseudoinverse technique is that it involves an analytic and not a numeric solution, and thus avoids many of the pitfalls of the inverse solution. This stems from the use of a priori knowledge from multiregistration with MRI and PET (Thatcher, Toro, et al., 1994; Wang et al., 1993).

It is important to emphasize that the point of this chapter is not simply to validate a multiple dipole source model or to use multimodal registration to determine model order; rather, the chapter concerns the exploitation of the time domain once dipole source locations are independently corroborated. The emphasis of "tomographic EEG" is precisely on the applications of time domain analyses of neural network dynamics, which is made possible through multimodal registration. This represents a departure from the conventional electrophysiological dipole analyses, where multiple source modeling and problems of source localization are the primary concern of researchers.

B. Competition between Dipoles

As described elsewhere, inverse relationships and/or 180° phase reversals in EEG coherence are believed to reflect competition between connected neural assemblies (Thatcher, Krause, & Hrybyk, 1986; Thatcher, Walker, & Giudice, 1987; Thatcher, 1992). For example, for three interconnected neural assemblies A, B, and C, increased coupling between A and B may be at the expense of coupling between A and C, B and C, or both. In the present study, increased coupling between the ipsilateral motor cortex dipole and the contralateral SMA dipole, was inversely related to the magnitude of coupling between the contralateral motor cortex dipole and the contralateral SMA dipole (see Fig. 4). This is indicative of dynamic competition between the ipsilateral and contralateral motor cortex and the SMA. Another example of possible competition was seen in the coherence relationships between the ipsilateral and contralateral motor cortex dipoles. In this case, there was a rapid decrease in coupling between the ipsilateral motor cortex (D2) and SMA (D3) immediately after motor movement (i.e., between 0 and 50 msec), which occurred simultaneously with an increase in coupling between the contralateral motor cortex dipole (D1) and the SMA (D3).

C. SMA as a Neural Network Switch Element

The SMA dipole was strongly coupled to the ipsilateral motor cortex dipole during the premovement period because these regions exhibited relatively high coherence and a zero phase lag (see Figs. 4C and 5C)[1]. In contrast, during the premovement period, the SMA dipole was weakly coupled to the contralateral motor cortex dipole with variable, but near 180° phase relationships (see Fig. 4B). Evidence for a SMA role as a neural network switching element was seen by the rapid (i.e., 20 to 50 msec) reversal in coherence values immediately after the motor movement (see Fig. 4). The label of the SMA dipole as a switching element is based upon the speed at which the coupling dynamics changed, and the primary relationship that the SMA dipole held with respect to the other dipoles, especially the contralateral motor cortex dipole (see Figs. 4 and 6). A more detailed analysis of the dynamics of the SMA changes in coupling, with respect to the ipsilateral and contralateral cortex, is shown in Figure 6. In

---

[1]Zero Phase lag cannot be explained by simple volume conduction because: (1) It is frequency specific. (2) Zero phase lag is maintained even while coherence radically changes. (3) Zero phase lag is spatially heterogeneous, involving longer interdipole distances than dipole distances with no zero phase lag.

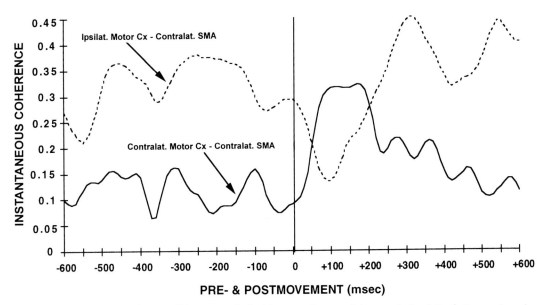

Figure 6 Instantaneous coherence (10 msec resolution) between the pseudoinverse derived dipole time series using a center frequency of 7 Hz and a bandwidth of 4 Hz. Coherence on the y-axis is plotted against pre- and postmovement time (msec) on the x-axis. The dotted line is instantaneous coherence between the time series from the ipsilateral motor cortex and the contralateral supplemental motor area or SMA. The solid line is instantaneous coherence between the time series from the contralateral motor cortex and the contralateral SMA. (Adapted from Thatcher et al., 1994.)

this figure, the center frequency of the filter was set to 7 Hz and the bandwidth was limited to 4 Hz. These filter settings provided a smoother picture of the time course of coherence changes.

D. Human Neural Network Dynamics and Zero Phase Coupling

The instantaneous coherence and phase analyses used in the present study may provide new information about the dynamics of neural interaction which occurred during the finger movement task. Three of the most significant dynamical features were: (1) The presence of oscillations in coherence and phase, (2) the duration and rate of large changes in coherence and phase, and (3) the presence of zero phase locking. The presence of oscillations in dipole coherence are a function of the bandwidth of the filter, that is oscillations diminish as the bandwidth narrows. This suggests that the oscillations are due to periodic shifts in frequency in one or both channels. The amplitude and frequency of these oscillations may be of relevance in dynamical modeling of the coupling phenomenon. We are currently conducting simulation analyses to learn more about the basis of the oscillations in the dipole coherence. The duration of the large changes in dipole coherence refers to the interval over which a relatively stable level of coherence suddenly changes to a new stable level. In the present study, this interval was ap-

proximately 50 msec to 100 msec (see Figs. 4 and 6). The rate of change in coherence between the pre- and postmovement periods was estimated by derivatives from approximately .001 to .003/msec. Finally, zero phase locking was present only between the SMA dipole and the contralateral motor cortex dipole. As mentioned previously, this is suggestive of strong coupling between these regions, which persists even though coherence may radically change (see Figs. 4 and 5). Although more analyses must be performed on a larger number of subjects, these findings tentatively suggest that the dynamics of neural network coupling observed in multiunit studies in animals (Gray et al., 1989; Eckhorn et al., 1988; Murthy and Fetz, 1992; Singer, 1995) may be similar to those observed in noninvasive human EEG studies.

E. Validity of the Technique in the Study of Human Neural Network Development

There was considerable evidence to validate the physiological foundations of the time domain analyses. First, the anatomical accuracy of the registration of the electrophysiological dipoles with the center of the PET activated regions varied from approximately 3 mm to 10 mm (see Plate 18). Second, the dipoles were located in cortical regions that are known to subserve finger movements (i.e., the anterior bank of the central sulcus and the SMA). Third, the time course of the dipole coherence events corresponded well with the time course of evoked potential (Toro et al., 1993, 1994) and event-related desynchronization events (Pfurtscheller, Steffan, & Maresch, 1986) obtained in similar, if not identical, motor movement tasks. Finally, the observed rapid changes in electrophysiological coupling between distributed brain regions was similar to that observed by Gevins and colleagues (Gevins et al., 1989a, 1989b) in subjects performing a motor movement task.

Although this technique was developed in adult normal subjects using PET and EEG, it is reasonable to assume that this technique can be applied to children using noninvasive fMRI and EEG. For example, if dipoles exist in children's brains as we know they do, then the development of human neural networks involved in perception and cognition may be studied over the human lifespan. Important developmental questions can be asked, such as: At what age does the time course of approximately 50 to 100 msec for SMA and motor cortex switching first appear? Are more spatially extensive networks involved in early child development in comparison to the adult? Is the development of self-paced or volitional movements the same as externally triggered movements? Do the spatial and temporal features of different neural networks develop linearly or nonlinearly over the human lifespan?

Acknowledgments

The author would like to gratefully acknowledge the collaboration of Dr. Camilo Toro, Dr. Mark Hallett, Dr. Binseng Wang, and Dr. Mark Pflieger for their assistance in various aspects of the tomographic EEG procedures. This work was supported by a grant from the Henry Jackson Foundation No. JFC36285006. R. W. Thatcher, Principal Investigator.

References

Eckhorn, R., Bauer, R., Jordan, W., Brosch, M., Kruse, W., Munk, M., & Reitboek, H. J. (1988). Coherent oscillations: A mechanism of feature linking in the visual cortex? *Biological Cybernetics, 60,* 121–130.

Gevins, A. S., & Bressler, S. L. (1988). Functional topography of the human brain. In G. Pfurtscheller (Ed.), *Functional Brain Imaging* (pp. 99–116). Berlin: Hans Huber.

Gevins, A. S., Cutillo, S. L., Bressler, S. L., Morgan, N. H., White, R. M., Illes, J., & Greer, D. S. (1989a). Event-related covariances during a bimanual visuomotor task. Part I: Methods & analysis of stimulus- and response-locked data. *Electroencephalography and Clinical Neurophysiology, 74*(1), 58–75.

Gevins, A. S., Cutillo, S. L., Bressler, S. L., Morgan, N. H., White, R. M., Illes, J., & Greer, D. S. (1989b). Event-related covariances during a bimanual visuomotor task. Part II: Preparation and feed-back. *Electroencephalography and Clinical Neurophysiology, 74*(2), 147–160.

Gevins, A., Cutillo, B., DuRousseau, D., Le J., Leong, H., & Smith, M. (1994). High-resolution evoked potential technology for imaging neural networks of cognition. In R. W. Thatcher, M. Hallett, T. Zeffiro, E. R. John, & M. Huerta (Eds.), *Functional Neuroimaging: Technical Foundations* (pp. 223–232). Orlando, Florida: Academic Press.

Gray, C. M., Konig, P., Engel, A. K., & Singer, W. (1989). Oscillatory responses in cat visual cortex exhibit inter-columnar synchronization which reflects global stimulus properties. *Nature (London), 338,* 334–337.

Murthy, V. N., & Fetz, E. E. (1992). Coherent 25- to 35Hz oscillations in the sensorimotor cortex of awake behaving monkeys. *Proceedings of the National Academy of Science U.S.A., 89,* 5670–5674.

Nunez, P. (1981). *Electrical Fields of the Brain.* New York: Oxford Univ. Press.

Otnes, R. K., & Enochson, L. (1988). *Applied Time Series Analysis.* New York: Wiley.

Pelizzari, C. A., Chen, G. T. Y., Spelbring, D. R., Weichselbaum, R. R., & Chen, C. T. (1989). Accurate three-dimensional registration of CT, PET, and/or MR images of the brain. *Journal of Computer Assisted Tomography, 13,* 20–29.

Penrose, R. (1955). A generalized inverse for matrices. *Proceedings of the Cambridge Philosophical Society, 51,* 406–413.

Pfurtscheller, G., Steffan, J., and Maresch, H. (1986). ERD mapping and functional topography: Temporal and spatial aspects. In G. Pfurtscheller (Ed.), *Functional Brain Imaging* (pp. 117–130). Berlin: Hans Huber.

Roth, B., Balish, M. S., Gorbach, A., and Sato, S. (1993). How well does a 3 sphere model predict positions of dipoles in a realistically shaped head? *Electroencephalography and Clinical Neurophysiology, 87,* 175–184.

Scherg, M. (1992). Functional imaging and localization of electromagnetic brain activity. *Brain Topography, 5*(2), 103–111.

Scherg, M., and Berg, P. (1991). Use of prior knowledge in brain electromagnetic source analysis. *Brain Topography, 4,* 143–150.

Simpson, G. V., Bellevue, J. W., Foxe, J. J., Baker, J. R., & Vaughan, H. G. (1993). Spatial imaging and temporal dynamics of visual brain-activation through integration of electrophysiological (ERP) and hemodynamic (fMRI) measures. *Society for Neuroscience, 19,* 1604.

Simpson, G. V., Foxe, J. J., Vaughan, H. G., Mehta, A. D., & Schroeder, C. E. (1996). Integration of electrophysiological source analyses, MRI and animal models in the study of visual processing and attention. *Electroencephalography and Clinical Neurophysiology,* in press.

Singer, W. (1995). Development and plasticity of cortical processing architectures. *Science, 270,* 758–764.

Talairach, J., & Tournoux, P. (1988). Co-planar Stereotaxic Atlas of the Human Brain: A 3-Dimensional Proportional System: An Approach to Cerebral Imaging. New York: Thieme.

Thatcher, R. W. (1992). Cyclic cortical reorganization during early childhood. *Brain and Cognition, 20,* 24–50.

Thatcher, R. W., Hallett, M., Zeffiro, T., John, E. R., & Huerta, M. (Eds.) (1994). *Functional Neuroimaging: Technical Foundations,* Orlando, FL: Academic Press.

Thatcher, R. W., Krause, P., & Hrybyk, M. (1986). Corticocortical association fibers and EEG coherence: A two compartmental model. *Electroencephalography and Clinical Neurophysiology, 64,* 123–143.

Thatcher, R. W., Toro, C., & Hallett, M. (1993a). Neural network switching during voluntary finger movements. *International Federation of Clinical Electroencephalography,* Vancouver, B. C., (abstract) 49, 233.

Thatcher, R. W., Toro, C., & Hallett, M. (1993b). Multimodal registration of EEG, PET and MRI: Analyses of Neural Network Switching. *Proceedings of the Society of Magnetic Resonance in Medicine: Functional MRI of the Brain, Arlington, VA, June 17–19,* 171–181.

Thatcher, R. W., Toro, C., Pflieger, M. E., & Hallett, M. (1994). Human neural network dynamics using multimodal registration of EEG, PET and MRI. In R. W. Thatcher, M. Hallett, T. Zeffiro, E. R. John, & M. Huerta (Eds.), *Functional Neuroimaging: Technical Foundations* (pp. 269–278). Orlando, FL: Academic Press.

Thatcher, R. W., Walker, R. A., & Giudice, S. (1987). Human cerebral hemispheres develop at different rates and ages. *Science, 236,* 1110–1113.

Toro, C., Matsumoto, J., Deuschl, G. Roth, B. J., & Hallett, M. (1993). Source analysis of scalp-recorded movement-related electrical potentials, *Electroencephalography and Clinical Neurophysiology, 86,* 167–175.

Toro, C., Wang, B., Zeffiro, T. A., Thatcher, R. W., & Hallett, M. (1994). Movement related cortical potentials: Source analysis and PET/MRI correlation. In R. W. Thatcher, M. Hallett, T. Zeffiro, E. R. John, & M. Huerta (Eds.), *Functional Neuroimaging: Technical Foundations* (pp. 259–267). Orlando, FL: Academic Press.

Wang, B., Toro, C., Wasserman, E. M., Zeffiro, T. A., Thatcher, R. W., & Hallett, M. (1994). Multimodal integration of electrophysiological data and brain images: EEG, MEG, TMS, MRI and PET. In R. W. Thatcher, M. Hallett, T. Zeffiro, E. R. John, & M. Huerta (Eds.), *Functional Neuroimaging: Technical Foundations.* (pp. 251–257). Orlando, FL: Academic Press.

Wang, J., Williamson, S. J., & Kaufman, L. (1992). Magnetic source images determined by a lead-field analysis: The unique minimum-norm least-squares estimation. *IEEE Transactions of Biology and Medicine, 39*(7), 665–675.Wang, J., Kaufman, L., & Williamson, S. J. (1993). Imaging regional changes in the spontaneopus activity of the brain: An extension of the minimum-norm least-squares estimate. *Electroencephalography and Clinical Neurophysiology, 86,* 36–50.

III

NEUROIMAGING
OF ABNORMAL
DEVELOPMENT

10

Functional Neuroimaging of Language in Children: Current Directions and Future Challenges

Susan Y. Bookheimer and Mirella Dapretto

Division of Brain Mapping, University of California School of Medicine, Los Angeles, California 90095

I. Introduction

Models of the neuroanatomical organization and modularity of language have developed slowly, primarily through the accumulation of single case studies of patients with cerebral lesions producing aphasia. It is not surprising, then, that relatively little information is available on the *development* of the neural organization of language functions, since conditions that produce focal lesions, especially strokes and tumors, are relatively rare in children. Neurobehavioral investigations of language functions following early hemispherectomies have also provided data on the neural bases of language in children, but these studies primarily address issues of neural plasticity and recovery of function, and they can tell us relatively little about how language is represented in the normally developing brain. A number of other techniques, such as electroencephalography (EEG), magnetoencephalography (MEG), and evoked potential recording (EP), have been used to investigate brain–language relationships, but the electrophysiological measures have limited spatial resolution, and direct cortical stimulation is extremely invasive.

The development of new neuroimaging technologies, in particular activation imaging with positron emission tomography (PET) and functional magnetic resonance imaging (fMRI), have had a profound impact on the study of language organization in the adult brain. In $H_2{}^{15}O$ PET studies, blood flow has been measured during ongoing performance on a variety of language tasks, including word generation (Frith, Friston, Liddle, & Frackowiak, 1991b; Petersen, Fox, Posner, Mintun, & Raichle, 1988), visual and auditory word processing (Petersen et al., 1988), phonological processing (Demonet, Chollet, Ramsay, Cardebat, Nespoulous, Wise, et al., 1992; Zatorre, Evans, Meyer, & Gjedde, 1992), and various aspects of semantic processing (Howard, Patterson, Wise, Brown, Friston, Weiller, et al., 1992). These studies have substantially expanded and refined the traditional models of language organization derived from lesion studies, leading to a dramatic increase in the number of brain regions implicated in language processing. The lesion literature primarily emphasized two basic language functions: speech comprehension and production. The major disorders of language were attributed to lesions in either of the two main regions implicated in these functions (Broca's and Wernicke's areas, respectively), or in the pathways connecting them. In contrast, activation imaging studies have focused on several key language functions (e.g., phonology, semantics, and syntax), identifying distinct cortical areas of activation subserving different aspects of language processing. While it is possible that lesions in some of these "activated" areas may not produce aphasia, the consistent pattern of activation found across studies suggests that these regions must, nevertheless, be considered part of the complex neural network subserving the processing of language.

143

While activation imaging technology has added much to our understanding of language organization in the adult brain, a number of constraints have limited its use with children. Until recently, functional neuroimaging was limited to PET, which requires injecting ionizing radiation. Although sick children have been administered radioisotopes typically used in resting metabolic studies, healthy children cannot be exposed to radiation for obvious ethical reasons. Furthermore, an acceptable dosimetry for the chief radioligand used in PET activation imaging—$H_2^{15}O$— has never been established for children. Thus, even sick children who might be good candidates for noninvasive language mapping (e.g., those about to undergo surgery to their language dominant hemisphere) have not been studied with this technology.

In the past few years, fMRI has emerged as a viable alternative for mapping brain functions, having clear advantages in spatial and temporal resolution, and an enhanced signal to noise ratio. More importantly, fMRI techniques are completely noninvasive, requiring no injection or inhalation of radioactive tracers. With this technology, it is now conceivable to examine the functional neuroanatomy of language in children, noninvasively and without radiation exposure. The development of fMRI to study brain function in children has far-reaching implications at both the theoretical and the applied levels. First, the mapping of specific brain–language relationships should foster our understanding of the mental processes underlying language itself. Second, detailed knowledge about the neural mechanisms associated with increasing levels of linguistic competence should prove extremely useful in the study of developmental language disorders, the single largest handicapping condition during childhood. Finally, fMRI can also provide a noninvasive alternative to brain mapping for surgical planning, which is usually accomplished by highly invasive techniques such as direct electrical stimulation or injection of sodium amytal into the cerebral hemisphere.

Performing fMRI studies with children presents several key challenges. First, while MRI is routinely performed in pediatric care, clinical MRI scans usually involve sedating the children; in contrast, activation imaging studies of cortical organization require fully alert and cooperative subjects. Thus, in order to conduct fMRI studies on a developmental population, effective and reliable techniques should be implemented to train the children to be in the scanner without being frightened or resistant, and to actively participate in the cognitive tasks while keeping their heads still. Second, fast, high resolution imaging methods are especially critical for functional mapping in children; while adults can easily take part in studies lasting two hours

or more, it is not reasonable to expect a similar study length for children. Third, there are issues of special theoretical concern when interpreting the results of neuroimaging studies of language in children. Language involves several different processes and linguistic structures, the mastery of which may be achieved according to different timetables. Finally, as with other cognitive processes, different levels of language competence can affect the characteristics of its neural representation, such as the size of the cortical regions involved (Ojemann, Ojemann, Lettich, & Berger, 1989). Thus, understanding the development of language organization in the brain will require a full understanding of how competence levels affect brain activation patterns, not only in terms of what regions may be active, but also in terms of the magnitude and spatial extent of the observed cortical activation.

In this chapter we will: (1) briefly review some well-known assumptions about the neural bases of language in the developing brain, (2) present recent neuroimaging data linking developmental language disorders to an abnormal representation of language in the brain, (3) describe the results of the few fMRI studies in children conducted thus far, (4) address some of the practical limitations in conducting functional neuroimaging of language in children, together with some possible solutions, and (5) describe some potential applications for the functional mapping of language in developmental clinical populations.

II. Neural Basis of Language Development

At present, we face a discouraging disparity between what we know about the normal course of language acquisition and what we know about the neural events that take place in the human brain during the years in which most children master their first language. The paucity of information on the neural mechanisms that accompany increasing levels of language competence is undoubtedly related to ethical and practical constraints that have limited the use of the most advanced tools of modern neuroscience with children. Thus, our understanding of how language skills are organized in the developing brain has been primarily derived from studies of children with focal brain damage. Unfortunately, however, the correlations between site of lesion and type of language breakdown are far from perfect even in adults, and a number of logical and empirical problems limit the interpretability of lesion data (Caramazza, 1986; Shallice, 1988). These problems are compounded when the lesion method is applied to the study of brain-injured children, because the effects of focal brain injury in children are much less severe and less consistent than in adults.

Theories of ontogenic specialization for language early in development have either emphasized the extreme notion of early equipotentiality and progressive lateralization, or the notion of invariance with adult-like specialization of the left hemisphere for language processing. Research on the neural bases of language development has initially been influenced strongly by Lenneberg's (Lenneberg, 1967) theory of early hemispheric equipotentiality. Based on data indicating that early left hemispherectomies did not preclude normal language development, and that right hemisphere lesions could give rise to aphasia in a significant proportion of aphasic children, Lenneberg suggested that lateralization of language to the left hemisphere is progressive until puberty, starting from an initial state of hemispheric equipotentiality. However, subsequent analyses of the old literature (Dennis & Whitaker, 1976; Hecaen, 1983; Witelson, 1987) challenged this notion and suggested that the early data were faulty due to a number of methodological problems. More recent, and better controlled, investigations of brain-injured children (Annett, 1973; Aram, 1988; Dennis & Kohn, 1975; Dennis, 1980; Woods & Carey, 1978), as well as electrophysiological studies in normally developing children (Molfese & Segalowitz, 1988), clearly indicate a greater role of the left hemisphere in the processing of most linguistic functions from the first months of life. Indeed, the anatomical asymmetry found in the planum temporale in neonates (Witelson & Pallie, 1973) and even fetuses (Wada, Clarke, & Hamm, 1975) suggests that the "blueprint" for language may be laid down prenatally during the period of neuronal cell formation and migration (Piatelli-Palmarini, 1989), a notion consistent with evidence linking congenital language disorders with aberrant migration and malformation of cells in the classical language areas (Geschwind & Galaburda, 1987).

It should be made clear, however, that the evidence of early left hemispheric specialization for language in children, as in adults, does not imply that the neural substrate of language in children mirrors that found in adults, or that the localization of language functions does not change over the course of development. An invariance model would not be able to account for the strikingly different outcomes observed in children and adults following focal brain lesions. Depending on the age of onset, left hemisphere lesions occurring during early childhood may lead to near complete, or substantial recovery of language functions, whereas corresponding lesions in adulthood lead to severe and permanent language impairments. However, the extraordinary degree of plasticity for language seen in

children is not complete, and careful testing shows persistent lexical and morphosyntactic deficits in children following left hemisphere lesions (Aram, 1988) or left hemispherectomy (Dennis, 1980; Dennis & Whitaker, 1976). Furthermore, while Lenneberg used the terms of progressive specialization to refer to a decreased participation of the right hemisphere for language processing, these notions may rightfully be invoked to describe the developmental changes in the neural representation of language within the language dominant hemisphere.

The ease with which speech may be supported by the right hemisphere in cases of left hemisphere damage or left hemispherectomies clearly indicates a high degree of plasticity in the young brain. This could also be taken as evidence of a greater role of the right hemisphere in language processing during childhood, a notion that is not necessarily at odds with evidence of early left hemispheric specialization. Indeed, some investigators have suggested that the normal pattern of asymmetric language processing may be contingent on interhemispheric inhibition, either of an early functioning or potentially functional secondary language substrate in the right hemisphere (Zaidel, 1990). While the role of the right hemisphere during language development has been downplayed since the fall of Lenneberg's theory of early hemispheric equipotentiality, recent evidence from functional neuroimaging studies indicates that the right hemisphere is also involved during language processing in adults (Cuenod, Bookheimer, Hertz-Pannier, Frank, Zeffiro, Theodore, et al., 1995; Price, Wise, Ramsay, Friston, Howard, Patterson, et al., 1992). Language is not a unitary phenomenon and language lateralization is not the same for all linguistic functions. Studies of commissurotomy or "split brain" individuals (Zaidel, 1985, 1990) have indicated very different linguistic profiles for the two hemispheres. The left hemisphere seems specialized for speech comprehension and production, and for processing phonological, morphological, and syntactic structures. In contrast, the right hemisphere seems unable to initiate any significant language production, though it seems adequate for comprehension of lexical items, perhaps by reliance on semantic and pragmatic cues, rather than on syntactic and phonological cues.

Further evidence that the brain regions mediating language acquisition in children differ from those mediating language processing in adults comes from data indicating different language deficits following damage to selective areas in the dominant hemisphere. Consistent with the literature on acquired aphasia in adults, young children with left hemisphere lesions tend to recover more slowly from expressive receptive deficits. Unlike adults, however, the expressive deficits are particularly persistent with lesions involving left posterior cortex early in life (Satz, Strauss, & Whitaker, 1990; Thal, Marchman, Stiles, Trauner, Nass, & Bates, 1991). This finding, paired with the lack of comprehension deficits following early posterior lesions, could be taken to reflect bilateral representation of some language functions early in life. Alternatively, the finding of different aphasic patterns in young children, compared to older children and adults, could index intrahemispheric reorganization of the language substrate during development with less focality of the anatomical substrate of language in the left hemisphere early in life (Hecaen, Perenin, & Jeannerod, 1984). This hypothesis is consistent with a growing body of research indicating that skill acquisition and skill maintenance may call upon different neural systems, and that mastery or "automatization" of a skill may actually result in a cutting back or sculpting of the neural substrate for that skill (Raichle, Fiats, Videen, MacLeod, Parde, Fox, et al., 1994). Finally, neuropsychological studies with normal children using electrophysiological measures (such as event-related potentials) indicate that the pattern of brain activity seen in children during language tasks does not become indistinguishable from the adult pattern until around puberty (Holcomb, Coffey, & Neville, 1992), probably reflecting significant changes in the nature of language processing (i.e., accessibility and automaticity of linguistic forms that have been acquired for considerable periods of time) (Marchman, Bates, Burkhardt, & Good, 1991) taking place throughout the school years.

III. Neuroimaging of Developmental Language Disorders

Two developmental language disorders have been studied using both structural and functional neuroimaging methods, including fMRI. Dyslexia represents the most common type of learning disability, and affects 2 to 8% of the school-aged population (American Psychiatric Association, 1987; Shaywitz, Shaywitz, Fletcher, & Escobar, 1990). Most typically, the diagnosis of dyslexia requires average or better intelligence, a significant discrepancy between intellectual ability and measured reading achievement, and an absence of any other handicapping condition that may produce difficulties in learning to read. The neurobiological basis of dyslexia has long been presumed, given both the similarity of symptoms in dyslexics and in patients with brain damage to the perisylvian and posterior regions, and the reported high familial risk rates (35–45%), suggesting a dominant, semidominant, or additive genetic transmission (Smith, Pennington,

Kimberling, & Ing, 1990). Developmental dysphasia affects an estimated 8 to 15% of all preschool-aged children (e.g., Aram & Nation, 1982). It is characterized by a failure to acquire language normally despite normal nonverbal intelligence, and implies a delay in language acquisition that exceeds the upper boundaries of the age for normal language acquisition, as well as deviance in some aspect of language. In later childhood, developmental language disorders may be manifested in reading and spelling deficits, and selective lowering of scores on tests of verbal intelligence (Aram, Ekelman, & Nation, 1984).

While most studies have usually focused on either language-impaired or dyslexic individuals, considerable evidence suggests that more than 85% of children with language disorders in the preschool years will later develop language-related learning disabilities (Tallal, 1987; Stark, Bernstein, Condino, Bender, Tallal, & Catts, 1984). Thus, children with developmental language disorders frequently become poor readers in the elementary school years (Silva, Williams, & McGee, 1987); conversely, poor readers are very likely to have histories of delayed language development (Ingram, Mason, & Blackburn, 1970). Although strong links exist between early language disorders and dyslexia, there is also evidence suggesting that dyslexics with and without histories of generalized language delay may show different profiles. For instance, while decoding is more impaired than reading comprehension in dyslexics (Conners & Olson, 1990), children with persistent language disorders are more likely to show poorer reading comprehension than phonological decoding skills (Bishop & Adams, 1990).

Although even the earliest descriptions of dyslexia attributed the problem to cerebral pathology, it is only recently that systematic neuroanatomical studies have attempted to link dyslexia to specific abnormalities in brain structure. *Postmortem* findings by Galaburda and associates reported increased symmetry of the plana temporale in the brains of several dyslexic individuals, due to an increase in size of the right planum (rather than the usual pattern of a larger planum temporale on the left side), as well as varying degrees of cortical abnormalities (e.g., dysplasia and ectopias), more common in the left perisylvian regions (inferior frontal and superior temporal areas) (Galaburda, Sherman, Rosen, Aboitiz, & Geschwind, 1985; Humphreys, Kaufmann, & Galaburda, 1990). Interestingly, the same cytoarchitectonic abnormalities were also observed in the brain of a dysphasic girl (Cohen, Campbell, & Yaghmai, 1989).

Structural neuroimaging studies of dyslexics (Larsen, Hoien, Lundberg, & Odegaard, 1990; Rumsey, Dorwart, Vermess, Denckla, Kruesi, & Rapoport, 1986)

and language-impaired children (Plante, Swisher, Vance, & Rapcsak, 1990; Jernigan, Hesselink, Sowell, & Tallal, 1991) have corroborated the neuropathological findings in these populations, although different studies have yielded somewhat different results with regard to the asymmetry of the plana temporale. For instance, one group reported that the lack of the usual asymmetry in dyslexics was due to a greater right planum length in this group than in normals (Larsen et al., 1990), whereas another investigation found a smaller planum in the left hemisphere than in the right hemisphere in dyslexics (Hynd, Semrud-Clikeman, Lorys, Novey, & Eliopulos, 1990). Yet another reported an exaggerated left asymmetry in the temporal planum in dyslexics, paired with an anomalous intrahemispheric asymmetry between the right temporal and parietal banks in some dyslexic subjects (Leonard, Voeller, Lombardino, Morris, Hynd, Alexander, et al., 1993). Moreover, a recent investigation found that the apparent differences in the size of left hemisphere structures and symmetry of the planum temporale between dyslexics and controls were not reliable after controlling for age and overall brain size (Schultz, Cho, Staib, Kier, Fletcher, Shaywitz, et al., 1994) This finding clearly indicates the need to consider these potential sources of variance when interpreting differences in morphological brain measures between different groups of individuals, especially in a developmental population. Finally, there is also evidence of abnormal callosal size in children with learning disabilities. In one study, thicker callosa were found in children with familial dysphasia and dyslexia (Njiokiktjien, de Sonneville, & Vaal, 1994), whereas another investigation of dyslexic children reported a smaller genu of the corpus callosum in this group, together with significant correlations between reading achievement and region-of-interest measurements for the genu and splenium (Hynd, Hall, Novey, Eliopulos, Black, Gonzalez, et al., 1995).

Recent functional neuroimaging studies have also shown abnormalities in the pattern of cortical activation in dyslexia and dysphasia. Using PET oxygen 15-labeled water as a tracer, Rumsey, Andreason, Zametkin, Aquino, King, Hamburger, et al. (1992) studied adults who had been diagnosed as dyslexic in childhood and who retained severe reading deficits in adulthood. In line with the neuroanatomical data, reliable differences were found between dyslexic and normal adults in the pattern of cortical activation during a phonological rhyme detection task, where subjects were presented with word pairs and had to judge whether or not they rhymed. More specifically, unlike the normal controls, the dyslexics failed to activate the left temporo–parietal cortex during this task, while

they showed activation in a more anterior temporal region, perhaps reflecting some compensatory strategy (Rumsey, Andreason, Zametkin, Aquino, King, Hamburger, Pikus, Rapoport, & Cohen, 1992). In contrast, dyslexic men did not differ from controls in their activation of left inferior frontal and middle to anterior temporal cortex during a syntactic task where subjects listened to pairs of sentences and had to judge whether or not they differed in meaning (Rumsey, Zametkin, Andreason, Hanahan, Hamburger, Aquino, et al., 1994). Abnormal patterns of activation in dyslexics were also observed in a different investigation using an oral reading task (Gross-Glenn, Duara, Barker, Loewenstein, Chang, Yoshii, et al., 1991). However, since the dyslexics were reading-impaired and their performance was below that of the controls, it is unclear whether differences in brain activation reflected differences in their neural organization of language, or differences in task performance during the language activation task.

A few functional neuroimaging studies of dysphasic children have shown that the abnormalities in cortical morphology of the left temporo–parietal and frontal regions seen in dysphasia are associated with corresponding abnormal patterns of activation during language tasks. For instance, using single photon emission computed tomography (SPECT) and hexamethylpropylene-amine oxime (HM–PAO) as a tracer, Denays, Tondeur, Foulon, Verstraeten, Ham, Piepsz, et al. (1989) found hypoperfusion in the left temporo–parietal regions and in the middle and superior regions of the right frontal lobe of dysphasic children with both receptive and expressive deficits. In contrast, a single hypoperfused area in the left inferior frontal gyrus was observed in dysphasic children with only expressive deficits. In a different study using xenon-133 inhalation and SPECT, dysphasic children failed to show activation in the left inferior parietal regions during a phoneme discrimination tasks, when compared to a control group of children with attention deficit/hyperactivity disorder (Tzourio, Heim, Zilbovicius, Gerard, & Mazoyer, 1994). Yet another SPECT study with xenon-133 reported hypoperfusion in the left central perisylvian region, compared to the right, in children with primarily lexical–semantic deficit, and hypoperfusion in left prefrontal region, compared to the right, in children with primarily phonological–syntactic deficits (Lou, Henriksen, & Bruhn, 1990).

Overall, the available empirical evidence provides support for the notion that developmental dysphasia and dyslexia are associated with subtle deviations in brain morphology, as well as with an abnormal pattern of cerebral organization for language processing. Furthermore, the cytoarchitectonic and neuroimaging data clearly indicate that the abnormal neurodevelopment thought to underlie these language disorders produces both structural and functional aberrations detectable with *in vivo* brain imaging. Beyond purely anatomical findings, functional neuroimaging tools can provide a window into the brain that promises to shed further insights into the biology of developmental language disorders. However, before one can assess how language is differentially processed and represented in the brains of dysphasic and dyslexic children, it is essential to determine (1) how language is organized in the brains of normally developing children, and (2) how much difference from norm can be tolerated before the neural substrate of language can be considered abnormal.

IV. Functional MRI in Children

A few recent reports have used fMRI to study the organization of cognitive skills in children. One is discussed in detail elsewhere in this volume (Shaywitz, Pugh, Constable, Shaywitz, Bronen, Fulbright, Shankweiler, Katz, Fletcher, Skudlarski, & Gore, 1995) and will not be discussed further here. A second investigation used fMRI to directly study language dominance in children. Using a word generation paradigm that has been well-studied in adult volunteers (Cuenod, Bookheimer, Hertz-Pannier, Frank, Zeffiro, Theodore, & Le Bihan, 1995), Hertz-Pannier, Gaillard, Mott, Cuenod, Bookheimer, & Weinstein, (1996). studied 11 children with epilepsy, aged 8 to 18, using fMRI. These children were under consideration for temporal lobectomy and five had also undergone a sodium amytal interview. Five children whose amytal exam indicated LH dominance showed concordant results on fMRI studies. Cerebral dominance was characterized by a larger spatial extent of activation associated with task performance. Blood flow changes were found largely in the inferior frontal gyrus, though related changes were also seen in middle and superior frontal gyri. In contrast, fewer subjects showed lateralized responses in temporal lobes, largely due to imaging artifacts. This study suggested that, at least among older children, language dominance similar to that seen in adults using the same methods (fMRI during word generation) could be demonstrated in children. This study used no special techniques to facilitate the scanning procedure for children; rather, only those subjects who were cooperative and comfortable with the procedure were selected. The authors did not attempt to demonstrate age-related changes in activation; rather, they suggested that the activation patterns found in the children were the same as those observed for adults.

A similar comparison was made between the performance of normal children and adults using a nonverbal working memory paradigm (Casey, Cohen, Jezzard, Turner, Noll, Trainor, et al., 1995). They also found a high degree of similarity between the brain activation patterns between adults and children. Most notably, they detected a trend toward increasing localization of function correlating with age. Though the sample of younger children was too small to draw firm conclusions, it would appear that nonverbal functions become increasingly focal with age, much in the same way that is hypothesized for language skills.

While laterality was found even among the younger children in both studies, it remains unclear how increased expertise in cognitive skills affects the dominance pattern, either the extent of laterality, or the spatial extent of activation. For example, Hertz–Pannier (Hertz-Pannier et al., 1996) found greater spatial extent of language areas in the dominant hemisphere, while Ojemann (1989), using direct cortical stimulation, found that the spatial extent of language areas decreases with higher levels of skill. The existing fMRI studies have not attempted to differentiate changes in spatial extent of activation associated with age vs expertise, and the variables are clearly easy to confound. A possible technique to differentiate these variables would present several difficulty levels within each task for both younger and older subjects, to determine age-independent effects of task performance on the spatial extent and magnitude of activated regions.

We have begun to study language skills in children with developmental language disorders and in those with normal language development. Results from children have been compared with adult normal volunteers as well. In this study, we examined both skills relevant to reading (nonword reading, rhyming, lexical decision and word–picture matching), and general language skills such as semantic processing and word generation. This is because a significant proportion of children with developmental dysphasia will later be diagnosed as dyslexic. While many of these patients will have caught up in other language skills, it is unknown whether their language organization is similar to other children who were never delayed.

Figure 1 presents the results of an adult normal volunteer on a spelling task, in which the subject sees the picture of an object and then chooses the correct spelling from one of two alternatives. The task is most similar to a lexical decision task, where the alternatives are close phonological possibilities (e.g., chare and chair). The semantic task required subjects to choose a word which was semantically related to a picture pre-

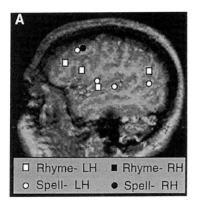
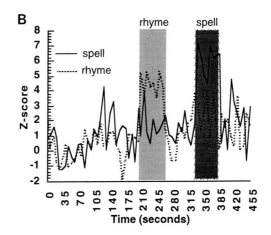

Figure 1 Adult normal volunteer performing rhyme matching and spelling tasks. Region locations are shown in the sagittal MR (A). Regions of interest (ROI) optimized for spelling and rhyming tasks are plotted separately in (B). Predominant activity is seen in the left hemisphere including superior temporal and angular gyri.

sented (e.g., apple–orange), and a rhyming task in which subjects chose a printed word which rhymed with a presented picture. Each activation task was compared to both a resting control condition and to the other activation tasks, in order to identify brain regions both shared by the language tasks and specific to individual tasks. MR images were collected on a GE Signa 1.5 tesla device using spoiled grass (SPGR) (TR = 45; TE = 30; Flip = 45; NEX = 0.75; thickness = 5mm). Images were corrected for head motion and were analyzed using pixel-wise comparisons with student's T. The corresponding maps of statistical significance were superimposed on the coplanar high resolution flow images for localization. The pixels achieving significance were converted to Z-scores and are

charted in the corresponding graph. The regions shown in Figure 1 were specifically activated during the spelling and rhyming tasks, and involve two general areas: the inferior frontal cortex, and the superior temporal and angular gyri in the dominant hemisphere. Performance of the same tasks produced right hemisphere (RH) activation only in the left premotor region. The region appears to be located near the dorsolateral prefrontal cortex and may be primarily involved in working memory, one important aspect of attending to this task. Figure 1(B) shows the left hemisphere regions plotted over time with respect to the task performed.

In contrast, Figure 2 presents data from a child (age 13) with severe dyslexia performing the same tasks.

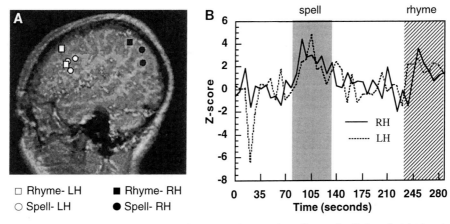

Figure 2 Dyslexic child performing rhyme matching and spelling tasks. Left and right hemisphere foci are identified in the sagittal slice (A). The time activity curves, measured in Z-units, for all significant pixels in each hemisphere are plotted in (B).

This child has a normal verbal IQ but functions several years below grade level in all reading tasks. Active regions around the inferior frontal lobe were similar to those found in the adult normal volunteer. This suggests that he performed (or attempted to perform) the task appropriately. There was a left frontal dominance pattern, which was also seen in a word generation task. This task has been reported by several others (Cuenod et al., 1995; McCarthy, Blamire, Rothman, Gruetter, & Shulman, 1993; Rueckert, Apollonio, Grafman, Jezzard, Johnson, Bihan, et al., 1994) and is a powerful activator of left frontal lobe. In contrast, the child shows no activation of the left superior temporal and angular regions in the dominant hemisphere, while the posterior temporal–angular gyri were active during task performance in the right hemisphere. These regions are plotted in time-activity curves in Figure 2(B).

Thus, the pattern of activation in the frontal lobe in this child was very similar to that of the adult for spelling and rhyme matching tasks. Both the child and adult showed a strong left hemisphere (LH) dominance as suggested by left inferior frontal gyrus (IFG) activation during all language tasks, while RH frontal activation was limited to dorsolateral prefrontal cortex (DLPFC). In the normal-reading adult, an LH bias was also found in the angular gyrus, a region implicated in phoneme to grapheme correspondence, and in ST, which is important in auditory processing. In contrast, only the right angular gyrus of the dyslexic child showed a corresponding level of activation. The absence of a normal LH dominance pattern in the temporal lobe is consistent with structural MR findings of either less asymmetry of the planum temporale (PT), or greater size of the right PT in dyslexic children. Finally, the regions of activations in the child were more focal than in the adult volunteer. This may be due to methodological differences (e.g., slice selection), differences in task difficulty, as well as differences in the degree of focal representation. Each of these confounding variables offers a conceptual challenge to comparing adults and children on cognitive activation paradigms.

A second subject, a 12 year old boy with normal reading and language (with right occipital epilepsy), was studied using the word generation paradigm and an auditory semantic task. Focal activation was found in the left IFG during word generation in a pattern identical to that seen in the adult normal volunteers and the dyslexic child. During semantic processing, focal activation was also found in the posterior temporal–inferior parietal junction, consistent with Wernicke's area. There were no discernible differences between the activation patterns seen in this child as compared with adult normal volunteers. Thus, in our

short experience, children in this age range show activation patterns in fMRI language paradigms indistinguishable from those found in normal adults, except in a region specifically associated with behavioral impairment in the dyslexic child. We tentatively suggest that fMRI may accurately map both normal and impaired language skills in children.

V. Limitations in Functional Imaging of Language in Children

A. Age and Relevance of Language Development

An argument may be made that, since the basic language structures are laid down by age 7, it is not meaningful to image language "development" after that age. However the limited data available suggest that while complete language reorganization may have a critical period of up to 7 years, substantial changes in language organization appear to continue until puberty. While the basic structures may be laid down, automaticity, or expertise in these basic structures, will continue to develop. What we may practically study, then, is how this development of expertise is represented in the brains of children through puberty. In the following we will discuss the dependent measures in fMR imaging and how they may be affected by performance factors including task difficulty, response automaticity, and practice.

B. Choice of Dependent Measures

In activation imaging, particularly fMRI, there are several possible dependent measures one can use to assess "organization" of a cognitive skills in the brain. These can be summarized as: (1) *regional*, those regions showing significant task-related changes, (2) *spatial extent*, the size of the activated region, (3) *magnitude*, the size of the activation, and (4) *correlational*, the pattern of activation in comparison to a second variable. Each of these dependent measures has been used in language activation studies in adults, and each has special advantages and disadvantages peculiar to studying children.

The *regional localization* approach is fundamental to activation, but indicating where significant cerebral blood flow (CBF) changes occur may not sufficiently describe the results. For instance, in lateralization experiments of language, it is common to find both right and left hemisphere activations in some key areas like Brodmann's area 44. In such cases, a second measure, such as magnitude, may indicate a higher percentage of change in the left hemisphere. A general problem with the localization approach is how to compare regions across subjects in brains which differ both anatomically and functionally. While all repeated studies require image registration to directly compare results, studies with children have the added difficulty of accounting for increasing brain size with age. Ideally, determining the course of development of language acquisition would entail longitudinal studies, which can effectively take into account individual differences in both precise locations of regional activation patterns and in rates of development. One of the current techniques for image registration, automated image registration (AIR) (Woods, Mazziotta & Cherry, 1993), has recently been modified to account for changes in brain size across the same individual. Such a program would seem necessary for accurate comparison of brain changes over time. Methods for combining activation data across individuals, such as image registration, are varied and are discussed at length elsewhere.

Magnitude of activation in critical regions has been reported as an important dependent variable in several fMRI studies. Such measures include percentage of signal intensity change in activation vs control, or magnitude of a statistical measure, such as Z or T. However, magnitude of activation as a dependent measure is peculiarly problematic in imaging children. Analyzing the cerebral glucose metabolic rates in children using PET, Chugani, Phelps, and Mazziotta (1987) found evidence for a well-characterized distribution of increasing and decreasing glucose metabolism over the first 20 years of life. At birth, infants had cerebral glucose metabolic (CGM) rates similar to those of adults. By age 3 these rates had increased dramatically to twice the adult rate, and returned gradually to adult levels over the next 20 years. Though blood flow has not been measured in a similar manner, a coupling between regional cerebral blood flow (rCBF) and CGM has been established for normal adult brains (Fox, Raichle, Mintun, & Dence, 1988) and one may presume that it follows a similar pattern in children. The reason for this change in rCGM has been posited as one of increasing synapses which are slowly pruned as ideal functional connections are made and reinforced. The changing rCGM patterns in childhood are problematic for activation imaging of the developing brain. Decreases in the magnitude of brain activation have been observed with increased practice and expertise in skills; this effect could easily be confounded with a decreased magnitude of activation due to fewer neurons as part of the normal course of synaptic pruning. Without a careful characterization of the relationship between synaptic density, rCGM, and activation-related changes in rCBF in development, it will be difficult to directly compare, for instance, the absolute magnitude of activation in adults vs children. Magnitude, for instance, measured as the percentage change in signal intensity during activation vs control tasks, may ultimately prove a poor measure for comparing age-related changes in skill development.

In PET studies, *spatial extent* of an area of activation is strongly confounded with magnitude due to this technique's relatively poor spatial resolution. With fMRI, several studies have attempted to use spatial extent as an independent variable, typically by counting the number of pixels exceeding a given threshold in a specified region. In language studies, region localization, magnitude, and spatial extent have all been demonstrated to vary with degree of task difficulty or practice. For instance, using direct cortical stimulation of the brain, Ojemann et al. (1989) found that the spatial extent of important language areas was greater in patients of less intelligence, while those with superior verbal skills tended to have small focal regions which were susceptible to speech arrest during electrical stimulation. Other tasks have demonstrated similar effects, indicating that experience or practice with the paradigm may reduce the spatial extent of the activation or the magnitude (Raichle et al., 1994).

Adult language activation studies have demonstrated that the automaticity of a skill can affect both the magnitude of cerebral activation and the pattern of activation (which areas are most active). This evidence generally comes from two sources: studies varying the rate, frequency, or difficulty of a task, and studies of learning and practice. Both have important implications for imaging in children, since degree of expertise or practice may be easily confused with age-dependent changes in brain activation patterns. It is therefore important to understand the effects of practice and performance level on the blood flow response for the specific paradigms under investigation. For example, Raichle et al. (1994) had subjects perform a learned motor sequence repeatedly, in an attempt to increase signal to noise ratio. After the task was repeated many times, the cortical regions showing maximal rCBF increases began to change. Whereas initially the primary motor cortex was very active, after practice this activity was reduced, while increases were seen in the insula. The authors suggested that the primary motor cortex was important for learning or acquiring a new motor pattern, while other regions were more important when that task became automatic.

We reported a related finding in a language paradigm (Bookheimer, Zeffiro, Blaxton, Gaillard, & Theodore, 1995). Subjects were required either to name objects or read single words. The rate of motor output, as well as the specific items, were identical across conditions, yet the active motor regions were different. While naming objects produced activation primarily in the insula, the reading task produced changes in the primary motor cortex (mouth area). The differences in motor output pathways may be attributed to the extent to which feedback is used to modify the response, a factor directly related to degree of expertise.

It is reported in the reading literature as well that separate pathways—whole-word reading vs sequential phoneme to grapheme correspondence—are differentially accessed according to expertise. In acquiring reading, a phonological route is emphasized, while in the practiced reader, a whole-word strategy may be used. While this is clearly the kind of critical information we hope that imaging in children will reveal, the pattern of activation within the MR experiment may be strongly affected by task parameters, including rehearsal and certain stimulus characteristics which may affect task difficulty.

C. Limitations on Verbal Output and Head Motion

One of the greatest advantages of fMRI—the enhanced spatial resolution—also produces one of its greatest limitations: susceptibility to head motion artifacts. Head motion is a serious issue in adult fMRI studies and is clearly a greater problem for children. This is discussed at length by Turner in this volume. For the study of language, head motion concerns have a particular significance: an easy source of head motion artifacts is motion caused by jaw movement when the subject speaks. Consequently, most fMRI studies, including those of language processing, have used paradigms requiring no vocal responses. The obvious disadvantage here is that speech is an important language function that one might want to study. Further, there is evidence that, at least in some experimental paradigms, silent performance produces differences in brain regions activated outside of primary motor regions. Using PET, which is less susceptible to contamination from head motion artifacts, several studies found differences in brain activation patterns depending upon whether language tasks were performed silently or aloud. For example, we conducted a study comparing silent and oral reading with silent and oral object naming. While silent object naming differed from oral naming almost exclusively in motor regions, silent and oral reading changed in several key language regions (Bookheimer et al., 1995). Oral word generation, which produces strong increases in several frontal lobe regions, was found by Frith et al. (1991a) to produce rCBF *decreases* in Wernicke's area. Finally, a cortical region

apparently important in phoneme monitoring (e.g., Zatorre et al., 1992; Demonet et al., 1992) has only been observed in silent language tasks. In contrast, when phoneme processing was measured by having subjects repeat a phoneme sequence aloud, we found activation only in the primary motor and superior temporal cortex (Bookheimer, Zeffiro, Gaillard, & Theodore 1992). Thus, the representation of some language processing regions can be strongly influenced by output demands. One fMRI study did have subjects generate words aloud (McCarthy et al., 1993) without too much head motion, and they reported frontal lobe activation like that reported in PET studies of oral word generation, but found no activation in silent generation. In contrast, several other silent generation studies using fMRI all found significant activation (Cuenod et al., 1995; Rueckert et al., 1994). Head motion is a problem even in silent performance (Cohen & Bookheimer, 1994), and most centers rely on silent tasks even for language processing experiments. Several approaches may be taken to minimize head motion or to correct it using postprocessing techniques. These are general issues affecting imaging of both adults and children, and are discussed at length by others in this volume.

One head motion control technique which has been adapted specifically for children was designed by the group at Johns Hopkins University (Slifer et al., 1993). This group has used well-established behavior modification techniques to control head motion and to desensitize children to the MR environment. The procedure is composed of two steps. In the first, children are exposed to a simulated MR environment which has been adapted (the front of the scanner is covered with a canvas painted in a childlike theme, such as a "Winnie-the-Pooh" picture or a spaceship). The child is able to watch a video or listen to an audiotape in the simulated scanner over several trials until he or she feels comfortable. A tape recording of the scanner noise is added to better simulate the MR environment. The child receives rewards for staying in the environment, and repeats this stage until he or she is comfortable. In the second phase, continued viewing of the movie is made contingent upon successively smaller head movements. These are recorded by mechanical potentiometers, which are attached to the child's head. When movement outside an acceptable range is detected, a signal is sent to the projection device and projection is terminated for a brief period. Using successive approximation, the criteria for head motion are gradually narrowed. This system, which was developed for structural MRI, was effective at reducing head motion to 1–2 mm; further, the vast majority of children entering the program were able to successfully complete their MR scans without sedation.

We are developing a similar system which works digitally instead of mechanically, using infrared detectors of head position over 9 degrees of freedom. The advantage of this system is that, in addition to providing subject feedback on head position, it can simultaneously record and store this information digitally. The data, in turn, can be used for image reconstruction for post hoc correction with extreme accuracy.

VI. Conclusions

There are several important potential clinical uses for functional MRI in mapping language skills in children: establishing hemispheric dominance and intra-hemispheric localization of language sites prior to surgery, and determining functional–neuroanatomical abnormalities in children with developmental language disorders, are foremost among them. These goals are hampered by a paucity of knowledge regarding the functional neuroanatomy of language processes in the normal brain, which is a necessity for interpretation of results in clinical populations. Potential confounding variables include the effects of difficulty vs developmental level on magnitude and spatial extent of results, necessity to account for changes in brain size and shape with development, difficulty in generalizing from adult imaging studies, as well as technical difficulties in providing a suitable environment for scanning children. Nevertheless, we have seen progress in each of these areas in the short time fMRI has been available. We can anticipate that future fMRI research will establish normative data on language organization in the developing brain which can serve as a basis to compare and contrast altered language development. Ultimately, fMRI may not only reveal how cognitive skills are organized in the developing brain, but may serve as a template by which we can diagnose early disorders and measure the efficacy of treatment interventions in children with developmental disabilities.

References

American Psychiatric Association, C. o. N. a. S. (1987). *Diagnostic and Statistical Manual of Mental Disorders, Revised Third Edition*. Washington, D.C., American Psychiatric Association.

Annett, M. (1973). Laterality of childhood hemiplegia and the growth of speech and intelligence. *Cortex, 9*, 4–33.

Aram, D. (1988). Language sequelae of unilateral brain lesions in children. *Language communication and the brain*. New York: Raven.

Aram, D. M., Ekelman, B. L., & Nation, J. E. (1984). Preschoolers with language disorders: 10 years later. *Journal of Speech and Hearing Research, 27*, 232–244.

Aram, D. M., & Nation, J. E. (1982). *Child Language Disorders*. St. Louis, MO: Mosby.

Bishop, D. V. M., & Adams, C. (1990). A prospective study of the relationship between specific language impairment, phonological disorders and reading retardation. *Journal of Child Psychology and Psychiatry, 31*, 1027–1050.

Bookheimer, S., Zeffiro, T., Blaxton, T., Gaillard, W., & Theodore, W. (1995). Regional cerebral blood flow during object naming and word reading. *Human Brain Mapping* 3(2), 93–106.

Bookheimer, S., Zeffiro, T., Gaillard, W., & Theodore, W. (1992). *Regional cerebral blood flow in premotor cortex during speech*. Paper presented at the Annual Meeting, American Academy of Neurology, Washington, D.C.

Caramazza, A. (1986). On drawing inferences about the structure of normal cognitive systems from the analysis of patterns of impaired performance: The case for single-patient studies. *Brain and Cognition, 5*, 41–66.

Casey, B., Cohen, J., Jezzard, P., Turner, R., Noll, D., Trainor, R., Giedd, J., Kaysen, D., Hertz-Pannier, L., & Rapoport, J. (1995). Activation of prefrontal cortex in children during a non-spatial working memory task with functional MRI. *Neuroimage, 2*, 221–229.

Chugani, H. T., Phelps, M. E., & Mazziotta, J. C. (1987). Positron emission tomography study of human brain functional development. *Annals of Neurology, 22*, 487–497.

Cohen, M., & Bookheimer, S. (1994). Localization of brain function using Magnetic Resonance Imaging. *Trends in Neurosciences, 17*(7), 268–277.

Cohen, M., Campbell, R., & Yaghmai, F. (1989). Neuropathological abnormalities in developmental dysphasia. *Annals of Neurology, 25*, 567–570.

Conners, F., & Olson, R. (1990). Reading comprehension in dyslexic and normal readers: A component skills analysis. *Comprehension Processes in Reading*. Hillsdale, NJ: Erlbaum.

Cuenod, C. A., Bookheimer, S. Y., Hertz-Pannier, L., Frank, J. A., Zeffiro, T. A., Theodore, W. H., & Le Bihan, D. (1995). Functional MRI during word generation using conventional equipment: A potential tool for language localization in clinical environment. *Neurology, 45*, 1821–1827.

Demonet, J. F., Chollet, F., Ramsay, S., Cardebat, D., Nespoulous, J.-L., Wise, R., Rascol, A., & Frackowiak, R. (1992). The anatomy of phonological and semantic processing in normal subjects, *Brain, 115*, 1753–1768.

Denays, R., Tondeur, M., Foulon, M., Verstraeten, F., Ham, H., Piepsz, A., & Noel, P. (1989). Regional Brain Blood Flow in Congenital Dysphasia: Studies with Technetium-99m HM-PAO SPECT. *Journal of Nuclear Medicine, 30*(11), 1825–1829.

Dennis, K., & Kohn, B. (1975). Comprehension of syntax in infantile hemiplegia after cerebral hemidecortication: Left hemisphere superiority. *Brain and Language, 2*, 472–482.

Dennis, M. (1980). Capacity and strategy for syntactic comprehension after left and right hemi-decortication. *Brain and Language, 10*, 287–317.

Dennis, M., & Whitaker, H. A. (1976). Language acquisition following hemi-decortication: Linguistic superiority of the left over the right hemisphere. *Brain and Language, 3*, 404–433.

Fox, P. T., Raichle, M. E., Mintun, M. A., & Dence, C. (1988). Nonoxidative glucose consumption during focal physilogic neural activity. *Science, 241*(4864), 462–464.

Frith, C. D., Friston, K., Liddle, P. F., & Frackowiak, R. S. (1991a). Willed action and the prefrontal cortex in man: A study with PET. *Proceedings of the Royal Society of London Biology, 244*(1311), 241–246.

Frith, C. D., Friston, K. J., Liddle, P. F., & Frackowiak, R. S. (1991b). A PET study of word finding. *Neuropsychologia, 29*(12), 1137–1148.

Galaburda, A. M., Sherman, G. F., Rosen, G. D., Aboitiz, F., & Geschwind, N. (1985). Developmental dyslexia: Four consecutive patients with cortical anomalies. *Annals of Neurology, 18,* 222–233.

Geschwind, N., & Galaburda, A. (1987). *Cerebral lateralization: Biological mechanisms, associations, and pathology.* Cambridge, MA: MIT Press.

Gross-Glenn, K., Duara, R., Barker, W. W., Loewenstein, D., Chang, J. Y., Yoshii, F., Apicella, A. M., Pascal, S., Boothe, T., Sevush, S., et al. (1991). Positron emission tomographic studies during serial word-reading by normal and dyslexic adults. *Journal of Clinical and Experimental Neuropsychology, 13,* 531–544.

Hecaen, H. (1983). Acquired aphasia in children: Revisited. *Neuropsychologia, 21,* 581–587.

Hecaen, H., Perenin, M., & Jeannerod, H. (1984). The effects of cortical lesions in children: Language and visual functions. *Behavioral biology of early damage.* New York: Academic Press.

Hertz-Pannier, L., Gaillard, W. D., Mott, S. H., Cuenod, C. A., Bookheimer, S. Y., Weinstein, S., Conry, J., Papero, P., Le Bihan, D., & Theodore, W. H. (1996). Functional MRI in children: Assessment of language hemispheric dominance in patients with epilepsy. under review.

Holcomb, P. J., Coffey, S. A., & Neville, H. J. (1992). Visual and auditory sentence processing: A developmental analysis using event-related brain-potentials. *Developmental Neuropsychology, 8,* 203–241.

Howard, D., Patterson, K., Wise, R., Brown, W. D., Friston, K., Weiller, C., and Frackowiak, R. (1992). The Cortical Localization of the Lexicons. *Brain, 115,* 1769–1782.

Humphreys, P., Kaufmann, W. E., & Balaburda, A. M. (1990). Developmental dyslexia in women: Neuropathological findings in three cases. *Ann Neurol., 28,* 727–738.

Hynd, G. W., Hall, J., Novey, E. S., Eliopulos, D., Black K., Gonzalez, J. J., Edmonds, J. E., Riccio, C., & Cohen, M. (1995). Dyslexia and corpus callosum morphology. *Archives of Neurology, 52,* 32–38.

Hynd, G. W., Semrud-Clikeman, M., Lorys, A. R., Novey, E. S., & Eliopulos, D. (1990). Brain morphology in developmental dyslexia and attention deficit disorder/hyperactivity. *Archives of Neurology, 47,* 919–926.

Ingram, T. T. S., Mason, A. W., & Blackburn, I. (1970). A retrospective study of 82 children with reading disability. *Developmental Medicine and Child Neurology 12,* 271–281.

Jernigan, T. L., Hesselink, J. R., Sowell, E., & Tallal, P. (1991). Cerebral structure on magnetic resonance imaging in language- and learning-impaired children. *Arch. Neurol., 48,* 539–545.

Larsen, J. P., Hoien, T., Lundberg, I., & Odegaard, H. (1990). MRI evaluation of the size and symmetry of the planum temporale in adolescents with developmental dyslexia. *Brain and Language, 39,* 289–301.

Lenneberg, E. (1967). *Biological Foundations of Language.* New York: Wiley.

Leonard, C. M., Voeller, K. K. S., Lombardino, L. J., Morris, M. K., Hynd, G. W., Alexander, A. W., Andersen, H. G., Garofalakis, M., Honeyman, J. C., Mao, J., Agee, O. F., & Staab, E. V. (1993). Anomalous cerebral structure in dyslexia revealed with magnetic resonance imaging. *Archives of Neurology, 50,* 461–469.

Lou, H. C., Henriksen, L., and Bruhn, P. (1990). Focal cerebral dysfunction in developmental learning disabilities. *The Lancet, 335,* 8–11.

Marchman, V., Bates, E., Burkhardt, A., & Good A. (1991). A functional constraints on the acquisition of the passive: Toward a model of the competence to perform. *First Language, 11,* 65–92.

McCarthy, G., Blamire, A. M., Rothman, D. L., Gruetter, R., & Shulman, R. G., (1993). Echo-planar magnetic resonance imaging studies of frontal cortex activation during word generation in humans. *Proceedings of the National Academy of Science, U.S.A., 90,* 4952–4959.

Molfese, D. T., & Segalowitz, S. J. (1988). *Brain lateralization in children: Developmental implications.* New York: Guilford.

Njiokiktjien, C., de Sonneville, L., & Vaal, J. (1994). Callosal size in children with learning disabilities. *Behavioral and Brain Research, 64*(1–2), 213–218.

Ojemann, G., Ojemann, J., Lettich, E., & Berger, M. (1989). Cortical language localization in left, dominant hemisphere. An electrical stimulation mapping investigation in 117 patients. *Journal of Neurosurgery, 71*(3), 316–326.

Petersen, S. E., Fox, P. T., Posner, M. I., Mintun, M., & Raichle, M. E. (1988). Positron emission tomographic studies of the cortical anatomy of single-word processing. *Nature (London), 331,* 585–589.

Piatelli-Palmarini, M. (1989). Evolution, selection, and cognition: From 'learning' to parameter setting in biology and in the study of language." *Cognition, 31,* 1–44.

Plante, E., Swisher, L., Vance, R., & Rapcsak, S. (1990). MRI findings in boys with specific language impairment. *Brain and Language, 40,* 52–66.

Price, C., Wise, R., Ramsay, S., Friston, K., Howard, D., Patterson, K., & Frackowiak, R. (1992). Regional response differences within the human auditory cortex when listening to words. *Neuroscience Letters, 146*(2), 179–182.

Raichle, M. E., Fiats, J. A., Videen, T. O., MacLeod, A. K., Pardo, J. V., Fox, P. T., & Peterson, S. E. (1994). Practice-related changes in human brain functional anatomy during nonmotor learning. *Cerebral Cortex, 4,* 8–26.

Rueckert, L., Apollonio, I., Grafman, J., Jezzard, P., Johnson, R., Le Bihan D., & Turner, R. (1994). MRI functional activation of left frontal cortex during covert word production. *Journal of Neuroimaging, 4,* 67–70.

Rumsey, J. M., Dorwart, R., Vermess, M., Denckla, M. B., Kruesi, M. J. P., & Rapoport, J. L. (1986). Magnetic resonance imaging of brain anatomy in severe developmental dyslexia. *Archives of Neurology, 43,* 1045–1046.

Rumsey, J. M., Andreason, P., Zametkin, A. J., Aquino, T., King, A. C., Hamburger, S. D., Pikus, A., Rapoport, J. L., & Cohen, R. M. (1992). Failure to activate the left temporoparietal cortex in dyslexia: An oxygen 15 positron emission tomography study. *Archives of Neurology, 49,* 527–534.

Rumsey, J., Zametkin, A., Andreason, P., Hanahan, A., Hamburger, S., Aquino, T., King, A., Pikus, A. & Cohen, R. (1994). Normal activation of frontotemporal language cortex in dyslexia, as measured with oxygen 15 positron emission tomography. *Archives of Neurology, 51*(1), 27–38.

Satz, P., Strauss, E., & Whitaker, H. (1990). The ontogeny of hemispheric specialization: some old hypotheses revisited. *Brain and Language, 38,* 596–614.

Schultz, R. T., Cho, N. K., Staib, L. H., Kier, L. E., Fletcher, J. M., Shaywitz, S. E., Shankweiler, D. P., Katz, L., Gore, J. C., Duncan, J. S., & Shaywitz, B. A. (1994). Brain morphology in normal and dyslexic children: The influence of sex and age. *Annals of Neurology, 35,* 732–742.

Shallice, T. (1988). *From neuropsychology to mental structure.* New York: Cambridge Univ. Press.

Shaywitz, S. E., Shaywitz, B. A., Fletcher, J. M., & Escobar, M. D. (1990). Prevalence of reading disability in boys and girls. *Journal of the American Medical Association, 264,* 998–1002.

Shaywitz, B., Pugh, K., Constable, R., Shaywitz, S., Bronen, R., Fulbright, R., Shankweiler, D., Katz, L., Fletcher, J., Skudlarski, P., & Gore, J. (1995). Localization of semantic processing using functional magnetic resonance imaging. *Human Brain Mapping, 2,* 149–158.

Silva, P. A., Williams, S., McGee, R. (1987). A longitudinal study of children with developmental language delay at age three: Later intelligence, reading and behaviour problems. *Developmental Medicine and Child Neurology, 29,* 630–640.

Slifer, K. J., Cataldo, M. F., Cataldo, M. D., Llorente, A. M., & Gerson, A. C. (1993). Behavior analysis of motion control for pediatric neuroimaging. *Journal of Applied Behavioral Analysis, 26*(4), 469–470.

Smith, S. D., Pennington, B. F., Kimberling, W. J., & Ing, P. S. (1990). Familial dyslexia: Use of genetic linkage data to define subtypes. *Journal of the American Academy of Child and Adolescent Psychiatry, 29,* 204–213.Stark, R. E., Bernstein, L. E., Condino, R., Bender, M., Tallal, P., & Catts, H. (1984). Four-year follow-up study of language impaired children. *Annals of Dyslexia, 34,* 49–68.

Tallal, P. (1987). Developmental Language Disorders. Interagency committee on learning disabilities—Report to the U.S. Congress.

Thal, D., Marchman, V., Stiles, J., Trauner, D., Nass, R., & Bates, E. (1991). Early lexical development in children with focal brain injury. *Brain and Language, 40,* 491–527.

Tzourio, N., Heim, A., Zilbovicius, M., Gerard, C., & Mazoyer, B. M. (1994). Abnormal regional CBF response in left hemisphere of dysphasic children during a language task. *Pediatric Neurology, 10*(1), 20–26.

Wada, J. A., Clarke, R., & Hamm, A. (1975). Cerebral hemispheric asymmetry in humans. *Archives of Neurology, 32,* 239–246.

Witelson, S. (1987). Neurobiological aspects of language in children. *Child Development, 58,* 653–688.Witelson, S. F., & Pallie, W. (1973). Left hemisphere specialization for language in the newborn. Neuroanatomical evidence of asymmetry. *Brain, 96,* 641–646.

Woods, B. T., & Carey, S. (1978). Language deficits after apparent clinical recovery from childhood aphasia. *Annals of Neurology, 6,* 405–409.

Woods, R. P., Mazziotta, J. C., & Cherry, S. R. (1993). MRI-PET registration with automated algorithm. *Journal of Computer Assisted Tomography, 17*(4), 536–546.

Zaidel, E. (1985). Right-hemisphere language. *The dual brain: Hemispheric specialization in humans.* New York: Guilford.

Zaidel, E. (1990). Language functions in the two hemispheres following complete cerebral commissurotomy and hemispherectomy. *Handbook of neuropsychology.* Amsterdam: Elsevier.

Zatorre, R., Evans, A., Meyer, E., & Gjedde, A. (1992). Lateralization of phonetic and pitch discrimination in speech processing. *Science 256,* 846–849.

11

Functional Magnetic Resonance Imaging as a Tool to Understand Reading and Reading Disability

Bennett A. Shaywitz,[*,†] Sally E. Shaywitz,[*] Kenneth R. Pugh,[*,‡]
Pawel Skudlarski,[§] Robert K. Fulbright,[§] R. Todd Constable,[§]
Richard A. Bronen,[§] Jack M. Fletcher,[¶] Alvin M. Liberman,[‡]
Donald P. Shankweiler,[‡] Leonard Katz,[‡] Cheryl Lacadie,[§]
Karen E. Marchione,[*] and John C. Gore[§,‖]

*Departments of Pediatrics, †Neurology and §Diagnostic Radiology, Yale University School of Medicine,
New Haven, Connecticut 06510; ‡Haskins Laboratories, New Haven, Connecticut 06510; ¶Department of
Pediatrics, University of Texas Medical School, Houston, Texas; and ‖Department of Applied Physics,
Yale University, New Haven, Connecticut 06510

I. Introduction

This chapter examines functional imaging, particularly the development of the methods critical in carrying out essentially *in vivo* studies in intact individuals as they are performing tasks engaging higher cognitive function, such as reading. We focus specifically on the newest of functional imaging methods, functional magnetic resonance imaging, first reviewing the theoretical basis for this technology and then examining the rationale for the tasks used in the study of reading. We conclude with examples from our own investigations.

II. The Cognitive Basis of Dyslexia

A. Neurolinguistic and Cognitive Mechanisms

Efforts to elucidate the underlying neural basis of reading and reading disability depend on our understanding of the cognitive basis of reading, and over the last two decades, investigators have made considerable progress in developing and validating a cognitive model of reading and reading disability (Gough & Tunmer, 1986; Gough, Ehri, & Treiman, 1992; Goswami & Bryant, 1992; Liberman, Shankweiler, & Liberman, 1989; Liberman, 1971; Perfetti, 1985). Evidence from several lines of investigation has now converged to identify and isolate phonological processing as the specific cognitive deficit responsible for reading disability (see reviews by Blachman, 1984; Wagner & Torgesen, 1987; Liberman & Shankweiler, 1991; Stanovich, 1988). Most recently, evidence from two large and well studied populations of children with reading disability (Fletcher, Shaywitz, Shankweiler, Katz, Liberman, Stuebing, et al., 1994; Shankweiler, Crain, Katz, Fowler, Liberman, Brady, et al., 1995; Stanovich & Siegel, 1994) confirms that a deficit in phonological processing represents the most robust correlate of reading disability. Furthermore, emerging studies in young adults support the notion that phonological processing deficits persist (Bell & Perfetti, 1994; Bruck, 1990, 1992, 1996). These deficits are most often demonstrated by difficulties (lack of automaticity) in word identification, particularly in pseudoword reading. Thus, not only does reading disability persist, but evidence now indicates that difficulties in reading across the full span of development are unified by reflecting a common deficit, phonological processing. Thus, a deficiency in phonological processing characterizes both older poor readers as well as poor beginning readers. With the identification of phonological processing as the core cognitive deficit in reading, we now know not only the particular cognitive system (linguistic), but which component of that system (phonological processing), to focus on in the search for the neural locus of dyslexia.

DEVELOPMENTAL NEUROIMAGING

III. Neurobiological Mechanisms in Reading and Reading Disability

A. Cerebral Localization of Reading

1. Studies Based on Subjects with Brain Injury

Reading can only be studied in people. There can be no animal models of reading. Thus, in contrast to other basic physiological processes which humans share with other species, studies of higher cognitive processes such as language and reading can only be studied in humans, a fact that significantly limits the range of scientific investigation. Historically, the concept of the cerebral localization of motor and sensory functions was first mentioned by a German physician, Joseph Baader, in 1763:

> By comparing pathological observations of the brain with the symptoms of the patient while living . . . it is possible to know and to predict which part of the brain gives to this or that limb its feeling or movement; so that, knowing which limb is affected, one can determine which part of the brain is affected, and, conversely, given a particular lesion of the brain, one can determine which limb is affected. (Joseph Baader, 1763, p. 116).

Studies of the cerebral localization of cognitive functions in humans are even more recent, beginning just two centuries ago with Gall's proposal that mental functions were localized in the cerebral hemispheres, rather than in other organs such as the liver or spleen (Young, 1990). Following Gall's hypotheses, others began to localize cognitive functions, including language, by studying the brains of individuals who suffered brain lesions from strokes or traumatic injury, and began to relate the loss of particular cognitive functions to damage to specific brain regions. Of the cognitive functions, language functions were the first to be characterized. Based on his study of an individual with a large lesion in the region of the inferior frontal gyrus of the left hemisphere, Broca proposed that this brain region was responsible for speech production. Other investigators followed, relating a range of cognitive functions to specific brain regions based on descriptions of patients with brain lesions. By the close of the 19th century, brain maps of the localization of cerebral function had become quite detailed (Plate 19) (Ferrier, 1890; Young, 1990).

Much has been learned from studies of cerebral localization of cognitive function based on studies of individuals with brain damage, and such studies continue to provide important information, particularly with the emergence of modern imaging methods which allow very fine-grained anatomical resolution (Damasio & Damasio, 1989). However, such studies, by necessity, can never fully address the question of brain function and organization in individuals without brain injury; clearly, reading disability in children is not the result of an injury but represents a subtle developmental disorder with effects that emanate through the language module. This means that ideally, in order to study and to understand reading disability, we must be able to measure brain function in the intact individual. In contrast, studies in brain damaged individuals address only indirectly the question of brain function and organization in healthy individuals.

More importantly, studies localizing cerebral function on the basis of damage to specific brain regions in brain injured individuals provide a static picture of brain anatomy, rather than a dynamic picture of brain function while individuals are performing a cognitive task. What is necessary is to be able to image, and then to identify, the functional units of the working nervous system, the neural networks that are engaged by specific cognitive functions. Functional imaging, the ability to measure brain function during performance of a cognitive task, meets such a requirement, and became possible in the early 1980s. For the first time, rather than being limited to examining the brain in an autopsy specimen, or measuring the size of brain regions using static morphometric indices based on computerized tomography (CT) or magnetic resonance imaging (MRI), scientists were able to think of studying brain metabolism while individuals were performing specific cognitive tasks.

2. Functional Imaging

When an individual is asked to perform a discrete cognitive task, that task places processing demands on particular neural systems in the brain. To meet those demands requires activation of neural systems in particular brain regions, and those changes in neural activity are, in turn, reflected by changes in brain metabolic activity (e.g., changes in cerebral blood flow or changes in cerebral utilization of metabolic substrates such as glucose. It is possible to measure those changes in metabolic activity in specific brain regions while subjects are engaged in cognitive tasks.

a. PET   The first studies of this kind used xenon 133 to measure cerebral blood flow, but more recent studies use positron emission tomography (PET). In practice, PET requires intraarterial or intravenous administration of a radioactive isotope to the subject, so that cerebral blood flow or cerebral utilization of glucose can be determined while the subject is performing the task. In order to minimize the risks to the subject, isotopes with very short biological half-lives are synthesized in a cyclotron immediately prior to the testing, a factor that mandates that the time course of the experiment conform to the short half-life of the radioisotope. Although much has been learned about language using PET technology (for reviews see Demonet, Price, Wise, & Frackowiak, 1994; Frackowiak, 1994; Petersen & Fiez, 1993), PET uses short-lived radioisotopes, requires a cyclotron and associated team of technicians, and suffers from poor spatial and temporal resolution and sensitivity. Particularly when considering studies in children, the invasive nature of the procedure, as well as the logistics of generating short-lived isotopes, limits the utility of PET.

b. Functional Magnetic Resonance Imaging (fMRI)

MRI, introduced into clinical practice in the early 1980s, has already become firmly established as the method of choice for imaging brain anatomy and providing information on tissue compositional changes in disease. With the development of functional MRI (fMRI), this strategy promises now to surpass other methods for its ability to map the individual brain's response to specific cognitive stimuli. Since it is noninvasive and safe, it can be used to repeatedly study humans, including children and neonates, without risk. This means that it can be used to investigate conditions that are uniquely human, such as reading and language.

The principle behind these methods is that the signal used to construct MRI images changes, by a small amount (typically of order 1–5%), in regions that are activated by a stimulus or task. The increase in signal results from the combined effects of increases in the tissue blood flow, volume, and oxygenation, though the precise contributions of each of these is still somewhat uncertain. At least in some conditions, the increase in activation produces a flow increase locally that introduces oxygenated blood to a degree that is greater than the increased metabolic demands, with the result that the tissue oxygen tension increases, and the venous blood becomes more oxygenated. The significance of this is that the intravascular magnetic susceptibility then more closely matches the surrounding tissue than when the vessels contain deoxyhemoglobin. In the deoxygenated state, the heme group in blood produces a significant paramagnetism that disturbs the homogeneity of the magnetic field in the environment of the vasculature, whereas in oxygenated blood the disturbance is much smaller. This, in turn, means that the magnetic field experienced by tissue water in the close vicinity of activated volumes is more uniform. The signal used to construct MR images is derived from the nuclear magnetization produced mainly by tissue water protons. This magnetization can be tipped away from its equilibrium alignment in the direction of an applied external field using radiofrequency pulses, and the resultant signal decays at a rate that is termed $1/T2^*$. The decay rate is slower, and the MR signal therefore stronger, when the magnetic field is uniform. Thus, MR image intensity increases when deoxygenated blood is replaced by oxygenated blood (Plate 20).

A variety of methods can be used to record the changes that occur, but one preferred approach makes use of so-called ultrafast imaging, such as echo-planar imaging (EPI), in which complete images are acquired in times substantially shorter than a second. These fast methods suffer fewer problems from motion artifacts and permit a greater variety of imaging paradigms. The spatial resolution is similar to that of conventional anatomic MRI; that is, of the order of a few millimeters or better. The temporal resolution is limited mainly by the hemodynamic response of the vasculature, since it takes a few seconds for the metabolic and flow changes to equilibrate after the onset of a stimulus, and to recover after the stimulus ends. Ultrafast MR techniques such as EPI can provide images at a rate fast enough to capture the time course of the hemodynamic response to neural activation and to permit a wide variety of imaging paradigms over large volumes of the brain. The spatial and temporal resolutions available with MR techniques go beyond the capabilities of PET, and are making new kinds of experiments possible. Furthermore, unlike PET, MR functional imaging does not require the use of exogenous agents and is completely noninvasive. This allows repeated scans of the same subject, and reduces or eliminates the need for intrasubject averaging.

The principal technical challenge of practical fMRI is to identify areas of true activation and to reject areas that appear to change but are actually artifacts. The most straightforward way to generate an activation image is simply to subtract an image acquired under baseline conditions from one acquired during the activation task. This may not be satisfactory for a number of reasons. The change in nuclear magnetic resonance (NMR) signal due to activation is small and of the order of the noise intensity in the original images. The ratio of the activation signal to noise (S/N) is improved if more than one pair of images is acquired. While this increases the ratio of the signal to random noise, it is less effective at eliminating other effects which can mimic an activation signal. Important sources of nonrandom noise are patient motion, "physiological" noise, and the effect due to relatively large vessels draining the activated parenchyma. If the patient moves between acquisition of the baseline and activated images, signal intensity will be misregistered in the two images. This can cause large errors in the subtraction image wherever the motion has a component perpendicular to steep intensity gradients (i.e., sharp edges) in the original images. In this case, thin regions around the periphery of the brain, sulci, and other cavities can appear to be "activated." Physiological noise is similar to bulk motion in that it arises from a time dependence of signal intensity which is unrelated to neural activity. In this case, the image intensity variations arise from the pulsation of cerebrospinal fluid (CSF) and blood in the major vessels, which are both driven by the cardiac cycle. A more subtle source of signal change is the cyclic variation of blood oxygen in the major vessels, which follows the respiratory cycle. These signal variations have been identified as the sources of several classes of activation map artifacts. Finally, a genuine effect can be due to venous drainage of the activated tissue. Although this is correlated with neural metabolism, it is not specific to the activated region, and can appear a centimeter or more from the functional focus. Since this "activation" signal is misplaced in the image, it may be considered an artifact. Some of these problems can be mitigated by the careful choice of imaging techniques. For example, EPI acquires data so quickly that patient motion is much less a problem than for conventional techniques.

To avoid the pitfalls of straightforward subtraction, several research groups have turned to mapping statistical parameters derived from image datasets. For example, we have used variations of the t statistic to locate brain activity. The t statistic is calculated for each pixel in a set of activation "on" and "off" images. The derived map of t values is thresholded at some level of significance (p value), and the pixels with t below this level are discarded. The threshold can be chosen so that the signal difference between the activation "on" and "off" cases is statistically highly significant. In effect, the t statistic normalizes the signal differences by their variations, so noisy pixels are less likely to be accepted. The retained pixels are assigned a color and superimposed on a grayscale anatomical image from the dataset to show the location of the active pixels.

Although this technique generally improves the specificity of activation images, it is not sufficient to eliminate all noise and motion artifacts. We have therefore sometimes employed spatial filtering of the t map, using a median filter applied to the t statistic image prior to overlaying this image on a high resolution T1-weighted image. The effect of this median filter can be to remove small isolated pixel clusters due to noise with minimal impact on activation resolution. We have also employed clustering criteria to establish significance. While these spatial criteria provide incremental improvements in the images, they may also degrade the resolution of the functional maps and are biased against isolated high t value pixels. Other groups have proposed significance tests which are based on the time dependence of individual pixel values across a series of images. The significance of the effect for a given pixel depends on how well its signal intensity matches the time dependence of the activation (which is assumed to be known). Bandettini and coworkers (Bandettini, Jesmanowicz, Wong, & Hyde, 1993) used the temporal correlation of the input function and activation signal to determine activation significance. They were able to reduce artifacts further by adding a second criterion which discriminated against large noise spikes in the data. In some of our studies we have used an alternating task paradigm and have then calculated the frequency spectrum of each pixel's signal intensity using a Fourier transform. By retaining only those pixels which have the same frequency components as the stimulation or activation task, we have successfully reduced the effect of noise at other frequencies.

Although a principal advantage of fMRI is its ability to detect changes in individuals, there are many instances where the change is still too small to be reliable in single subjects, so that intersubject averaging of some sort is required. Superposition of MR images using image normalization and warping can be used, and a common approach employs the coordinate system of Talairach and Tournoux (1988) to achieve this coregistration. A further approach uses region of interest analyses that result in lower spatial resolution information but avoid the constraint that all brains appear identical in normalized space. In this method, regions of interest are defined in individual subjects from anatomic landmarks, and the degree of activation (the change in signal or number of activated pixels) measured for each condition is compared. Conventional analyses of variance (ANOVA) can then be used to look for correlations and interactions of factors in studies involving multiple subjects and tasks. This approach can be especially useful for looking for how multiple regions covary in their behaviors.

B. Issues in Task Design

1. Overview

We take as a starting premise the view, well-supported within cognitive psychology, that printed word recognition in reading consists of several dissociable stages or operations, each of which might be associated with different neural substrates. In attempting to identify the anatomical correlates, we have employed a hierarchically organized set of tasks. These tasks progressively emphasize each one of these component operations. A critical aspect of our approach is to make careful use of the principle of converging operations in doing subtractions among these tasks, in order to be able to more confidently ascribe function to different cortical sites. This emphasis on converging subtractions must be an essential component of any systematic attempt to relate brain and cognitive function, and its employment distinguishes the current investigations in our laboratory from previous imaging studies. In the following section, we discuss the theoretical overview of word identification in reading that motivates our research strategy. After this, we describe in detail, the structure and logic of the specific tasks and subtractions employed in recent studies of the functional organization of the brain for reading.

2. Word Identification in Reading

When considering the process of word identification in reading, cognitive psychologists tend to focus their research on questions about the relative contributions of at least three component operations: Orthographic coding, phonological coding, and lexical–semantic coding. Difficulty with printed word identification is a defining characteristic of dyslexia. Further, basic problems with phonological processing in print perception (decoding) seems to be both a central deficit, and the single best predictor of later performance, for these individuals. Why early decoding skill and later reading performance should be so strongly linked suggests to many researchers a particular view of reading development (Share, 1995). On this view, for the beginning reader, the process of mapping from graphemes to phonemes is the primary means of lexical access (finding the word's representation in the mental lexicon). The child must initially learn to associate visual symbols (graphemes) with corresponding parts of spoken words (phonemes) in order to integrate the two modalities and learn to recognize printed words. To accomplish this, the child must first learn to decompose speech into parts (e.g., syllables, onsets and rimes, and/or phonemes) in order make the appropriate associations. This has been referred to as phonological awareness (Liberman et al., 1989). Performance on tasks which tap phonological awareness has been shown to be the single best predictor of later reading development (Bradley & Bryant, 1983; Brady & Shankweiler, 1991; Shankweiler, Liberman, Mark, Fowler, & Fischer, 1979). Many researchers assume that with increased reading experience, the child establishes direct orthographic to lexical associations, at least for more familiar words, and that for these readers access to the lexicon may represent some combination of both orthographic and phonological coding (Coltheart, 1978). From this so-called dual-coding per-

spective many researchers have suggested that, for skilled readers at least, lexical access is primarily orthographic; phonological processing is relegated to a secondary route for coping with unfamiliar letter strings (Coltheart, Curtis, Atkins, & Haller, 1993). From this perspective, initial difficulties in establishing orthographic to phonological correspondences in poor readers makes this developmental transition toward greater reliance on orthographic coding in lexical access difficult or impossible (Bruck, 1990). Further, Bruck notes that younger skilled readers, after approximately four years of reading instruction, begin to shift toward the orthographic route (regularity effects are observed only for low frequency words similar to older skilled readers). However, dyslexic children fail to show evidence of this shift (Seidenberg, Bruck, Fornarolo, & Backman, 1985). Thus, the dual note model suggests that continued problems at the level of word recognition, which in turn makes higher level processing all the more effortful and error prone, is a consequence of failure to develop orthographic skill. This, however, is thought to be the consequence of initial failure to develop adequate decoding skills.

The phonologic and orthographic routes are usually thought to be functionally independent; if so, then we should observe cases where overt neurological damage (lesions) interferes with the operation of one route but spares the other. Such evidence has been obtained over the years (Marshall & Newcombe, 1973; Patterson, Marshall, & Coltheart, 1985; Shallice and Warrington, 1980). One type of acquired dyslexia, called surface dyslexia, is characterized by a preserved ability to read aloud both nonwords (which clearly require the phonologic route) and regular words, but extreme difficulties with exception words (words such as "pint" tend to be given regularized pronunciations). In this case, it appears that the phonologic route is preserved while the direct (orthographic) route is damaged. By contrast, phonological dyslexia is associated with a diminished ability to read nonwords, relative to the reading of real words. In this latter case, the evidence seems to suggest that the direct route is spared while the phonologic route is damaged.

Another prediction from dual coding models, predicated on the notion that the two routes are independent, is that skilled readers can selectively tune their performance, depending on task demands, to either use or bypass the phonologic route. Evidence of context dependent shifts in the relative contributions of orthography and phonology has been reported (Shulman, Hornak, & Sanders, 1978; Monsell, Patterson, Graham, Hughes, & Milroy, 1992; Pugh, Rexer, & Katz, 1994a, 1994b). Each of these studies may be interpreted within the dual coding framework as suggesting that two independent routes, each of which can mediate word recognition, can be traded off in order to meet the demands of the reading context. Further, with increased reading skill, the extent to which word recognition is constrained, in general, by orthographic coding, is increased. Persistent problems with word recognition skill can be hypothesized to be the consequence of failure to establish the two types of coding processes to a sufficient degree (Bruck, 1990, 1992). The notion that phonologic coding plays little or no role in skilled adult reading has been challenged by work on word recognition (Lukatela & Turvey, 1994a, b). It is nonetheless also strongly suggested that with developing skill, the contribution or constraint made by orthographic knowledge steadily increases (Bruck, 1990, Oney, Peter, & Katz, 1996). Several researchers have proposed that orthographic and phonologic coding are not independent; rather, they constitute strongly intercorrelated dimensions within the lexical system (Lukatela & Turvey, 1994a, 1994b; Seidenberg & McClelland, 1989; Van Orden, Pennington, & Stone, 1990), which mutually constrain one another, and ultimately mutually constrain word identification.

We are most comfortable with the view that printed word identification represents some combination of both phonological and orthographic coding processes; the relative weighting of one or the other may well differ from reader group to reader group. Further, it may well be the case that phonological processes continue to contribute substantially at all stages of reading development (Lukatela & Turvery, 1994). In order to ultimately use neuroimaging data to address this issue in the brain, the critical first step is to begin the process of mapping out the anatomical correlates of these three basic components: orthographic, phonological, and lexical–semantic coding. Whatever the relative contributions of orthographic and phonological knowledge in lexical processing may be in different populations of readers, any serious investigation must begin with localizing these cognitive operations.

In order to derive hypotheses about functional anatomical differences between dyslexic and non-impaired readers, we must consider what the behavioral literature tells us about how reading differs in these two groups. As noted a number of studies have suggested that phonological deficits in pseudoword naming persist beyond early stages for dyslexic readers (Bell, & Perfetti, 1994, Bruck, 1990, 1992, Scarborough, 1984). Bell and Perfetti (1994) found that college age poor readers showed evidence of persistent difficulties with both pseudoword and real word processing on accuracy and particularly, latency measures. Further, these deficits predicted comprehension performance when the texts were unfamiliar or difficult.

Bruck (1990, 1992) found persistent problems with decoding in college age poor readers. Further, this pattern of results did not differ among previously diagnosed reading disabled subjects who scored high or low on tests of comprehension. In summary, it appears that phonological difficulties do not diminish appreciably with increased reading experience. Hence, we have reason to hypothesize that abnormalities in cortical regions associated with phonological processing will be characteristic of dyslexia, irrespective of whether younger or older dyslexic readers are studied. Differences on both orthographic and lexical–semantic dimensions are not anticipated. Again, in order to test these hypotheses we must make use of tasks which are designed to specifically isolate each of these functions.

3. Hierarchical Subtractions and Converging Operations

Like most previous functional neuroimaging studies, our studies use a subtraction methodology in attempting to isolate brain/cognitive function relations (Friston, Frith, Liddle, & Frackowiak, 1993; Petersen & Fiez, 1993; Sergent, 1994). To briefly review the logic of this approach: Patterns of metabolic activity are monitored while subjects perform a cognitive task which involves a given process, X, among others. A control task is designed which, in principle, shares all cognitive operations with the experimental task save X. By subtracting the activation produced in the control task from the activation produced in the experimental task, regions associated with process X can be isolated.

One assumption inherent in this approach is that adding or deleting a given cognitive operation when changing the task leaves the other operations unchanged. A good deal of research in cognitive psychology has demonstrated that information processing systems, even those likely to consist of series or stages of processing, are not simply serial and unidirectional (McClelland, 1979). As new stages are added to a task, feedback from these later stages will be likely to modify the operation of earlier stages. Thus, changing the parameters of a task may not simply add or delete a stage; it may also change the way that the other stages are functioning. This notion of forward and backward communication suggests highly interactive systems. This view is central in the advent of connectionist models of cognitive function (McClelland & Rumelhart, 1981). The implication of all of this is that when using subtractions, the activation seen may not only reflect the operation of the distinct process, it may also reflect changes in the putatively shared processes.

Another difficulty is the lack of control over how subjects actually perform tasks. While we may assume that two tasks differ only on a single process, the experimental demands on subjects might well encourage task specific strategies, unrelated to the critical function, and thus interpretation of activation patterns is problematic. Thus, a given control task which, in principle, differs from the experimental task on a single dimension, may differ on any number of uncontrolled dimensions. This is nicely illustrated in a study by Sergent Zuck, Levesque, and MacDonald (1992). These investigators compared a common experimental task (judging whether a letter rhymed with "ee") with two controls (one required a judgment of whether the letter was normal or inverted, the second whether a given single object was "natural"). Activation in the left prefrontal cortex was observed in both conditions, while superior temporal activation was observed only with the naturalness control. Clearly, while both controls differed from the experimental task on a phonological dimension (the dimension of interest), other differences between them gave somewhat divergent results in some regions. This illustrates the supreme importance of choosing the "right" control task, and establishing just what is right is certainly no mean feat. In short, adding or deleting cognitive processes can change the way other processes operate; task specific strategies are difficult to control; and differences between tasks on uncontrolled dimensions might well make interpretation of activation results problematic.

4. Our Approach to Task Design

Since subtraction methods are at present the best available approach, our means of dealing with potential confoundings are to: (1) employ a carefully constructed hierarchical set of tasks which should differentially tap language processes, while sharing as many secondary operations as possible; and (2) to use a variety of subtractions in order to *converge* on a conclusion about the relative function of a given cortical region. Thus, we have built into the tasks a consistent means of validity checking, and in principle, we can put the logic of the hierarchical design to a careful test. We use a hierarchical subtraction technique to isolate orthographic, phonological, and lexical–semantic foci. Subjects perform four distinct same–different tasks. The decision (same vs different) and response components (press a response bulb for same pairs) of these tasks are comparable, although in each the type of linguistic information engaged differs. In a line judgment task, subjects view two sets of four lines with right or left orientations, one above the other, and determine whether the upper and lower displays have the same pattern of left–right alternation (see Table 1). This task should primarily engage visual–spatial feature information processing. In a letter case judgment task, two sets of consonant strings are displayed, and subjects determine whether they contain the same pattern of case (upper and lower) alternation. This task engages both visual–spatial and orthographic (letter) processing. In a rhyme judgment task, subjects determine whether two nonsense word strings rhyme. This task engages visual–spatial, orthographic, and assembled phonological processing (subjects must map the letter strings onto appropriate phonological representations). Finally, in a semantic category task, subjects determine whether two words come from the same semantic cate-

Table 1   Tasks and Subtractions

Task	Stimuli	Processes engaged
Line	//\/ //\/	Visual–spatial
Case	BtBT BtBT	Visual–spatial+Orthographic
Rhyme	LETE JEAT	Visual–spatial+Orthographic+Phonological
Category	CORN RICE	Visual–spatial+Orthographic+Phonological+Semantic

Subtractions	Processes isolated
Case−Line	Orthographic
Rhyme−Line	Orthographic+Phonological
Rhyme−Case	Phonological
Category−Line	Orthographic+Phonological+Semantic
Category−Rhyme	Semantic
Category−Case	Phonological+Semantic

gory. This task engages visual, orthographic, phonological, and semantic information.

a. One Step Subtractions

By subtracting the line task from the case task, activation in regions associated with orthographic processing can be isolated, since the two tasks both engage visual–spatial processing, but only the latter task engages letter processing (see Table 2). By subtracting the case task from the rhyme task, regions associated with assembled phonological processing (i.e., mapping from orthography to phonology) can be isolated, since the tasks differ primarily on that dimension. Finally, by subtracting the rhyme task from the semantic category task, regions associated with lexical semantic processing can be isolated, since only the latter task engages this type of processing (i.e., by using nonsense word stimuli in the rhyme task, spurious activation of semantic sites should be minimized).

b. Common Baseline Subtractions

The experimental paradigm also allows us to test additional hypotheses concerning the relative demands made by each task on a given region, by comparing the activation produced by each with respect to a common baseline. This is accomplished by using the line judgment task as a baseline for the case, rhyme, and semantic category tasks respectively. For instance, if a given region of interest is associated with phonological processing to some extent and semantic processing to a greater extent, while the activation observed should be greater in the rhyme−line (read rhyme **minus** line) than in the case−line subtraction, the semantic category−line should be associated with even greater activation than rhyme−line. Similarly, if a region is associated uniquely with phonological processing, then both rhyme−line and semantic category−line should produce greater activation than case−line; however, the semantic and rhyme conditions should not differ. (Semantic−line activation should be strong, on the view that a word's phonological form needs to be recovered in reading.)

c. Additional Subtractions

By examining additional subtractions, converging evidence regarding function can also be obtained. For example, if a given region shows stronger activation in the case−line subtraction compared to the rhyme−case or semantic category−rhyme conditions, we would assume that region is associated primarily with orthographic processing. If this is so, then by extension, a comparison of the rhyme−line (two step) and rhyme−case (one step) subtractions should show greater activation in the former condition. This is expected, since only in the

rhyme−line subtraction, but not the rhyme−case subtraction, do the tasks differ on an orthographic dimension.

To summarize, by using both the hierarchical subtraction method together with multiple comparisons in this experiment, we can evaluate the hypothesis that a given region serves a particular functional role in reading. This, in our view, provides a significant methodological advantage over many previous studies of language foci. If a consistent pattern of findings is observed across different subtractions (using different experimental and/or control tasks but logically isolating the same function), our confidence in the validity of our findings will be greatly increased.

C. Recent Progress Using Functional MRI to Study Reading

Our current research program, focused on elucidating the functional organization of the brain for reading and language, has several related goals. First, we seek to identify for skilled readers the cortical regions associated with various subcomponent operations in reading. Second, with these findings as a foundation, we seek to ascertain whether the brain activation patterns of individuals with specific reading disability differ from these normal readers on either qualitative or quantitative dimensions. And finally, we seek to examine the relationship between brain organization and reading strategies. We have made progress in all three areas.

Our first studies examined normal readers, and in a recent article we reported findings from 19 neurologically normal right-handed men and 19 women performing the tasks just described (Pugh, Shaywitz, Shaywitz, Constable et al., in press; Shaywitz, Pugh et al ., 1995; Shaywitz, Shaywitz et al., 1995). We focused on those brain regions which previous neuropsychological and neuroimaging investigations indicated were of relevance for language function (Demonet et al., 1994; Frackowiak, 1994; Petersen & Fiez, 1993). Our initial analyses identified one region uniquely associated with orthographic processing (extrastriate, ES). A second region, located within the superior aspect of the inferior frontal gyrus, roughly encompassing Brodmann's areas 44–45 (which we term IFG), and previously shown to be activated in speech tasks when phonetic decisions are required (Demonet et al., 1992, 1994), was found to be uniquely associated with phonological processing on rhyme judgments. The rhyme judgment task was also associated with activation at sites in both the superior temporal gyrus and middle temporal gyrus, areas which fall within traditional language regions. However, the semantic task activated both of these areas significantly more strongly than the rhyme task, suggesting that these regions subserved both phonological and lexical semantic processing. The IFG, by contrast, was *uniquely* associated with phonological processing. Of particular interest were differences in brain activation during phonological processing in men compared to women. Activation during the performance of the rhyming task in men was lateralized to the left IFG; in contrast, activation during this same task in women resulted in bilateral activation of this region.

These findings provide the first clear evidence of sex differences in the functional organization of the brain for language, and indicate that these differences exist at the level of phonological processing. At one level, they support and extend a long held hypothesis which suggests that language functions are more likely to be highly lateralized in males but represented in both cerebral hemispheres in females (Halpern, 1992; Hampson & Kimura, 1992; Harshman, Remington, & Krashen, 1983; Hines, 1990; Hellige, 1993; Iaccino, 1993; McClone, 1980; Witelson & Kigar, 1992).

On another level, and of particular relevance to the scientific study of reading and reading disability, these data indicate that it is now possible to isolate specific components of language and, at the same time, to relate these language processes to distinct patterns of functional organization in brain. These data suggest that the activation of the IFG region during the performance of a rhyming task may provide a neural "signature" for phonological processing, the core cognitive component in reading and reading disability.

Thus, this initial study indicated to us that it is now possible to carry out studies linking cognitive function and brain organization, not only in non-reading-impaired individuals, but in subjects with histories of dyslexia. And, in fact, we have most recently used these same tasks in men and women with a lifelong history of severe reading difficulty and are now analyzing our results. We have also begun to address questions relating to the relationship between the functional organization of the brain as demonstrated during fMRI and reading strategies. We used individual differences in the magnitude of phonological effects in word recognition, as measured by spelling-to-sound regularity effects on lexical decision latencies, and related these data to brain activation patterns during the four tasks described previously (Pugh, Shaywitz, Shaywitz, Shankweiler et al., in press). Our findings indicate that the regularity effects (measured out of magnet) are strongly related to differences in the degree of hemispheric lateralization during fMRI. These relations imply systematic links between neurobiologic measures of brain activation and reading strategies.

D. Studies in Progress

The discovery of a biological signature for reading and, potentially, for reading disability, has significant implications; implications not only for our understanding of the fundamental neural mechanisms underlying reading and reading disability, but for the identification and diagnosis of dyslexia and for assessing the effects of interventions in dyslexia. For example, it will now be possible to examine the development over time of the neural mechanisms serving reading in both dyslexic and non-reading-impaired subjects. In the study just described, we have established that, for nonimpaired readers, the neural systems engaged by mature men and women during phonological processing differ significantly. But it is not known whether there are differences in these neural systems in boys and girls, or at what age these differences emerge. Studies in progress are designed to address just this question; that is, how the neural locus of reading changes over the course of development in boys and girls individually, to determine for the first time what happens in the brain as children mature. These studies address not only this development in non-reading-impaired boys and girls, but the development of the functional organization of the brain for phonological processing in boys and girls with well-defined dyslexia.

The discovery of a biological signature or marker for reading (and potentially for dyslexia) offers the promise of a unique opportunity to identify and diagnose dyslexia in older individuals. Thus, studies in progress are examining the functional organization of the brain for phonological processing in three groups of older individuals: (1) non-reading-impaired, (2) dyslexics, and (3) those adults who have compensated, either wholly or partially, for their reading deficits. We hypothesize that the functional organization of phonological processing will differ among groups, not only between nonimpaired and dyslexics but between compensated and noncompensated dyslexic readers. It is possible that the neural signature for phonological processing may provide the most sensitive index of dyslexia in individuals who appear to have compensated for their reading disability. Finally, the discovery of a biological signature for reading offers an unprecedented opportunity to assess the effects of interventions on reading in nonimpaired readers as well as dyslexics. Thus, using brain activation patterns obtained while subjects engage in tasks tapping phonological processing as the most precise measure of phonological processing, it is now possible to determine the functional organization of the brain in dyslexic individuals, impose an intervention, and measure the effects of that intervention on the brain. If there are measurable effects on brain organization following the intervention, it will be possible to repeat the fMRI to determine whether these differences persist after the intervention ends.

Acknowledgments

The work at the Yale Center for the Study of Learning and Attention described in this chapter was supported by grants from the National Institute of Child Health and Human Development (HD21888 and HD25802). We thank Carmel Lepore and Hedi Sarofin for their assistance.

References

Baader, J. (1763). *Observationes Medicae incisionibus cadaverum anatomicis illustratae.* Augsburg & Freiburg: Ignatius & Anton Wagner.

Bandettini, P. A., Jesmanowicz, A., Wong, E. C., & Hyde, J. S. (1993). Processing strategies for time-course data sets in functional MRI of the human brain. *Magnetic Resonance in Medicine, 30,* 161–173.

Bell, L. C., & Perfetti, C. A. (1994). Reading skill: Some adult comparisons. *Journal of Educational Psychology, 86,* 244–255.

Blachman, B. (1984). The relationship of rapid naming ability and language analysis skills to kindergarten and first grade reading achievement. *Journal of Educational Psychology, 76,* 610–622.

Bradley, L., & Bryant, P. E. (1983). Categorizing sounds and learning to read—a causal connection. *Nature (London), 301,* 419–421.

Brady, S. A., & Shankweiler, D. P., eds. (1991). *Phonological processes in literacy: A tribute to Isabelle Y. Liberman.* Hillsdale, NJ: Erlbaum.

Bruck, M. (1990). Word-recognition skills of adults with childhood diagnoses of dyslexia. *Developmental Psychology, 26,* 439–454.

Bruck, M. (1992). Persistence of dyslexics' phonological awareness deficits. *Developmental Psychology, 28,* 874–886.

Bruck, M. (1996). Outcomes of adults with childhood histories of dyslexia. In R. M. Joshi, ed., *Cognitive and linguistic bases of reading, writing, and spelling,* in press.

Coltheart, M. (1978). Lexical access in simple reading tasks. In G. Underwood (Ed.), *Strategies of information processing.* London: Academic Press.

Coltheart, M., Curtis, B., Atkins, P., & Haller, M. (1993). Models of reading aloud: Dual-route and parallel-distributed-processing approaches. *Psychological Review, 100,* 589–608.

Damasio, H., & Damasio, A. (1989). *Lesion analysis in neuropsychology.* New York: Oxford University Press.

Demonet, J. F., Chollet, F., Ramsey, S., Cardeloat, D., Nespoulous, J. L., Wise, R., Rascol, A., & Frackowiak, R. (1992). The anatomy of phonological and semantic processing in normal subjects. *Brain, 115,* 1753–1768.

Demonet, J. F., Price, C., Wise, R., & Frackowiak, R. S. J. (1994). A PET study of cognitive strategies in normal subjects during language tasks; Influence of phonetic ambiguity and sequence processing on phoneme monitoring. *Brain, 117,* 671–682.

Ferrier, D. (1890). *The Croonian lectures on cerebral localization.* London: Smith, Elder, and Co.

Fletcher, J. M., Shaywitz, S. E., Shankweiler, D. P., Katz, L., Liberman, I. Y., Stuebing, K. K., Francis, D. J., Fowler, A. E., & Shaywitz, B. A. (1994). Cognitive profiles of reading disability: Comparisons of discrepancy and low achievement definitions. *Journal of Educational Psychology, 86,* 6–23.

Frackowiak, R. S. J. (1994). Functional mapping of verbal memory and language. *Trends in the Neurosciences, 17,* 109–115.

Friston, K. J., Frith, C. D., Liddle, P. F., & Frackowiak, R. S. J. (1993). Functional connectivity: The principal-component analysis of large (PET) data sets. *Journal of Cerebral Blood Flow and Metabolism, 13,* 5–14.

Goswami, U., & Bryant, P. (1992). Rhyme, analogy, and children's reading. In P. B. Gough, L. C. Ehri, & R. Treiman (Eds.), *Reading acquisition* (pp. 49–64). Hillsdale, N. J.: Erlbaum.

Gough, P. B., Ehri, L. C., & Treiman, R., eds. (1992). *Reading acquisition.* Hillsdale, N. J.: Erlbaum.

Gough, P. B., & Tunmer, W. E. (1986). Decoding, reading, and reading disability. *Remedial and Special Education, 7,* 6–10.

Halpern, D. F. (1992). *Sex differences in cognitive abilities* (2nd ed.). Hillsdale, N. J.: Erlbaum.

Hampson, E., & Kimura, D. (1992). Sex differences and hormonal influences on cognitive function in humans. In J. B. Becker, S. M. Breedlove, & D. Crews (Eds.), *Behavioral endocrinology* (pp. 357–398). Cambridge, MA: MIT Press.

Harshman, R., Remington, R., & Krashen, S. (1983). *Evidence from dichotic listening for adult sex differences in verbal lateralization.* Ontario, Canada: University of Western Ontario.

Hellige, J. (1993). Hemispheric asymmetry: What's right and what's left. pp. 1–396. Cambridge, MA: Harvard University Press.

Iaccino, J. (1993). Left brain–right brain differences: Inquiries, evidence, and new approaches, pp. 1–284. Hillsdale, N. J.: Lawrence Erlbaum Associates.

Hines, M. (1990). Gonadal hormones and human cognitive development. In J. Balthazart, ed., *Hormones, Brain and Behavior in Vertebrates. 1. Sexual Differentiation, Neuroanatomical Aspects, Neurotransmitters and Neuropeptides* (Vol. 1, pp. 51–63). Basel: Karger.

Liberman, I. Y. (1971). Basic research in speech and lateralization of language: Some implications for reading disability. *Bulletin of the Orton Society, 21,* 71–87.

Liberman, I. Y., & Shankweiler, D. (1991). Phonology and beginning to read: A tutorial. In L. Rieben & C. A. Perfetti, eds., *Learning to read: Basic research and its implications.* Hillsdale, N. J.: Erlbaum.

Liberman, I. Y., Shankweiler, D., & Liberman, A. M. (1989). The alphabetic principle and learning to read. In D. Shankweiler & I. Y. Liberman, eds., *International Academy for Research in Learning Disabilities Monograph Series: Number 6. Phonology and Reading Disability, Solving the Reading Puzzle* (pp. 1–33). Ann Arbor: Univ. of Michigan Press.

Lukatela, G., & Turvey, M. T. (1994a). Visual lexical access is initial phonological: 1) Evidence from associative priming words, homophones, and pseudohomophones. *Journal of Experimental Psychology, 123,* 107–128.

Lukatela, G., & Turvey, M. T. (1994b). Visual lexical access is initially phonological: 2) Evidence from phonological priming by homophones and pseudohomophones. *Journal of Experimental Psychology, 123,* 331–353.

Marshall, J. C., & Newcombe, F. (1973). Patterns of paralexia: A psycholinguistic approach. *Journal of Psycholinguistic Research, 2,* 175–200.

McClelland, J. L. (1979). On the time-relations of mental processes: An examination of systems in cascade. *Psychological Review, 86,* 287–330.

McClelland, J. L., & Rumelhart, D. E. (1981). An interactive activation model of context effects in letter perception. Part 1. An account of basic findings. *Psychological Review, 88,* 375–407.

McClone, J. (1980). Sex differences in human brain assymetry: A critical survey. *The Behavior and Brain Sciences, 3,* 215–263.

Monsell, S., Patterson, K., Graham, A., Hughes, C. H., & Milroy, R. (1992). Lexical and sublexical traslations of spelling to sound:

Strategic anticipation of lexical status. *Journal of Experimental Psychology: Learning, Memory, and Cognition, 18,* 452–467.

Oney, B., Peter, M., & Katz, L. (1996). Printed Word Naming as a Function of Age and Orthographic Transparency, in press.

Patterson, K. E., Marshall, J. C., & Coltheart, M. (1985). *Surface dyslexia: Neuropsychological and cognitive studies of phonological reading.* Hillsdale, N. J.: Erlbaum.

Perfetti, C. A. (1985). *Reading ability.* New York: Oxford Univ. Press.

Petersen, S. E., & Fiez, J. A. (1993). The processing of single words studied with positron emission tomography. *Annual Review of Neuroscience, 16,* 509–530.

Pugh, K., Rexer, K., & Katz, L. (1994a). Evidence for flexible coding in visual word recognition. *Journal of Experimental Psychology, HPP20,* 807–825.

Pugh, K., Rexer, K., & Katz, L. (1994b). Neighborhood effects in visual word recognition: Effects of letter delay and nonword context difficulty. *Journal of Experimental Psychology: Learning, Memory, and Cognition, 20,* 639–648.

Pugh, K. R., Shaywitz, B. A., Shaywitz, S. E., Constable, R. T., Skudlarski, P., Fulbright, R. K., Bronen, R. A., Shankweiler, D. P., Katz, L., Fletcher, J. M., & Gore, J. C. (in press). Cerebral organization of component processes in reading. *Brain.*

Pugh, K. R., Shaywitz, B. A., Shaywitz, S. E., Shankweiler, D. P., Katz, L., Fletcher, J. M., Skudlarski, P., Fulbright, R. K., Constable, R. T., Bronen, R. A., & Gore, J. C. (in press). Predicting reading performance from neuroimaging profiles: The cerebral basis of phonological effects in printed word identification. *Journal of Experimental Psychology.*

Scarborough, H. S. (1984). Continuity between childhood dyslexia and adult reading. *British Journal of Psychology, 75,* 329–348.

Seidenberg, M. S., Bruck, M., Fornarolo, G., & Backman, J. (1985). Word recognition processes of poor and disabled readers: Do they necessarily differ? *Applied Psycholinguistics, 6,* 161–180.

Seidenberg, M. S., & McClelland, J. L. (1989). A distributed developmental model of word-recognition and naming. *Psychological Review, 96,* 523–568.

Sergent, J. (1994). Brain-imaging studies of cognitive function. *Trends in the Neurosciences, 17,* 221–227.

Sergent, J., Zuck, E., Levesque, M., & MacDonald, B. (1992). Positron emission tomography study of letter and object processing: Empirical findings and methodological considerations. *Cerebral Cortex,* 268–280.

Shallice, T., & Warrington, E. K. (1980). Single and multiple component central dyslexic syndromes. In M. Coltheart, K. Patterson, & J. C. Marshall, eds., *Deep dyslexia* (pp. 326–380). London: Routledge & Kegan Paul.

Shankweiler, D., Liberman, I. Y., Mark, L. S., Fowler, C. A., & Fischer, F. W. (1979). The speech code and learning to read. *Journal of Experimental Psychology: Human Learning and Memory, 5,* 531–545.

Shankweiler, D., Crain, S., Katz, L., Fowler, A. E., Liberman, A. M., Brady, S. A., Thornton, R., Lundquist, E., Dreyer, L., Fletcher, J. M., Stuebing, K. K., Shaywitz, S. E., & Shaywitz, B. E. (1995). Cognitive profiles of reading-disabled children: Comparison of language skills in phonology, morphology, and syntax. *Psychological Science, 6,* 149–156.

Share, D. L. (1995). Phonological recoding and self-teaching: Sine qua non of reading acquisition. *Cognition, 55,* 151–218.

Shaywitz, B. A., Shaywitz, S. E., Pugh, K. R., Constable, R. T., Skudlarski, P., Fulbright, R. K., Bronen, R. T., Fletcher, J. M., Shankweiler, D. P., Katz, L., Fletcher, J. M., and Gore, J. C. (1995). Sex differences in the functional organization of the brain for language. *Nature, 373,* 607–609.

Shaywitz, B. A., Pugh, K. R., Constable, R. T., Shaywitz, S. E., Bronen, R. A., Fulbright, R. K., Shankweiler, D. P., Katz, L., Fletcher, J. M., Skudlarski, P and Gore, J. D. Localization of semantic processing using functional magnetic resonance imaging. *Human Brain Mapping, 2,* 149–158, 1995.

Shulman, H. G., Hornak, R., & Sanders, E. (1978). The effect of Graphemic, phonetic, and semantic relationships on access to lexical structure. *Memory and Cognition, 6,* 115–123.

Stanovich, K. E. (1988). Explaining the differences between the dyslexic and the garden-variety poor reader. The phonological-core variable difference model. *Journal of Learning Disabilities, 21*(10), 590–604.

Stanovich, K. E., & Siegel, L. S. (1994). Phenotypic performance profile of children with reading disabilities: A regression-based test of the phonological-core variable-difference model. *Journal of Educational Psychology, 86,* 24–53.

Talairach, J., & Tournoux, P. (1988). *Co-planar stereotaxic atlas of the human brain. 3-dimensional proportional system: An approach to cerebral imaging.* New York: Thieme.

Van Orden, G. C., Pennington, B. F., & Stone, G. O. (1990). Word identification in reading and the promise of subsymbolic psycholinguistics. *Psychological Review, 97,* 488–522.

Wagner, R. K., & Torgesen, J. K. (1987). The nature of phonological processing and its causal role in the acquisition of reading skills. *Psychological Bulletin, 101,* 192–212.

Witelson, S. F., & Kigar, D. L. (1992). Sylvian fissure morphology and asymmetry in men and women: Bilateral differences in relation to handedness in men. *Journal of Comparative Neurology, 323,* 323–326.

Young, R. (1990). Mind, brain, and adaptation in the nineteenth century. Oxford, UK: Oxford University Press.

12

Structural Variations in Measures in the Developmental Disorders

Pauline A. Filipek

Departments of Pediatrics and Neurology
University of California, College of Medicine
Irvine, California 92717

I. Introduction

Our current understanding of brain–behavior relationships is based on correlations between behavior and associated variations in brain structure. The majority of our conventional localization knowledge has resulted from lesion studies in adults, where presumably previously intact mature neural systems have been destroyed. Because of the relative absence of focal lesions, this approach has shed little light on the localization and pathophysiology of the developmental disorders (Filipek, Kennedy, & Caviness, 1992). Rather, these disorders can be presumed to result from anomalies in neuronal–glial development. The location, extent, and age of occurrence of such anomalies within the developmental trajectory, and the resulting effects of plasticity, will all have variable implications for the resulting behavioral deficit (Filipek, 1995a, 1995b; Filipek & Kennedy, 1991; Filipek, Kennedy, et al., 1992). With the advent of neuroimaging technology, especially magnetic resonance imaging (MRI), much effort has been made to find characteristic brain anomalies in these disorders.

This review will address how the available *structural* imaging techniques have improved our understanding and confirmed anatomic localization theories in the developmental disorders, specifically the autistic spectrum and developmental language disorders, dyslexia, and attention deficit hyperactivity disorder

(ADHD). Many neuroimaging studies have been performed with children or adult subjects with developmental disorders. The reader should clearly understand that these studies collectively include a wide variety of methods of computerized tomography (CT) or MR image acquisition and subsequent image analysis, which contributes to the many inconsistent findings outlined in the following sections. In general, the studies reported for each of the disorders represent relatively small heterogeneous subject cohorts, who were diagnosed by variable criteria, with collective ages ranging from early childhood through adulthood. In addition, control subjects were either medical controls who were imaged for a variety of clinical indications, and therefore cannot be considered "normal," or normal volunteers, neither of whom have been uniformly matched, nor resulting data routinely analyzed, for the effects of age, gender, handedness, socioeconomic status (SES), psychiatric codiagnoses, intellectual ability (IQ), or educational setting. The end result moves beyond the comparison of "apples and oranges" and approaches the comparison of "apples and camels."

Reasons behind the often conflicting and contradictory results will be discussed in greater detail after the current neuroimaging findings are reviewed. Finally, the future directions of correlation studies in the developmental disorders will be explored, to address the potential benefits to be gained towards a greater understanding of brain–behavior relationships in the developmental disorders. Until larger homogeneous

169

matched cohorts can replicate the prior and current studies, the findings described here should be considered as suggesting, rather than indicating, characteristic structural differences in any of the developmental disorders based on current imaging studies (Filipek, 1995a; Filipek, Kennedy, et al., 1992).

II. Autistic Spectrum and Developmental Language Disorders

A. Autistic Spectrum Disorders

Over the past 20 years, since Hauser, DeLong, and Rosman (1975) first reported ventricular dilatation in autistic subjects, particularly of the temporal horns, by pneumoencephalography, many investigators have used neuroimaging techniques to look *in vivo* at the brain in autism. Few investigators reported neuropsychological or diagnostic data, making specific diagnostic differentiation difficult. Therefore, this section will consider the autistic spectrum disorders (ASD) as a whole, to include the DSM III-R (American Psychiatric Association, 1987) and DSM IV (American Psychiatric Association, 1994) diagnoses under the umbrella of *pervasive developmental disorders.*

Williams, Hauser, Purpura, DeLong, and Swisher (1980) first reported neuropathologic studies in four retarded individuals with "autistic behaviors" and noted essentially normal gross neuroanatomy. The only noted microscopic abnormality was a decreased density of Purkinje cells in the cerebellum of only one case, without evidence of nerve cell loss or gliosis in the hippocampus, parahippocampus, thalamus, hypothalamus, anterior striatum, or midbrain tectum. Coleman, Romano, Lapham, and Simon (1985) found no differences in neuronal cell counts in the cerebral cortex of a single autistic patient. In 1985, Bauman and Kemper (1985) reported additional microscopic, but again, not gross anatomic, abnormalities in postmortem studies, which now total 3 children and 3 adult autistic subjects (Bauman & Kemper, 1994). Microscopic study of the cerebral cortex found only mild cytoarchitectonic abnormalities, which were confined to the anterior cingulate gyrus in 5 subjects, without evidence for abnormalities in the basal forebrain, thalamus, hypothalamus, or basal ganglia. The only forebrain abnormalities were found in the limbic system, where reduced neuron size and increased cell-packing density were found in the hippocampus, subiculum, entorhinal cortex, amygdala, mammillary bodies, anterior cingulate, and septum.

Arin, Bauman, and Kemper (1991) and Bauman and Kemper (1994) also noted a 50 to 60% reduction in the number of Purkinje and granular cells in the cerebellar *hemispheres* without significant gliosis or other evidence of an atrophic or degenerative process, which was most prominent posteriorly and inferiorly. A milder (~25%) reduction of Purkinje cells was noted in the posterior vermis. However, these findings were only microscopic, and the vermis lobules were not grossly hypoplastic. These investigators also reported mild abnormalities in the inferior olivary nuclei, with small and pale neurons, but without the retrograde cell loss and atrophy usually seen with perinatal or postnatal Purkinje cell loss (Bauman & Kemper, 1994). Ritvo, Freeman, Scheibel, Duong, Robinson, Guthrie, et al. (1986) also noted a mild general reduction in Purkinje cell number in the cerebellar hemispheres and vermis. Therefore, the available postmortem data provides evidence of *microscopic* pathology, predominantly localized to the cerebellar hemispheres and to a lesser extent to the cerebellar vermis, but not to a degree sufficient to account for the structural changes reported in the following neuroimaging studies.

In contrast to the grossly normal neuroanatomy noted in these pathologic studies (Bauman & Kemper, 1985; Williams et al., 1980), Piven, Berthier, Starkstein, Nehme, Pearlson, and Folstein (1990) reported qualitative cortical malformations in 7 of 13 high functioning autistic adolescents and adults, including 5 with polymicrogyria, 1 with schizencephaly and macrogyria, and 1 with macrogyria, which were noted in either hemisphere, without prevalence in a particular lobe. Berthier, Starkstein, and Leiguarda (1990) reported cortical dysplasias in the frontal, temporal, and frontal opercular regions in 2 male adolescents with Asperger's syndrome, and Berthier, Bayes, and Tolosa (1993) also noted cortical defects in the right central perisylvian, right temporo–occipital, or posterior parietal regions in 4 of 7 male adolescents and adults with concurrent Asperger's and Tourette's syndrome. Berthier (1994) subsequently reported qualitatively small gyri and increased sulcal widths in the anterior perisylvian, posterior parietal, or parietal–occipital regions in 7 of 19 adolescents and adults with Asperger's syndrome, with concurrent posterior thinning of the corpus callosum noted in 3 patients. It is presently unclear whether these findings of cortical dysplasias are more prevalent in autism than is currently recognized. Additional systematic evaluations of cortical architecture in larger cohorts will be needed to address this issue.

1. Posterior Fossa

a. Cerebellar Vermis The initial quantitative neuroimaging report from Courchesne, Yeung–Courchesne, Press, Hesselink, and Jernigan (1988) noted a significantly smaller area (greater than 1 standard deviation) of vermal lobules VI and VII (see Fig. 1) in 16 male and 2 female autistic children and adults, which was unrelated to IQ. These findings were felt to represent a consistent anatomic abnormality in most autistic subjects, and to possibly be responsible for the characteristic behavioral deficits. Courchesne, Saitoh, Yeung–Courchesne, Press, Lincoln, Haas, and Schreibman (1994) subsequently reported similar vermal pathology in a cohort of 41 male and 9 female autistic subjects (including the original 18 subjects), aged 2 to 40 years.

By 1993, eight studies (Filipek, Richelme, Kennedy, Rademacher, Pitcher, Zidel, et al., 1992; Garber & Ritvo, 1992; Hashimoto, Murakawa, Miyazaki, Tayama, & Kuroda, 1992; Hashimoto, Tayama, Miyazaki, Murakawa, & Kuroda, 1993; Hashimoto, Tayama, Miyazaki, Murakawa, Shimakawa, Yoneda, et al., 1993; Holttum, Minshew, Sanders, & Phillips, 1992; Kleinman, Neff, & Rosman, 1992; Piven, Nehme, Simon, Barta, Pearlson, & Folstein, 1992), using similar techniques, had reported finding no differences in area measures of vermal lobules VI–VII in a total of 111 male and 21 female autistic subjects, collectively aged 2 to 53 years. Each study was composed of a different age group, with variable nonautistic comparison groups who were not equivalently matched to the autistic subjects for IQ or SES. For example, Piven et al. (1992) used two volunteer control groups: Group I was matched for IQ to the autistic subjects, while Group II was matched for SES only. Kleinman et al. (1992) matched the retarded autistic and medical control children only for age. Filipek, Richelme, et al. (1992) used one normal control and four comparison groups: two

autistic groups (with IQ ≥ 80 and IQ < 80), nonautistic language disordered (with IQ ≥ 80), and nonautistic mentally deficient (with IQ < 80). Holttum et al. (1992) matched their autistic and control subjects for age, gender, IQ, race, and SES. Hashimoto, Murakawa, et al. (1992) compared mentally retarded autistics (IQ < 80) with nonautistic retarded and normal controls, as well as high functioning autistics (IQ ≥ 80) with normal controls matched for age and gender (Hashimoto, Tayama, Miyazaki, Murakawa, Shimakawa, et al., 1993).

Courchesne et al. (1994) then reported that the vermal abnormalities in their 50 subjects consisted of two subtypes: 43 with the previously noted hypoplasia, and 7 with *hyper*plasia of vermal lobules VI–VII. The authors concluded that the combination of these two subtypes within the subject populations was responsible for the apparently "normal" mean vermal areas noted in the other studies in autistic subjects (Filipek, Richelme, et al., 1992; Garber & Ritvo, 1992; Holttum et al., 1992; Kleinman et al., 1992; Piven et al., 1992). To further test this hypothesis, Courchesne, Townsend, and Saitoh (1994b) statistically reanalyzed the measures of vermal lobules VI–VII from their two previous studies (Courchesne et al., 1994a; Courchesne et al., 1988) plus two of the contradictory studies (Kleinman et al., 1992; Piven et al., 1992). Although there were no significant interstudy area differences in the autistic subjects, the collective measures were statistically smaller than those of the normal controls used in three of the autism studies (Courchesne, Saitoh, et al., 1994; Courchesne et al., 1988; Piven et al., 1992, Group II only) and a fourth study comprised of only normal volunteers (Raz, Torres, Spencer, White, & Acker, 1992). A bimodal distribution across the collective autistic subjects was also noted, composed of 68 (87%) with vermal hypoplasia and 10 subjects (13%) with vermal hyperplasia, as compared with the normal controls. Courchesne, Townsend, and Saitoh (1994) also plotted mean vermal areas from the collective hypoplastic subgroup (Courchesne, Saitoh, et al., 1994; Courchesne et al., 1988; Kleinman et al., 1992; Piven et al., 1992) plus a fifth cohort of autistic subjects (Holttum et al., 1992) as a function of "verbal or social intelligence" (Courchesne, Townsend, et al., 1994, p. 220), resulting in what appeared to be a virtually linear correlation (see Fig. 2). This further implicates IQ as contributing to size of vermal lobules VI–VII (Piven & Arndt, 1995), and strengthens the call for IQ matched subjects and controls in morphometric analyses (Filipek, 1995b).

In contrast to their previous reports, Hashimoto, Tayama, Murakawa, Yoshimoto, Miyazaki, Harada, and Kuroda (1995) recently reported that cerebellar

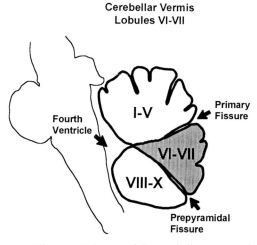

Figure 1 Midline sagittal view of the cerebellar vermis, showing lobules I–V, VI–VII, and VIII–X. Reproduced and adapted with permission from Filipek (1995b).

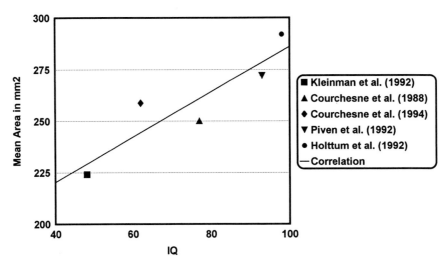

Figure 2 Mean area of vermal lobules VI–VII as a function of IQ from five MRI studies (Courchesne, Saitoh, et al., 1994; Courchesne et al., 1988; Holttum et al., 1992; Kleinman et al., 1992; Piven et al., 1992). Courchesne, Townsend, et al. (1994) plotted the mean areas of the hypoplastic subgroups on a similar graph. This figure represents the mean areas of all subjects, as reported in the original papers. Reproduced and adapted with permission from Filipek (1995b).

vermal lobules I–V, VI–VII, and VIII–X were significantly smaller in area in 102 autistic (75% male) and 112 control (58% male) subjects, aged 3 months to 20 years, although the size of the vermis significantly increased with age in both groups. The autistic group included 11 infants ranging in age from 6 to 23 months, who were identified as having developmental delay, poor eye contact, and facial expression, who were imaged when identified and formally diagnosed as autistic at age 3 years. It should be noted that the entire cohort was imaged using two substantially differing imaging systems and pulse sequence protocols, and that the control group (64% of whom were medical controls) were *not* matched for gender or IQ (autistic mean IQ was 60, with a standard deviation of 25; controls were not measured). In addition, because statistical corrections were apparently not performed for the *nonrepeated* measures of variance, some of the group differences reported for vermal lobules VI–VII may well represent Type I error.

Courchesne recently concluded that "16 quantitative MR and autopsy studies involving 240 cases of autism from nine laboratories have reported evidence of cerebellar abnormalities" (Courchesne, 1995, p. 20). However, despite the recent monumental efforts of Hashimoto et al. (1995), unresolved issues persist concerning differing imaging and study methods and the matching of autistic and control subjects for age, IQ, handedness, and SES. To date, all neuropathological cerebellar abnormalities have been noted only with microscopic analyses. Therefore, the "jury is still out"

concerning the presence of characteristic cerebellar structural anomalies as visualized by neuroimaging studies in all subjects with autism. The interested reader is referred to a recent review for further details (Filipek, 1995b).

b. Cerebellar Hemispheres and Brainstem Gaffney, Tsai, Kuperman, and Minchin (1987) noted smaller cerebellar hemisphere areas when evaluated with a cerebellar–posterior fossa ratio in 14 autistic children and adolescents, as compared with 35 medical controls. Rumsey, Creasey, Stepanek, Dorwart, Patronas, Hamburger, and Duara (1988) reported the lack of qualitative cerebellar atrophy in ASD based on normal sulcal widths in 15 autistic adults. Murakami, Courchesne, Press, Yeung-Courchesne, and Hesselink (1989), also noting the absence of sulcal widening, reported significantly smaller cumulative areas of the medial 6.5 cm of the cerebellar hemispheres, which correlated with decreased areas of vermal lobules VI–VII. These findings may be indicative of cerebellar hemispheric hypoplasia, but represent a mixture of qualitative and quantitative measures of areas on a single or a few selected sagittal MRI slices using a variety of measurement techniques. Therefore, it cannot yet be concluded that the smaller cerebellar hemisphere areas reported in these studies are indicative of generalized cerebellar hypoplasia in autism.

The brainstem has also been a focus of neuroimaging studies, in an attempt to identify *in vivo* the anatomic correlates of potential functional disturbances in autistic subjects (Courchesne, Yeung-Courchesne, Hicks, & Lincoln, 1985; Ornitz, Atwell, Kaplan, & Westlake, 1985). Gaffney, Kuperman, Tsai, and Minchin (1988) initially reported smaller areas of the pons and entire brainstem in 13 high functioning autistic children and adolescents (IQ ≥ 60), as compared with 35 medical controls. Hsu, Yeung–Courchesne, Courchesne, and Press (1991) reported finding no differences in area measurements of the midbrain and pons, including ventral division, in 34 autistic and 44 unmatched control subjects ranging in age from 2 to 39 years. Hashimoto, Tayama, Miyazaki, Murakawa, Sakurama, Yoshimoto, and Kuroda (1991), and Hashimoto, Tayama, Miyazaki, Sakurama, Yoshimiti, Murakawa, and Kuroda (1992) found shorter midsagittal midbrain and pontine widths in 29 autistic children, with the shorter measures associated with lower IQ (Hashimoto, Tayama, Miyazaki, Sakurama, Yoshimiti, Murakawa, et al., 1992). These investigators noted smaller midbrain and medulla areas in *both* 14 retarded autistic and 16 retarded nonautistic children, as compared with normal controls. A smaller pontine area was noted only for the retarded nonautistic controls, with no differences between the two retarded groups for total brainstem area (Hashimoto, Murakawa, et al., 1992). Hashimoto, Tayama, (1993) then reported smaller areas of the midbrain, pons, and medulla in 21 autistic children (IQ range 20 to 129), as compared with normal children (mean IQ 109), and smaller areas of the midbrain and medulla, but not the pons, in 13 high functioning autistic children (IQ ≥ 80) matched with normal controls for IQ and gender (Hashimoto, Tayama, Miyazaki, Murakawa, Shimakawa, 1993). Most recently, Hashimoto et al. (1995) reported smaller areas of the midbrain, pons, and medulla in 102 autistics than in 112 controls, whose subject characteristics are as described above. As with the cerebellar measures, a positive correlation with age was seen for midbrain, pontine, and medullary area measurements. These conflicting reports, most of which originate from the same group of investigators, used variably matched control groups and differing MRI methods, and suggest potential dependence of these measures on IQ. Therefore, no definitive conclusions can be made concerning the presence of midbrain, pontine, or medullary structural anomalies by MRI as being characteristic in autism.

2. Cerebral Hemispheres

a. Hemispheres Although early neuroimaging studies using CT scans in autistic subjects reported a reversal of the normally asymmetric posterior hemispheric widths (Hier, LeMay, & Rosenberger, 1979), subsequent reports have found the incidence of reversed posterior cerebral asymmetry in ASD to be no different from the normal population (Damasio, Maurer, Damasio, & Chui, 1980; Harcherik, Cohen, Ort, Paul, Shaywitz, Volkmar, et al., 1985; Prior, Tress, Hoffman, & Boldt, 1984; Rumsey et al., 1988; Tsai, Jacoby, Stewart, & Beisler, 1982), or from children with other neurological diagnoses (Tsai, Jacoby, & Stewart, 1983). Using MRI, Gaffney, Kuperman, Tsai, and Minchin (1989) reported narrower left frontal lobes, with normal appearing temporal lobes and opercular regions as compared with medical controls.

Midsagittal hemisphere areas on MRI scans have been reported as being similar in 13 autistic and 35 medical controls, aged 4 to 22 years (Gaffney, Kuperman, Tsai, Minchin, & Hassanein, 1987). Qualitative parietal lobe volume loss was also reported on MRI scans in 9 of 21 autistic subjects, aged 6 to 32 years, based on enlarged sulcal widths (Courchesne, Press, & Yeung-Courchesne, 1993). In contrast, larger hemispheric size has been reported in autism, based on autopsy studies (Bailey, Luthert, Bolton, Le Couteur, Rutter, & Harding, 1993; M. L. Bauman, personal communication, 1994) and quantitative MRI (Filipek, Richelme, et al., 1992, see Section II.C below; Piven et al., 1992).

b. Hemispheric Substructures Subsequent CT studies analyzed volumes of hemispheric gray and white matter, including the deep gray nuclei, where no differences were found (Creasy, Rumsey, Schwartz, Duara, Rapoport, & Rapoport, 1986). Jacobson, LeCouteur, Howlin, and Rutter (1988) first implicated subcortical rather than cortical abnormalities in ASD, reporting normal frontal lobe CT densities, which were higher in the left thalamus and lower in both caudate nuclei. The lateral ventricles of ASD subjects have been variously reported to be wider and larger than in control populations (Campbell, Rosenbloom, Perry, George, Kricheff, Anderson, et al., 1982; Gaffney et al., 1989), but these findings did not correlate with clinical variables, including birth weight, head circumference, language development scores, adaptive behavior scores, congenital anomalies, or severity of asocial symptoms (Campbell et al., 1982). Other investigators have reported normal ventricular size (Creasey et al., 1986; Garber, Ritvo, Chiu, Griswold, Kashanian, Freeman, & Oldendorf, 1989; Nowell, Hackney, Muraki, & Coleman, 1990; Prior et al., 1984; Rosenbloom, Campbell, George, Kricheff, Taleporos, Anderson, et al., 1984). Ventricular enlargement, a nonspecific indication of possible cerebral injury or maldevelopment, cannot be related specifically to the neuroanatomic basis of ASD. Nowell et al. (1990) also noted qualitatively normal amygdala and limbic systems.

The limbic system has often been implicated in the pathogenesis of autism, particularly in microscopic neuroanatomic studies (Bauman, 1991; Bauman & Kemper, 1985, 1990, 1994). Most recently by MRI, the cross-sectional area of the posterior hippocampus, including the subiculum and the dentate gyrus, was measured in 30 male and 3 female autistic subjects, aged 6 to 42 years (mean 13.8 ± 9.1 years) (Saitoh, Courchesne, Egaas, Lincoln, & Schreibman, 1995). These measures were found to be similar in autistic and control subjects, differing only by approximately 1.5%, and were independent of IQ or presence of seizures in the autistic subjects.

B. Developmental Language Disorders

Few postmortem studies have been performed in patients with developmental language disorders. In a young boy with probable verbal auditory agnosia, which is analogous to word deafness in adults (Rapin & Allen, 1987), Landau, Goldstein, and Kleffner (1960) reported bilateral perisylvian cystic lesions with surrounding cortical dysplasias. In a 7 year old girl with developmental dysphasia, Cohen, Campbell, and Yaghmai (1989) found symmetric plana temporale and a single dysplastic microgyrus in the left insular cortex.

1. Diencephalon and Caudate

Jernigan, Hesselink, Stowell, and Tallal (1991) performed volumetric MRI measurements of the cerebral hemispheres on a cohort of 13 male and 7 female mixed language and learning-impaired children, with a mean age of 8.9 ± 0.7 years. Comparisons were made with 8 male and 4 female age-matched controls, who demonstrated normal language development and academic achievement. Measurements included caudate, lenticulate, and diencephalic gray matter (including

mammillary bodies, hypothalamus, septal nuclei, and thalamus). Volumes of right diencephalic gray matter were decreased in the total group of subjects. In the right-handed subjects ($N = 18$), bilateral caudate volumes were also significantly reduced, relative to the right-handed controls ($N = 11$). No group differences were noted in volumetric symmetry of these subcortical structures.

2. Perisylvian Regions

Several groups of investigators have measured MRI-based *en bloc* hemispheric brain regions in language-disordered children. In a pilot study, Filipek, Kennedy, Caviness, Klein, and Rapin (1987) reported bilaterally reduced posterior temporal volumes in 4 male adolescents with verbal auditory agnosia (word deafness) (Rapin & Allen, 1987). Plante, Swisher, and Vance (1989), in 4 year old dizygotic twins, subsequently reported atypical perisylvian configuration, which was symmetric in the language-impaired male. They subsequently noted atypical perisylvian asymmetry in 6 of 8 mixed language-impaired boys, aged 4 to 9 years, with a larger right and normal left perisylvian regional volume. In addition, various extraperisylvian regions were occasionally different in the language-impaired children, although none proved characteristic for language impairment (Plante, Swisher, Vance, & Rapcsak, 1991). They also reported atypical perisylvian asymmetries in the parents and siblings of 4 of the language-impaired boys, which were associated with disordered language skills in these family members (Plante, 1991).

In addition to the structural morphometric measures reported above, Jernigan et al. (1991) also divided the cerebral hemispheres into *en bloc* subdivisions. They noted diminished volumes of the left posterior perisylvian language regions in the total group of 20 mixed language and learning-impaired

Table 1 Characteristics of Subjects with AD, DLD, and NALIQ

Subjects	NVIQ criteria[a]	N	NVIQ	Males/females	Mean age ± SD
High AD	≥80	13	98 ± 17[b]	11/2	9.3 ± 1.0
Low AD	<80	16	49 ± 19[b]	14/2	8.8 ± 1.6
DLD	≥80	25	101 ± 23[b]	17/8	8.1 ± 1.6[c]
NALIQ	<80	9	42 ± 26[b]	4/5	8.1 ± 2.2
Controls	—	30	—	15/15	9.1 ± 1.2

Notes: AD = autistic disorder (American Psychiatric Association, 1987); DLD = developmental language disorder; NALIQ = nonautistic low IQ; and SD = standard deviation. Data from Filipek, Richelme, et al. (1992).

[a]Based on the traditional nonverbal IQ (NVIQ) criteria for DLD in preschoolers (Aram, Morris, & Hall, 1992).

[b]No group differences in NVIQ.

[c]Group difference in age ($p < .01$).

children relative to the controls. In the right-handed subjects, both posterior perisylvian language areas were reduced in volume.

3. Corpus Callosum

Njiokiktjien, de Sonneville, and Vaal (1994) measured the ratio of area of the entire corpus callosum as a function of midsagittal brain area in 25 boys and 12 girls with developmental dysphasia/dyslexia, aged 3 to 14 years, as compared with 42 medical controls. These investigators reported similar total callosal areas for the dysphasic/dyslexic and control children. However, they noted significantly larger callosal areas in the "familial" cases (with first-degree relatives with learning disabilities) than in the "nonfamilial" cases.

C. Morphometric Analysis in a Mixed AD and DLD Cohort

MRI-based morphometry was performed on 63 developmentally disordered school aged children diagnosed with autistic disorder (AD, $N= 29$) by DSM III–R criteria (American Psychiatric Association, 1987),

developmental language disorder (DLD, $N= 25$), or nonautistic low IQ (NALIQ, $N= 9$) as preschoolers (Filipek, Richelme et al., 1992) through NINDS (National Institute of Neurologic Disorders and Stroke) Program Project NS 20489 (Rapin, 1996). The normal control children had headaches or were volunteers, with normal histories, examinations, and school achievement. See Table 1 for characteristics. Measures included global cerebral hemispheres, cerebellum, and brainstem, individual hemispheric substructures, and *en bloc* hemispheric regions, as previously described (see Fig. 3) (Filipek, Kennedy et al., 1992; Filipek, Kennedy, Caviness, Rossnick, Spraggins, & Starewicz, 1989; Filipek, Richelme, Kennedy, & Caviness, 1994).

1. Global Hemispheric and Structural Measures

AD and DLD cerebral hemispheres were unexpectedly larger in volume than the controls, with a significant volumetric hierarchy noted across most measures, where High AD > DLD > Low AD > controls > NALIQ. This larger volume was principally due to greater volumes of diencephalon and white matter, with a corpus callosum similar in size to childhood

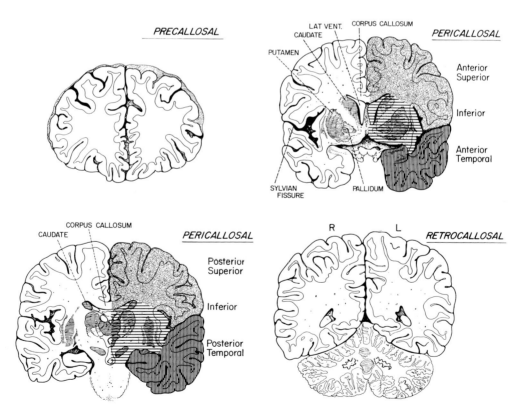

Figure 3 "Callosal" regions used for morphometric analysis. The *precallosal* (prefrontal) and *retrocallosal* (posterior parietal–occipital) regions are those positionally normalized anterior and posterior coronal slices, respectively, which do not visualize the corpus callosum. The *anterior* and *posterior pericallosal* regions are defined by the appearance of the anterior commissure. The *superior, inferior,* and *temporal pericallosal* regions are defined by hand-drawn borders. Figure by Edith Tagrin, Medical Art Resources, Boston, MA. Reproduced and adapted with permission from Filipek, Kennedy, et al. (1992).

controls. No morphometric abnormalities were identified in the AD or DLD subjects in the hippocampus (in concordance with Saitoh et al. (1995) and M. L. Bauman, personal communication, 1994), amygdala, or ventricular system. All five groups were similar only in volumes of the ventricles and hippocampus. In contrast, all NALIQ structures were smaller than the controls, except for the hippocampus and surprisingly, the ventricular system.

2. Hemispheric Regions

In AD, the larger hemispheric volumes were disproportionately localized to the posterior temporal and parietal–occipital regions, with High AD also showing enlarged volumes in the prefrontal, anterior temporal, and parietal regions. The larger white matter volumes were disproportionately localized to the anterior and posterior temporal (which includes the primary auditory and auditory association cortices), and, in High AD, the prefrontal and posterior parietal association regions (which includes the superior and inferior parietal lobules).

In DLD children, who share similar language deficits with AD children, the larger hemispheric volumes were localized to the posterior temporal and parietal–occipital regions, also seen in the AD children. The larger white matter volumes were also localized to the anterior and posterior temporal and parietal association regions, as seen with the High AD children. In contrast, despite significantly smaller hemispheric volumes, NALIQ subjects had relatively preserved prefrontal, temporal, and parietal association regions, which differed considerably from the High and Low AD volumetric profiles.

3. Posterior Fossa

In AD subjects, the volumes of the cerebellar hemispheres and areas of vermal lobules I–V were larger than the controls, while areas of lobules VI–VII were similar to controls. No differences were noted for the proportion of area of verbal lobules VI–VII to cerebellar hemispheric volume. There was also no evidence for a bimodal distribution of vermal area measures in this AD cohort, as suggested by Courchesne, Saitoh, et al. (1994) as the cause of apparently normal mean areas of vermal lobules VI–VII.

III. Dyslexia

Galaburda, Sherman, Rosen, Aboitiz, and Geschwind (1985) and Humphreys, Kaufmann, and Galaburda (1990) have performed the only comprehensive postmortem studies of the brains of 4 male and 3 female severe adult dyslexics, many of whom were referred by the Orton Dyslexia Society Brain Bank. They found a very high frequency of microdysgenesis, particularly in the frontal and temporal opercula, and more prominent in the left hemisphere. They also measured the planum temporale, a triangular landmark located within the superior plane of the temporal lobes, just posterior to Heschl's gyrus within the depth of the sylvian fissure. The left planum is larger than the right in approximately 65% of normal brains, the right is larger than the left ("reversed" asymmetry) in 11%, with the remaining 24% being symmetric, according to a previous autopsy study of 100 brains (Geschwind & Levitsky, 1968). Galaburda et al. (1985) and Humphreys et al. (1990) found symmetric areas of the plana temporale in all 7 subjects studied (100% prevalence in this dyslexic sample vs 24% in the normal population), which were uniformly due to larger areas of the right rather than smaller areas of the left planum temporale. These findings in dyslexic brains suggested anomalous brain development during the late stages of corticogenesis, potentially leading to improved neuronal survival, and subsequent redefinition of cortical architecture, underlying asymmetry and cerebral dominance (Galaburda, 1988; Galaburda, 1992).

A. Cerebral Hemispheres

1. Symmetry Measurements

Hynd, Semrud-Clikeman, Lorys, Novey, and Eliopulos (1990) reported normal posterior (temporal–parietal–occipital) but smaller right anterior (frontal) width measurements on a single horizontal MRI slice, the latter producing symmetric frontal regions in 10 dyslexic children. In contrast, Duara, Kushch, Gross-Glenn, Barker, Jallad, Pascal, et al. (1991) reported a reversal (right > left) of the normal posterior asymmetry on single horizontal MRI slices in 21 dyslexic adults, who demonstrated larger right and similar left areas when compared with the controls. In contrast to Hynd et al. (1990), the anterior regions were similar in the dyslexics and controls, demonstrating the expected right > left asymmetry. The area of the right occipital polar region in the dyslexic subjects, although not different from the controls, correlated with the severity of reading disability. One of the dyslexic cohorts in these studies was limited to late childhood and the other to adults, which may contribute to the divergent data. Additional considerations of the image analysis methods used are discussed below, all of which probably play a role in this discrepancy.

2. Corpus Callosum

Three fairly recent MRI studies have focused on measurements of the corpus callosum in dyslexic subjects. The underlying hypotheses were that previously reported findings of frontal and/or temporal–parietal symmetry in dyslexics may be related to anomalous interhemispheric pathways through the callosum to the known language regions. These studies are composed of subjects in differing age ranges, one each in adults, adolescents, and children. Each study used differing methods of performing the area measurements, and differing methods of reporting the data obtained.

Duara et al. (1991) noted a larger splenial (posterior) area of the midsagittal corpus callosum in 12 male and 9 female dyslexic adults, as compared with 19 nondyslexic adult controls who were matched only for age. Many of the dyslexic subjects also had a codiagnosis of ADHD. The 9 female dyslexics also had larger genu and total callosal areas than the male dyslexic or mixed control subjects. In contrast, using an apparently similar technique, Larsen, Høien, and Ödegaard (1992) reported no differences or gender effects in the areas of the total callosum or the splenium between 15 male and 4 female adolescent dyslexic subjects and 17 controls matched for age, gender, IQ, SES and educational environment. They also reported no significant effects of dividing the dyslexics on the basis of specific linguistic deficiencies or symmetry measurements of the planum temporale.

Hynd, Hall, Novey, Eliopulos, Black, Gonzales, et al. (1995), using a different callosal segmentation technique, noted smaller measurements of the genu in 11 male and 5 female dyslexic children, as compared with 16 control children matched for age, gender, and handedness but with significantly higher IQs. In the dyslexics, 37.5% had psychiatric codiagnoses. Small but significant positive correlations were found between reading ability and the areas of the genu and splenium in these children, without evidence for gender effects.

In summary, these studies of the corpus callosum in dyslexia provide conflicting structural information: total callosal measurements are reported to be both larger in females and similar in both genders; the "splenium" region is reported to be both larger and similar in size; and the genu is reported to be both smaller and similar in size. In part, these contradictions may be due to the divergent age ranges and differing matching of controls. It should also be noted that each study used differing MRI and morphometric methods to obtain the measurements, which significantly confounds the results. Figure 4 shows the various methods used in these studies to subdivide the callosum into regions (Filipek, 1995a). Also shown is the Witelson (1989) postmortem method, which is the basis of the majority of existing studies of normal corpus callosum morphology, as well as the effects of gender and handedness. The subdivided callosal regions are obviously not equivalent across the methods. There-

fore, caution is urged in interstudy comparisons of these "typical" callosal anomalies in developmental dyslexia.

B. Temporal Lobes

1. Temporal Lobes and "Language" Regions

Hynd et al. (1990) noted bilaterally shortened insular regions in 8 dyslexic male and 2 female children. The authors concluded that the smaller (shorter) insulae were responsible for the reported bilaterally decreased insular glucose utilization in dyslexics during reading tasks (Gross-Glenn, Duara, Barker, Loewenstein, Chang, Yoshii, et al., 1991). Kushch, Gross-Glenn, Jallad, Lubs, Rapin, Feldman, et al. (1993) reported symmetrical posterior and total superior temporal lobe surface areas in 9 male and 8 female dyslexic adults, and 21 controls matched only for handedness. Three dyslexics reported symptoms of ADHD. The symmetry noted in the dyslexics was seemingly due to smaller left temporal lobe measures, while the controls demonstrated the expected larger regions on the left side. There were no effects of gender or gender-by-diagnosis in these measurements. In the dyslexics, the degree of leftward asymmetry of the posterior temporal regions positively correlated with reading comprehension abilities. In the controls, none of the laterality indices were associated with any of the measures from the psychoeducational battery.

2. Planum Temporale

The planum is an anatomic landmark and not a discrete structure with clearly defined boundaries (Filipek, 1995a; Filipek, Kennedy, et al., 1992; Galaburda, 1988, 1993). As measured postmortem, the planum represents solely the bidimensional area of *visualized* cortex on the superior surface of the temporal lobe, and does not include measurements into sulcal depths (Galaburda, 1993). In postmortem studies, the parietal lobe is cut away, leaving a full view of the planum temporale from the superior aspect of the hemisphere. Even with this advantage, accurate identification of the planum boundaries is often difficult in postmortem studies. In any neuroimaging study producing a single imaging plane (coronal, sagittal, or horizontal), it is very difficult to clearly define the borders of this relatively small region (Galaburda, 1993; Filipek, 1995a).

Ideally, the sagittal plane should be used to define the posterior border, and the coronal plane to define the medial and lateral borders; accurate border definition in the axial plane is extremely limited (Galaburda, 1993). Newer software can alleviate this problem, by permitting simultaneous visualization of three-dimensional (3D) MRI scans in all three planes, with border markers superimposed from one plane to another (Galaburda, 1993; Kennedy, Meyer, Filipek, & Caviness, 1994). However, even with this technological support, definition of the plana temporale is one of the most difficult tasks in MRI-based morphometry (Filipek, 1995a). Also, mathematical computations must be used to account for the superior angulation of the sylvian fissure (Galaburda, 1993). This "structural" ambiguity has led to neuroimaging measurements of only unidimensional lengths, to the creation of often discrepant criteria for plana boundaries, or to the avoidance of this landmark altogether (Jernigan et al., 1991). Therefore, direct comparisons across the published studies of the plana temporale in dyslexia, which are summarized in Table II, cannot be made at present (Filipek, 1995a). The interested reader is referred to a recent review for a detailed discussion of these and other issues (Filipek, 1995a).

Hynd et al. (1990) reported shorter left and similar right planum length in 8 male and 2 female dyslexic children, leading to symmetric or reversed asymmetry of planum measures in 90% of the dyslexics. Larsen, Høien, & Ödegaard (1990) also measured lengths, and found symmetric plana due to longer right lengths, in 70% of 15 male and 4 female dyslexic adolescents, as compared with 17 matched controls (3 with phonologic deficiencies). The remaining 30% of the dyslexics showed the normal left > right symmetry, as did 70% of the control subjects. Four dyslexic subjects with pure phonologic deficits had symmetric plana, leading to the conclusion that a close relationship exists between phonologic deficiencies and planum symmetry.

Leonard, Voeller, Lombardino, Morris, Hynd, Alexander, et al. (1993) divided the planum into temporal [the traditional planum measured by Galaburda (1988)] and parietal banks in 7 male and 2 female adult

dyslexics, 4 male and 6 female unaffected relatives, and 5 male and 7 female adult controls. They reported a leftward asymmetry of the temporal bank, and a rightward asymmetry of the parietal bank, in all three groups. The dyslexic subjects had larger right parietal than temporal banks, relative to both comparison groups; the investigators concluded that the dyslexics showed a "transfer" of planar tissue from the right temporal to parietal bank. They also found anomalous sylvian fissures and multiple Heschl's gyri in all 9 dyslexics (bilateral in 7) and in 7 unaffected relatives (bilateral in 2). In comparison, such anomalies were noted in only 1 of the controls. They also questioned whether bilateral anomalies were less prevalent in females, leaving them less vulnerable to the complete syndrome of dyslexia.

Schultz, Cho, Staib, Kier, Fletcher, Shaywitz, et al. (1994) reported no differences in the *convolutional* surface area of the planum temporale, the superior surface area, and volume of the temporal lobes in 10 male and 7 female dyslexic children and 14 normal controls, matched for age and IQ. The majority (76%) of the dyslexics had a left-predominant planum measure. Filipek, Pennington, Holmes, Lefly, Kennedy, Meyers, et al. (1995), also found a L>R asymmetry of the planum temporale in 30 pairs of monozygotic and dizygotic twins (see Table 3), using methods according to Galaburda (1993), Galaburda, Corsiglia, Rosen, and Sherman (1987), and Geschwind and Levitsky (1968). These collectively reviewed studies appear to report widely variable results on measurements of the planum temporale. However, it should be understood that the definitions of the "planum temporale" and methods used for measurements differ considerably in all of these studies, thereby making direct comparisons impossible.

Table 2   Summary of Planum Temporale (PT) Measures in Dyslexics

Authors	Subjects	PT Measurement	Finding	Lateralization
Galaburda, 1988	adults (postmortem)	area	symmetric	larger right
Hynd et al., 1990	children	length	right ≥ left	shorter left
Larsen et al., 1990	adolescents	length	symmetric	longer right
Leonard et al., 1993	adolescents and adults	length, temporal/ parietal banks	—	—
Schultz et al., 1994	children	area, temporal/ parietal banks	left > right	—
Filipek et al., 1995	adolescents and adults	area	left > right	—

Note: Reproduced and adapted with permission from Filipek (1995a).

Table 3 MRI-Based Morphometric Twin Study of Dyslexia

	N	MZ/DZ	Age (yrs)[a]	Gender	FSIQ[b]	DISCR[b,c]	Handedness
Dyslexic	36	21/15	21 ± 3	17M/18F	101 ± 10	−1.2 ± 0.6	1.1 ± 0.2
DZ siblings	5	0/5	19 ± 2	3M/2F	112 ± 10	0.5 ± 0.4	1.1 ± 0.4
Controls	18	8/10	19 ± 3	9M/9F	121 ± 8	2.4 ± 0.7	1.1 ± 0.2

Notes: MZ = monozygotic; DZ = dizygotic; FSIQ = full scale IQ; and DISCR = composite reading score from the Peabody Individual Achievement Test (PIAT) (Dunn & Markwardt, 1970), reading recognition, reading comprehension, and spelling subscores.
[a]Group differences significant ($p < .05$).
[b]Dyslexic $\leq 0 <$ nondyslexic.
[c]Group differences significant ($p < .001$).

C. Morphometric Analyses in Dyslexic Twins

Filipek, Pennington, Holmes, Lefly, Kennedy, Meyers, et al., (1995) performed full MRI-based morphometric analyses on the brains of the 30 twin pairs (see Table 3) and noted significant differences in the perisylvian language regions, white matter, basal ganglia, thalamus, and parietal association regions (Fig. 3). Smaller volumes were noted in the diencephalon and both perisylvian language regions of both male and female dyslexics. However, female dyslexics had larger volumes of parietal hemispheric regions than did the female controls. Significantly greater monozygotic than dizygotic correlations were noted for total cerebral volume and diencephalon, suggesting genetic influence, whereas monozygotic and dizygotic correlations were similar for the perisylvian language regions.

IV. Attention Deficit Hyperactivity Disorder

Based on numerous adult lesion (Damasio & Damasio, 1989; Kertesz, 1983; Mesulam, 1985) and functional imaging studies (Corbetta, Miezin, Dobmeyer, Shulman, & Petersen, 1991; Corbetta, Miezin, Shulman, & Petersen, 1993; Petersen, Corbetta, Miezin, & Shulman, 1994; Petersen, Robinson, & Morris, 1987; Posner & Dehaene, 1994; Posner, Petersen, Fox, & Raichle, 1988), many cognitive neuroscientists hypothesize three attentional networks: the *orienting/shifting (selective) attention network*, localized to both superior parietal lobules, thalamus, and midbrain; the *executive network*, localized to the anterior cingulate and basal ganglia; and the *alerting/arousal (vigilance) network*, localized to the right frontal lobe, especially the superior region of Brodmann area 6 (Posner & Petersen, 1990; Posner & Raichle, 1994). Experimental lesions to the head of the caudate in animals have been associated with hyperactivity and deficient attentional abilities (Iversen, 1977).

Casey, Giedd, Vauss, Vaituzis, & Rapoport (1992) have also shown that the development of selected and divided attention in normal children and adolescents correlated with MRI morphometric measures of the anterior cingulate (particularly the right), but not with whole brain area. Imaging studies have focused on these regions in an attempt to localize structural anomalies in ADHD.

A. Cerebral Hemispheres

1. Hemispheric Asymmetries

In one of the earliest CT studies, Nasrallah, Loney, Olson, McCalley–Whitters, Kramer, and Jacoby (1986) noted a 58% prevalence of mild to moderate qualitative cortical atrophy in 24 young male adults with ADHD, all of whom had received an unspecified trial of methylphenidate during childhood. The prevalence of atrophy in those reporting the single psychiatric codiagnosis of alcohol abuse rose to 71%. Therefore, this association was felt to possibly be related as much to concurrent psychiatric codiagnoses as to the presence of ADHD or to the use of methylphenidate. Nasrallah et al. (1986) and Shaywitz, Shaywitz, Byrne, Cohen, and Rothman (1983) have also reported normal ventricular size, while Hynd et al. (1990) noted normal midsagittal brain areas and normal lengths and symmetries of the planum temporale and insular regions. Using linear measurements on CT, Shaywitz et al. (1983) noted symmetric frontal lobe widths in 35 ADHD children as compared with medical controls.

2. Caudate Measures

With MRI, Hynd et al. (1990) also reported symmetric frontal lobe widths, due to narrower right frontal measurements. Hynd, Hern, Novey, Eliopulos, Marshall, Gonzalez, and Voeller (1993) also reported that 64% of 8 male and 3 female ADHD children demonstrated a reversal of the normal (found in 73% of controls) left > right caudate asymmetry, which was due to a significantly smaller left caudate area. The investigators felt these findings were suggestive of anomalies in the frontal–striatal systems in ADHD.

In contrast, Castellanos, Giedd, Eckburg, Marsh, Vaituzis, Kaysen, et al. (1994) reported symmetric caudate volumes in 50 ADHD males, aged 6 to 19 years, who were matched for age, weight, height, Tanner stage (Tanner, 1962), and handedness to 48 normal controls, but were not matched for scores of Wechsler Intelligence Scale for Children–Revised (WISC–R) vocabulary and block design subtests (Wechsler, 1974). In contrast to Hynd et al. (1993) and Filipek, Semrud-Clikeman, Steingard, Renshaw, Kennedy, and Biederman (in press), the normal controls in this study demonstrated a right > left asymmetry of the caudate nucleus. In addition, the ADHD cohort had specific math or reading learning disabilities (26%) and psychiatric codiagnoses of conduct (16%) or oppositional (42%) disorder.

Filipek, Semrud-Clikeman, Steingard, Renshaw, Kennedy, and Biederman (in press), also measured caudate volumes in 15 male adolescents with "pure" ADHD (*without* psychiatric codiagnoses or learning disabilities), as compared with normal controls matched for age, IQ, and handedness. The left caudate head was significantly smaller in the ADHD subjects, with similar measures noted for the right caudate. The smaller left caudate resulted in a reversal in ADHD (left < right) of the caudate asymmetry found in the normal controls (left > right), which replicates the caudate area and symmetry findings reported by Hynd et al. (1993), but not of Castellanos et al. (1994).

In an MRI-based study of 15 male and 15 female normal children aged 6 through 11 years (Caviness, Kennedy, Richelme, Rademacher, and Filipek, in press), caudate symmetry was found to be slightly sexually dimorphic: left > right in the boys, and right > left in the girls, with absolute caudate volumes similar to those reported by Castellanos et al. (1994) for their similarly aged normal control subgroup. In the morphometric analysis of the brains of 10 male and 10 female normal young adults (Filipek et al., 1994), the caudate was symmetric in both the males and females, in contrast to the right > left asymmetry reported by Castellanos et al. (1994) in normal child and adolescent males, and by Breier, Buchanan, Elkashef, Munson, Kirkpatrick, and Gellad (1992), and Peterson, Riddle, Cohen, Katz, Smith, and Leckman (1993), in 20 male and 9 female, and in 16 male and 3 female normal adults, respectively. These apparently discrepant caudate asymmetries in normal cohorts do not appear to be gender-dependent. Handedness, not uniformly noted in these studies, may contribute to these variable results.

3. Corpus Callosum

Assuming a correlation between the narrower right frontal regions and the size of the corpus callosum in ADHD, Hynd, Semrud-Clikeman, Lorys, Novey, Eliopulos, and Lyytinen (1991) subsequently measured the areas of 5 callosal regions in 5 male and 2 female ADHD children, using the methods described in Figure 4. All 7 ADHD subjects had psychiatric codiagnoses. In the ADHD group, they found smaller areas of the genu, splenium, and region just anterior to the splenium. These callosal abnormalities are localized to regions connecting the prefrontal–orbital, peri- and juxtastriate, and insular–temporal–posterior–parietal hemispheric regions, respectively, and possibly reflect variations of structure and processing of the frontal lobes and right hemisphere (Hynd et al., 1991).

Using a differing image analysis method (Filipek et al., 1994) according to Witelson (1989, see Fig. 4), Semrud-Clikeman, Filipek, Biederman, Steingard, Kennedy, Renshaw et al, (1994), replicated the similar total callosal, but smaller splenium, areas in 15 male adolescents with "pure" ADHD (without psychiatric codiagnoses or learning disabilities), as compared with normal controls matched for age, IQ, and handedness. In this cohort, there was also a tendency noted for smaller areas of the two regions just anterior to the splenium in ADHD, but the genu regions were similar to controls. In addition, the 5 subjects who did not respond to stimulant medication had the smallest total and posterior callosal measurements, providing the first evidence for a potential structural basis for response to stimulant medications.

Giedd, Castellanos, Casey, Kozuch, King, Hamburger, et al. (1994) also used the Witelson (1989) method to evaluate the corpus callosum in 18 boys, ranging in age from 7 to 15 years, who also were codiagnosed with conduct disorder (11%) or oppositional disorder (89%). The ADHD cohort was matched for age, weight, height, handedness, and Tanner stage (Tanner, 1962) with 18 normal controls, but differed significantly from the controls in scores of WISC–R vocabulary and block design subtests (Wechsler, 1974). The rostrum and rostral body (labelled as Regions 1 and 3 in Fig. 4), but not the genu or splenium, were smaller in the ADHD cohort. In addition, the rostral body areas, serving the premotor and supplementary motor cortical regions (Witelson, 1989), negatively correlated only with factor IV (impulsivity/hyperactivity) scores from the Connors questionnaires (Goyette, Connors, & Ulrich, 1978).

Again, these three studies represent differing age groups, differing MRI and image analysis methods, differing subject and control matching (particularly of

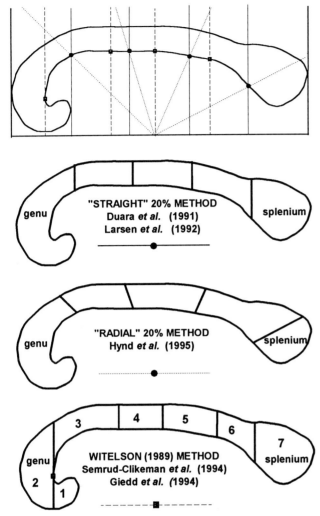

Figure 4 Author's reconstruction of the three conventional methods to subdivide the corpus callosum for morphometric analysis. Note the variable regional definitions leading to variable area measurements. The MRI studies in dyslexia which utilized these methods are referenced in the figure. The method of Witelson (1989) generated the majority of the existing postmortem data in normal subjects. Reproduced and adapted with permission from Filipek (1995a).

IQ), and differing concurrent psychiatric codiagnoses, all in relatively small cohorts. *These studies therefore cannot be directly compared.* However, the findings raise interesting implications about the possibility of anomalous corpus callosum morphology in ADHD.

B. Morphometric Analyses in ADHD Adolescents

Filipek et al. (1996), also performed full morphometric analyses of the brain in the adolescent ADHD cohort described above (Semrud-Clikeman, Filipek, Biederman, Steingard, Kennedy, Renshaw, et al., 1994). Of all the global brain measures, only the right hemispheric white matter volume tended to be smaller in the ADHD subjects ($p < .07$). The volumes of the total caudate, including the head and tail, were similar to the controls. When the hemispheres were subdivided into *en bloc* regions (Filipek, Kennedy, et al., 1992) (Fig. 3), the differences in the volume of the head of the caudate were noted, as described above. In addition, significantly smaller volumes were noted in the ADHD subjects in the right frontal (anterior superior pericallosal) and bilateral posterior parietal–occipital (retrocallosal) regions (see Fig. 3). These findings are consistent with earlier reports of symmetric unidimensional widths of the frontal regions.

The slightly reduced volume of white matter in the ADHD right hemisphere was not evenly distributed throughout the hemispheric regions, but rather was localized to the right frontal and both posterior parietal–occipital regions, and to a lesser degree to the frontal basal ganglia region. These *en bloc* hemispheric regions are coarse, and encompass multiple neural systems while splitting others. In general, the right frontal hemispheric region includes posterior prefrontal cortex, motor association area, Brodmann area 6, and midanterior cingulate; the posterior parietal–occipital region includes superior and inferior parietal lobules and angular gyri, in addition to primary visual and visual association cortices (Mesulam, 1985). These morphometric findings are analogous with the many prior positron emission tomography (PET) studies (Corbetta et al., 1991; Corbetta et al., 1993; Petersen et al., 1987; 1994; Posner & Dehaene, 1994), and the attentional networks postulated by Mesulam (1985) and Posner & Dehaene (1994). The lower posterior parietal–occipital white matter volumes are also consistent with the findings of a smaller splenium of the corpus callosum in these subjects.

V. Why the Inconclusive Findings in the Developmental Disorders?

A. Subject and Control Characteristics

These composite studies included relatively small heterogeneous cohorts, with little diagnostic or neuropsychological data reported, particularly concerning handedness, IQ, SES, educational setting, or psychiatric codiagnoses. The collective controls were not adequately matched for these variables, or for gender and age. As a result, the results are inconsistent within a given developmental disorder. The use of only medical controls (subjects needing imaging studies for clinical indications, including seizures) is no longer suitable given the lack of risk inherent in MRI (Consensus Conference. Magnetic Resonance Imaging, 1988). Larger *homogeneous* subject groups with well-matched *normal* control groups are needed to unravel the current confusion from neuroimaging studies in the developmental disorders. Larger cohorts require longer and larger *parallel* studies, with *comparable* anatomic definitions, imaging, and image analysis methods, to verify characteristic anomalies in the developmental disorders (Filipek, 1995a; Filipek, Kennedy, et al., 1992).

B. Variability from MRI and Image Analysis Methods

The available studies used a variety of qualitative and quantitative imaging methods, which collectively are most responsible for the inconsistent results. Several factors in MRI-based analyses, particularly slice thickness, partial volume effects, slice orientation, and position, should be considered (Filipek, 1995a; Filipek, Kennedy et al., 1992).

1. Slice Thickness

Conventional MRI (and CT) scan slices are usually 3–10 mm in thickness; *skip serial* scans have interslice gaps of 10–100% of the slice thickness, where the brain is not imaged. Some skip serial analyses ignore the gaps to produce two-dimensional (2D) areas on a single selected slice, or "cumulative areas" across multiple slices; others interpolate volume through the gaps. Both approaches result in larger error. The current generation of 1.5 tesla MRI scanners are capable of producing thin (1–3 mm) contiguous 3D slices of the entire brain (Filipek, 1995a; Filipek, Kennedy et al., 1992).

2. Partial Volume Effects

"Partial volume" or "volume averaging" effects are intrinsic to any imaging method: the anatomic borders on any 2D slice actually represent borders *averaged* through the depth (thickness) of that slice. Therefore, three contiguous 3 mm slices will more closely approximate the actual neuroanatomy than a single 9 mm slice. These effects are significant for both qualitative and quantitative studies, as *in vivo* brain–behavior correlations are performed on a 3D brain constructed from 2D planar images (Filipek, 1995a; Filipek, Kennedy et al., 1992).

3. Slice Orientation and Position

Slice orientation (e.g., coronal vs axial vs sagittal), and the angle at which the slices are obtained, contribute to the neuroanatomic variability across subjects, despite the conventional use of a laser cross-beam to position the head prior to imaging. This is particularly relevant for unidimensional or 2D measurements of structures or regions on single selected slices, where the given slice may significantly differ across subjects. For example, positional variability may result in significantly different "midsagittal" planes for measurement of corpus callosum or cerebellar vermis across subjects. Volumetric measurements across contiguous thin slices are also affected, although to a lesser extent (Filipek, 1995a; Filipek, Kennedy et al., 1992).

C. Future Directions

Despite these relatively inexact composite methods, these current findings validate the use of quantitative MRI in the developmental disorders. With the ability to image the entire brain *in vivo* within an acceptable imaging time for children, a cognitive approach to the developmental disorders is now plausible. Analyses should no longer be limited to single or a few structures, but rather expanded to include the multitude of neural systems residing in the entire brain. Measurements of developmental trajectories in normal children are now plausible without associated risk. These are critical not only as comparison measures for children under study, but also to improve our understanding of the normal variability of the developing brain (Caviness, Filipek, & Kennedy, 1989; Filipek, 1995a; Filipek, Kennedy et al., 1992).

Computerized MRI-based morphometric methods have essentially replaced hand-drawn methods, and traditional planimetric analysis is virtually obsolete. Objective mathematical approaches are being developed in many centers to further decrease investigator interaction, with associated subjectivity and error. These approaches aim to create a given contour automatically, perhaps even off line, and markedly decrease the still tedious effort required for a full morphometric analysis of the entire brain (Worth, 1993; Worth & Kennedy, 1993).

Techniques have been developed to reformat 3D MRI image data into any plane, which allows positional normalization of the entire brain within an MRI regardless of the original position of the head in the scanner (Alpert, Bradshaw, Kennedy, & Correia, 1990; Filipek, Kennedy, & Caviness, 1991; Filipek et al., 1994). These techniques are capable of producing essentially identical image planes, and also permit more accurate cross-scan anatomic comparisons. Although some anatomic resolution is indeed compromised with positional normalization methods (Courchesne, Yeung-Courchesne, & Egaas, 1994), the superior quality of reformatted images resulting from conventional

3D MRI pulse sequences far outweighs the multiple liabilities of repeatedly repositioning children in the MRI scanner gantry (Filipek, 1995a; Filipek, Kennedy et al., 1992).

With MRI, actual neural systems are only grossly related to the behavioral–anatomic correlations in the developing brain. *En bloc* cerebral hemispheric subdivisions, used by many centers, include regions assigned differing neuropsychological functions, and often separate functional regions across subdivisions. Methods which parcellate the cerebral cortex (Rademacher, Galaburda, Kennedy, Filipek, & Caviness, 1992), although still approximate and based on the extremely variable human surface topology, will considerably improve the ability to localize cognitive function using traditional brain–behavior nomenclature based on the adult model (Damasio & Frank, 1992; Damasio & Damasio, 1989; Heilman & Valenstein, 1985; Mesulam, 1985). As an example, consider potential implications of morphometric differences reported in the "posterior temporal region" vs the "primary auditory and auditory association cortices" in dyslexic, language-disordered, or autistic children. With larger studies in the pediatric population, comprising normal and developmentally disordered children, age-appropriate structural parameters may be included within the traditional adult model, based on actual structural–functional correlation data (Caviness et al., 1989; Caviness, Filipek, & Kennedy, 1993; Filipek, 1995a; Filipek, Kennedy, et al., 1992).

Because of relatively poor anatomic localization, functional imaging methods have generally relied upon anatomic atlases of brain structure for localization. Such methods of cortical parcellation now permit precise anatomic localization with functional imaging modalities, providing direct correlations between the individual's structural MRI and functional imaging scan (functional MRI, single proton emission computed tomography or PET), for individualized, and therefore more accurate, localization. These collective approaches can now accommodate the challenge of brain–behavior correlations in the developing brain (Caviness et al., 1989, 1993; Filipek, 1995a; Filipek, Kennedy et al., 1992).

Acknowledgments

This work was supported in part by HD 27802 from the National Institute of Child Health and Human Development, National Institutes of Health, Bethesda, MD, USA.

This author wishes to thank Dr. Jack Fletcher for methodological advice and Ms. Jennifer Holmes for assistance with manuscript preparation.

References

Alpert, N. M., Bradshaw, J. F., Kennedy, D. N., & Correia, J. A. (1990). The principle axis transformation-A method for image registration. *Journal of Nuclear Medicine, 31,* 1717–1722.

American Psychiatric Association (1987). *Diagnostic and Statistical Manual of Mental Disorders. (3rd ed., revised).* Washington, D.C.: American Psychiatric Association.

American Psychiatric Association (1994). *Diagnostic and Statistical Manual of Mental Disorders. (4th ed.).* Washington, D.C.: American Psychiatric Association.

Aram, D. M., Morris, R., & Hall, N. E. (1992). The validity of discrepancy criteria for identifying children with developmental language disorders. *Journal of Learning Disabilities, 25,* 549–554.

Arin, D. M., Bauman, M. L., & Kemper, T. L. (1991). The distribution of Purkinje cell loss in the cerebellum in autism. *Neurology, 41*(Suppl. 1), 307.

Bailey, A., Luthert, P., Bolton, P., Le Couteur, A., Rutter, M., & Harding, B. (1993). Autism and megalencephaly. *Lancet, 341,* 1225–1226.

Bauman, M. L. (1991). Microscopic neuroanatomic abnormalities in autism. *Pediatrics, 87*(5 Part 2), 791–796.

Bauman, M. L., & Kemper, T. L. (1985). Histoanatomic observations of the brain in early infantile autism. *Neurology, 35,* 866–874.

Bauman, M. L., & Kemper, T. L. (1990). Limbic and cerebellar abnormalities are also present in an autistic child of normal intelligence. *Neurology, 40* (Suppl. 1), 359.

Bauman, M. L., & Kemper, T. L. (1994). Neuroanatomic observations of the brain in autism. In M. L. Bauman & T. L. Kemper (Eds.), *The neurobiology of autism* (pp. 119–145). Baltimore: Johns Hopkins Univ. Press.

Berthier, M. L. (1994). Corticocallosal anomalies in Asperger's syndrome [letter]. *American Journal of Roentgenology, 162,* 236–237.

Berthier, M. L., Bayes, A., & Tolosa, E. S. (1993). Magnetic resonance imaging in patients with concurrent Tourette's disorder and Asperger's syndrome. *Journal of the American Academy of Child and Adolescent Psychiatry, 32,* 633–639.

Berthier, M. L., Starkstein, S. E., & Leiguarda, R. (1990). Developmental cortical anomalies in Asperger's syndrome: Neuroradiological findings in two patients. *Journal of Neuropsychiatry and Clinical Neurosciences, 2,* 197–201.

Breier, A., Buchanan, R. W., Elkashef, A., Munson, R. C., Kirkpatrick, B., & Gellad, F. (1992). Brain morphometry and schizophrenia: A magnetic resonance imaging study of limbic, prefrontal cortex, and caudate structures. *Archives of General Psychiatry, 49,* 921–926.

Campbell, M., Rosenbloom, S., Perry, R., George, A., Kricheff, I., Anderson, L., Small, A., & Jennings, S. (1982). Computerized axial tomography in young tuistic children. *American Journal of Psychiatry, 139,* 510–512.

Casey, B. J., Giedd, J., Vauss, Y., Vaituzis, C. K., & Rapoport, J. L. (1992). Selective attention and the anterior cingulate: A developmental neuroanatomical study. *Society for Neuroscience Abstracts, 18*(Part I), 332.

Castellanos, F. X., Giedd, J. N., Eckburg, P., Marsh, W. L., Vaituzis, A. C., Kaysen, D., Hamburger, S. D., & Rapoport, J. L. (1994). Quantitative morphology of the caudate nucleus in attention deficit hyperactivity disorder. *American Journal of Psychiatry, 151,* 1791–1796.

Caviness, V. S., Filipek, P. A., & Kennedy, D. N. (1989). Magnetic resonance technology in human brain science: A blue print for a program based upon morphometry. *Brain and Development, 11,* 1–13.

Caviness, V. S., Filipek, P. A., & Kennedy, D. N. (1993). The neurobiology of learning disabilities: Potential contributions from magnetic resonance imaging. In A. M. Galaburda (Ed.), *Dyslexia & development: Neurobiological aspects of extraordinary brains* (pp. 257–268). Cambridge, MA: Harvard Univ. Press.

Caviness, V. S., Kennedy, D. N., Richelme, C., Rademacher, J., & Filipek, P. A. (1996). The human brain age 6–11 years. A volumetric analysis based upon magnetic resonance images. *Cerebral Cortex,* in press.

Cohen, M., Campbell, R., & Yaghmai, F. (1989). Neuropathological abnormalities in developmental dysphasia. *Annals of Neurology, 25,* 567–570.

Coleman, P. D., Romano, J., Lapham, L., & Simon, W. (1985). Cell counts in cerebral cortex of an autistic patients. *Journal of Autism and Developmental Disorders, 15,* 245–255.

Consensus Conference. Magnetic Resonance Imaging (1988). *Journal of the American Medical Association, 259,* 2132–2138.

Corbetta, M., Miezin, F. M., Dobmeyer, S., Shulman, G. L., & Petersen, S. E. (1991). Selective and divided attention during visual discriminaton of shape, color, and speed: Functional anatomy by positron emission tomography. *Journal of Neuroscience, 11,* 2383–2402.

Corbetta, M., Miezin, F. M., Shulman, G. L., & Petersen, S. E. (1993). A PET study of visuospatial attention. *Journal of Neuroscience, 13,* 1202–1226.

Courchesne, E. (1995). New evidence of cerebellar and brainstem hypoplasia in autistic infants, children and adolescents: The MR imaging study by Hashimoto and colleagues. *Journal of Autism and Developmental Disorders, 25,* 19–22.

Courchesne, E., Press, G. A., & Yeung-Courchesne, R. (1993). Parietal lobe abnormalities detected with MR in patients with infantile autism. *American Journal of Roentgenology, 160,* 387–393.

Courchesne, E., Saitoh, O., Yeung-Courchesne, R., Press, G. A., Lincoln, A. J., Haas, R. H., & Schreibman, L. (1994). Abnormalities of cerebellar vermian lobules VI and VII in patients with infantile autism: Identification of hypoplastic and hyperplastic subgroups by MR imaging. *American Journal of Roentgenology, 162,* 123–130.

Courchesne, E., Townsend, J., & Saitoh, O. (1994). The brain in infantile autism: Posterior fossa structures are abnormal. *Neurology, 44,* 214–223.

Courchesne, E., Yeung-Courchesne, R., & Egaas, B. (1994). Methodology in neuroanatomic measurement (editorial). *Neurology, 44,* 203–208.

Courchesne, E., Yeung-Courchesne, R., Hicks, G., & Lincoln, A. (1985). Functioning of the brain-stem auditory pathway in nonretarded autistic individuals. *Electroencephalography and Clinical Neurophysiology, 61,* 491–501.

Courchesne, E., Yeung-Courchesne, R., Press, G. A., Hesselink, J. R., & Jernigan, T. L. (1988). Hypoplasia of cerebellar vermal lobules VI and VII in autism. *New England Journal of Medicine, 318,* 1349–1354.

Creasey, H., Rumsey, J., Schwartz, M., Duara, R., Rapoport, J., & Rapoport, S. (1986). Brain morphometry in autistic men as measured by volumetric computed tomography. *Archives of Neurology, 43,* 669–672.

Damasio, A. R., & Frank, R. (1992). Three-dimensional *in vivo* mapping of brain lesions in humans. *Archives of Neurology, 49,* 137–143.

Damasio, H., & Damasio, A. R. (1989). *Lesion analysis in neuropsychology.* New York: Oxford Univ. Press.

Damasio, H., Maurer, R., Damasio, A. R., & Chui, H. (1980). Computerized tomographic scan findings in patients with autistic behavior. *Archives of Neurology, 37,* 504–510.

Duara, R., Kushch, A., Gross-Glenn, K., Barker, W. W., Jallad, B., Pascal, S., Loewenstein, D. A., Sheldon, J., Rabin, M., Levin, B., & Lubs, H. (1991). Neuroanatomic differences between dyslexic and normal readers on magnetic resonance imaging scans. *Archives of Neurology, 48,* 410–416.

Dunn, L. M., & Markwardt, F. C. (1970). *Peabody Individual Achievement Test.* Circle Pines, MN: American Guidance Service.

Filipek, P. A. (1995a). Neurobiological correlates of developmental dyslexia-What do we know about how the dyslexics' brains differ from those of normal readers? *Journal of Child Neurology, 10*(suppl. 1), S62–S69.

Filipek, P. A. (1995b). Quantitative magnetic resonance imaging in autism: The cerebellar vermis. *Current Opinion in Neurology, 8,* 134–138.

Filipek, P. A., & Kennedy, D. N. (1991). Magnetic resonance imaging: Its role in the developmental disorders. In D. Gray & D. Duane (Eds.), *The reading brain: The biological basis of dyslexia* (pp. 133–160). Parkton, MD: York Press.

Filipek, P. A., Kennedy, D. N., & Caviness, V. S., Jr. (1991). Volumetric analysis of central nervous system neoplasm based on MRI. *Pediatric Neurology, 7,* 347–351.

Filipek, P. A., Kennedy, D. N., & Caviness, V. S. (1992). Neuroimaging in child neuropsychology. In I. Rapin & S. Segalowitz (Eds.), *Volume 6: Child Neuropsychology* (pp. 301–329). Amsterdam: Elsevier.

Filipek, P. A., Kennedy, D. N., Caviness, V. S., Klein, S., & Rapin, I. (1987). *In vivo* MRI-based volumetric brain analysis in subjects with verbal auditory agnosia [abstract]. *Annals of Neurology, 22,* 410.

Filipek, P. A., Kennedy, D. N., Caviness, V. S., Rossnick, S. L., Spraggins, T. A., & Starewicz, P. M. (1989). MRI-based brain morphometry: Development and application to normal subjects. *Annals of Neurology, 25,* 61–67.

Filipek, P. A., Pennington, B. F., Holmes, J. F., Lefly, D., Kennedy, D. N., Meyers, J. M., Lang, J. E., Gayan, J., Galaburda, A. M., Simon, J. M., Filley, C. M., Caviness, V. S., & DeFries, J. C. (1995). Developmental dyslexia: Cortical and subcortical anomalies by MRI-based morphometry [abstract]. *Annals of Neurology, 38,* 509.

Filipek, P. A., Richelme, C., Kennedy, D. N., & Caviness, V. S. (1994). The young adult human brain: An MRI-based morphometric analysis. *Cerebral Cortex, 4,* 344–360.

Filipek, P. A., Richelme, C., Kennedy, D. N., Rademacher, J., Pitcher, D. A., Zidel, S. Y., & Caviness, V. S. (1992). Morphometric analysis of the brain in developmental language disorders and autism [abstract]. *Annals of Neurology, 32,* 475.

Filipek, P. A., Semrud-Clikeman, M., Steingard, R. J., Renshaw, P. F., Kennedy, D. N., & Biederman, J. (1996). Volumetric MRI analysis comparing attention-deficit hyperactivity disorder and normal controls. *Neurology,* in press.

Gaffney, G. R., Kuperman, S., Tsai, L. Y., & Minchin, S. (1988). Morphological evidence for brainstem involvement in infantile autism. *Biological Psychiatry, 24,* 578–586.

Gaffney, G. R., Kuperman, S., Tsai, L. Y., & Minchin, S. (1989). Forebrain structure in infantile autism. *Journal of the American Academy of Child and Adolescent Psychiatry, 28,* 534–537.

Gaffney, G. R., Kuperman, S., Tsai, L. Y., Minchin, S., & Hassanein, K. M. (1987). Midsaggital magnetic resonance imaging of autism. *British Journal of Psychiatry, 151,* 831–833.

Gaffney, G. R., Tsai, L. Y., Kuperman, S., & Minchin, S. (1987). Cerebellar structure in autism. *American Journal of Diseases of Children, 141,* 1330–1332.

Galaburda, A. M. (1988). The pathogenesis of childhood dyslexia. *Research Publications—Association for Research in Nervous and Mental Disease, 66,* 127–138.

Galaburda, A. M. (1992). Neurology of developmental dyslexia. *Current Opinion in Neurology and Neurosurgery, 5,* 71–76.

Galaburda, A. M. (1993). The planum temporale (editorial). *Archives of Neurology, 50,* 457.

Galaburda, A. M., Corsiglia, J., Rosen, G. D., & Sherman, G. F. (1987).

Planum temporale asymmetry: Reappraisal since Geschwind and Levitsky. *Neuropsychologia, 25,* 853–868.

Galaburda, A. M., Sherman, G. F., Rosen, G. D., Aboitiz, F., & Geschwind, N. (1985). Developmental dyslexia: Four consecutive patients with cortical anomalies. *Annals of Neurology, 18,* 222–233.

Garber, H. J., Ritvo, E. R., Chiu, L. C., Griswold, V. J., Kashanian, A., Freeman, B. J., & Oldendorf, W. H. (1989). A magnetic resonance imaging study of autism: Normal fourth ventricle size and absence of pathology. *American Journal of Psychiatry, 146,* 532–534.

Garber, J. H., & Ritvo, E. R. (1992). Magnetic resonance imaging of the posterior fossa in autistic adults. *American Journal of Psychiatry, 149,* 245–247.

Geschwind, N., & Levitsky, W. (1968). Human brain: Left–right asymmetry in temporal speech region. *Science, 161,* 186–187.

Giedd, J. N., Castellanos, F. X., Casey, B. J., Kozuch, P., King, A. C., Hamburger, S. D., & Rapoport, J. L. (1994). Quantitative morphology of the corpus allosum in attention deficit hyperactivity disorder. *American Journal of Psychiatry, 151,* 665–669.

Goyette, C. H., Connors, C. K., & Ulrich, R. F. (1978). Normative data on revised Connors parent and teacher rating scales. *Journal of Abnormal Child Psychology, 6,* 221–236.

Gross-Glenn, K., Duara, R., Barker, W. W., Loewenstein, D., Chang, J. Y., Yoshii, F., Apicella, A. M., Pascal, S., Boothe, T., Sevush, S., Jallad, B. J., Novoa, L., & Lubs, H. A. (1991). Positron emission tomographic studies during serial word reading by normal and dyslexic adults. *Journal of Clinical and Experimental Neuropsychology, 13,* 531–544.

Harcherik, D. F., Cohen, D. J., Ort, S. H., Paul, R., Shaywitz, B. A., Volkmar, F. R., Rothman, S. L. G., & Leckman, J. F. (1985). Computed tomography brain scanning in four neuropsychiatric disorders of childhood. *American Journal of Psychiatry, 142,* 731–734.

Hashimoto, T., Murakawa, K., Miyazaki, M., Tayama, M., & Kuroda, Y. (1992). Magnetic resonance imaging of the brain structures in the posterior fossa in retarded autistic children. *Acta Paediatrica, 81,* 1030–1034.

Hashimoto, T., Tayama, M., Miyazaki, M., Murakawa, K., & Kuroda, Y. (1993). Brainstem and cerebellar vermis involvement in autistic children. *Journal of Child Neurology, 8,* 149–153.

Hashimoto, T., Tayama, M., Miyazaki, M., Murakawa, K., Sakurama, N., Yoshimoto, T., & Kuroda, Y. (1991). Reduced midbrain and pons size in children with autism. *Tokushima Journal of Experimental Medicine, 38,* 15–18.

Hashimoto, T., Tayama, M., Miyazaki, M., Murakawa, K., Shimakawa, S., Yoneda, Y., & Kuroda, Y. (1993). Brainstem involvement in high functioning autistic children. *Acta Neurologica Scandinavica, 88,* 123–128.

Hashimoto, T., Tayama, M., Miyazaki, M., Sakurama, N., Yoshimiti, T., Murakawa, K., & Kuroda, Y. (1992). Reduced brainstem size in children with autism. *Brain and Development, 14,* 94–97.

Hashimoto, T., Tayama, M., Murakawa, K., Yoshimoto, T., Miyazaki, M., Harada, M., & Kuroda, Y. (1995). Development of the brainstem and cerebellum in autistic patients. *Journal of Autism and Developmental Disorders, 25,* 1–18.

Hauser, S. L., DeLong, G. R., & Rosman, N. P. (1975). Pneumographic findings in the infantile autism syndrome. *Brain, 98,* 667–688.

Heilman, K. M., & Valenstein, E. (Eds.). (1985). *Clinical neuropsychology.* New York: Oxford Univ. Press.

Hier, D., LeMay, M., & Rosenberger, P. B. (1979). Autism and unfavorable left–right asymmetries of the brain. *Journal of Autism and Developmental Disorders, 9,* 153–157.

Holttum, J. R., Minshew, N. J., Sanders, R. S., & Phillips, N. E. (1992). Magnetic resonance imaging of the posterior possa in autism. *Biological Psychiatry, 32,* 1091–1101.

Hsu, M., Yeung-Courchesne, R., Courchesne, E., & Press, G. A. (1991). Absence of magnetic resonance imaging evidence of pontine abnormality in infantile autism. *Archives of Neurology, 48,* 1160–1163.

Humphreys, P., Kaufmann, W. E., & Galaburda, A. M. (1990). Developmental dyslexia in women: Neuropathological findings in three patients. *Annals of Neuroology, 28,* 727–738.

Hynd, G. W., Hall, J., Novey, E. S., Eliopulos, D., Black, K., Gonzales, J. J., Edmonds, J. E., Riccio, C., & Cohen, M. (1995). Dyslexia and corpus callosum morphology. *Archives of Neurology, 52,* 32–38.

Hynd, G. W., Hern, K. L., Novey, E. S., Eliopulos, D., Marshall, R., Gonzalez, J. J., & Voeller, K. K. (1993). Attention deficit-hyperactivity disorder and asymmetry of the caudate nucleus. *Journal of Child Neurology, 8,* 339–347.

Hynd, G. W., Semrud-Clikeman, M., Lorys, A., Novey, E. S., & Eliopulos, D. (1990). Brain morphology in developmental dyslexia and attention deficit disorder/hyperactivity. *Archives of Neurology, 47,* 919–926.

Hynd, G. W., Semrud-Clikeman, M., Lorys, A. R., Novey, E. S., Eliopulos, D., & Lyytinen, H. (1991). Corpus callosum morphology in attention-deficit hyperactivity disorder (ADHD): Morphometric analysis of MRI. *Journal of Learning Disabilities, 24,* 141–146.

Iversen, S. D. (1977). Behavior after neostriatal lesions in animals. In I. Divac & R. G. E. Oberg (Eds.), *The Neostriatum* (pp. 195–210). Elmsford, NY: Pergamon.

Jacobson, R., LeCouteur, A., Howlin, P., & Rutter, M. (1988). Selective subcortical abnormalities in autism. *Psychological Medicine, 18,* 39–48.

Jernigan, T. L., Hesselink, J. R., Stowell, E., & Tallal, P. (1991). Cerebral structure on magnetic resonance imaging in language- and learning-impaired children. *Archives of Neurology, 48,* 539–545.

Kennedy, D. N., Meyer, J. W., Filipek, P. A., & Caviness, V. S. (1994). MRI-based topographic segmentation. In R. W. Thatcher, M. Hallet, T., Zeffiro, E. R. John, & M. Huerta (Eds.), *Functional neuroimaging: Technical foundations* (pp. 201–208). San Diego: Academic Press.

Kertesz, A. (1983). *Localization in Neuropsychology.* New York: Academic Press.

Kleinman, M. D., Neff, S., & Rosman, N. P. (1992). The brain in infantile autism: Are posterior fossa structures abnormal? *Neurology, 42,* 753–760.

Kushch, A., Gross-Glenn, K., Jallad, B., Lubs, H., Rapin, M., Feldman, E., & Duara, R. (1993). Temporal lobe surface area measurements on MRI in normal and dyslexic readers. *Neuropsychologia, 31,* 811–821.

Landau, W., Goldstein, R., & Kleffner, F. (1960). Congenital aphasia: A clinico-pathologic study. *Neurology, 10,* 915–921.

Larsen, J. P., Høien, T., & Ödegaard, H. (1990). MRI evaluation of the size and symmetry of the planum temporale in adolescents with developmental dyslexia. *Brain and Language, 39,* 289–301.

Larsen, J. P., Høien, T., & Ödegaard, H. (1992). Magnetic resonance imaging of the corpus callosum in developmental dyslexia. *Cognitive Neuropsychology, 9,* 123–134.

Leonard, C. M., Voeller, K. K. S., Lombardino, L. J., Morris, M. K., Hynd, G. W., Alexander, A. W., Andersen, H. G., Garofalakis, M., Honeyman, J. C., Mao, J., Agee, O. F., & Staab, E. V. (1993). Anomalous cerebral structure in dyslexia revealed with magnetic resonance imaging. *Archives of Neurology, 50,* 461–469.

Mesulam, M.-M. (1985). Patterns in behavioral neuroanatomy: Association areas, the limbic system, and hemispheric specialization. In M.-M. Mesulam (Ed.), *Principles and behavioral neurology* (pp. 1–70). Philadelphia, PA; Davis.

Murakami, J. W., Courchesne, E., Press, G. A., Yeung-Courchesne, R., & Hesselink, J. R. (1989). Reduced cerebellar hemisphere size and its relationship to vermal hypoplasia in autism. *Archives of Neurology, 46,* 689–694.

Nasrallah, H. A., Loney, J., Olson, S. C., McCalley-Whitters, M., Kramer, J., & Jacoby, C. G. (1986). Cortical atrophy in young adults with a history of hyperactivity in childhood. *Psychiatry, 17,* 341–346.

Nijiokiktjien, C., de Sonneville, L., & Vaal, J. (1994). Callosal size in children with learning disabilities. *Behavioral Brain Research, 64,* 213–218.

Nowell, M. A., Hackney, D. B., Muraki, A. S., & Coleman, M. (1990). Varied MR appearance of autism: fifty-three pediatric patients having the full autistic syndrome. *Magnetic Resonance Imaging, 8,* 811–816.

Ornitz, E. M., Atwell, C. W., Kaplan, A. R., & Westlake, J. R. (1985). Brain stem dysfunction in autism. *Archives of General Psychiatry, 42,* 1018–1025.

Petersen, S. E., Corbetta, M., Miezin, F. M., & Shulman, G. L. (1994). PET studies of parietal involvement in spatial attention: Comparison of different task types. *Canadian Journal of Experimental Psychology, 48,* 319–338.

Petersen, S. E., Robinson, D. L., & Morris, J. D. (1987). Contributions of the pulvinar to visual spatial attention. *Neuropsychology, 25,* 97–105.

Peterson, B. S., Riddle, M. A., Cohen, D. J., Katz, L. D., Smith, J. C., & Leckman, J. F. (1993). Human basal ganglia volume asymmetries on magnetic resonance images. *Magnetic Resonance Imaging, 11,* 493–498.

Piven, J., & Arndt, S. (1995). The cerebellum and autism [letter]. *Neurology, 45,* 398–399.

Piven, J., Berthier, M. L., Starkstein, S. E., Nehme, E., Pearlson, G., & Folstein, S. E. (1990). Magnetic resonance imaging evidence for a defect of cerebral cortical development in autism. *American Journal of Psychiatry, 147,* 734–739.

Piven, J., Nehme, E., Simon, J., Barta, P., Pearlson, G., & Folstein, S. E. (1992). Magnetic resonance imaging in autism: Measurement of the cerebellum, pons, and fourth ventricle. *Biological Psychiatry, 31,* 491–504.

Plante, E. (1991). MRI findings in the parents and siblings of specifically language-impaired boys. *Brain and Language, 41,* 67–80.

Plante, E., Swisher, L., & Vance, R. (1989). Anatomical correlates of normal and impaired language in a set of dizygotic twins. *Brain and Language, 37,* 643–655.

Plante, E., Swisher, L., Vance, R., & Rapcsak, S. (1991). MRI findings in boys with specific language impairment. *Brain and Language, 41,* 52–66.

Posner, M. I., & Dehaene, S. (1994). Attentional networks. *Trends in Neuroscience, 17,* 75–79.

Posner, M. I., & Petersen, S. E. (1990). The attention system of the human brain. *Annual Review of Neuroscience, 13,* 25–42.

Posner, M. I., Petersen, S. E., Fox, P. T., & Raichle, M. E. (1988). Localization of cognitive operations in the human brain. *Science, 240,* 1627–1631.

Posner, M. I., & Raichle, M. E. (1994). Networks of attention. In M. I. Posner & M. E. Raichle (Eds.), *Images of mind* (pp. 153–179). New York: Scientific American Library.

Prior, M., Tress, B., Hoffman, W., & Boldt, D. (1984). Computed tomographic study of children with classic autism. *Archives of Neurology, 41,* 482–484.

Rademacher, J., Galaburda, A. M., Kennedy, D. N., Filipek, P. A., & Caviness, V. S. (1992). Human cerebral cortex: Localization, parcellation, and morphometry with magnetic resonance imaging. *Journal of Cognitive Neuroscience, 4,* 352–374.

Rapin, I. (Ed.). (1996). *Preschool children with inadequate communication: Developmental language disorder, autism, mental deficiency.* Clinics in Developmental Medicine, Volume 139. London: McKeith Press.

Rapin, I., & Allen, D. A. (1987). Syndromes in developmental dysphasia and adult aphasia. *Research Publications—Association for Research in Nervous and Mental Disease, 66,* 57–75.

Raz, N., Torres, I. J., Spencer, W. D., White, K., & Acker, J. D. (1992). Age-related regional differences in cerebellar vermis observed *in vivo. Archives of Neurology, 149,* 412–416.

Ritvo, E. R., Freeman, B. J., Scheibel, A. B., Duong, T., Robinson, H., Guthrie, D., & Ritvo, A. (1986). Lower Purkinje cell counts in the cerebella of four autistic subjects: Initial findings of the UCLA-NSAC Autopsy Research Report. *American Journal of Psychiatry, 143,* 862–866.

Rosenbloom, S., Campbell, M., George, A., Kricheff, I., Taleporos, E., Anderson, L., Reuben, R., & Korein, J. (1984). High resolution CT scanning in infantile autism: A quasntitative approach. *Journal of the American Academy of Child and Adolescent Psychiatry, 23,* 72–77.

Rumsey, J. M., Creasey, H., Stepanek, J., Dorwart, R., Patronas, N., Hamburger, S., & Duara, R. (1988). Hemispheric asymmetries, fourth ventricular size, and cerebellar morphology in autism. *Journal of Autism and Developmental Disorders, 18,* 127–137.

Saitoh, O., Courchesne, E., Egaas, B., Lincoln, A. J., & Schreibman, L. (1995). Cross-sectional area of the posterior hippocampus in autistic patients with cerebellar and corpus callosum abnormalities. *Neurology, 45,* 317–324.

Schultz, R. T., Cho, N. K., Staib, L. H., Kier, L. E., Fletcher, J. M., Shaywitz, S. E., Shankweiler, D. P., Katz, L., Gore, J. C., Duncan, J. S., & Shaywitz, B. A. (1994). Brain morphology in normal and dyslexic children: The influence of sex and age. *Annals of Neurology, 35,* 732–742.

Semrud-Clikeman, M., Filipek, P. A., Biederman, J., Steingard, R., Kennedy, D. N., Renshaw, P., & Bekken, K. (1994). Attention deficit hyperactivity disorder: Difference in the corpus callosum by MRI morphometric analysis. *Journal of the American Academy of Child and Adolescent Psychiatry, 33,* 875–881.

Shaywitz, B. A., Shaywitz, S. E., Byrne, T., Cohen, D. J., & Rothman, S. (1983). Attention deficit disorder: quantitative analysis of CT. *Neurology, 33,* 1500–1503.

Tanner, J. M. (1962). *Growth at adolescence. 2nd ed.* Oxford: Blackwell.

Tsai, L., Jacoby, C., & Stewart, M. (1983). Morphological cerebral asymmetries in autistic children. *Biological Psychiatry, 18,* 317–326.

Tsai, L., Jacoby, C., Stewart, M., & Beisler, J. (1982). Unfavourable left–right asymmetries of the brain and autism: A question of methodology. *British Journal of Psychiatry, 140,* 312–319.

Wechsler, D. (1974). *Wechsler intelligence scale for children—revised.* New York: Psychological Corporation.

Williams, R. S., Hauser, S. L., Purpura, D. P., DeLong, G. R., & Swisher, C. N. (1980). Autism and mental retardation: Neuropathologic studies performed in four retarded persons with autistic behavior. *Archives of Neurology, 37,* 749–753.

Witelson, S. F. (1989). Hand and sex differences in the isthmus and genu of the human corpus callosum: A postmortem morphological study. *Brain, 112,* 799–835.

Worth, A. J. (1993). *Neural networks for automated segmentation of magnetic resonance images.* Unpublished doctoral dissertation, Boston University, Boston.

Worth, A. J., & Kennedy, D. N. (1993). *Employing shape to aid magnetic resonance brain segmentation.* Paper presented at the International Conference on Neural Networks, San Francisco.

13

Neuroimaging of Developmental Nonlinearity and Developmental Pathologies

Harry T. Chugani

*Director, Positron Emission Tomography Center,
Children's Hospital of Michigan; and Departments of Pediatrics, Neurology, and Radiology,
Wayne State University School of Medicine,
Detroit, Michigan 48201*

I. Introduction

Recent advances in neuroimaging have made it possible to study noninvasively a number of physiological and biochemical processes in the developing human brain. Results from these studies indicate that, at least with regard to energy utilization and blood flow, the brain does not follow a linear course during its maturation. In this chapter, the neurobiological correlates of nonlinearity in brain energy requirement are discussed in relation to synaptogenesis and plasticity of the central nervous system. The clinical implications of this nonlinearity are presented, followed by several examples of developmental brain pathologies which are best detected with functional imaging.

II. Nonlinearity of the Developing Brain

In most species, including humans, brain development follows a pattern consisting of phases during which there is an exuberance of neuronal populations and their elements, followed by phases during which there is elimination or regression of the excessively produced cells and connections (Cowan, Fawcett, O'Leary, & Stanfield, 1984). The timing of these phenomena are different for neurons and their processes and synaptic contacts. In addition, differences in timing exist for various brain regions and for different species. The proliferation and overproduction of neurons in humans occur prenatally, whereas the elimination phase of excessively proliferated neuronal populations begins prenatally and continues until about the second postnatal year (Rabinowicz, 1979).

In contrast, the overproduction and subsequent elimination (also referred to as "pruning") of neuronal processes and their synaptic contacts in humans is largely a postnatal phenomenon with a rather protracted course (Huttenlocher, 1979; Huttenlocher, & de Courten, 1987; Huttenlocher, de Courten, Gary, & van der Loos, 1982). For example, synaptic density in human frontal cortex of children up to 11 years of age has been shown to exceed that in adults (Huttenlocher, 1979). The process of transient exuberant connectivity as a general rule in brain development is believed to be biologically advantageous in reducing the genetic load that would otherwise be required for specifically programming the enormous numbers of synaptic contacts in the nervous system (Changeux & Danchin, 1976; Jacobson, 1978). Furthermore, the individual is given the opportunity to retain and increase the efficiency of connections that, through repeated use during a critical period, are deemed to be important, whereas connections that are used to a lesser extent are more susceptible to be eliminated. This allows for a fine tuning of neuronal circuits, based on early exposure and environmental nurturing, that makes the neuronal architecture of each individual unique.

These phases of exuberance and elimination do not parallel the general growth of the brain as measured by weight. For example, at birth, the average weight of the brain for a full-term male is about 370 gm. By the third postnatal year, average brain weight has tripled to 1080 gm, and by 6–14 years, the average weight is 1350 gm.

III. PET Methodology

The development of positron emission tomography (PET) has allowed the measurement of local chemical functions in various body organs to be made noninvasively in humans (Ter-Pogossian, Phelps, Hoffman, & Mullani, 1975; Phelps, Hoffman, Mullani, & Ter-Pogossian, 1975). This technique employs positron cameras which are sensitive to coincidence detection of photons released from positron–electron annihilations. Application of tracer kinetic mathematical modeling of the *in vivo* behavior of compounds labeled with positron-emitting isotopes, which are administered to the patient, allows for the quantification of functional activity in various organs. There has been a proliferation of PET tracers produced for the study of various neurological disorders, some of which are suitable for the study of human brain development. The most widely applied tracer for PET imaging in the brain has been for the study of local cerebral metabolic rates for glucose utilization, but cerebral blood flow, oxygen utilization, protein synthesis, and the release and binding of various neurotransmitters have also been measured with PET (Mazziotta & Gilman 1992).

IV. Brain Glucose Metabolism in Infants

Since glucose and oxygen are the principal substrates used under normal circumstances for meeting the energy demands of the brain, the rates at which these substrates are utilized in various brain regions provide a measure of brain regional energy demands. This strategy was used by Sokoloff and colleagues, who developed the ^{14}C-2-deoxyglucose (2DG) autoradiography method for the quantitative measurement of local cerebral metabolic rates for glucose (LCMRglc) in laboratory animals (Sokoloff, Reivich, Kennedy, Desrosie, Patlak, Pettigre, et al., 1977). The Sokoloff method, which involves sacrificing the animal, was later adapted for human use with PET and 2-deoxy-2[^{18}F]-fluoro-D-glucose (FDG), and the Sokoloff tracer kinetic model modified for the PET method (Huang, Phelps, Hoffman, Sideris, Selin, & Kuhl, 1980).

Using PET with FDG in children of various ages, we found that the pattern of brain glucose utilization in the human newborn differed markedly from that of normal young healthy adults. In the newborn, four brain regions showed the most prominent glucose metabolism: primary sensorimotor cortex, thalamic nuclei, brainstem, and cerebellar vermis (Chugani & Phelps, 1986; Chugani, Phelps, & Mazziotta, 1987; Chugani, 1994, pp. 153–175). More recent studies using higher resolution scanners indicate that the cingulate cortex, hippocampal region, and occasionally the basal ganglia also show a relatively high metabolic rate for glucose consumption in the newborn period (Chugani H. T., Da Silva, E., & Chugani, D. C., unpublished observations) (Fig. 1). This pattern of glucose metabolism in the newborn, characterized by highest activity in phylogenetically old structures, is in keeping with the relatively limited behavioral repertoire of neonates. For example, it is likely that reflex behaviors, such as the Moro, root, and grasp responses present in newborns are mediated by these brain regions which are functionally active during this period (Andre-Thomas & Saint-Anne Dargassies, 1960). More sophisticated activity, such as visuomotor integration required in

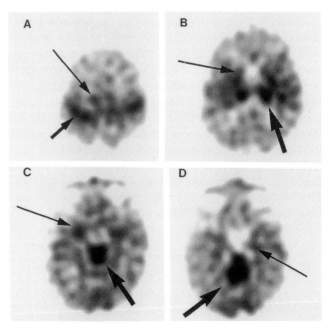

Figure 1 Neonatal pattern of brain glucose metabolism. (A) Sensorimotor cortex (short arrow) and cingulate cortex (long arrow); (B) Thalamus (thick arrow) and basal ganglia (thin arrow); the latter is only occasionally seen in neonates; (C) Brainstem (thick arrow) and mesial temporal region (thin arrow); (D) Cerebellar vermis (thick arrow) and mesial temporal (hippocampal) region. Note the relatively low glucose metabolic rate in most of the cerebral and cerebellar cortex.

reaching out towards a target and other eye-hand co-ordination tasks, are at a relatively primitive level in the newborn (von Hofsten, 1982); this is not unexpected judging from the relatively simple pattern of brain glucose metabolism.

Beyond the neonatal period, the ontogeny of glucose metabolism also follows a phylogenetic order, with functional maturation of older anatomical structures preceding that of newer areas (Chugani & Phelps, 1986; Chugani et al., 1987; Chugani, 1994, pp. 153–175). Moreover, the sequence of functional brain development as determined by regional glucose metabolism correlates well with the maturation of behavioral, neurophysiological, and neuroanatomical events in the infant. As visuospatial and visuosensorimotor integrative functions are acquired in the second and third months of life (Bronson, 1974), and primitive reflexes become reorganized (Andre-Thomas & Saint-

Anne Dargassies, 1960; Parmelee & Sigman, 1983), increases in glucose metabolism are observed in parietal, temporal, and primary visual cortical regions, basal ganglia, and cerebellar hemispheres (Fig. 2). Increasing glucose metabolism in cerebral cortex during the second and third months of life presumably reflects maturation of the cortex, and is consistent with the dramatic maturation of electroencephalogram (EEG) activity seen during the same period (Kellaway, 1979).

Between 6 and 8 months, the frontal cortex begins to show a maturational rise in glucose metabolism, at first in the lateral portion (Fig. 3), subsequently in the mesial, and lastly in the dorsal prefrontal areas (Fig. 4). Functional maturation of these frontal cortical regions coincides with the appearance of higher cortical and cognitive abilities. For example, the infant now shows more sophisticated interaction with its surroundings and exhibits the phenomenon of stranger anxiety (Kagan, 1972). Performance on the delayed response task, which is a commonly used neuropsychological

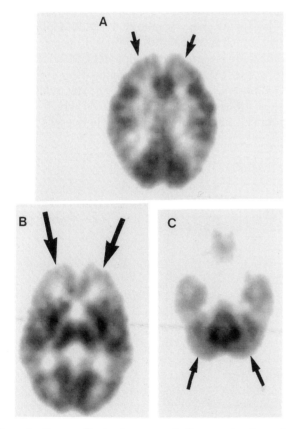

Figure 2 Pattern of brain glucose metabolism seen in a 3 month old infant. (A & B) Compared to newborns, there is now considerable glucose metabolic activity in the cerebral cortex including parietal, temporal, and occipital cortex, but not the frontal cortex, which still shows relatively low activity (arrows). Basal ganglia metabolism have increased to the level seen in the thalamus; (C) In the cerebellum, glucose metabolism has increased in the cortex (arrows) as compared to the newborn pattern.

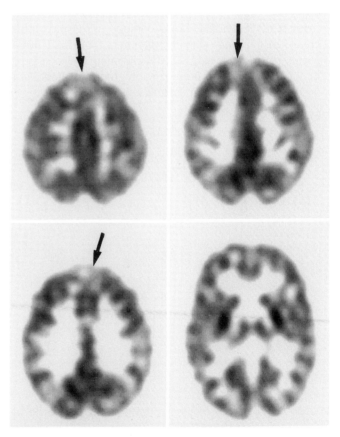

Figure 3 Pattern of brain glucose metabolism seen in an 8 month old infant. Most of the cerebral cortex shows a pattern that is similar to adults, with the exception of frontal cortex, where glucose metabolism has risen in the lateral and inferior aspects, but not the dorsal mesial portion (arrows).

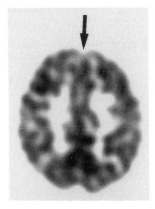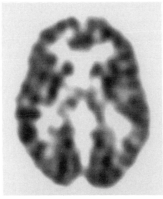

Figure 4 Pattern of brain glucose metabolism seen in a 10 month old infant. An adult pattern of glucose metabolism is almost present, except for the most rostral portion of the mesial prefrontal cortex (arrow).

paradigm for evaluating prefrontal lobe integrity (Fuster, 1984; Goldman-Rakic, 1984), markedly improves during this period of frontal lobe metabolic maturation. Neuroanatomical studies in human infants have shown that there is an expansion of dendritic fields (Schade & van Groenigen, 1961) and an increase in capillary density (Diemer, 1968) in frontal cortex during this stage of development. By one year of age, the overall pattern of brain glucose metabolism is similar to that seen in adults.

V. Glucose Metabolic Rates: Developmental Nonlinearity

PET studies in normal children have shown that, although a pattern of brain glucose metabolism similar to adults is reached by about one year of age, dynamic changes of LCMRglc occur in a nonlinear fashion, whereby they exceed adult levels during much of the first two decades of life. These changes are most marked for the neocortex (Fig. 5), show an intermediate magnitude for basal ganglia and thalamus, and are probably not present in brainstem and cerebellum. In other words, there appears to be a hierarchical ordering of structures in terms of the degree to which maturational increases in LCMRglc exceed adult values.

The typically low neonatal values of LCMRglc, which are about 30% lower than adult rates, rapidly increase from birth and reach adult values by about the second year. Thereafter, LCMRglc values continue to increase and begin to exceed adult values during the third postnatal year. By about 4 years, a plateau is reached which extends until about 9–10 years; following this, there is a gradual decline in LCMRglc to reach adult values by about 16–18 years (Chugani et al., 1987; Chugani, 1994, pp. 153–175). The relative increase of LCMRglc over adult values, which is most pronounced in neocortical regions between 4 and 10

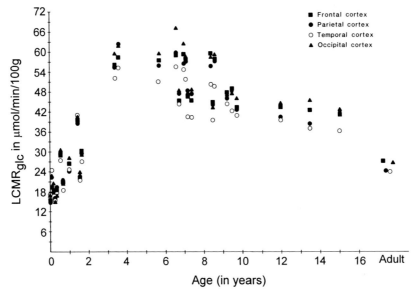

Figure 5 Absolute values of local cerebral metabolic rates for glucose (LCMRglc) for cortical brain regions, plotted as a function of age in normal infants and children, and corresponding adult values. In the infants and children, points represent individual values of LCMRglc; in adults, points are mean values from 7 subjects, in which the size of the symbols equals the standard error of the mean.

years, reaches a peak LCMRglc of over twice the LCMRglc levels seen in adults.

These studies replicate and expand upon earlier observations by Kennedy and Sokoloff (1957), who demonstrated that the average global cerebral blood flow in 9 normal children (aged 3 to 11 years) was approximately 1.8 times that of normal young adults. Similarly, average cerebral oxygen utilization was approximately 1.3 times higher in children than in adults. In other words, there appears to be a transient phase during development when the human brain requires more nutrients to support its activities. Because of methodological limitations, however, these measurements were obtained only for the brain as a whole, and not for individual brain regions as can now be achieved with PET.

VI. Developmental "Hypermetabolism" in Animal Models

In order to explore the significance of developmental nonlinearity of brain glucose metabolism, we have studied this phenomenon in the cat and in the monkey. Both models also show a developmental phase during which LCMRglc exceeds adult levels, but the timing appears to differ for each species.

In the kitten, very low LCMRglc levels were seen during the first 15 days of life, with phylogenetically older brain regions being generally more metabolically mature than newer structures (Chugani, Hovda, Villablanca, Phelps, & Xu, 1991). After 15 days of age, many brain regions (particularly telencephalic structures) underwent sharp increases of LCMRglc to reach, or exceed, adult rates by 60 days. At 90 and 120 days, a slight decline of LCMRglc was observed, but this was followed by a second, larger peak occurring at about 180 days. Only after 180 days did LCMRglc decrease to reach final adult values. Thus, the cat showed an even more complex nonlinear pattern of glucose metabolism during development than humans.

Analysis of the relationship between LCMRglc and synaptogenesis in the kitten visual cortex suggests that LCMRglc measured in the resting state may be an indirect measure of synaptic density. During the immediate newborn period, synapses in area 17 are sparse (Voeller, Pappas, & Purpura, 1963; Winfield, 1981) and LCMRglc values are low. Subsequently, a rapid rise in synaptic density is seen, with a peak occurring by about 70 days postnatally (Winfield 1981, 1983). This period of rapid synaptic proliferation coincides with the period of rapid LCMRglc increase in the visual cortex, reaching an initial peak at about 60 days. However, the second LCMRglc peak in the cat, occurring at about 180 days, did not appear to have a neuroanatomical correlate. Instead, this is the time of puberty in the cat (Kling, 1965) and, therefore, it is possible that the high LCMRglc seen during this period may be related to hormonal influences.

A similar relationship between LCMRglc and synaptogenesis occurs in the rhesus monkey. The LCMRglc of cerebral cortex in infant rhesus remains at about 60% of adult levels until after 2 months postnatally, when LCMRglc rises steeply to about 155% of adult values (Jacobs, Chugani, Allada, Chen, Phelps, Pollack, & Raleigh, 1995). This rise is coincident with transient synaptic overproduction in this species (Rakic, Bourgeois, Eckenhoff, Zecevic, & Goldman-Rakic, 1986). After 6 months, LCMRglc in cortex gradually declines to reach adult values, following a time course similar to that of synaptic pruning in rhesus (Jacobs et al., 1995).

Thus, in both the cat and rhesus monkey, the nonlinear developmental profile of LCMRglc seems to run parallel to the profile for synaptogenesis. This is not surprising considering the fact that, under normal circumstances, the major portion of glucose utilized by the brain postnatally goes towards the maintenance of resting membrane potentials in the dendritic arborization, rather than for processes occurring in the cell bodies (Mata, Fink, Gainer, Smith, Davidsen, Savaki, et al., 1980; Kadekaro, Crane, & Sokoloff, 1985; Nudo & Masterton, 1986). Therefore, in the resting state, the cerebral energy demand must be related to synaptic numbers and will increase or decrease depending upon developmental regulation of synaptic production and regression.

The relationship between LCMRglc and synaptogenesis also holds for humans, where there is an overproduction of synapses in the first several years of life (Huttenlocher, 1979; Huttenlocher & de Courten, 1987) coincident with a rapid rise of LCMRglc (Chugani et al., 1987; Chugani, 1994). Subsequently, at about 8–10 years of age, LCMRglc in cerebral cortex begins slowly to decline, corresponding approximately to the phase of synaptic elimination and dendritic pruning (Huttenlocher, 1979; Huttenlocher & de Courten, 1987). Studies measuring the volume of gray matter using magnetic resonance imaging volumetry have found that the cerebral cortex, particularly frontal and parietal cortex, diminish in volume during adolescence, presumably in relation to the pruning process (Jernigan, Trauner, Hesselink, & Tallal 1991). The "plateau" period during which LCMRglc exceeds adult values corresponds to the period of increased cerebral energy demand as a result of transient exuberant connectivity in children.

VII. Brain Plasticity and "Window of Opportunity"

It is well known that following brain injury, compensatory reorganization or plasticity is greater in the nervous system that is still developing compared to one that is fully mature (Kolb & Whishaw, 1989; Irle, 1987; Finger & Wolf, 1988). The degree of plasticity following injury depends upon the species involved, brain regions damaged, size of lesion, state of maturation at the time of injury, and other factors.

There is evidence to suggest that the developmental period of exuberant connectivity is one which is characterized by a relatively high degree of plasticity in response to injury. For example, in the kitten, the period of excessive connectivity during development coincides with a period of considerable brain plasticity in response to physiologic and environmental manipulation, and to injury (Morest, 1969). Thus, in the feline visual system, the gradual regression of excessive cellular processes and connections after day 70 is accompanied by diminishing plasticity of the visual cortex (Barlow 1975; Hirsch & Leventhal, 1978; Sherman & Spear, 1982). The timing of these regressive phenomena coincide with the end of a "critical period" between 4 weeks and about 3 months postnatally, during which various experimental manipulations in the feline visual system (e.g., monocular deprivation by suturing one eyelid closed) can cause neuroanatomical changes resulting in altered connectivity (Hubel & Wiesel, 1970; Spinelli, Hirsch, Phelps, & Metzler, 1972). This window of neural plasticity corresponds well to that segment of the LCMRglc developmental curve between the onset of rapid increase in LCMRglc (15–30 days) and the beginning of a downward trend in LCMRglc (60–90 days) after reaching the initial 60 day peak (Chugani et al., 1991). Therefore, it appears that the transient maturational changes of LCMRglc not only predict periods of synaptic excess, but also indicate when plasticity in the nervous system is at a maximum.

Clinically, there also appears to be a relationship between diminishing brain plasticity in children and the gradual decline of LCMRglc, with its onset between 8 and 10 years of age measured with PET (Chugani et al., 1987; Chugani, 1994). For example, in the human visual system, the decline of LCMRglc in visual cortex beginning at about 8–10 years coincides with a notable decrease in plasticity, as judged by the development of amblyopia (irreversible loss of vision from one eye) in the presence of monocular occlusion or certain kinds of strabismus (Awaya, 1978; Vaegan & Taylor, 1979; Marg, 1982). In addition, patients enucleated prior to 8 years of age perform better on depth perception tasks than individuals whose enucleation occurs after 8 years (Schwartz, Linberg, Tillman, & Odom, 1987).

Language acquisition and reorganization in response to dominant hemisphere damage in children are clearly most efficient during a critical period ending at about 10 years (Basser, 1962; Lenneberg, 1967; Curtiss, 1977). Children who have been isolated since birth in the wilderness, away from all civilization and exposure to language, (so-called "feral" children), acquire language most successfully if intervention is initiated in early childhood prior to about 10 years of age (Curtiss, 1981). This is not to say that there is no language plasticity after 10 years, but clearly there appears to be a "window of opportunity" during which the brain is particularly efficient in learning. With this in mind, one cannot help but wonder why second language is still taught in high school rather than prior to 10 years when it is best acquired.

VIII. Developmental Pathologies

The observations and hypotheses developed in this chapter suggest that measurements of LCMRglc obtained noninvasively with PET may provide an important index of brain plasticity in children. In fact, concepts derived from this approach are already being applied in children undergoing epilepsy surgery. These children suffer from medically refractory epilepsy and ultimately undergo large resections of the cortical epileptogenic zone for seizure relief (Hoffman, Hendrick, Dennis, & Armstrong, 1979; Chugani, Shewmon, Peacock, Shields, Mazziotta, & Phelps, 1988; Chugani, Shields, Shewmon, Olson, Phelps, & Peacock, 1990;

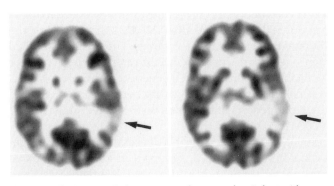

Figure 6 Positron emission tomography scan of an infant with uncontrolled seizures and no evidence of focal abnormalities on magnetic resonance imaging. A focus of decreased glucose metabolism is clearly seen in the left temporal cortex (arrows), corresponding to the location of interictal epileptiform discharges and seizure onset documented on the electroencephalogram. Pathological examination of the surgically excised epileptic brain tissue showed disturbances of neuronal lamination consistent with cortical dysplasia.

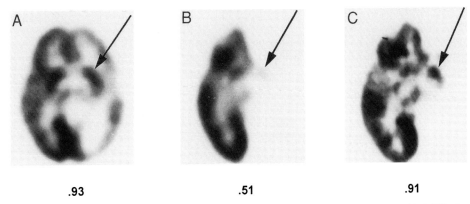

Figure 7 Serial positron emission tomography scans of glucose utilization in a 4 year old child before and after left hemidecortication. (A) Just prior to surgery, ratio of glucose metabolism in caudate nucleus of affected hemisphere (arrow) to that in the normal hemisphere was .93; (B) 3 months following left hemidecortication, glucose metabolism was severely depressed in the left caudate (arrow) and the ratio decreased to .51; (C) 2 years after surgery, there has been recovery and the left caudate once again shows glucose metabolism comparable to preoperative levels with a ratio of .91 (arrow).

Chugani, Shewmon, Shields, Sankar, Comair, Vinters et al., 1993). Although a focus of epileptogenicity is suggested on the EEG, the epileptogenic area often is not visible on structural neuroimaging such as computed tomography or magnetic resonance imaging. Here again, PET seems to play an important role, because it is sensitive in detecting the abnormal glucose metabolism (Fig. 6) associated with disturbances of neuronal lamination and organization commonly present in seizure foci of young children (Chugani et al., 1988, 1990, 1993).

Although the severity of motor and cognitive deficits after surgery is related to multiple factors, including the age of the child when damage to the brain resulting in epilepsy occurred, duration of epilepsy, extent and topography of epileptogenic region, and whether or not there is bilateral homotopic injury, it is clear that the age of the child when surgery is performed is an important factor relating to outcome. These children provide important opportunities for the study of developmental brain plasticity. Recently, it was observed that deprivation of ipsilateral cortical input to the basal ganglia by hemidecortication in young children is initially associated with a loss of glucose metabolism in basal ganglia, but with time, there is a recovery of metabolism in caudate (Fig. 7). These findings suggest that anatomical reorganizational changes, presumably from contralateral cortex, as seen with similar lesions in animal models, may have occurred (Chugani and Jacobs, 1995).

IX. Conclusion

In this chapter, we have demonstrated that studies with FDG–PET, which is but one of many potential PET probes, have offered important insight into our understanding of human brain development and plasticity. As PET technology continues to expand and new tracers are developed, there will be a plethora of probes suitable for the study of the many biochemical processes which distinguish the developing brain from one that is fully mature. Such studies will continue to modify our concepts of human brain maturation, neuronal plasticity, developmental disorders, and brain reorganization following injury, and will continue to impact decision making in clinical practice as has occurred in epilepsy surgery.

References

Andre-Thomas, C. Y., & Saint-Anne Dargassies, S. (1960). *The neurological examination of the infant.* London, Medical Advisory Committee of the National Spastics Society.

Awaya, S. (1978). Stimulus vision deprivation amblyopia in humans. In R. D. Reinecke (Ed.), *Strabismus* (pp. 31–44). New York: Grune & Stratton.

Barlow, H. B. (1975). Visual experience and cortical development. *Nature (London), 258,* 199–203.

Basser, L. S. (1962). Hemiplegia of early onset and the faculty of speech with special reference to the effects of hemispherectomy. *Brain, 85,* 427–460.

Bronson, G. (1974). The postnatal growth of visual capacity. *Child Development, 45,* 873–890.

Changeux, J. P., & Danchin, A. (1976). Selective stabilization of developing synapses as a mechanism for the specification of neuronal networks. *Nature (London), 264,* 705–712.

Chugani, H. T. (1994). Development of regional brain glucose metabolism in relation to behavior and plasticity. In G. Dawson & K. W. Fischer (Eds.), *Human behavior and the developing brain* (pp. 153–175). New York: Guilford.

Chugani, H. T., Hovda, D. A., Villablanca, J. R., Phelps, M. E., & Xu, W. F. (1991). Metabolic maturation of the brain: A study of local cerebral glucose utilization in the developing cat. *Journal of Cerebral Blood Flow and Metabolism, 11,* 35–47.

Chugani, H. T., & Jacobs, B. (1995). Metabolic recovery in caudate nucleus of children following cerebral hemispherectomy. *Annals of Neurology 36,* 794–797.

Chugani, H. T., & Phelps, M. E. (1986). Maturational changes in cerebral function in infants determined by [18]FDG positron emission tomography. *Science, 231,* 840–843.

Chugani, H. T., Phelps, M. E., & Mazziotta, J. C. (1987). Positron emission tomography study of human brain functional development. *Annals of Neurology, 22,* 487–497.

Chugani, H. T., Shewmon, D. A., Peacock, W. J., Shields, W. D., Mazziotta, J. C., & Phelps, M. E. (1988). Surgical treatment of intractable neonatal onset seizures: The role of positron emission tomography. *Neurology, 38,* 1178–1188.

Chugani, H. T., Shewmon, D. A., Shields, W. D., Sankar, R., Comair, Y., Vinters, H. V., & Peacock, W. J. (1993). Surgery for intractable infantile spasms: Neuroimaging perspectives. *Epilepsia, 34,* 764–771.

Chugani, H. T., Shields, W. D., Shewmon, D. A., Olson, D. M., Phelps, M. E., & Peacock, W. J. (1990). Infantile spasms: I. PET identifies focal cortical dysgenesis in cryptogenic cases for surgical treatment. *Annals of Neurology, 27,* 406–413.

Cowan, W. M., Fawcett, J. W., O'Leary, D. D. M., & Stanfield, B. B. (1984). Regressive events in neurogenesis. *Science, 225,* 1258–1265.

Curtiss, S. (1977). *Genie: A psycholinguistic study of a modern-day "wild child."* New York: Academic Press.

Curtiss, S. (1981). Feral children. In J. Wortis (Ed.), *Mental retardation and developmental disabilities XII* (pp. 129–161). New York: Brunner/Mazel.

Diemer, K. (1968). Capillarisation and oxygen supply of the brain. In D. W. Lubbers, U. C., Luft, G., Thews, & E. Witzleb, (Eds.), *Oxygen transport in blood and tissue* (pp. 118–123). Stuttgart: Thieme.

Finger, S., & Wolf, C. (1988). The 'Kennard effect' before Kennard: The early history of age and brain lesions. *Archives of Neurology, 45,* 1136–1142.

Fuster, J. M. (1984). Behavioral electrophysiology of the prefrontal cortex. *Trends in Neuroscience, 7,* 408–414.

Goldman-Rakic, P. S. (1984). The frontal lobes: Uncharted provinces of the brain. *Trends in Neuroscience, 7,* 425–429.

Hirsch, H. V. B., & Leventhal, A. G. (1978). Functional modification of the developing visual system. In M. Jaconson (Ed.), *Handbook of Sensory Physiology, Volume IX: Development of Sensory Systems* (pp. 279–335). Berlin and Heidelberg: Springer-Verlag.

Hoffman, H. J, Hendrick, E. B., Dennis, M., & Armstrong, D. (1979). Hemispherectomy for Sturge-Weber syndrome. *Child's Brain, 5,* 233–248.

Huang, S. C., Phelps, M. E., Hoffman, E. J., Sideris, K., Selin, C. J., & Kuhl, D. E. (1980). Noninvasive determination of local cerebral metabolic rate of glucose in man. *American Journal of Physiology 238,* E69–E82.

Hubel, D. H., & Wiesel, T. N. (1970). The period of susceptibility to the physiological effects of unilateral eye closure in kittens. *Journal of Physiology (London), 206,* 419–436.

Huttenlocher, P. R. (1979). Synaptic density in human frontal cortex-developmental changes and effects of aging. *Brain Research, 163,* 195–205.

Huttenlocher, P. R., & de Courten, C. (1987). The development of striate cortex in of man. *Human Neurobiology, 6,* 1–9.

Huttenlocher, P. R., de Courten, C., Gary, L. J., & van der Loos, H. (1982). Synaptogenesis in human visual cortex-evidence for synapse elimination during normal development. *Neuroscience Letters, 33,* 247–252.

Irle, E. (1987). Lesion size and recovery of function: Some new perspectives. *Brain Research and Review, 12,* 307–320.

Jacobs, B., Chugani, H. T., Allada, V., Chen, S., Phelps, M. E., Pollack, D. B., & Raleigh, M. J. (1995). Developmental changes in brain metabolism in sedated rhesus macaques and vervet monkeys revealed by positron emission tomography. *Cerebral Cortex, 3,* 222–233.

Jacobson, M. (1978). *Developmental neurobiology* (2nd ed., pp. 302–307). New York: Plenum.

Jernigan, T. L., Trauner, D. A., Hesselink, J. R., & Tallal, P. A. (1991). Maturation of human cerebrum observed *in vivo* during adolescence. *Brain, 114,* 2037–2049.

Kadekaro, M., Crane, A. M., & Sokoloff, L. (1985). Differential effects of electrical stimulation of sciatic nerve on metabolic activity in spinal cord and dorsal root ganglion in the rat. *Proceedings of the National Academy of Sciences USA, 82,* 6010–6013.

Kagan, J. (1972). Do infants think? *Scientific American, 226,* 74–82.

Kellaway, P. (1979). An orderly approach to visual analysis: Parameters of the normal EEG in adults and children. In D. W. Klass, & D. D. Daly (Eds.), *Current practice of clinical electroencephalography* (pp. 69–147). New York: Raven.

Kennedy, C., & Sokoloff, L. (1957). An adaptation of the nitrous oxide method to the study of the cerebral circulation in children; normal values for cerebral blood flow and cerebral metabolic rate in childhood. *Journal of Clinical Investigation, 36,* 1130–1137.

Kling, A. (1965). Behavioral and somatic development following lesions of the amygdala in the cat. *Journal of Psychiatric Research, 3,* 263–273.

Kolb, B., & Whishaw, I. Q. (1989). Plasticity in the neocortex: Mechanisms underlying recovery from early brain damage. *Progress in Neurobiology, 32,* 235–276.

Lenneberg, E. (1967). *Biological foundations of language* (pp. 125–187). New York: Wiley.

Marg, E. (1982). Prentice Memorial Lecture: Is the animal model for stimulus deprivation amblyopia in children valid or useful? *American Journal of Optometry and Physiological Optics, 59,* 451–464.

Mata, M., Fink, D. J., Gainer, H., Smith, C. B., Davidsen, L., Savaki, H., Schwartz, W. J., & Sokoloff, L. (1980). Activity-dependent energy metabolism in rat posterior pituitary primarily reflects sodium pump activity. *Journal of Neurochemistry, 34,* 213–215.

Mazziotta, J. C., & Gilman, S. (1992). *Clinical brain imaging: Principles and applications,* Contemporary Neurology Series. Philadelphia, PA: Davis.

Morest, D. K. (1969). The growth of dendrites in the mammalian brain. *Zeitschrift fur Anatomie und Entwicklungsgeschichte, 128,* 290–317.

Nudo, R. J., & Masterton, R. B. (1986). Stimulation-induced [14C]2-deoxyglucose labeling of synaptic activity in the central auditory system. *Journal of Comparative Neurology, 245,* 553–565.

Parmelee, A. H., & Sigman, M. D. (1983). Perinatal brain development and behavior. In M. Haith & J. Campos. (Eds.), *Biology and Infancy, Volume II* (pp. 95–155). New York: Wiley.

Phelps, M. E., Hoffman, E. J., Mullani, N. A., & Ter-Pogossian, M. M. (1975). Application of annihilation coincidence detection to transaxial reconstruction tomography. *Journal of Nuclear Medicine 16,* 210–224.

Rabinowicz, T. (1979). The differentiated maturation of the human cerebral cortex. In F. Falkner & J. M. Tanner (Eds.), *Human Growth, Volume 3. Neurobiology and Nutrition* (pp. 97–123). New York: Plenum.

Rakic, P., Bourgeois, J. P., Eckenhoff, M. F., Zecevic, N., & Goldman-Rakic, P. S. (1986). Concurrent overproduction of synapses in diverse regions of the primate cerebral Cortex. *Science, 232,* 232–235.

Schade, J. P., & van Groenigen, W. B. (1961). Structural organization of the human cerebral cortex. *Acta Anatomica, 47,* 74–111.

Schwartz, T. L., Linberg, J. V., Tillman, W., & Odom, J. V. (1987). Monocular depth and vernier acuities: A comparison of binocular and uniocular subjects. *Investigative Ophthalmology Visual Science, 28*(Suppl.), 304.

Sherman, S. M., & Spear, P. D. (1982). Organization of visual pathways in normal and visually deprived cats. *Physiological Review 62,* 738–855.

Sokoloff, L., Reivich, M., Kennedy, C., Desrosie, M. H., Patlak, C. S., Pettigre, K. D., Sakurada, O., & Shinohara, M. (1977). The [^{14}C] deoxyglucose method for the measurement of local cerebral glucose utilization: Theory, procedure, and normal values in the conscious and anesthetized albino rat. *Journal of Neurochemistry, 28,* 897–916.

Spinelli, D. N., Hirsch, H. V. B., Phelps, R. W., & Metzler, J. (1972). Visual experience as a determinant of the response characteristics of cortical receptive fields in cats. *Experimental Brain Research, 15,* 289–304.

Ter-Pogossian, M. M., Phelps, M. E., Hoffman, E. J., Mullani, N. A. (1975). A positron emission transaxial tomograph for nuclear imaging (PETT). *Radiology, 114,* 89–98.

Vaegan, & Taylor, D. (1979). Critical period for deprivation amblyopia in children. *Transactions of the Ophthalmological Societies of the United Kingdom, 99,* 432–439.

Voeller, L., Pappas, G. D., & Purpura, D. P. (1963). Electron microscope study of development of cat superficial neocortex. *Experimental Neurology, 7,* 107–130.

Von Hofsten, C. (1982). Eye-hand coordination in the newborn. *Developmental Psychology, 18,* 450–461.

Winfield, D. A. (1981). The postnatal development of synapses in the visual cortex of the cat and the effects of eyelid suture. *Brain Research, 206,* 166–171.

Winfield, D. A. (1983). The postnatal development of synapses in different laminae of the visual cortex in the normal kitten and in kittens with eyelid suture. *Developmental Brain Research, 9,* 155–169.

14

Event Related Potential Correlates of Glucose Metabolism in Normal Adults during a Cognitive Activation Task

Frank B. Wood, Amy S. Garrett, Lesley A. Hart, D. Lynn Flowers, and John R. Absher

Section on Neuropsychology, Bowman Gray School of Medicine, Wake Forest University, Winston-Salem, North Carolina 27157

I. Introduction

Scientific opportunities both complex and rich arise inevitably when measurement techniques of widely different scales are employed to examine the same phenomenon. In geology, for example, the seismologist measuring the moment by moment tremors of the earth operates on a geographical and temporal scale vastly different from that of the geologist, who documents the drift of continents. In this example, the task of theory is to achieve a unified understanding of how a single process like plate tectonics can generate movements of separate pieces of the earth's crust, resulting in one set of events that is measurable as momentary tremors in short time, or in another set of events that is measurable as continental drift in geologic time. In contrast, it would be a scientifically unenlightening and theoretically sterile exercise simply to attempt an explanation of how the relatively molecular processes involved in small earth tremors are integrated in some way to result in the macro-level processes of earthquakes, or the still larger integrative processes of continental drift. Even if such a description were possible, it would not really explain "what" is actually "going on." Plate tectonics does just that.

The above example may be useful in more than superficial ways as an analogy to neuroscience and to the problems of converging measurement techniques that are confronted in this chapter. First, it reminds us that the system being measured, whether earth or brain, is substantially bigger and more complex than the measurements applied to it, so important events may be happening that are invisible to any limited set of measurements. It is therefore likely the rule, not the exception, that the directly measured processes will ultimately prove to be less interesting than the inferred processes that they indirectly reflect. A second useful feature of the analogy is its reminder that small scale measurements are inherently no more or less accurate for describing the system than large scale measurements, and "clinical" events (like earthquakes) are as inherent to the system being described as "basic" events (like earth tremors).

In applying the above analogy to the two techniques described in this chapter, we note that the higher temporal resolution is afforded by scalp recordings of the electrophysiological event related potential (ERP) during repeated performance of a stimulus recognition task. By contrast, glucose metabolic rate by positron emission tomography (PET), summed over approximately 40 minutes of time during which the task performance was continuously underway, has the coarsest possible temporal resolution—only one value is computed for the entire 40 minute session. However, PET spatial resolution is on the order of millimeters, whereas ERP spatial resolution is far coarser and subject to considerable distortion (as with seismic recordings, which are temporally resolute but spatially indistinct). The interpretive challenge is obviously to combine the high resolution information from both techniques in an informative way. Equally obvious, however, is the inherent difficulty in understanding a correlation between a time series and a single spatial manifold. The two measurement domains—because they differ so widely in their temporal and spatial resolutions—could not directly measure each other's primary events of interest. In turn, that requires us to assume, consistent with the analogy, that they could only separately and indirectly reflect an underlying process.

It is fair enough to remark in the above context that quests for mechanisms "behind" the data, particularly for mechanisms that explain measurements of widely different spatial and temporal scales, are new and unfamiliar in neuroscience. We are perhaps still too close to our particular measurement techniques to permit us to flexibly consider what kind of processes may be giving rise to our separate and sometimes disparate measurements. Nonetheless, as we shall see, data of the type presented in this chapter can be combined in ways that could stimulate new theoretical interpretive possibilities.

II. Methods

A total of N=40 healthy adults were recruited randomly from the surrounding communities by advertisement. Each person was interviewed by telephone to screen for a history of pertinent neurologic or psychiatric illness. Each person reported to be free of relevant medications and to have no history of head injury, diabetes, heart of neurological disease, seizures, or drug abuse. All suitable volunteers abstained from

nicotine and caffeine for 24 hours prior to the study, and had no food or drink except water past midnight before the day of the study. The study required approximately 8 hours to complete. All subjects were paid $50 for participation, and an additional $150 for a drug-free urine specimen. Lunch was provided.

The subjects ranged in age from 20 to 69 (mean = 38.1, sd = 12.5). The group was 52.5% male and 76% Causasian. Table 1 provides further demographic and psychometric information for the sample.

All subjects arrived at 7:00 AM on the day of the study. Data were collected using four methods: (1) An MRI scan for localization of regions of interest (ROIs) on the PET scan; (2) A PET scan using the tracer F-18-fluorodeoxyglucose (FDG), during a letter recognition task; (3) ERPs collected during the glucose uptake period; and (4) Performance, in terms of hits and false alarms, for the letter recognition task. Control measures of cognitive ability were also taken at a separate time.

Before the physiological measures were made, an individually molded, thermosetting plastic mask was made for each subject to stabilize and standardize head position for PET and MRI scans. A 1.5 tesla GE Signa MRI scanner was used to acquire 3D Fourier transform spoiled gradient echo T1 weighted images (2.5 mm thickness, no interslice gap, TR = 45 msec, TE = 5 msec, Flip angle = 45 degrees, NEX = 1). Subjects were placed in the scanner using the thermoplastic head holder. Earplugs were used to protect subjects from scanner noise. Scanning time was approximately 20 minutes.

Prior to isotope injection for PET scanning, a transmission scan was acquired for 2 bed positions and used to correct for attenuation during reconstruction

Table 1 Descriptive Variables for the $N = 40$ Adult Sample

Variable	Mean	Standard deviation	Minimum	Maximum
Age	38.1	12.5	20.8	69.0
Education	15.5	1.9	13.0	20.0
Spielberger state anxiety	30.1	8.9	20.0	64.0
WAIS vocabulary	11.2	2.4	5.0	16.0
WAIS block design	10.3	2.7	5.0	15.0
Percentage of hits	97.3	4.0	79.0	100.0
Hit reaction time (msec)	474.7	53.6	379.0	630.0
Percentage of false alarms	4.6	4.8	0.0	20.0
False alarm reaction time (msec)	428.0	93.8	247.0	654.0
Task D-prime	4.2	1.0	2.2	5.6

Note: WAIS = Wecshler Adult Intelligence Scale.

of the emission scan. Emission scanning acquired 62 planes, each 3.375 mm thick, imaged parallel to the canthomeatal line. Transmission and emission scanning were performed using a Siemens ECAT 951/31 PET scanner.

An indwelling venous line was placed in the dorsal hand vein of the left arm, which was then wrapped in a hot pack to provide arterialized venous blood. A winged infusion set was placed in the right antecubital vein. These intravenous (IV) lines were started well in advance of glucose injection to allow time for anxiety due to needle stick to abate. After the subject practiced the computer task (described below), 10 mCi of FDG was pushed as an IV bolus into the right antecubital vein. The subject then performed the computer task for 35 minutes. State anxiety was measured using the Spielberger State Anxiety Inventory (Spielberger, Gorsuch, Luchene, Vagg, & Jacobs, 1983), both prior to injection and at the end of the 35 minute activation task. The subject was allowed to void before being placed, using the thermoplastic head holder, inside the PET scanner. Images were acquired in two bed positions, each lasting 15 minutes.

FDG input function was calculated using 2 cc blood samples drawn from the IV line every 15 seconds over the first 2 minutes, as well as 9 later samples (at 3, 4, 6, 8, 13, 18, 28, and 38 minutes, and at the end of the 30 minute scan). Five samples were taken over the course of uptake and analyzed for blood glucose levels. All samples were centrifuged and counted in a well counter in duplicate. Functional images of glucose metabolic rate were calculated using the method of Phelps, Huang, Hoffman, Selin, Sokoloff, and Kuhl (1979).

Collection of ERPs began simultaneously with FDG injection. Prior to the placement of the IV lines, an electrode cap (International Electro-cap, Inc.) for acquiring evoked potentials was positioned on the scalp using the 10/20 International System. An electrode gel reduced skin resistance to less than 3 kohms. ERPs were amplified by 16 Grass Model 8A5 amplifiers of a Grass Electroencephalograph Model 8-16E. Averaged activity was recorded at occipital (O1, O2), parietal (P3, P4), central (C3, C4), frontal (F3, F4), temporal (T3, T4, T5, T6), and midline (PZ, CZ, and FZ) sites. To control for eye movement artifact, the electro-oculogram (EOG) was also recorded from electrodes placed 2 cm to the right and 2 cm below the right eye. The electrode site Fpz served as a ground and reference electrodes were the linked ears. The criterion for rejection of a trial due to artifact was a voltage value above 80 millivolts in any channel, including the eye channel.

Filters for half amplitude high and low frequencies were set at 70 and .3 Hz, respectively. Each channel was digitized at a rate of every 4 ms for each 1000 ms epoch, and processed by a Gateway 2000 (386/25 processor) computer. Data was collected over 35 minutes, accumulating 538 response trials (a range of 332 to 732 trials). The first 50 ms of the waveform served as the baseline.

During simultaneous FDG uptake and ERP recording, subjects performed a letter recognition task presented in a computer game format by a Zenith Z-200 PC (286 processor), time locked to the data acquisition Gateway computer. Subjects responded by lifting their fingers from a computer mouse according to instructions. The visual stimuli subtended a .7 degree visual angle. Each stimulus was flashed for 50 msec with a 1.5 to 2.0 second interstimulus interval, depending on whether or not the subject made a behavioral response to the preceding stimulus. A black dot fixation point was displayed continuously in the center of the screen.

The subject controlled the pace of the game by pressing and holding the mouse button to start a trial. They were instructed to lift their fingers from the mouse button as quickly as possible when a target stimulus was presented. Probability of target versus nontarget items was 50/50. The stimuli included 12 letters and 12 symbols, both presented in either black or white on the contrasting background. The target was any letter, whether black or white. The computer provided auditory feedback for correct responses, and auditory and visual feedback for incorrect responses. The total number of hits, false alarms, misses, and correct rejections was recorded. Reaction times were also recorded. Event related trials in response to both target and nontarget stimuli were averaged, but only correct response trials, hits, or correct rejections were included.

III. Data Analysis

The MRI scans were registered to the average normal brain MRI of Evans, Marrett, and Collins (1989) using a cross-correlation minimization procedure developed by Louis Collins (Montreal Neurological Institute). The register program uses a Procrustes method to minimize root mean squared (RMS) error between two sets of homologous points (one from the PET and the other from the MRI from the same subject). The PET-to-MRI transformation was combined with the MRI-to-stereotaxic space transformation to resample the PET data in stereotaxic space. The result was 60–70 matched MRI–PET pairs, all linearly scaled and oriented along the bicommissural line of Talairach (AC–PC) in a standard stereotaxic coordinate space (Talairach & Tournoux, 1988).

The metabolism in each of the fourteen ROIs was measured using the following method:

1. Each subject's MRI image was segmented into ranges of values for gray matter, white matter, and cerebral spinal fluid (CSF) by finding the median pixel value in the corpus callosum, caudate nucleus, and cerebral spinal fluid, respectively. The range of values for gray matter was determined by finding the midpoint between tissue medians. These values set the upper and lower thresholds for delineating gray matter.

2. For each subject's brain scan, each ROI was located first on that subject's MRI and enclosed in a sphere. The diameter of the spheres ranged from 2.0 to 3.0 cm and was standard across all brains within a given locus, but varied with anatomical site. The size of a given sphere was chosen to take in as much as possible of the area of interest without impinging on other, distinctly separate anatomical regions. Only MRI im-

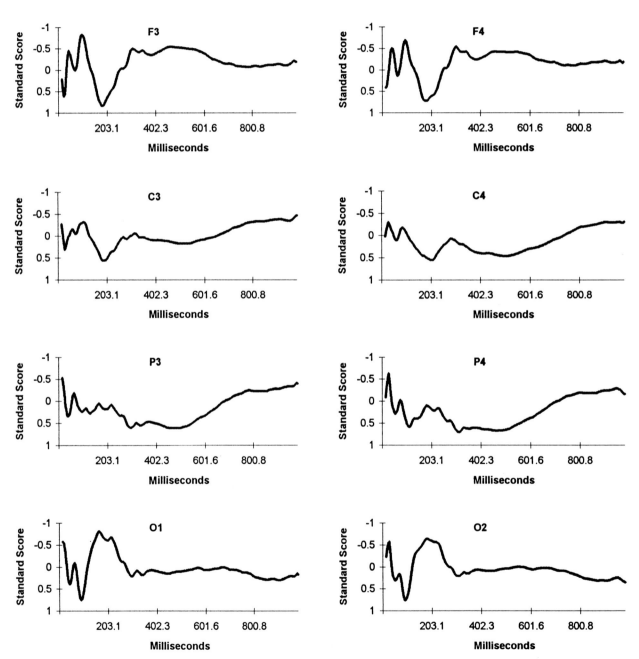

Figure 1 Average normalized ERP waveforms for occipital (O1, O2), parietal (P3, P4), central (C3, C4), and frontal (F3, F4) sites across a 1000 ms epoch. (Negative voltage is up.)

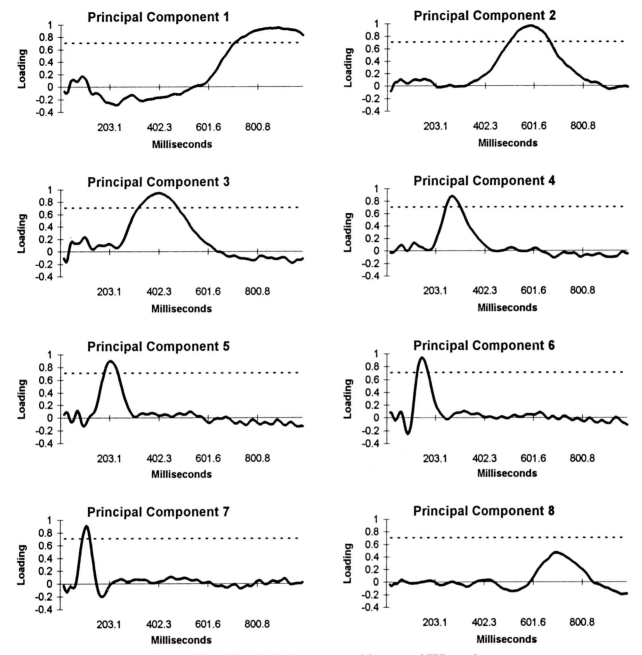

Figure 2 Plots of the principal components of the averaged ERP waveform.

age pixels having values within the gray matter range are included in the analysis.

3. The pixels on the PET image which correspond to the gray matter values within the sphere on the MRI image were selected and plotted as a histogram of PET (glucose) quantitative values versus number of pixels having that value.

4. The 95 or 99.5 percentiles of the resulting PET histogram, for a given spherical ROI, were taken as the glucose metabolic values for the the ROI. By this method, only the most metabolically active PET voxels within a region were included in the calculation of regional metabolism. The resulting values are shown in Table 2.

The individual ERP trials at each electrode site were submitted to a 60 Hz notch filter and averaged separately for color (black/white), symbol (letter/nonletter), and response (correct/incorrect). Only correct responses (correct hits, correct rejections) were

Table 2 Glucose Metabolic Values for the Regions of Interest

	95%ile[a]		99.5%ile[a]	
	Mean	Std Dev	Mean	Std Dev
Left thalamus	13.1	2.8	14.0	2.9
Right thalamus	12.8	2.6	13.8	2.8
Left occipital	14.5	3.0	15.3	3.0
Right occipital	14.7	3.3	15.4	3.5
Left area 37	12.2	2.3	13.0	2.4
Right area 37	12.0	2.6	12.8	2.8
Left angular gyrus	12.1	3.0	12.7	3.1
Right angular gyrus	12.1	2.7	12.7	2.9
Bilateral anterior cingulate	12.6	3.1	13.3	3.2
Left inferior dorsal lateral frontal	12.9	3.1	13.7	3.3
Right inferior dorsal lateral frontal	13.3	3.4	14.2	3.6
Left caudate	12.2	2.6	13.1	2.8
Right caudate	11.9	2.8	12.8	3.0

[a]Percentile of MRI-classified gray matter voxels, within a single spherical region of interest.

considered in subsequent analyses. The records were then as follows: 42 subjects × 2 color conditions × 2 symbol conditions × 15 electrodes = 2520 records. All 2520 records were submitted to a factor analysis of the 256 data points, to identify components. Eight varimax-rotated factors were kept, with eigenvalues ranging from 81.91 to 5.56 (17 had eigenvalues greater than one). The resulting factor scores could then be averaged over symbol type to get summed waveforms for each subject. Two subjects' data were dropped because of technically unsatisfactory PET scans, leaving a total of 40 subjects. Figure 1 shows the standardized waveforms for each electrode; figure 2 shows the eight principal components.

IV. Results and Discussion

A straightforward way to present the data is to cross the temporal dimension of the ERP data with the spatial dimension of the PET data. Correlations between these two dimensions can then be calculated. Notably, this method isolates the high resolution information in both domains. Table 3 presents the data in this fashion, as a correlation matrix between the PET and ERP measurements. In considering this table, it is natural to look for correlations that could be expected on *a priori* grounds. Thus, one might expect the earlier components [P1 (positive peak around 100 ms) and N1 (negative peak around 100 ms)] to correlate best with glucose levels in the primary visual pathway; for example, in the occipital pole. Later "cognitive" components such as the P3 (positive peak around 300 ms) might be expected to correlate best with metabolism in secondary extrastriate visual association areas such as area 37, or tertiary multimodal areas such as the angular gyrus. A rising negativity, represented by the latest components, has sometimes been associated with frontal activation, so dorsolateral inferior frontal metabolism might be expected to correlate with these components. We note in passing that expectations of this type are inherently simple. In contrast to the considerations in the introduction to this chapter, they imply a process that is relatively straightforward and directly measurable by both measurement techniques. Terms like "neural processing" or "brain activation" are often used to convey this expectation of a process that is more or less interchangeably measurable by either method.

Even a casual glance at Table 3 disconfirms these simple, albeit straightforward, expectations. At least one of the conventionally expected relationships is indeed found in a general way: the N1 component is rather strongly associated with left posterior occipital activation. This invites interpretations involving left lateralization of verbal processes (even at this early sensory and visual level), and the possibility that the actual generators of the N1 may either be concentrated in this cortex or in a region with such close functional connections to this cortex that the regions would be highly correlated metabolically.

Most simple expectations, however, are not only disconfirmed but explicitly refuted—by inverse rather than positive correlations. Thus, the extrastriate visual association cortex in area 37 of the left hemisphere has metabolic activity that is inversely, not positively, correlated with the classic P3 component of the ERP, so that greater area 37 activity is related to reduced P3 amplitude. Were there other positive correlations between P3 and regional glucose metabolism, we could treat the area 37 results as an interesting exception. Instead, area 37 has the only significant metabolic correlation with P3, either positive or inverse. Moreover, 10 of the 13 significant PET–ERP correlations are inverse, and this preponderance of inverse correlations is itself a significant finding, at $p < .05$, by the frequency of the tail category of the binomial distribution. In other words, on the assumption that the analyzed regions are a representative subset of the larger set of possible regions of interest, it is likely that more than half of their significant correlations would show inverse, not positive, relationships between between glucose metabolism and amplitude of ERP components. Furthermore, since there are 104 correlations in this table, and

Table 3 Pearson Product–Movement Correlations between Principal Components of the Evoked Related Potential and Localized Measurements of Glucose Utilization

	PC7 100ms "P1"	PC6 160ms "N1"	PC5 200ms "P2"	PC4 280ms "N2"	PC3 400ms "P3"	PC2 600ms "N6"	PC8 700ms "N7"	PC1 900ms "late N"
L thalamus								
R thalamus						−34		
L occipital		43[a]						
R occipital								
L area 37					−35			34
R area 37								46[b]
L ang gyrus								−33
R ang gyrus	−38	−34						
B ant cing[c]		−32					−32	−36
L inf front							−33	
R inf front								
L caudate		−32						
R caudate	−38							

Note. All entries are significant at $p<.05$.
[a] $p<.01$.
[b] $p<.005$.
[c] Bilateral; the measured sphere is centered on the midline.

only 5 or 6 of them would be expected by chance to be significant, we may provisionally interpret these 13 significant correlations as an existence proof that inverse correlations between PET and ERP measurements are not only possible, but likely. Our particular selection of regions may well have omitted those which actually contain measurable concentrations of the generators of the measured electrophysiological components, so that we "missed" the positive correlations, but that does not relieve us of the burden of interpreting inverse relationships of the type seen in the present data. We cannot feasibly explain them by chance alone, and must seek the beginnings of an explanation that is more complex than the simple notion that glucose metabolism and ERP amplitude both reflect a simple process of neuronal activity.

Negative correlations involving brain metabolism or blood flow are not unfamiliar, but they have tended to deal mostly with task or subject variables. (See Wood, 1990, for a review of this question.) The logic is generally that skilled, accurate, or well-practiced performance may well be metabolically less demanding than clumsy, inaccurate, or unpracticed performance. The present data, however, are the first report of inverse correlations between metabolism and ERPs, so the logic of unskilled performance may be difficult to apply. P3 amplitudes are well known to reflect novel, hence less well-practiced, events, so the logic can reach as far as to explain the fact that smaller P3s imply more familiar

stimuli, which in turn evoke smaller electrophysiological responses. However, this explanation does not in any way explain why low P3 amplitude should be accompanied by high locally measured metabolism.

The preceeding question is sharpened by the strong inverse correlation between area 37 metabolism and accuracy of performance of the task done during glucose uptake—the same task for which the ERPs were measured. Left area 37 is the only region measured which shows any significant correlation with task accuracy. Properly, such a correlation should partial out the variance due to whole brain metabolism as well as the variance due to age, so neither of them is confounded. So partialled, the Pearson correlation between left area 37 metabolism and percent hits on the task is strong and inverse ($r = −.51$, $p<.005$). The corresponding partial correlation with false alarms is also significant and positive ($r = +.35$, $p<.05$), however this is found to be due to correlated variance with percentage of hits. By itself, free of confound by inverse relation to percentage of hits, the percentage of false alarms is not correlated with glucose metabolism in left area 37, whereas percentage of hits remains strongly correlated with left area 37 metabolism when this control is imposed. Hits on the task (independent of false alarms) are also correlated with the P3, though the correlation is confined mostly to the posterior electrodes.

The above considerations suggest that P3 amplitude is inversely correlated with left area 37 metabolism because they have opposite signed correlations with task performance. In this context, it is worth remembering that ERPs measure the activity of a select population of neurons, largely pyramidal, whose lengthwise orientation is similar. In a given local region, the synaptic activity of these neurons, at a high rate or in great number, is presumably metabolically demanding. Without considering what the other neurons in the region are doing, however, we cannot be sure that the increased metabolic demand from pyramidal neurons would be enough to raise the metabolic average for the whole region. However, if the activity of other neurons (stellate sensory cells, for example) was either synchronized with pyramidal synaptic activity or—if uncorrelated—was not so noisy as to "swamp" the pyramidal activation, then the area-wide metabolic measure could reflect the impact of increased pyramidal cell activity, leading to a positive correlation between PET and ERP. By contrast, if the activity of stellate neurons were actually diminished during accurate task performance, in reciprocity with the increased activity of the pyramidal neurons, and if that diminished stellate metabolism outweighed the increased pyramidal metabolism, then task relevant activation that evokes pyramidal activity (and is measured by increases in ERP amplitude) could result in decreased overall glucose metabolic demand and glucose consumption in a local region. One mechanism of reduced stellate cell activity is obvious: the suppression of attention to irrelevant or random environmental stimuli would reduce the aggregate firing of these neurons over time. Furthermore, if these stellate neurons are responding to irrelevant stimuli, then their activity might not even issue in a pyramidal cell discharge from a given cortical column. In that case, there would be a double dissociation: excess stellate activation disengages pyramidal activation, whereas pyramidal activation is facilitated by diminished, that is, less noisy, stellate activation.

The foregoing attentional rationale is one approach to explaining the P3 data, but in the present data postresponse processes appear even more salient and in need of explanation. The first principal component of the ERP, peaking at 900 ms, which by definition explains a larger amount of electrophysiological variance than any other component, also correlates with PET data in more ROIs than any other component. Yet, this component peaks long after the stimulus presentation and well after the subject's behavioral response. This late component may reflect anticipation of the computer feedback about correctness of response, which is provided at 1100 ms after the stimulus. Alternatively, it could represent an internalized evaluative response of satisfaction or consternation, such as "Good, I got it right" or "Darn, I missed it." Whatever its detailed

content, it is by definition a postresponse process and is quite unlikely to be simply a lingering stimulus process. Its multiplicity of correlations with glucose metabolism suggests that it may reflect a variety of processes. The particularly strong positive correlation with area 37, this time on the right, is interesting in light of the previously discussed left area 37 inverse correlations with P3 and with task accuracy.

The location of area 37 is shown on MRI and PET in Figure 3. It is also instructive to map the distribution of ERP principal component scores at each electrode site and the interpolated areas between sites. Plate 21 shows such a mapping of the P3 and "late N" components across a stylized representation of the scalp surface. This mapping shows the typical concentration of the amplitude of the P3 evoked potential in the parietal regions of the scalp and a left-central-posterior concentration of the "late N" component. Plate 22 then maps the correlations between left or right area 37 metabolism and P3 or "late N" component scores, distributed across the scalp. Only the upper left (P3 with left area 37) and lower right ("late negativity" with right area 37) maps show significant correlations.

It is not plausible that left area 37 is the location of most of the generators of P3 in this task. All we know about P3 suggests its wide distribution, and the unilateral feature (left but not right area 37), essentially precludes left area 37 as the major locus of the generators of the rather symmetrical, slightly rightward, P3 topography. On the other hand, correlated activation between area 37 and the source generators of P3 is essentially what the data indicate. The map of P3 correlation with left area 37 (upper left of Plate 21) is similar to, but certainly not identical with, the map of the P3 distribution itself (top of Figure 3). This requires the conclusion that not all of the P3 generators are linked metabolically to left area 37; the glass is half empty. On the other hand, there is also a considerable overlap, whereby a bilateral subset of the generators of the P3 is indeed affected by the metabolic activity in left area 37; the glass is half full. The existence proof of such modulation of a robust electrophysiological component by task related activity in an associated but distinct region is a major implication of our method and our findings.

Interpretation of the "late N" findings is necessarily more speculative, since we have little firm evidence of what kind of process is reflected by this component. We can, however, assume that it is likely to be a postresponse process in content, not just in timing. Regardless of that assumption, the anatomy invites at least one speculation. There appears to be lateral specialization in the contributions of area 37 to task performance. The correlation of task accuracy with only left area 37 may be another instance of left hemisphere verbal specialization, since the task requires letter recognition. More

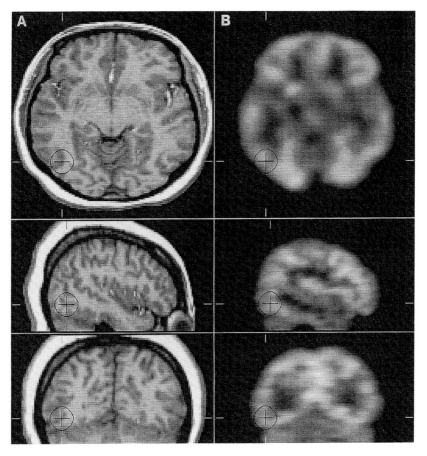

Figure 3 Registered MRI and PET metabolic images showing the spherical region of interest at left Brodmann's area 37 from the axial, sagittal, and coronal views (top to bottom).

precisely, in line with other considerations developed previously, we might say that left area 37 could be a place where random sensory activity must be suppressed in order for accurate task performance to take place (and for the P3 amplitude to be optimally maximized). By contrast, then, the contribution of the homologous right area 37 is much later and more evaluative. (Note that the topography of the N9 is also inconsistent with its generation solely in right area 37, as was the case with the left area 37 linkage to P3.) What makes this neurobehaviorally interesting is that it could be assumed that the capabilities of left and right area 37 are similar, so that both can detect letters. The specialization would be that execution is guided by the letter detection done in left area 37, whereas the internal monitoring of the correctness of response is guided by the letter detection in right area 37. Such monitoring would be relevant to the anticipation of feedback about correctness of response, and serve as the basis for improving performance on subsequent trials.

While speculative, this account can address the other major difference between the left correlation with P3 and the right correlation with the "late N"—the differences in the signs of the correlations. Suppression of stellate activity, leading to an inverse PET–ERP correlation, is relevant only when the processing involves attention to stimuli for recognition purposes, and the transmission of that recognition elsewhere for purposes of informing the response. That is the extent of what has been proposed for left area 37, so an inverse correlation between glucose and P3 amplitude is consistent. In contrast, a positive correlation between right area 37 metabolism and the "late N" amplitude suggests that there is an additional processing demand on the stellate neurons that overcomes the suppression brought about by stimulus recognition. In this present speculative account, that additional demand is imposed by the dual task of maintaining the image of the stimulus and matching it to the response that has just occurred, thus leading to the formulation of an internal evaluative response.

The foregoing speculation is an example of what was proposed in the introduction: the convergence of data from disparate measurement techniques, in different scales, to yield an account of an underlying process that is only indirectly and partially represented by either technique. It is only one example; however, most of the correlations reported here have not even been discussed and each could generate equally extensive speculations. The limited discussion presented here may nevertheless suffice to suggest a few simple points about PET–ERP correlations, as follows:

1. While some correlations can be positive, many will be inverse. When they are, their interpretations may require a consideration of differential activity of separate neuronal populations within a given region.
2. While some correlations can be attributed to neural events that occur in the same location, many correlations will reflect synchronous events occuring in widely different brain locations.
3. While some correlations can be informative standing alone, regardless of task or subject variables, most correlations will probably not be interpretable except by reference to task or subject variables.

References

Evans, A. C., Marrett, S. & Collins, L. (1989). Anatomical-functional correlative analysis of the human brain using three dimensional imaging systems. *Proceedings SPIE. 1092,* 264–274.

Phelps, M. E., Huang, S. C., Hoffman, E. J., Selin, C., Sokoloff, L., & Kuhl, D. E. (1979). Tomographic measurement of local cerebral glucose metabolic rate in humans with [18F]2-Fluoro-2-deoxy-2-D-glucose: Validation of method. *Annals of Neurology, 6,* 371–388.

Spielberger, C. D., Gorsuch, R. L., Luchene, R., Vagg, P. R., & Jacobs, G. (1983). *Manual for the state trait anxiety inventory.* Palo Alto, CA: Consulting Psychologists Press.

Talairach, J. & Tournoux, P. (1988). *Co-planar stereotaxic atlas of the human brain.* New York: Thieme.

Wood F. (1990). Functional neuroimaging in neurobehavioral research. In A. A. Boulton, G. B. Baker, & M. Hiscock (Eds.), *Neuromethods: (Vol. 17, pp. 107–125).* Clifton, NJ: Human.

15

Structural Variation in the Developing and Mature Cerebral Cortex: Noise or Signal?

Christiana M. Leonard

*Department of Neuroscience, University of Florida Health Science Center,
Gainesville, Florida 32610*

I. Introduction

Due to recent advances in magnetic resonance imaging technology (MRI), the brains of living children can be visualized with a detail unimaginable a decade ago (Fig. 1). At last it is possible to ask and answer questions about structural correlates of normal brain development, minimal brain damage, handedness, intelligence, and brain lateralization for language.

A. Problem

This technological revolution in neuroimaging has caught the developmental community unawares. Because the brains of young children have never been available for study, developmental psychologists have few paradigms that include brain structure as a variable (Torres, 1995). Human neuroanatomy is not a required subject for developmentalists, and even if it were, most courses do not discuss cerebral cortex in sufficient depth to be helpful to the psychologist interested in cognitive, motor, or emotional development.

There are only a handful of neurologists, neuroanatomists, and psychologists who have been willing to immerse themselves in the threatening study of the human cerebral cortex. Many of these scientists have been somewhat isolated and have not sailed in the mainstream of neuroscience or psychology. In contrast, in other fields, such as visual perception, motor control or learning, charismatic scientists with good communication skills and a keen understanding of the value of hypothesis testing have spawned schools of disciples and ushered in explosive scientific development (Gazzaniga, 1995).

In the field of human cortical neuroanatomy, there are currently few shared paradigms and techniques and virtually no common body of data. Fundamental questions on which there is no agreement include: (1) terminology for cortical regions, (2) area number and boundaries, (3) the relation between structural and functional variables, and (4) appropriate goals and techniques. A dominant view, expressed by one neuroscientist attending the second annual meeting of the Cognitive Neuroscience Society, is "Convince me that the cortex is more than a bowl of spaghetti!" It is widely believed that the advent of functional MRI has obviated the need for careful structural analysis—because it is the function, not the structure, that is ultimately of interest. This chapter will argue an opposing view. I believe that anatomy is destiny and the cortical sulci should be treated like a valuable geological fossil record. A better understanding of sulcal architecture can open a window into genetic and developmental history.

B. Background

The first suggestion that regional differentiation might be related to function is attributed to Paul Broca

DEVELOPMENTAL NEUROIMAGING

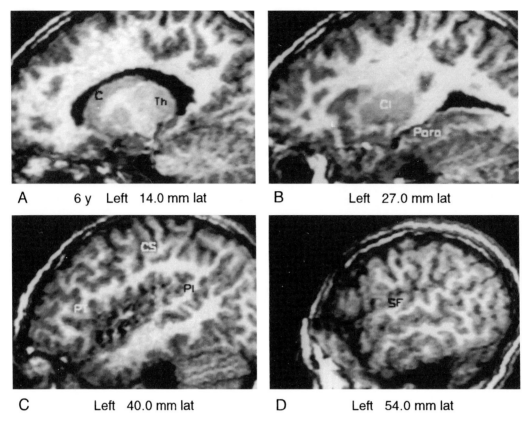

Figure 1 Four parasagittal images in the left hemisphere of a 6 year old female control. In this and the subsequent figures, the images are photographs of 1 mm thick sagittal sections that have been rotated into the AC–PC plane and reformatted to correct for head tip in the coronal and axial planes. The images were acquired in a Seimens 1T Magnetom with an MPRage "Turboflash" gradient echo, volumetric sequence with the following parameters: repetition time = 10 ms, echo time = 4 ms, flip angle 10°, matrix 130 × 256, field of view = 25 cm, 1 acquisition, 1.25 or 1.4 mm thick sections. The scan time for this sequence is 6 minutes and sedation is seldom necessary to keep children still. C: caudate nucleus; Cl: claustrum; CS: central sulcus; lat: lateral to the midline; Para: parahippocampal gyrus; Pl: planum temporale (Wernicke's area); PT: pars triangularis (Broca's area); SF: sylvian fissure; Th: thalamus; y: years of age.

(Heilman & Valenstein, 1993). Five successive right-handers with aphasia had damage anteriorly in the left hemisphere. Broca proposed that righthanders had language in the left hemisphere, while lefthanders had a mirror-image arrangement. A century of subsequent research has supported the first but not the second prediction. In almost all righthanders, the left hemisphere is "eloquent" and the right "silent." There is also clinical evidence that the left hemisphere can be further divided into an anterior fluent "Broca's area," and a posterior receptive "Wernicke's area" (Fig. 2). The brains of lefthanders, however, are not organized in a reciprocal fashion. Very few people, at most 5% of the population, have language limited to the right hemisphere (Strauss, Gaddes, & Wada, 1987).

For a century, this dramatic functional asymmetry was unaccompanied by any accepted evidence of structural asymmetry. Although the German literature contained references to anatomical asymmetries in the

lower bank of the sylvian fissure, the consensus in the English speaking world came down on the side of the spaghetti view (Witelson, 1982). Most American psychologists assumed that function was diffusely represented in the cortex and unaccompanied by structural specializations. A paradigmatic shift in thinking was initiated by a landmark *Science* paper that reported on a sample of 100 autopsy specimens of whole brain (Geschwind & Levitsky, 1968). Geschwind and Levitsky measured the length of the posterior sylvian fissure, the planum temporale that forms the core of Wernicke's area (Figs. 2 and 3). They made one simple linear measurement on the external surface of the left and right hemispheres (probably using a piece of string). In 65% of the brains, the planum was longer on the left; in 25% of the brains, there was no difference. However, only 10% of the brains had a significant right-sided asymmetry (arbitrarily designated as a greater than 1 mm difference).

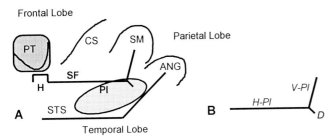

Figure 2 (A) Schematic diagram of structures surrounding the sylvian fissure as they appear on the surface of the left hemisphere. The square dark-stippled area indicates the region called Broca's area, the oval light-stippled area indicates Wernicke's area. These terms are concepts, rather than locations (Bogen & Bogen, 1976). ANG: angular gyrus; CS: central sulcus; H: Heschl's transverse gyrus (primary auditory cortex); Pl: planum temporale (H-planum); PT: pars triangularis; SF: sylvian fissure; SM: supramarginal gyrus; STS: superior temporal sulcus. (B) Detail of posterior termination of sylvian fissure. H-planum: horizontal bank of the planum temporale; V-planum: vertical bank of planum temporale (posterior ascending ramus); D: posterior descending ramus.

Although the distribution of handedness and language lateralization was unknown, the percentage of right-larger brains was comparable to the expected percentage of right dominance for language. Geschwind therefore proposed that a macroscopic feature, planar asymmetry, could be used as an indicator of functional localization for language. The study caught the popular imagination, and confirmation of a robust anatomical asymmetry followed quickly, in newborns, children, and even fetuses (Witelson & Paillie, 1973; Wada & Clarke, 1975; Chi, Dooling, & Gilles, 1977). This early structural asymmetry suggested that leftward superiority for language is established prenatally, rather than induced by experience.

One of the remarkable features of these papers is that none was, strictly speaking, a replication, for each used a different method for measuring the planum (Witelson, 1982). The average coefficient of asymmetry (the difference between the two sides divided by the average) seemed to hover around 35%, whether investigators measured area or length. This is particularly noteworthy because planar structure is variable, and it is sometimes no simple matter to identify the anterior and posterior boundaries (Fig. 4).

Autopsies are decreasing, postmortem specimens are available to only a few investigators, and few scientists are willing to make the investment and compromises necessary to study the postmortem human brain. There were thus few studies in the subsequent decades that tried to test Geschwind's hypothesis that structural asymmetry predicted lateralization for lan-

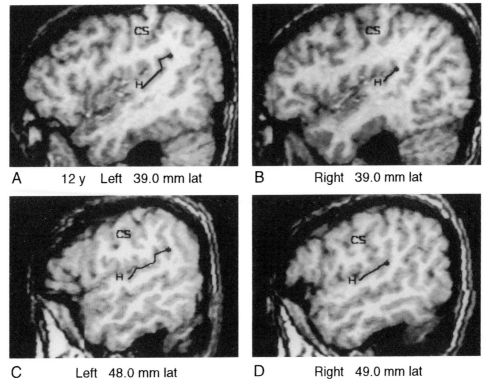

Figure 3 Leftward asymmetry of the H-planum (outlined in black) at two different parasagittal positions in a 12 year old male control. CS: central sulcus; H: Heschl's transverse gyrus.

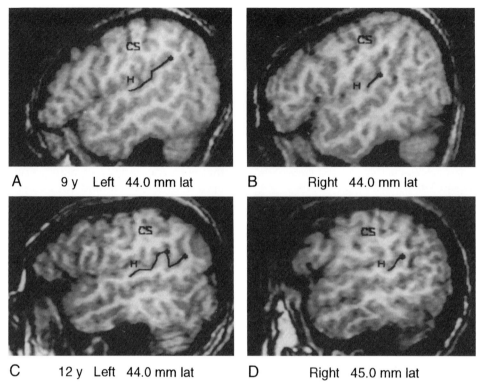

Figure 4 Variation in structure of the left and right H-plana in two control children. (A) No V-planum, stepwise elevation in the horizontal bank. (B) Stepwise elevation, but origin of V-planum unambiguous. (C) Posterior bulge in horizontal bank, origin of V-planum ambiguous. (D) Bifurcation at termination of sylvian fissure, origin of V-planum unambiguous; CS: central sulcus; H: Heschl's transverse gyrus.

guage. One notable exception is the pioneering work of Albert Galaburda, who, like Levitsky, was a neurology resident trained by Geschwind. Galaburda's findings with respect to planar symmetry in cases of developmental dyslexia invented a field, for they provided the first evidence that learning disabilities could arise from anomalous brain development (Galaburda, 1989).

The advent of imaging caused an explosion of studies investigating asymmetry, with somewhat mixed results due to the absence of accepted paradigms for experimental design, diagnosis, brain scan, and measurement techniques. The cortical structure of human beings is variable. There are few living anatomists who have made a study of this variability. Fewer are involved in magnetic resonance imaging studies. By default, the investigations have been shaped by the medical model of the neurologist or the computer model of the psychologist and cognitive scientist.

The brain model of the neurologist has evolved from clinical observations in patients. There has historically been no means of untangling the confounding factors of individual variation in premorbid cognitive function and brain structure from variability due to disease. The brain model of the computer scientist and psychologist, in contrast, is a network of linked computer modules. Individual variation is attributed to software (experience), not hardware, differences. There has been a strong drive in many laboratories to eliminate, or at least reduce, variation in brain structure by warping, distorting, and averaging in order to produce an average or normative brain. When brains are averaged, almost all the cortical sulci disappear (Evans, 1992), submerging the fossil record.

II. Mapping Function to Structure

Once Fritsch and Hitzig had established that electrical stimulation of different regions of the cortex produced different movements (Penfield & Roberts, 1959), it seemed reasonable to try to map other behaviors to the brain. But as Hans-Lucas Teuber always opened his graduate seminar on brain and behavior by asking "What brain? What behavior?" Should cerebral structure be described in terms of (1) Brodmann's areas, (2) anatomically visible gyri and sulci, or (3) standardized (Talairach) coordinates?

A. Anatomical Landmarks

1. Brodmann's Areas

Brodmann's areas are based on cytoarchitectonic criteria, that is, differences in cell size, packing density, laminar width, and myelination that are not visible in current MRI technology. But boundaries between many major Brodmann's areas (primary and secondary visual cortex, primary motor and primary sensory cortex), lie in the fundi (depths) of primary sulci that are visible on MRI. Thus, a general idea of cytoarchitecture can be gleaned from an examination of major sulci. This is important because Brodmann's areas are not just structural entities. Many of Brodmann's areas contain cortical maps of stimulus dimensions in the external environment. Area 17 (striate cortex) lies on the banks of the calcarine fissure and contains a map of the contralateral visual field as transmitted by the retina. Area 42 covers the first transverse gyrus of Heschl (Figs. 2–4) and contains a map of the frequency dimension as transmitted by the cochlea (Merzenich & Brugge, 1973). Area 3 lies in the posterior bank of the central sulcus (Figs. 2–4) and contains a complete map of the muscles and joints of the contralateral body. Area 4 lies in the anterior bank and contains a map of movements (Paxinos, 1990). Although the size of these maps varies among individuals (Stensaas, 1974), their location in major fissures does not. It is safe to assume that Heschl's gyrus will contain auditory cortex, although the exact boundaries may be in question (Liegeois-Chauvel, Musolino, & Chavel, 1991). Theoretically, then, a high resolution MRI scan in a suitable plane of section should be adequate for localization of major functions. Practically, however, this method has limited application. Clinical scans are acquired in standard planes of section in which even major sulci, like the sylvian fissure and the central sulcus, can be difficult to identify. Sulci are also quite variable in structure (Ono, Jubik, & Abernathy, 1990) among individuals. Furthermore, Positron Emission Tomography (PET), the major functional imaging method in use during the last two decades, does not even provide structural information.

2. The Talairach Proportional Coordinate System

An alternative system for describing location is the coordinate system described in the atlas of Talairach and Tournoux (1988). In this method, the image is rotated so that the anterior and posterior commissure lie in the horizontal plane (Fig. 5). Every point in the brain is described in terms of three normalized coordinates, with the anterior commissure as origin. The atlas brain has a left hemisphere that is 69 mm wide and a right hemisphere that is 67 mm wide. Thus, all brains have a Talairach coordinate of 69 at the widest point of the left hemisphere and one of 67 at the widest point of the right hemisphere, no matter whether their real widths are 54 mm or 73 mm (the range found in our MRI studies).

A few studies have shown that major sulci vary by about a centimeter from their atlas coordinates (Steinmetz, Furst, & Freund, 1989). Comparable data have not been published for minor sulci. For PET studies, where the resolution is of the order of a centimeter, Talairach coordinates are an ideal way of dealing with individual variation (Fox, Perlmutter, & Raichle, 1985; Friston, Passingham, Nutt, Heather, Sawle, & Frakowiak, 1989). The method is also useful for choosing comparable slice positions in different brains (Leonard, Voeller, Lombardino, Morris, Alexander, Andersen, et al., 1993). As the ability to measure the structural correlates of function becomes more precise, it will be interesting to see whether the Talairach coordinates continue to be useful, for sulci in association cortex vary considerably with respect to these coordinates (Figs. 5 and 6). Whether eliminating individual variation by normalizing to a standard coordinate system is a better tool for understanding brain function than preserving it by describing function mapped to sulci, remains an open question.

B. Cortical Maps: Why Might Sulci Be Important?

A major advance in our understanding of the principles of cortical functional organization was provided by Allman and Kaas (1971). Prior to their study, sensory modalities were thought to integrate in "association" cortex, making the connections on which learning and behavioral development were based. There were few hints as to the rules governing this integration. It was vaguely assumed that percepts lost their local signs and acquired more complex properties (multimodality, for example) as they progressed serially through association cortex. Allman and Kaas discovered a simple principle of organization which has proven to be a very powerful tool for the investigation of cortical function. They found a retinotopic map of the visual field far away from striate cortex in the bank of the superior temporal sulcus, the middle temporal area (MT). Subsequent studies demonstrated primary and secondary visual cortex maps to many separate "association" areas, producing at least 32 separate retinotopic maps of the visual field in each hemisphere. Brodmann's area 19 is thus a mosaic of many repeated maps of the visual field (Sereno, Dale, Tootell, Reppas, Kwong, Belliveau, et al., 1995).

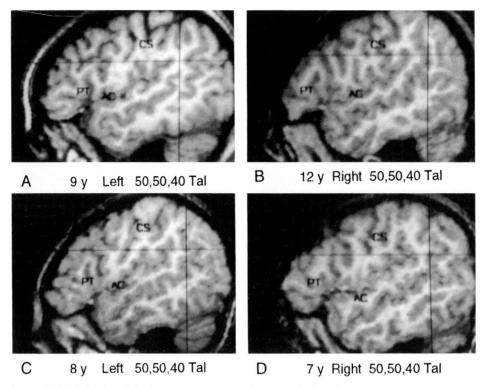

Figure 5 Variation in sylvian fissure structures as a function of Talairach (tal) coordinates at lateral 50 in 4 control children. In this and subsequent figures, the perpendicular lines indicate tal posterior (P) 50 and superior (S) 40. In (A) through (D), the V-planum terminates in increasingly superior positions. (A) No V-planum. (B) and (C) V-planum ascends considerably anterior to the cross hairs. (D) V-planum angles anteriorly. These four panels illustrate the difficulty of applying the "knife cut" technique described by Witelson (1982). The origin of the V-planum might not coincide with the point at which a knife cut would pass through the horizontal bank in (B) and (C). AC: anterior commissure; CS: central sulcus; PT: pars triangularis.

Each time the sensory field is remapped to a new area of cortex, the cells specialize in discriminations along a new stimulus dimension. Cells in MT, for example, are sensitive to the speed and direction of motion and are active during the motion aftereffect visual illusion (Tootell, Reppas, Dale, Look, Sereno, Brady, et al., 1995). Localized damage to MT interferes with the ability to track moving visual stimuli in particular parts of the visual field (Newsome, Wurtz, Dursteler, & Mikami, 1985). Cells in other regions specialize in color, pattern perception and even, it seems, recognizing faces (Allison, Ginter, McCarthy, Nobre, Luby, & Spencer, 1994). The principle of cortical mapping has been extended to other sensory and motor areas, and it is now a generally accepted principle that most, if not all, cortical areas contain a topographic map of some stimulus dimension (Allman, 1987). Walter Schneider, a cognitive psychologist at the University of Pittsburgh, has expanded this concept to the totality of human cortex (Schneider, W. S., personal communication, April, 1995). Comparing cortical measurements in monkey and human, he proposes that there may be

1000 brain areas in the human, each of which specializes in a particular task. He challenges other cognitive scientists to provide tasks that will differentially challenge each area. I would like to challenge cognitive neuroanatomists to search for these areas in cortical sulci.

Differences in the size and shape of sulci could provide insight into cognitive differences among individuals. For example, if the sylvian fissure in one individual extends horizontally 2 cm farther than another, this could be a valuable clue that the functions performed in this region are different both qualitatively and quantitatively. We have preliminary supporting evidence. In our March of Dimes study conducted with Linda Lombardino (Leonard, Lombardino, Mercado, Browd, Breier, & Agee, 1996), we found that 5 to 9 year old children with planar asymmetry due to small H-plana on the right had significantly better phonemic awareness (the metalinguistic ability to manipulate the building blocks of language) than children with large right (symmetrical) plana. In contrast, children with large plana performed better on a spatial patterns test.

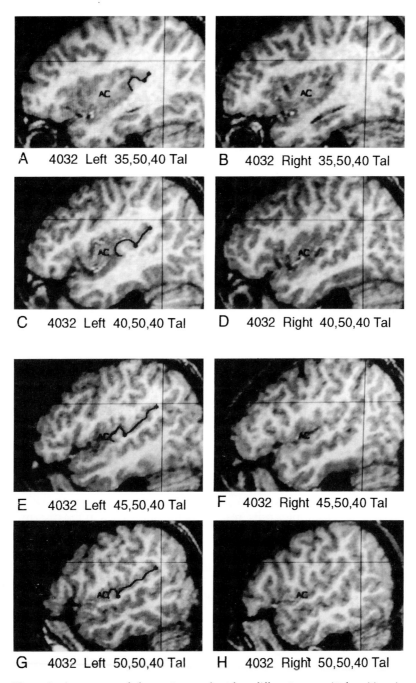

A 4032 Left 35,50,40 Tal   B 4032 Right 35,50,40 Tal

C 4032 Left 40,50,40 Tal   D 4032 Right 40,50,40 Tal

E 4032 Left 45,50,40 Tal   F 4032 Right 45,50,40 Tal

G 4032 Left 50,50,40 Tal   H 4032 Right 50,50,40 Tal

Figure 6 Appearance of planum temporale at four different parasagittal positions in the left and right hemispheres in a 12 year old male control. Heschl's gyrus and the H-planum are outlined on the left. On the left (A,C,E,G), the sylvian fissure extends more posteriorly at more lateral positions, while on the right (B,D,F,H), the fissure angles superiorly. It is this difference in the course of the left and right sylvian fissures that is responsible for the typical leftward asymmetry of the planum.

In a separate Veterans Administration study of schizophrenia directed by John M. Kuldau, we are finding that patients who have the normal number of sulci and gyri in the region of the sylvian fissure have better phonemic awareness and verbal fluency than patients with extra or missing gyri.

C. Anatomical Specializations for Function

Is there any experimental background for the idea that macroscopic anatomical differences actually reflect individual differences in functional specialization, or is sulcology just rewarmed phrenology (Calvin

& Ojemann, 1994)? There is some suggestive evidence. In animals, functional areas frequently have distinguishing macroscopic characteristics. Vision is our most highly developed sense, and primary visual cortex has a thick band of myelinated fibers and a very thick band of tiny granule cells, that can be distinguished with the naked eye, giving it the name "striate cortex" (Paxinos, 1990). Area MT (the motion sensitive area) can be identified by a thick band of myelinated fibers, and this anatomically defined area coincides with a particular functional specialization (Tootell et al., 1995). The region of the central sulcus that contains the receptors and upper motor neurons for the thumb and fingers can be recognized by a posterior bulge (Yousry, Schmid, Jassoy, Schmidt, Eisner, Reulen, et al., 1995). No other species depends on auditory input to the extent that we do for social and intellectual development. And no other species has such a prominent Heschl's gyrus for receiving auditory information (Seldon, 1985).

1. Animal and Experimental Data

Even complex cognitive functions can be accompanied by visible specializations. The most dramatic is the case of learned bird song. The species and the sex (male) in which song structure is dependent on environmental input have a unique set of brain structures that are easily visible to the naked eye (Nottebohm, Stokes, & Leonard, 1976). In females, the structures are small or missing (Gurney & Konishi, 1980). Damage to these nuclei severely compromises the ability to sing. In a less thoroughly documented example, cells responsive to faces cluster in a heavily myelinated bulge in the upper bank of the superior temporal sulcus of the monkey (Baylis, Rolls, & Leonard, 1985). Elsewhere in the temporal lobe, face-sensitive cells are more sparsely distributed (Baylis, Rolls, & Leonard, 1987).

The relative sizes of cortical areas also reflect their degree of functional specialization. The foveal projection of diurnal species is much larger than that of the periphery in visual areas devoted to form perception (Allman, 1987). The periphery of the visual field has a larger representation in areas devoted to motion perception. The projection areas for the thumb and the mouth are larger than those for the trunk and the foot (Shepherd, 1994). Thus, within an individual, it is possible to predict the relative importance of a function by measuring the size of its projection area. Between species, the variation in the size of cortical areas explains differences in functional dependence on specific functions. The olfactory area is large in nocturnal animals that need to identify predators, prey, and sexual partners by smell. It is small in humans who depend on vision for these tasks. There is now increasing evidence that the size of areas devoted to the representation of specific stimuli grows while the animal is learning to attend to those stimuli (Recanzone, Schreiner, & Merzenich, 1993). It seems only a slight extrapolation to suggest that differences in the relative size of cortical projection areas might explain some of the variance in cognitive function between individuals. Such differences could be due to an epigenetic interaction between genetic constitution and the environment (Brauth, Hall, & Dooling, 1991).

In order to test these hypotheses, one needs to have reliable and valid measuring instruments for both brain and behavior, as well as a sophisticated understanding of brain–behavior maps. Arguing from analogy with vision, it seems likely that the banks of the sylvian fissure contain a mosaic of areas, each specialized to discriminate stimuli along a particular auditory dimension. A current working hypothesis in many laboratories is that children and adults with learning and language disabilities have anomalous development of these auditory areas. Unfortunately, scientific understanding of the organization of these areas, what stimulus dimensions they map, and how their functional properties might differ in the left and right hemispheres is primitive compared to that for vision (Rauschecker, Tian, & Hauser, 1995; Steinschneider, Schroeder, Arezzo, & Vaughan, 1993).

Tallal and her colleagues have marshaled a body of compelling evidence that one important difference between the auditory capacities of the left and right hemispheres lies in the discrimination of small temporal intervals (Tallal, Miller, & Fitch, 1993). This ability is degraded in children with specific language impairment (Tallal, Stark, & Mellits, 1985), and differences in this ability predict differences in the rate of language development in normal children (Benasich, Spitz, & Tallal, 1995). Our laboratory is investigating the hypothesis that structural differences between the shape and size of the sylvian fissures in the left and right hemisphere are correlated with these functional differences, and may provide insight into the developmental sources of language disability.

III. MRI Technology

The possibility of examining brain–behavior correlations in individual children has only emerged recently, due to dramatic improvements in imaging technology. Notwithstanding these improvements, there are still many technical pitfalls that may trap the unwary. The major debate in the field is between the use of anatomical landmark-based manual drawing and automatic segmentation methods. The difference between these two approaches has been beautifully captured by Andreason, as the difference between a medieval monk and the word processor (Andreason, 1994a). But this may be too simplistic. Actually, the two approaches can be complementary, for they ask and answer different questions. A method should not be chosen on the basis of technology but on the basis of results. Do the methods result in anatomical measurements that are sensitive and specific for the variable of interest, namely, disease, age, sex, handedness, or cognitive function?

A. Brain Structure Sampler

To frame the discussion, Table 1 provides a list of the most frequently measured structures in anatomical MRI investigations, the theoretical rationale for their choice, and the measurement problems that have been encountered.

B. Physics and Biology

1. What Can Be Measured or Counted in a Brain Scan?

Variation between groups is quantified with means and standard deviations. But means and standard deviations can only be calculated when something has been counted. Voxels are easy to count in brain images. Thus volumes, areas, lengths, and widths can be measured using "semiautomated" computerized techniques. But volumes, areas, lengths, and widths of what? Should structures be anatomically defined, functionally defined, arbitrarily defined, or thresholded by automatic segmentation? What are appropriate units of measurement?

2. Digital Image Processing

Modern scans appear so similar to neuropathological specimens that it is easy to forget that the image is a synthetic one. The numbers are only indirectly related to traditional histological elements such as Nissl substance, membranes, or myelin. Voxel signal intensities reflect the relative reactivity of water molecules trapped in different environments. The data are originally wave forms that are reconstructed into images by digital sampling techniques. Since the reconstructed data are numbers, not abstract visual percepts like cells or dendrites, they can be manipulated with mathematical operations such as averages, histograms, scaling functions, filters, and Fourier transforms. But although scan images are frequently referred to as data, the digitized gray levels are not the traditional data of the anatomist. Neuroanatomical structure boundaries in the mammalian brain, even at the microscopic level, are frequently ambiguous. The mathematical tools currently available may be inappropriate for analyzing

Table 1A   Gross Anatomical Regions That Have Been Measured, Rationale for Their Measurement, Technical Difficulties, and Sample References[a]

Structure	Rationale	Problems
Total brain volume	Affected by sex (Filipek et al., 1994), socioeconomic status (Barta, Pearlson, Powers, Richards, & Tune, 1990), IQ (Giedd, Castellanos, Kozuch, Casey, Kaysen, Casey, et al., 1995), and disease (Andreason, 1994b).	Should cerebellum be included? Manual measurement tedious. Automatic methods tend to include extracerebral tissue because signal characteristics of brain and nonbrain tissue are similar. Wide range of sizes compatible with normal function (Filipek et al., 1994; Giedd et al., 1995).
Gray matter, white matter, CSF	Gray-white ratios are different in the two hemispheres (Breier, Leonard, Bauer, Roper, & Gilmore, 1996), change with development (Harris et al., 1994), and disease (Zipursky, Lim, Sullivan, Brown & Pfefferbaum, 1992). Could be related to intelligence and psychological function.	Voxel misclassification because (1) no sharp boundary between gray and white matter in most regions, (2) noisy signal, (3) partial volume averaging, and (4) no reliable relation between voxel signal and tissue characteristics.
Volumes of frontal and temporal lobes	Neuropsychological evidence that various psychological functions are localized in different regions.	A multitude of independent functions are influenced by these lobes. Lobes do not function as a unit. No defined caudal boundary for the temporal or parietal lobes. No good evidence that disease or development affect lobes as units (Jernigan et al., 1990; Wible, Shenton, Hokama, Kikinis, Jolesz, Metcalf, et al., 1995).

[a]No attempt has been made to provide an exhaustive bibliography. Refer to other chapters in this volume for additional examples.

Table 1B   Landmark-Based Measurements of Anatomically Defined Structures[a]

Structure	Rationale	Problems
Hippocampus	Many psychological functions have been related to the hippocampus. It is damaged in epilepsy and the side with shrinkage can be used to predict the side of the epileptic focus.	Manual measurement tedious but reliable and valid in many independent studies. Automatic segmentation difficult because boundaries with amygdala and cortex are unclear. Initial studies used arbitrary anterior and posterior cutoffs. Although reported absolute sizes vary greatly among studies, all studies agree in the clinical utility of asymmetry coefficient in predicting seizure focus in temporal lobe epilepsy (Jack, Sharbrough, & Twomey, 1990; McCarthy & Luby, 1994; Gilmore, Childress, Leonard, Quisling, Roper, Eisenchenk, et al., 1995).
Corpus callosum	Boundaries easy to define. Size (and, sometimes, shape) related to disease, development, IQ, language lateralization, sex, and handedness.	No rationale exists for subdivision definition. Although fibers from different brain regions are topographically distributed in the corpus callosum, no methods for defining the location of fibers from defined regions have been developed. Few replicated findings (Witelson, 1989; Steinmetz, Jancke, Kleinschmidt, Schlaug, Volkmann, & Huang, 1992; Rowe, Kuldau, Gautier, Lombardino, Kranzler, & Leonard, 1995; Giedd, Castellanos, Casey, Kozuch, King, Hamburger, et al., 1994).
Caudate	Related to frontal function, size and asymmetry related to drugs, development, sex, and disease.	Ventral and caudal boundaries must be arbitrarily defined. Lateral boundary difficult to distinguish from white matter (Filipek et al., 1994; Giedd et al., 1995).
Amygdala	Related to emotion and memory, size related to disease.	Boundary with hippocampus must be arbitrarily defined. Other boundaries difficult to distinguish (Watson, Andermann, Gloor, Jones-Gotman, & Peters, 1992).
Other basal ganglia —and thalamic nuclei	Related to motor and cortical function.	Relatively small. Boundaries difficult to distinguish.
Cerebellum	Related to numerous cognitive and motor functions. Size of midsagittal section, vermal subdivisions related to disease.	No accepted methods of establishing structure function correlations.
Planum temporale	Asymmetry related to language lateralization and learning disabilities.	No consensus on boundaries or measurement method (Morgan & Hynd, 1995; Leonard et al., 1993; Kulynych et al., 1994; Schultz et al., 1994).
Heschl's gyrus	Asymmetry related to language lateralization.	Boundary between Heschl's gyrus and planum must be determined arbitrarily when gyrus is divided by sulci. Position and depth of dividing sulci are variable (Musiek & Reeves, 1990).
Sylvian fissure	Asymmetry related to language lateralization.	Anterior and posterior termination points not well defined.
Superior temporal —gyrus	Asymmetry and atrophy related to disease (Barta et al., 1990; Shenton, Kikinis, Jolesz, Pollak, LeMay, , Wible et al., 1992).	Posterior boundary not well defined (Loftus et al., 1993; Ide et al., 1995).
Other sulci and gyri	Related to specific information processing, language, and motor functions.	Tremendous variability of sulci makes identification of sulci, variants, and boundaries difficult (Ono et al., 1990; Steinmetz et al., 1990).

[a]See other chapters in this volume for additional studies.

anatomical abstractions such as "the sylvian fissure" and the "supramarginal gyrus."

3. Voxel Biology

Biological tissue is made up of cells with different chemical compositions. The cell's composition is regionally specific and there are many different types and sizes of cells in the brain. Cells and fibers range in size by many orders of magnitude. The myelin in two neighboring fibers may be thin or thick. A cell may have many long, wavy dendrites or a few stubby ones. The tissue contributing to one voxel's signal could contain 600,000 cells and fibers of all varieties. There are no areas restricted to either cell bodies or fibers, notwithstanding the neurologist's colloquial references to white and gray matter. Cells and fibers of different sizes and chemical composition intermingle with different packing densities. Regions of white and gray matter rarely have sharp boundaries, but shade indistinguishably into one another. Since there are no real edges, automatic segmentation into binary categories of "white" and "gray" has questionable validity.

C. Measurement Issues

1. Partial Volume Effect

The fact that the brain is a biological tissue with regional patterning poses a problem for digital interpretation. A high resolution scan with many little cubes provides a weak, noisy signal. Although amplification of the signal can be achieved by combining cubes, such amplification is accompanied by a loss of information concerning local tissue properties. This is known as the partial volume effect (Plante & Turkestra, 1991). The intensity of the signal registered at the receiving coil is an average of all tissue within a certain range. If the tissue contains a border between a region of heavily myelinated fibers and neuronal cell bodies, the emitted signal intensity may be indistinguishable from that of a region of lightly myelinated fibers. Error introduced by the partial volume effect increases as a function of the thickness of the slice. In the early days of magnetic resonance scanning, 5 and 7 mm thick sections separated by 2.5 mm gaps were standard. More recently, most groups have switched to gapless series of 1 to 3 mm thick sections. This reduces, but does not eliminate, the partial volume effect.

2. Automatic White–Gray Segmentation

Many studies using automated methods have divided the brain tissue into three segments: cerebrospinal fluid (CSF), gray matter, and white matter (Fletcher, Barsotti, & Hornak, 1993; Harris, Barta,

Peng, Lee, Brettschneider, Shah, et al., 1994). This method can produce useful results (Jernigan, Hesselink, Sowell, & Tallal, 1990; Filipek, Richelme, Kennedy, & Caviness, 1994). Our laboratory (Breier, Leonard, Bauer, Roper, & Gilmore, 1994) found that an automated segmentation method produced clinically significant information. Control subjects had a "white matter" asymmetry, in that the left temporal lobe had a relatively greater percentage of voxels with high signal intensities than the right. This asymmetry was exaggerated in patients with right hemisphere seizure foci and reduced in patients with left hemisphere foci. The paper describing these findings was rejected, however, for lack of validation. The appearance of a bimodal distribution in the histogram was not considered adequate evidence of validity. The reviewer was dissatisfied with the arbitrary nature of the thresholding algorithm, which simply divided the distribution at the minimum between the two peaks. We had argued that the algorithm divided the intensity levels into clinically meaningful subdivisions, and that the location of the voxels in the high signal peak was rationally related to the apparent white matter distribution on the displayed image (see Figures 7–9 for examples).

We became more sympathetic to the reviewer's point after trying binary segmentation of localized cortical regions in our developing population. We discovered that small adjustments in the location of the threshold in small volumes produced great variation in the percentages of white and gray. A change of four intensity levels in the location of the threshold in the 6 year old, shown in Figure 7, changed the white–gray ratio from .64 to .88, for example. In Figure 7, Panel A is the original image and Panel B shows the histogram of signal intensities in the scan as it was reconstructed by the scanner software (i.e., unmodified by filters or other image processing). The distribution is clearly bimodal. The images in Panels C and D demonstrate the effect of lowering the "white matter" threshold from 57 to 53. Note how sharp the edge between white and gray seems in all three images, even though the location of the boundary is quite different. This suggests that neither regional minima nor visual inspection are reliable guides for binary segmentation.

A more promising method of segmenting the distribution is demonstrated in Figures 8 and 9. During the examination of data collected with binary segmentation methods, we noticed that the relation between the heights of the peaks appeared to change reliably with age. The gray peak dropped with age while the white peak rose, as would be expected if there were increases in myelination (Benes, Turtle, Khan, & Farol, 1994). This reversal was not reliably reflected in the proportions of voxels in the upper and lower parts of the dis-

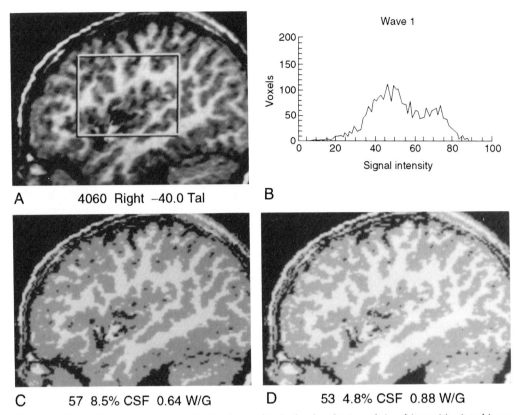

A   4060 Right −40.0 Tal   B

C   57 8.5% CSF 0.64 W/G   D   53 4.8% CSF 0.88 W/G

Figure 7   Effect of using a single threshold value to divide the distribution of signal intensities into binary partitions. Scan was acquired as 1.25 mm sections. (A) Original (unprocessed) image displayed with 90 gray levels. (B) Bimodal distribution of voxel signal intensities in region marked by box in (A). (C) Thresholded image displayed with three gray levels: Voxels with intensities that are above the threshold (W) are displayed in white, those below in gray (G), and CSF in black. %CSF: percentage of voxels with signal intensities below 28. (D) The thresholds for both white and gray are lowered by four. This relatively small change in the location of the threshold has a dramatic effect on the W–G ratio.

tribution. When voxels in the trough between the two peaks were eliminated, however, the white–gray ratio increased steadily with age (W+/G, see Figure 8), and reliably reflected the difference in height of the two peaks. We are encouraged to conclude that the voxels at the low and high ends of the distribution reflect true differences in the proportions of relatively homogeneous gray and white matter. The voxels in the trough, however, come from regions of the gray–white inter-

face where partial volume effects render small changes in signal level and are uninformative about histological characteristics of the tissue. More importantly, including partial volume voxels can obscure important physiological relationships.

Most of the voxels in the basal ganglia, thalamus, and hippocampus fall in this intermediate range: that is they are neither gray or white. It is thus difficult to pick out the boundaries of structures and to perform

Figure 8   Effect of removing an intermediate signal region (trough) from the "white matter" and "gray matter" estimates in the right hemisphere of 4 controls aged 6 to 49. Scans were acquired as 1.25 mm sections. The white–gray ratio measured in this way (i.e., without the partial volume voxels in the trough) is robust to changes in the width of the removed region. (A),(E),(I), and (M) show the unprocessed image. (B), (F), (J), and (N) show histograms of the area enclosed by the box on the left. %CSF: percentage of voxels with signal intensities between 0 and 23. The two numbers represent the boundaries of the trough for image on lower left. (C),(D),(G),(H),(K),(L),(O), and (P) represent the thresholded images displayed with four gray levels. G: gray, voxels between 24 and lower bound of trough; W−: voxels in the trough; W+: voxels in the higher intensity peak. Left: 8 signal level band in light gray. Right: trough widened by two signal levels in each direction. The light gray voxels tend to be located in regions where fibers enter and leave the white matter. These voxels are composed of varying proportions of fibers and cells (partial volume effect).

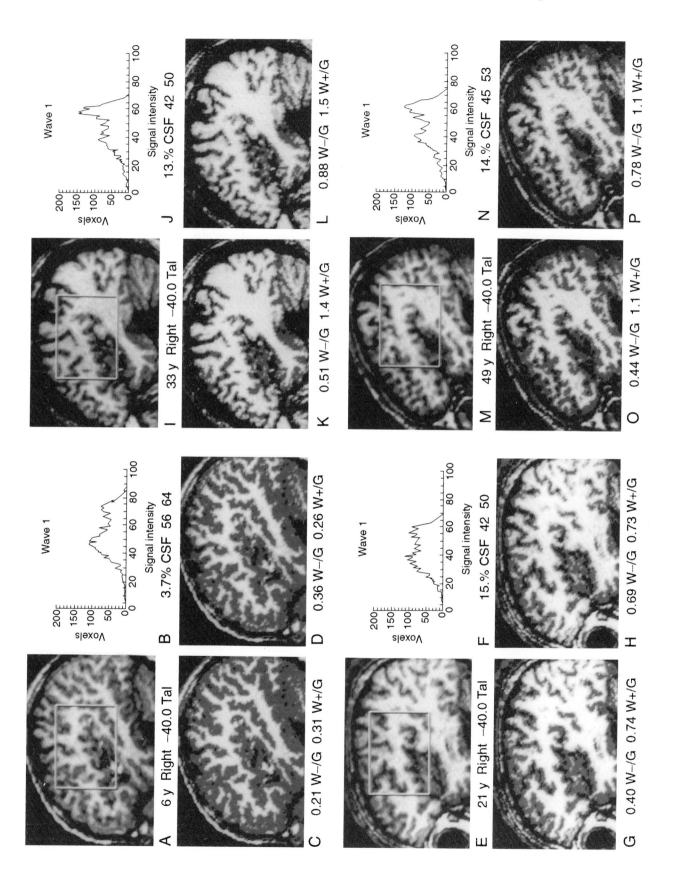

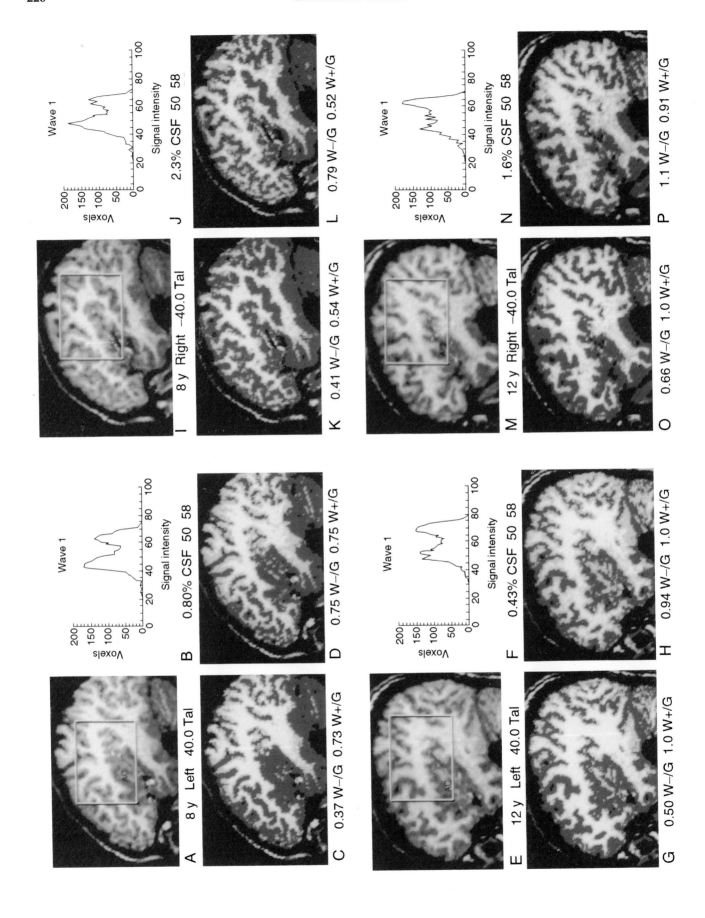

automatic segmentation. This is not only due to partial volume effects, but to the actual histological structure. If voxel values in the intermediate region of the distribution represent unknowable proportions of gray and white matter, it seems somewhat risky to average these values among brains. Interpretation of the meaning of differences among groups becomes difficult.

It is well known that ventricular size and intrasulcal CSF increases as a function of age and disease (Pearlson, Garbacz, Ahn, & DePaulo, 1984). It is therefore of great interest to accurately measure CSF. We have recently been surprised to find that a presumably minimal 15% increase in image thickness had a significant effect on the number of voxels identified as CSF in thin sagittal images of children (compare Figs. 8 and 9). There is much less CSF apparent in both the original and segmented images in Figure 9 (slice thickness originally 1.4 mm) than in Figure 8 (slice thickness originally 1.25). In further corroboration, the midsagittal 1.25 mm thick images (not shown) contained a population of very low signal voxels that was absent in the 1.4 mm thick images. In adults with significant atrophy, such a difference in section thickness may not be as critical as it is in children.

3. Identifying Comparable Sulci among Brains

The preceding sections describe some pitfalls of automatic segmentation. But manual methods are equally perilous, and certainly less elegant. How can brains with different fissure patterns be compared? If the sylvian fissure ascends 3 cm on the right, but continues horizontally on the left, are the posterior segments performing comparable functions? If regional variation in information processing is the foundation of neural organization and is related to developmental structural adjustments, then regional variation in structure is likely to be significant. Ideally, we would like to quantitate aspects of nervous tissue that could reasonably be related to behavioral function or biobehavioral risk factors. How can sulcal irregularities that are simply the result of mechanical forces (noise) be differentiated from ones that arise as the result of behaviorally genetic or environmental pressures?

It is conventional to rely on three-dimensional reconstructions, in particular, surface renderings, to present anatomical MRI findings (Schlaug, Jancke, Huang, & Steinmetz, 1995; Kulynych, Vladar, Jones, & Weinberger, 1994; Schultz, Cho, Staib, Kier, Fletcher, Shaywitz, et al., 1994). This rationale rests on the assumption that the important anatomical information is visible on the surface, but this assumption may be incorrect. At least ⅔ of the surface area of the cortex is actually hidden in sulci. A view of the surface provides scant information about those hidden depths. In fact, it may provide misinformation, because it is impossible to distinguish between surface dimples and deep chasms (Ono et al., 1990). Furthermore, a great deal of data smoothing and filtering is necessary to render a surface that resembles reader's expectations. Many published renderings are unaesthetic and difficult to reconcile with conventional anatomy. The pars triangularis, or the central sulcus, is frequently missing, for example.

Recently, there has been progress (Carman, Drury, & Van Essen, 1995; Dale & Sereno, 1993) in the use of graphical map making techniques to unfold the cortical gyri in a manner which maintains information about size and shape. These systems are not yet available for general use and may be computationally expensive, but they have great potential for comparing individual sulci among brains. It should ultimately be possible to code individual variability in sulcal depth as a probability map.

While waiting for these methods to become available for general use, we are taking a different approach, one pioneered by Helmuth Steinmetz and Sandra Witelson. Steinmetz has made a convincing case for the value of thin sagittal images in visualizing the sylvian fissure. In this plane, all the details of Broca's and Wernicke's areas are visible (Figs. 2–6). We have found that individual variation in these features is related to genetic history (Leonard, Weintraub, Martinez, & Hauser, 1995; Leonard, Williams, Nicholls, Agee, Voeller, Honeyman, et al., 1993), diagnosis (Leonard et al., 1993; Mercado, Browd, Leonard, Lombardino, Voeller, Ross, et al., 1994), language lateralization (Foundas, Leonard, Gilmore, Fennell, & Heilman, 1994), handedness (Foundas, Leonard, & Heilman, 1995), and cognitive ability (Leonard et al., 1996). In the remaining space I will review the principal features of sylvian fissure anatomy and present preliminary results on the use of a rating scheme for quantifying the presence of qualitative features. This scheme is an adaptation of the published methods (Steinmetz, Ebeling, Huang, & Kahn, 1990; Witelson & Kigar, 1992; Ide, Rodriguez, Zaidel, & Aboitiz, 1996).

Figure 9 White–gray ratios in the left and right hemispheres of an 8 year old female and a 12 year old male control. Labels as in Figure 8. These scans were acquired as 1.4 mm thick sections. There are many fewer pure CSF voxels.

IV. The Sylvian Fissure

A. Gross Anatomy

When viewing the brain from the sagittal aspect, the boundaries of the frontal lobe are clearly visible. Posteriorly, the frontal lobe is bounded by the central sulcus or fissure of Rolando; its inferior boundary is the lateral or sylvian fissure (Figure 2). The other lobes have no real boundaries, but fade into one another in the region where the sylvian fissure terminates. In thin parasagittal slices, the frontal and temporal lobes, together with the inferior parietal lobe, are well visualized. A number of sylvian fissure branches are visible: pars triangularis in the frontal operculum, the superior temporal sulcus in the temporal lobe, and the supramarginal and angular gyrus in the parietal lobe. Heschl's gyrus, which contains primary auditory cortex, is clearly visible in the lower bank of the sylvian fissure. Posterior to Heschl's gyrus is the auditory association cortex of the planum temporale. Anteriorly, the planum merges with Heschl's sulcus, a deep groove that separates Heschl's gyrus form the superior temporal gyrus (Figures 2–6).

Posteriorly, the planum may terminate in a bifurcation into a vertically oriented V-planum and descending ramus, or ascend in a series of short steplike segments. A series of variably sized "pseudo" branches sometimes arises from the upper bank, making identification of the V-planum difficult (Ono et al., 1990; Ide et al., 1996). Witelson suggested the "knife cut" technique for identifying the origin of the V-planum in these ambiguous cases (Witelson, 1982), but as the examples in Figures 3–7 demonstrate, it is no trivial matter to position the figurative knife.

B. Structure–Function Correlations

In a minority of cases, a second bulge appears in the planum immediately posterior to Heschl's gyrus giving rise to what appears to be multiple Heschl's gyri. When Heschl's gyrus splits, however, it is not referred to as multiple Heschl's gyri. The planum, not withstanding its name, has a very irregular surface. A major unanswered question is the relation of functional auditory areas to these bumps. Are multiple Heschl's gyri anatomical noise arising from mechanical distortion during development, or do they represent areas of extra growth or particular cytoarchitectonic or functional regions? Does the V-planum ascend in a superior direction simply because of pressure from parietal lobe structures, or is it a separate functional entity from the H-planum?

We have found that multiple Heschl's gyri are more frequent in families with genetic disorders (Leonard, Williams et al., 1993; Leonard, et al., 1995) and learning disabilities (Leonard, Voeller et al., 1993; Mercado et al., 1994). Risk factors are not associated with split Heschl's gyri or with bulges in other parts of the planum. The size and asymmetry of the H-planum, however, predict musical ability (Schlaug et al., 1995), handedness (Witelson & Kigar, 1992; Steinmetz, Volkmann, Jancke, & Freund, 1991; Foundas et al., 1995), language lateralization (Foundas et al., 1994), and phonemic awareness in early childhood (Leonard et al., 1996). In reports of symmetry in women, learning disability and schizophrenia are conflicting (Galaburda, 1989; Hynd & Semrud-Clikeman, 1989; Leonard, Voeller, et al., 1993; Schultz et al., 1994; Kulynych et al., 1994).

In Foundas' study, 11 patients with language localization limited to the left hemisphere had longer left plana. All 11 were dextral. The one patient with right hemisphere language was adextral and had a significantly longer *right* H-planum (reversed asymmetry). Two additional adextral Wada patients with right hemisphere language were measured. One had symmetrical plana (C. M. Leonard, unpublished data, 1994) and the other, reversed asymmetry (Gilmore, Childress, Leonard, Quisling, Roper, Eisenschenk, et al., 1995). Right hemisphere language and adextrality associated with reversed asymmetry has also been reported in a case study by Blonder, Pettigrew, and Smith (1994). These findings are important for two reasons. First, they provide evidence that structural lateralization is functionally significant. Second, they provide validation for treating the horizontal and vertical banks of the planum separately.

It is actually surprising how many studies have produced similar results, given the difficulty of identifying the boundary between the H- and V-planum. When the H-planum on the left ends in a clear bifurcation into ascending and descending rami, the posterior boundary is unambiguous (Figures 1(D), 3(A),(C), and (D), 5(D), and 6(G)). In this case, the ascending ramus or V-planum forms the core of the supramarginal gyrus (area 40), an structure implicated in praxis (Heilman & Gonzalez-Rothi, 1993). In contrast to the H-planum, the V-planum is generally shorter on the left than on the right (Steinmetz, Rademacher, Jancke, Huang, Thron, & Zilles, 1990; Witelson & Kigar, 1992; Leonard Voeller et al., 1993). This rightward asymmetry has led Witelson to propose that it is involved in visuospatial functions on the right. Due to the difficulty of separating H- and V-plana, some groups have included both structures in one measurement, with a resulting failure to find asymmetry (Loftus, Tramo, Thomas, Green, Nordgren, & Gazzaniga, 1993). Given the many relations between H-planar length and functional variables that have been described, this is probably not an optimal solution. It is to be hoped that functional imaging studies will provide some guidelines as to appropriate boundaries between fissure structures involved in language, and those involved in visuospatial function.

For the present, it is necessary to rely on local anatomical criteria. Rademacher (Rademacher, Galaburda, Kennedy, Filipek, & Caviness, 1992) has published a method for parcellating cortex based on Ono's comprehensive description of cerebral sulci (Ono et al., 1990). Although Ono and Rademacher have made valuable contributions, both studies depend on a small number of brains. We have found that the range of variability in sulcal anatomy is so large, and the number of subject variables that contribute to variation in sylvian fissure structure is so great, that the rules described by Rademacher are not always easy to follow. The cortex cannot be parcellated into standard divisions unless one can consistently recognize the landmarks used for the parcellation. We have found that the identification of standard landmarks, such as the termination of the sylvian fissure, is far from straightforward in many brains.

1. Classification of Sylvian Fissure Anatomy

The sylvian fissure is more likely to bifurcate in the left hemisphere than the right (Von Economo & Horn, 1930; Rubens, Mahwold, & Hutton, 1976). Steinmetz and colleagues performed the first classification study on MRI images (Steinmetz et al., 1990). They called the bifurcating fissure Type 1, and reported that the posterior ascending ramus (V-planum) was absent (Type 2), or ascended posteriorly to the supramarginal gyrus (Type 3), more frequently on the left than the right, while the ascending ramus ascended anteriorly to the supramarginal gyrus more frequently on the right (Type 4). Thus the horizontal branch of the fissure tended to extend too posteriorly on the left (Type 2–3), while it had a tendency to terminate too abruptly on the right (Type 4). Steinmetz and colleagues proposed that these hemispheric differences in fissure development were probably responsible for leftward asymmetry in the length of the planum. In these studies, no information was available on the handedness, sex, or psychological characteristics of the subjects.

At the same time, Witelson and Kigar were completing one of the few prospective postmortem studies ever performed. They analyzed 67 brains whose sex and handedness were known and reported findings consistent with those of Steinmetz. Their classification scheme differs somewhat, in that it focuses on the presence or absence of the H- and V-plana rather than

the relation of these structures to parietal lobe sulci. They found that the V-planum was more likely to be absent on the left (Type H) while the H-planum was more likely to be absent on the right (Type V). The proportions of H and V fissures found in this study are remarkably close to the proportions of Type 2–3 and Type 4 of Steinmetz. Witelson and Kigar found an interaction between sex and handedness. A majority of right-handed men had H fissures on the left, and a majority of nonright-handed men had Type V fissures on the right. Women had HV fissures, that is fissures with both H- and V-plana, regardless of handedness.

Ide and his colleagues have recently performed a study of 40 postmortem brains for whom sex but not handedness was known. They challenge the Steinmetz et al. (1990) and Witelson & Kigar (1992) view that the ascending ramus (V-planum) is absent on the left in 30% of cases. They maintain that the ramus is always present, but that it is angled anteriorly (inverted) and can be missed. They call Witelson's Type H Type I (for inverted), and find that females rather than males are more likely to have the inverted type. As described later, our data are compatible with all of the above schemes. In some of our cases, the sylvian fissure has no clear terminal branches (Type 2 or H); in others, an ascending ramus branches off considerably anteriorly to the termination (Type I). Although we do not yet have enough subjects matched on sex and handedness to make firm conclusions, our data at present suggest that female controls have Types H and I, while male patients have Type I. A very large sample of brains balanced for sex and handedness will be necessary to settle this issue.

C. Variation in Health and Disease: Pilot Data

As reported above, we have used the Steinmetz scheme in a number of published studies, where we found that anomalous (less frequent) fissure types are more frequent in populations with genetic mutations or family histories of learning disabilities, particularly in males. The relation of handedness to anomalies could not be determined in these previous studies because almost all subjects were right-handed. We did not find either the Steinmetz or the Witelson scheme a sensitive indicator of diagnosis as distinct from family history (Mercado et al., 1994; Leonard, Weintraub, et al., 1995). We have now identified a number of additional features that are sensitive to diagnosis using a more elaborate rating scheme (see Figure 10). The fissures are classified on each of eight sections 2 mm apart between Talairach 40 and 52 mm. The anomalies include absent H- and V-plana, extra gyri between the postcentral gyrus and supramarginal gyrus, the in-

Normal Fissure Features

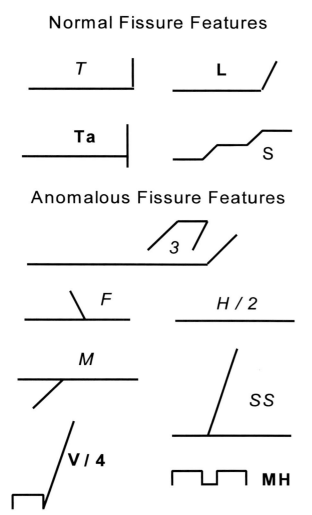

Anomalous Fissure Features

Figure 10 Schematic illustration of normal and anomalous fissure features. See text and Table 2 for explanation.

pects of sylvian fissure structure which are affected separately by sex, handedness, age, and diagnosis. The definitions for the fissure types are given in Table 2.

The main conclusions from this study were that: (1) the two hemispheres have different frequencies of fissure types; (2) no anomaly type is specific for diagnosis, sex, or handedness; (3) patients are more likely to have anomalies and more likely to have more than one anomaly, and (4) There may be developmental changes in the frequency of anomalies. We conclude that anomalous fissure types are evidence of genetic or developmental risk factors that increase the probability of a diagnosis. Since the same types of anomaly occur in schizophrenia, specific language impairment, and a variety of genetic diseases, specific fissure features are not predictive of a particular diagnosis. It is possible, however, that a common factor in many behavioral disorders is a compromised auditory processing ability, as Tallal has suggested for specific language impairment (Tallal et al., 1993). Phonemic awareness depends on sophisticated auditory processing, and many patients in our studies, regardless of diagnosis, are deficient in this ability.

Figures 11–14 give examples of normal and anomalous fissure features. Figure 11 shows a dramatic case of the S (step) type fissure on the left and right sides of an adextral adult. Figure 12 shows multiple Heschl's gyri in two children with specific language impairment. Figure 13 shows the only two individuals in the sample who had bilateral F-fissures. One was a boy with a severe word finding disorder that caused him to stutter, while the other was an adult man with schizophrenia. The child had multiple Heschl's gyri on the right, while the adult had multiple Heschl's bilaterally. Note the symmetry of the fissures in the adult with schizophrenia. It is possible that the absence of a substantial V-planum in either hemisphere was an additional risk factor for this disease.

In Figure 14, the brains of two additional patients with schizophrenia are shown. The patient depicted in (A) has an H and F on the left (absence of a clear V-planum or descending ramus), and a Heschl's sulcus that merges with the superior temporal sulcus, a feature that has not been found on the right in our sample. In Panel (B), the patient lacks an H-planum. It is this kind of multiple anomaly that we think increases the risk for schizophrenia. We presume that such multiple anomalies are an index of the severity of developmental alterations in neuronal migration or axonal pathfinding (Rakic, 1991). The patient in Panels (C) and (D) had an H and an F on the left, and a normal L type fissure on the right. This combination of fissure types was seen in several left-handed female controls,

verted ascending ramus of Ide (which we call a split-sensory strip), multiple Heschl's gyri, and a sylvian fissure that merges with the superior temporal sulcus.

This scheme has been used to classify 144 new scans, 111 controls (56 male and 55 female), 22 patients with schizophrenia (17 M, 5 F) and 11 children with specific language impairment (7 M, 4 F). Trained raters had 90% reliability on a subset of 50 of these scans. The controls were recruited to match the patient sample and represent a mix of university and nonuniversity personnel. The schizophrenic patients were diagnosed by two psychiatrists using published research criteria, while the children with language impairments were diagnosed by two speech pathologists on the basis of a battery of neurolinguistic tests. Figure 10 presents a schematic depiction of the 11 fissure features that are classified. Although this classification system is elaborate, the complexity is necessary to characterize as-

Table 2 Definition of Feature Types

Normal features	Definition
T (Rotated Letter T)	*The posterior horizontal ramus ends in a bifurcation into short and approximately equal posterior ascending (PAR) and posterior descending rami (PDR).*
L (Rotated letter L shape)	**The posterior horizontal ramus (main branch of the sylvian fissure) ends in a PAR. PDR minimal and appears more than 5 mm lateral to PAR.**
Ta (Nonbifurcating T)	PDR appears at least 4 mm long, but appears 5 or more mm laterally to origin of PAR.
S (Step)	The origin of the PAR is ambiguous because the posterior horizontal ramus consists of a series of right-angle steps and there is no clear PAR.

Anomalous Features: More common in groups with behavioral and genetic diagnoses	
Type 3 (PAR too posterior, Steinmetz et al., 1990)	*The posterior horizontal ramus continues posteriorly past the supramarginal gyrus (SMG). The PAR ascends posteriorly to the SMG.*
F (Flat)	*The posterior horizontal ramus continues >1 cm posteriorly past the origin of a "pseudo" posterior ascending ramus that enters the postcentral gyrus.*
H (Missing V-planum, Witelson and Kigar, 1992)	*No posterior ascending ramus (pseudo PAR is no longer than other branches of the upper bank of PHR, Steinmetz Type 2).*
M (Merge)	*The posterior horizontal ramus merges with the superior temporal sulcus (STS) anterior to or at Heschl's sulcus.*
SS (Split Sensory Gyrus)	*A sulcus descends through the postcentral gyrus and joins the posterior horizontal ramus. [Sometimes this sulcus can be confused with PAR (pseudo PAR).]*
V (Missing H-planum, Witelson)	**The PHR terminates caudal to Heschl's gyrus. The PDR is equivalent either to Heschl's sulcus or the sulcus defining the caudal border of the second Heschl's gyrus.**
MH (Multiple Heschl's gyri)	**A second gyrus appears directly posterior to Heschl's gyrus, just lateral to the insula.**

Notes: Each feature is counted as present or absent on a series of 8 serial sagittal images 2 mm apart between Talairach coordinates 40 and 54. Ratings can be performed either on films or digitized images on a computer. Features that are more frequent in the left hemisphere are in italics. Features that are more frequent in the right hemisphere are in bold.

but no male controls. This implies that women can tolerate more anomalous sylvian fissure structure than men. Men with these anomalies may have cognitive and learning problems, and therefore do not appear in our normal sample. There may be other brain regions which are more critical for normal female function. The female patients with schizophrenia had lower frequencies of anomalies than the men, although the sample is much too small to make much of this difference. It does suggest, however, that a search for other dysfunctional brain regions may prove fruitful in the female patients.

Now that functional MRI is becoming a more conventional technique, it is at last possible to describe the anatomy underlying functional activation—not in the language of cytoarchitectonics or Talairach, but in terms of macroscopic neuroanatomy. The results presented here suggest that it might be fruitful to treat cortical structure as an independent variable, and to choose subjects or patients with particular configurations of sulci for the investigation of particular cognitive functions or dysfunctions. This might be a strategy for reducing the individual variability that plagues so much human clinical research.

1. Implications for Development and Plasticity

A century of research suggests that sylvian fissure organization differs in the left and right hemispheres.

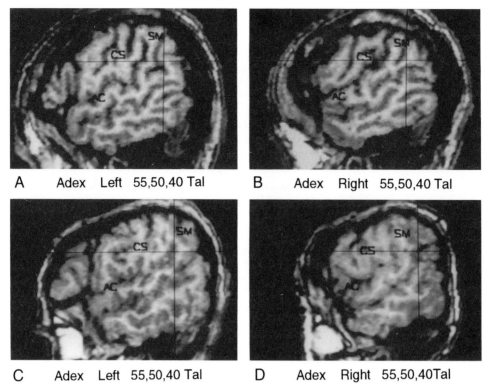

Figure 11   Normal and anomalous features in two left-handed male controls. (A),(B) Adult. High rating for feature S. (C) Child. Moderate ratings for features L and Ta. (D) Child. High rating for feature V. V-planum ascends directly posterior to Heschl's gyrus (unlabeled). AC: anterior commissure; CS: central sulcus; SM: supramarginal gyrus.

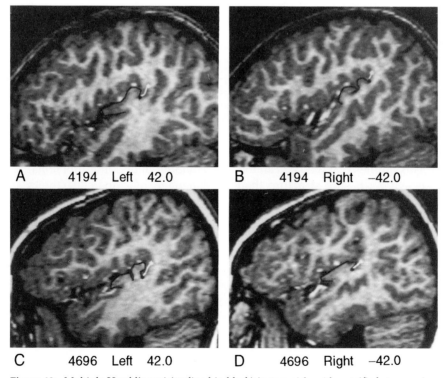

Figure 12   Multiple Heschl's gyri (outlined in black) in two girls with specific language impairment. H-planum is outlined in white.

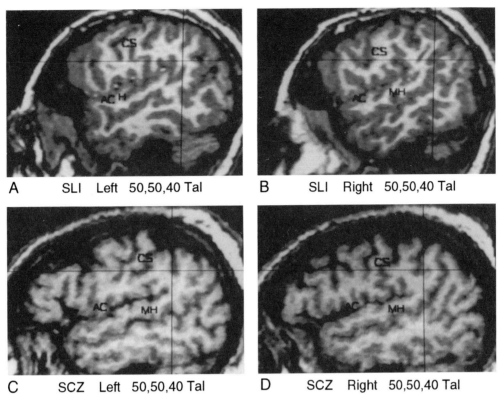

Figure 13 Examples of anomalous fissure features. (A) and (B) represent a 12 year old boy with specific language impairment (SLI). (A) Ambiguous V-planum, no descending ramus at posterior termination of sylvian fissure (near cross hairs). High rating for features F and MH, moderate rating for H. (B) Multiple Heschl's gyri (MH), no H-planum posterior to MH, no descending ramus, V-planum ascends just posteriorly to the central sulcus (CS). High ratings on features MH and V, moderate rating on F. This boy's fissures are asymmetrical, both in shape and in relation to Talairaich coordinates. It is also remarkable that pars triangularis is not visible on either side [compare with (C),(D), and Figures 5(A)–(D)]. This suggests that the frontal lobes are narrow for the width of the parietal lobes. (C) and (D) represent a 25 year old man with schizophrenia (SCZ). (C),(D) Multiple Heschl's gyri, ambiguous V-plana and no descending ramus in either hemisphere. High ratings on features MH and F. This man's fissures are remarkably symmetrical, both in shape and in relation to Talairach coordinates.

What role does development play in establishing or minimizing these differences? At what points do gender and handedness exert their influence? Is handedness a result or a cause? The developmental history of girls and boys may affect fissure development differently with important consequences for behavior. We speculate that the bilateral organization of female brains (Shaywitz, Shaywitz, Pugh, Constable, Skudlarski, Fulbright, et al., 1995) allows a shift in responsibilities from the left hemisphere and an escape from possibly detrimental effects of anomalous fissure patterns. Males with anomalous fissure patterns may be less able to shift cognitive functions to the right hemisphere (perhaps because the male right hemisphere is preoccupied with spatial functions). This lack of flexibility may explain why boys and men run a greater risk of diagnosis. These speculations arise out of longstanding theoretical arguments (Teuber, 1974; Satz & Whitaker, 1990; Kinsbourne, 1988). High resolution MRI has the potential to reveal the anatomical substrate for such theoretical concepts as "crowding," "sparing," and "transfer of function." Such studies may also help explain why some children with left hemisphere damage early in development are able to shift linguistic functions to the right hemisphere (Aram, 1988; Thal, Marchman, Stiles, Aram, Trauner, Nass, et al., 1991). Some anatomical patterns of sylvian fissure organization in the right hemisphere may be more conducive than others to accepting language functions. It is to be hoped that the institutes that funded the workshop on which this volume is based will be able to fund longitudinal developmental studies that can put these ideas to experimental test.

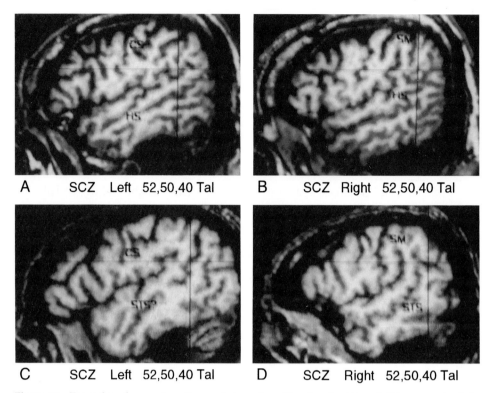

Figure 14 Examples of anomalous fissure features in schizophrenia. (A) and (B) represent a left-handed 55 year old man with schizophrenia. (A) The anterior segment of the superior temporal sulcus merges with Heschl's sulcus (HS), the V-planum is ambiguous, and there is no descending ramus. High ratings on features F, H, and M. In addition, the sylvian fissure is excessively long. (B) No H-planum, fissure is excessively short. High rating for feature V. (C) and (D) represent a 50 year old man with schizophrenia. (C) Anomalous sulcus entering Heschl's gyrus (not labeled), ambiguous V-planum, no descending ramus. High ratings on features H and F, moderate rating on feature M. AC: anterior commissure; CS: central sulcus; HS: Heschl's sulcus; SM: supramarginal gyrus; STS: superior temporal sulcus.

Acknowledgments

The work described in this chapter was supported in part by the March of Dimes Social and Behavioral Research Services Grant #93–551, the National Science Foundation, and a RAG grant from the Veterans Administration to John M. Kuldau. It is a pleasure to thank the colleagues, students, and research subjects who participated in these experiments, in particular, John M. Kuldau, Linda J. Lombardino, Anne L. Foundas, Janice C. Honeyman, Douglas Jones, Mary Ellen Bentham, Chrissy Meyer, Laurie R. Mercado, Mark Eckert, Lisa Rowe, Sean Robins, Erin Gautier, Sam Browd, Melissa Mahoney, Tim Lucas, and Ralph Rios.

References

Allison, T., Ginter, H., McCarthy, G., Nobre, A. P., A., Luby, M., & Spencer, D. (1994). Face recognition in human extrastriate cortex. *Journal of Neurophysiology, 71,* 821–825.

Allman, J. (1987). Maps in context: Some analogies between visual cortical and genetic maps. In L. Vaina (Ed.), *Matters of intelligence* (pp. 369–393). Dordrecht, The Netherlands: Reidel.

Allman, J., & Kaas, J. (1971). A representation of the visual field in the caudal third of the middle temporal gyrus of the owl monkey *(Aotus Trivirgatus). Brain Research, 31,* 85–101.

Andreason, N. A. (1994a). Interview. *Science, 266,* 275.

Andreason, N. A. (1994b). The neural mechanisms of mental phenomena. In N. A. Andreason (Ed.), *Schizophrenia, From Mind to Molecule* (pp. 49–92). Washington, DC: American Psychiatric Press.

Aram, D. (1988). Language sequelae of unilateral brain lesions in children. In F. Plum (Ed.), *Language, communication and the brain* (pp. 171–198). New York: Raven.

Barta, P., Pearlson, G., Powers, R., Richards, S., & Tune, L. (1990). Auditory hallucinations and smaller temporal gyral volume in schizophrenia. *American Journal of Psychiatry, 147,* 1457–1462.

Baylis, G., Rolls, E., & Leonard, C. (1985). Selectivity between faces in the responses of a population of neurons in the cortex of the superior temporal sulcus of the monkey. *Brain Research, 342,* 91–102.

Baylis, G., Rolls, E., & Leonard, C. (1987). Functional subdivisions of temporal lobe neocortex. *Journal of Neuroscience, 7,* 330–342.

Benasich, A., Spitz, R., & Tallal, P. (1995). Relationships among infant auditory temporal processing, perceptual cognitive abilities and early language development. *Cognitive Neuroscience Society Abstracts, 2,* 91.

Benes, F., Turtle, M., Khan, Y., & Farol, P. (1994). Myelination of a key relay zone in the hippocampal formation occurs in the human brain during childhood, adolescence, and adulthood. *Archives of General Psychiatry, 51,* 477–484.

Blonder, L., Pettigrew, C., & Smith, C. (1994). Anomalous cerebral dominance: Neurobehavioral studies and three-dimensional magnetic resonance imaging. *Neuropsychiatry, Neuropsychology, and Behavioral Neurology, 7,* 41–50.

Bogen, J. B., & Bogen, G. (1976). Wernicke's region—where is it? *Annals of the New York Academy of Sciences, 280,* 834–843.

Brauth, S. E., Hall, W. S., & Dooling, R. J. (1991). *Plasticity of development.* Cambridge, MA: Bradford–MIT.

Breier, J., Leonard, C., Bauer, R., Roper, S., & Gilmore, R. (1994). Quantified volumes of temporal lobe structures; seizure variables in patients with epilepsy. *Epilepsia, 35* (abstract).

Breier, J., Leonard, C., Bauer, R., Roper, S., & Gilmore, R. (1996). Quantified volumes of temporal lobe structures: Seizure variables in patients with epilepsy. *Journal of Neuroimaging.*

Briggs, G. N., & Nebes R. D. (1974). Patterns of hand preference in a student population. *Cortex, 11,* 230–238

Calvin, W., & Ojemann, G. (1994). *Conversations with Neil's brain: The neural nature of thought and language.* Reading, MA: Addison-Wesley.

Carman, G., Drury, H., & Van Essen, D. (1995). Computational methods for reconstruction and unfolding of the cerebral cortex. *Cerebral Cortex, 5,* 506–517.

Chi, J., Dooling, E., & Gilles, F. (1977). Left-right asymmetries of the temporal speech areas of the human fetus. *Archives of Neurology, 34,* 346–348.

Dale, A., & Sereno, M. (1993). Improved localization of cortical activity by combining MEG and EEG with MRI cortical surface reconstruction: A linear approach. *Journal of Cognitive Neuroscience, 5,* 162–176.

Evans, A.C., Marrett, S., Neelin, P., Collins, L., Worsley, K., Dai, W., Milot, S., Meyer, E., and Bub, D., (1992). Anatomical mapping of functional activation in stereotactic coordinate space. *Neuroimage, 1,* 43-53.

Filipek, P., Richelme, C., Kennedy, D., & Caviness, V. (1994). The young adult human brain: An MRI-based morphometric analysis. *Cerebral Cortex, 5,* 344–360.

Fletcher, L., Barsotti, J., & Hornak, J. (1993). A multispectral analysis of brain tissues. *Magnetic Resonance in Medicine, 29,* 623–630.

Foundas, A., Leonard, C. M., Gilmore, R., Fennell, E., & Heilman, K. (1994). Planum temporale asymmetry and language dominance. *Neuropsychologia, 32,* 1225–1231.

Foundas, A., Leonard, C. M., & Heilman, K. (1995). Morphological cerebral asymmetries and handedness; the pars triangularis and planum temporale. *Archives of Neurology, 52,* 501–508.

Fox, P., Perlmutter, J., & Raichle, M. (1985). A stereotactic method of anatomical localization for positron emission tomography. *Journal of Computer Assisted Tomography, 9*(1), 141–153.

Friston, K., Passingham, R., Nutt, J., Heather, J., Sawle, G., & Frakowiak, R. (1989). Localization in PET images: Direct fitting of the intercommissural (AC-PC) line. *Journal of Cerebral Blood Flow and Metabolism, 9,* 690–695.

Galaburda, A. M. (1989). Ordinary and extraordinary brain development: Anatomical variation in developmental dyslexia. *Annals of Dyslexia, 39,* 67–79.

Gazzaniga, M. (1995). *The cognitive neurosciences.* Cambridge, MA: MIT Press.

Geschwind, N., & Levitsky, W. (1968). Human brain: Left-right asymmetries in temporal speech region. *Science, 161,* 186–187.

Giedd, J., Castellanos, F., Casey, B., Kozuch, P., King, A., Hamburger, S. & Rapoport, J. (1994). Quantitative morphology of the corpus callosum in attention deficit hyperactivity disorder. *American Journal of Psychiatry, 151,* 665–669.

Giedd, J., Castellanos, F., Kozuch, P., Casey, B., Kaysen, D., Casey, B. J., Vaitusis, C. K., Vauss, Y. C., Hamburger, S., Kozuch, P., & Rapoport, J. L. (1996). Quantitative magnetic resonance imaging of human brain development: Ages 5–18. *Cerebral Cortex,* in press.

Gilmore, R., Childress, M., Leonard, C., Quisling, R., Roper, S., Eisenschenk, S., & Mahoney, M. (1995). Hippocampal volumetrics differentiates patients with temporal lobe epilepsy and extratemporal lobe epilepsy. *Archives of Neurology, 52,* 819–824.

Gurney, M., & Konishi, M. (1980). Hormone induced sexual differentiation of brain and behavior in zebra finches. *Science, 208,* 1380–1383.

Harris, G., Barta, P., Peng, L., Lee, S., Brettschneider, P., Shah, A., Hendered, J., Schlaepfer, T., & Pearlson, G. (1994). MR Volume segmentation of gray matter and white matter using manual thresholding; dependence on image brightness. *American Journal of Neuroradiology, 15,* 225–230.

Heilman, K., & Gonzalez-Rothi, L. (1993). Apraxia. In K. Heilman & E. Valenstein (Eds.), *Clinical neuropsychology, Third edition* (pp. 141–163). New York: Oxford Univ. Press.

Heilman, K., & Valenstein, E. (1993). *Clinical neuropsychology.* New York: Oxford Univ. Press.

Hynd, G. W., & Semrud-Clikeman, M. (1989). Dyslexia and brain morphology. *Psychological Bulletin, 106,* 447–482.

Ide, A., Rodriguez, E., Zaidel, E., & Aboitiz, F. (1996). Bifurcation patterns in the human sylvian fissure: Hemispheric and sex differences. *Cerebral Cortex, 6,* in press.

Jack, C., Sharbrough, F., & Twomey, C. (1990). Temporal lobe seizures: Lateralization with MR volume measurements of the hippocampal formation. *Radiology, 175,* 423–429.

Jernigan, T., Hesselink, J., Sowell, E., & Tallal, P. (1990). Cerebral morphology on MRI in language and learning-impaired children. *Archives of Neurology, 48,* 539–545.

Kimura, D. (1993). Sex differences in the brain. *Mind and brain* (pp. 78–89). New York: Freeman.

Kinsbourne, M. (1988). Sinistrality, brain organization, and cognitive deficits. In D. Molfese & S. Segalowitz (Eds.), *Brain lateralization in children: Developmental implications* (pp. 259–280). New York: Guildford.

Kulynych, J., Vladar, K., Jones, D., & Weinberger, D. (1994). Gender differences in the normal lateralization of the supratemporal cortex-MRI surface-rendering morphometry of Heschl's gyrus and the planum temporale. *Cerebral Cortex, 4,* 107–118.

Leonard, C. M., Martinez, P., Weintraub, B., & Hauser, P. (1995). Magnetic resonance imaging of cerebral anomalies in subjects with resistance to thyroid hormone. *American Journal of Medical Genetics, 60,* 238–243.

Leonard, C., Lombardino, L., Mercado, L., Browd, S., Breier, J., & Agee, O. (1996). Cortical asymmetry and cognitive development: A magnetic neuroimaging study. *Psychological Science, 7,* 89–95.

Leonard, C., Williams, C., Nicholls, R., Agee, O., Voeller, K., Honeyman, J., & Staab, E. (1993). Angelman and Prader–Willi syndrome. A magnetic resonance imaging study of differences in cerebral structure.. *American Journal of Medical Genetics, 46,* 26–33.

Leonard, C. M., Voeller, K. K., Lombardino, L., Morris, M. K., Alexander, A., Andersen, H., Garofalakis, M., Hynd, G., Honeyman, J., Mao, J., Agee, O., & Staab, E. (1993). Anomalous cerebral structure in dyslexia revealed with magnetic resonance imaging. *Archives of Neurology, 50,* 461–469.

Liegeois-Chauvel, C., Musolino, A., & Chavel, P. (1991). Localization of the primary auditory area in man. *Brain, 114,* 139–153.

Lindamood, C., & Lindamood, P. (1979). *Lindamood auditory conceptualization test.* Hingham MA: Teaching Resources.

Loftus, W., Tramo, M., Thomas, C., Green, R., Nordgren, R., & Gazzaniga, M. (1993). Three-dimensional quantitative analysis of hemispheric asymmetry in the human superior temporal region. *Cerebral Cortex, 3,* 348–355.

McCarthy, G., & Luby, M. (1994). Imaging the structural changes associated with human epilepsy. *Clinical Neuroscience, 2,* 82–88.

Mercado, L., Browd, S., Leonard, C., Lombardino, L. J., Voeller, K., Ross, J., Noffzinger, K., & Agee, O. (1994). Sylvian fissure anomalies in children with learning disabilities. *Society for Neuroscience Abstracts, 22,* 1481.

Merzenich, M., & Brugge, J. (1973). Representation of the cochlear partition of the superior temporal plane of the macaque monkey. *Brain Research, 50,* 275–276.

Morgan, A., & Hynd, G. (1996). Dyslexia, neurolinguistic ability, and anatomical variation of the planum temporale. *Brain Imaging and Behavior,* in press.

Musiek, F., & Reeves, A. (1990). Asymmetries of the auditory areas of the cerebrum. *Journal of the American Academy of Audiology, 1,* 240–245.

Newsome, W., Wurtz, R., Dursteler, M., & Mikami, A. (1985). Deficits in visual motion processing following ibotenic acid lesions of the middle temporal visual area of the macaque monkey. *Journal of Neuroscience, 5,* 825–840.

Nottebohm, F. F., Stokes, T. M., & Leonard, C. M. (1976). Central control of song in the canary. *Journal of Comparative Neurology, 165,* 457–486.

Ono, M., Jubik, S., & Abernathy, C. (1990). *Atlas of the Cerebral Sulci.* New York: Thieme.

Paxinos, G. (1990). *The human nervous system.* New York: Academic Press.

Pearlson, G., Garbacz, D. B., W. R., Ahn, H., & DePaulo, J. (1984). Lateral ventricular enlargement associated with persistent unemployment and negative symptoms in both schizophrenia and bipolar disorder. *Psychiatry Research, 12,* 1–19.

Penfield, W., & Roberts, L. (1959). *Speech and brain-mechanisms.* Princeton, NJ: Princeton Univ. Press.

Plante, E., & Turkestra, L. (1991). Sources of error in the quantitative analysis of mri scans. *Magnetic Resonance Imaging, 9,* 589–595.

Rademacher, J., Galaburda, A., Kennedy, D., Filipek, P., & Caviness, V. (1992). Human cerebral cortex: Localization, parcellation, and morphometry with magnetic resonance imaging. *Journal of Cognitive Neuroscience, 4,* 352–374.

Rakic, P. (1991). Plasticity of cortical development. In S. Brauth, W. Hall & R. Dooling (Eds.), *Plasticity of development* (pp. 127–161). Cambridge, MA: MIT Press.

Rauschecker, J., Tian, B., & Hauser, M. (1995). Processing of complex sounds in the macaque nonprimary auditory cortex. *Science, 268,* 111–114.

Recanzone, G., Schreiner, C., & Merzenich, M. (1993). Plasticity in the frequency representation of primary auditory cortex following discrimination training in adult owl monkeys. *Journal of Neuroscience, 13,* 87–103.

Rowe, L., Kuldau, J., Gautier, E., Lombardino, L., Kranzler, J., & Leonard, C. (1995). MRI of the corpus callosum: Measurement issues in children and schizophrenia. *Society for Neuroscience Abstracts, 23,* 439.

Rubens, A., Mahwold, M., & Hutton, J. (1976). Asymmetry of the lateral sylvian fissures in man. *Neurology, 26,* 620–624.

Satz, P. S., E., & Whitaker, H. (1990). The ontogeny of hemispheric specialization: Some old hypotheses revisited. *Brain and Language, 38,* 596–614.

Schlaug, G., Jancke, L., Huang, Y., & Steinmetz, H. (1995). In vivo evidence of structural brain asymmetry in musicians. *Science, 267,* 699–701.

Schultz, R., Cho, N., Staib, L., Kier, L., Fletcher, J., Shaywitz, S., Shankweiler, D., Katz, L., Gore, J., Duncan, J., & Shaywitz, B. (1994). Brain morphology in normal and dyslexic children: The influence of sex and age. *Annals of Neurology, 35,* 732–742.

Seldon, H. (1985). The anatomy of speech perception: Human auditory cortex. In A. Peters & E. Jones (Eds.), *Cerebral cortex* (pp. 273–327). New York: Plenum.

Sereno, M., Dale, A., Tootell, R., Reppas, J., Kwong, K., Belliveau, J., Brady, T., & Rosen, B. (1995). Human visual areas identified by visual field sign on the cortical surface using phase-encoded retinotopic stimulation. *Science, 268,* 889–993.

Shaywitz, B., Shaywitz, S., Pugh, K., Constable, R., Skudlarski, P., Fulbright, R., Bronen, R., Fletcher, J., Shankweiler, D., Katz, L., & Gore, J. (1995). Sex differences in the functional organization of the brain for language. *Nature (London), 373,* 607–609.

Shenton, M., Kikinis, R., Jolesz, F., Pollak, S., LeMay, M. Wible, C. G., Hokama, H., Martin, J., Metcalf, D., Coleman, M., & McCarley, R. (1992). Abnormalities of the left temporal lobe and thought disorder in schizophrenia; a quantitative magnetic resonance imaging study. *New England Journal of Medicine, 327,* 604–612.

Shepherd, G. (1994). *Neurobiology.* New York: Oxford Univ. Press.

Steinmetz, H., Ebeling, U., Huang, Y., & Kahn, R. (1990). Sulcus topography of the parietal opercular region; An anatomic and MR study. *Brain & Language, 38,* 414–433.

Steinmetz, H., Furst, G., & Freund, H. (1989). Cerebral localization: Application and validation of the proportional grid system in MR imaging. *Journal of Computer Assisted Tomography, 13,* 10–19.

Steinmetz, H., Jancke, L., Kleinschmidt, A., Schlaug, G., Volkmann, J., & Huang, Y. (1992). Sex but no hand difference in the isthmus of the corpus callosum. *Neurology, 42,* 749–752.

Steinmetz, H., Rademacher, J., Jancke, L., Huang, Y., Thron, A., & Zilles, K. (1990). Total surface of temporoparietal intrasylvian cortex: Diverging left-right asymmetries. *Brain & Language, 39,* 357–372.

Steinmetz, H., Volkmann, J., Jancke, L., & Freund, H. (1991). Anatomical left-right asymmetry of language related temporal cortex is different in left- and right-handers. *Annals of Neurology, 29,* 315–319.

Steinschneider, M., Schroeder, C., Arezzo, J., & Vaughan, H. J. (1993). Temporal encoding of phonetic features in auditory cortex. *Annals of the New York Academy of Sciences, 682,* 415–417.

Stensaas, S. (1974). The topography and variability of primary visual cortex in man. *Journal of Neurosurgery, 40,* 747–755.

Strauss, E., Gaddes, W., & Wada, J. (1987). Performance on a free-recall verbal dichotic listening task and cerebral dominance determined by the carotid amytal test. *Neuropsychologia, 25*(5), 747–753.

Talairach, J., & Tournoux, P. (1988). *Coplanar stereotaxic atlas of the human brain: Three-dimensional proportional system: An approach to cerebral imaging.* New York: Thieme.

Tallal, P., Miller, S., & Fitch, R. H. (1993). Temporal processing in the nervous system; implications for the development of phonological systems. *Annals of the New York Academy of Sciences, 682,* 27–47.

Tallal, P., Stark, R., & Mellits, D. (1985). Identification of language-impaired children on the basis of rapid perception and production skills. *Brain and Language, 25,* 314–322.

Teuber, H. (1974). Why two brains? In F. Schmidt & F. G. Wordern (Eds.), *The neurosciences: Third study program* (pp. 71–74). Cambridge, MA: MIT Press.

Thal, D., Marchman, V., Stiles, J., Aram, D., Trauner, D., Nass, R., & Bates, E. (1991). Early lexical development in children with focal brain injury. *Brain and Language, 40,* 491–527.

Tootell, R., Reppas, J., Dale, A., Look, R., Sereno, M., Brady, T., & Rosen, B. (1995). Functional MRI evidence for a visual motion aftereffect in human cortical area MT/V5. *Nature, 375,* 139–141.

Torres, I. (1995). Review of *Human behavior and the developing brain. American Journal of Psychiatry, 152,* 637–638.

Von Economo, C., & Horn, L. (1930). Gyral relief, size and cortical architectonics of the suprotemporal surface: Their individual and lateral differences. *Zeitschrift Geselschaft fur Neurologie und Psychiatrie, 130,* 687–757.

Wada, J., & Clarke, R. H., A. (1975). Cerebral hemispheric asymmetry in humans. *Archives of Neurology, 32,* 239–246.

Watson, C., Andermann, F., Gloor, P., Jones-Gotman, M., & Peters, T. (1992). Anatomic basis of amygdaloid and hippocampal volume measurement by magnetic resonance imaging. *Neurology, 42,* 1743–1750.

Wible, C., Shenton, M., Hokama, H., Kikinis, R., Jolesz, F., Metcalf, D. M., & McCarley, R. W. (1995). Prefrontal cortex and schizophrenia. *Archives of Psychiatry, 52,* 279–288.

Witelson, S. (1982). Bumps on the brain: Right–left asymmetries in temporal speech region. In S. Segalowitz (Ed.), *Language functions and brain organization* (pp. 117–144). Orlando, FL: Academic Press.

Witelson, S. (1989). Hand and sex differences in the isthmus and genu of the human corpus callosum. *Brain, 112,* 799–835.

Witelson, S., & Kigar, D. (1992). Sylvian fissure morphology and asymmetry in men and women: Bilateral differences in relation to handedness in men. *Journal of Comparative Neurology, 323,* 326–340.

Witelson, S., & Paillie, W. (1973). Left hemisphere specialization for language in the newborn: Neuroanatomical evidence of asymmetry. *Brain, 96,* 641–646.

Yousry, T., Schmid, U., Jassoy, A., Schmidt, D., Eisner, W., Reulen, H., Reiser, M., & Lissner, J. (1995). Topography of the cortical motor hand area: Prospective study with functional MR imaging and direct motor mapping at surgery. *Neuroradiology, 195,* 23–29.

Zipursky, R., Lim, K., Sullivan, E., Brown, B., & Pfefferbaum, A. (1992). Widespread cerebral gray matter volume deficits in schizophrenia. *Archives of General Psychiatry, 49,* 195–205.

IV

NEUROIMAGING DEVELOPMENT OF BRAIN–BEHAVIOR RELATIONSHIPS

16

Conceptual and Methodological Issues in the Interpretation of Brain–Behavior Relationships

F. Gonzalez-Lima* and A. R. McIntosh[†]

*Institute for Neuroscience and Department of Psychology, University of Texas, Austin, Texas 78712; and
[†]Rotman Research Institute of Baycrest Centre, University of Toronto, Toronto, Ontario M6A 2E1, Canada

I. Introduction

Brain imaging studies of learning and behavioral functions during the past decade have permitted the visualization of a whole brain at work during behavioral change (for recent review books see Gonzalez-Lima, Finkenstädt, & Scheich, 1992; Roland, 1993). These neuroimaging studies support a basic neurophysiological concept developed decades ago, based on electrophysiological analysis of behavioral change (John & Schwartz, 1978). This concept, as we define it, states that it takes multiple parallel neuroanatomical pathways acting together in the brain to achieve an observed behavioral change. The experimental origins of this basic concept may be traced back to the work of Franz (1912). But it was taken to an extreme position by Franz's student Lashley, (1950) with his equivocal principle of "equipotentiality." Lashley attempted to explain cortical lesion studies of learning by proposing that cortical regions are mostly equipotential for learning, in the sense that one region could usually compensate for the loss of another. This line of work has often been misquoted to an unfortunate extreme by suggesting that learning functions cannot be localized to specific brain regions and pathways (Weiskrantz, 1968). Our interpretation of behavioral change in terms of brain activity patterns is based on adaptive views of the brain, in which functional brain activity is viewed as dynamically related to the specific behavioral demands rather than a static property (Gonzalez-Lima, 1992; John & Schwartz, 1978; McIntosh & Gonzalez-Lima, 1994a, 1994b; Merzenich & Sameshima, 1993; Pascaul-Leone, Gaufman, & Hallett, 1992; Scheich, Simonis, Ohl, Thomas, & Tillen, 1992; Zohary, Celebrini, Britten, & Newsome, 1994; and others).

In this chapter, we review a new methodological approach combining behavior, functional neuroimaging, and neural network analysis within the conceptual framework that behavioral change is linked to how multiple brain regions interact in different behaviors (McIntosh & Gonzalez-Lima, 1994a). Based on this concept, the design of a functional neuroimaging experiment of behavioral change may take advantage of two conditions: (1) the ability to map distributed activity in the brain specifically linked to the behavioral change, and (2) the ability to analyze how the distributed patterns of brain activity are functionally integrated to bring about the behavioral change. We refer to the first kind of information as task-related regional variations (univariate increase or decrease) in neural activity. The second type is referred to as task-related interregional covariations (multivariate covariance) in brain activity (McIntosh & Gonzalez-Lima, 1994b). The first kind of information is related to the distributed nature of brain functioning, where multiple neural regions participate in any particular behavioral task (Gonzalez-Lima, 1989). The second kind of information is related to the

DEVELOPMENTAL NEUROIMAGING

basic principle of neural interactions that allows the brain to act together to mediate a behavioral change (Gonzalez-Lima & McIntosh, 1994).

In order to relate a behavioral change with brain functioning, the behavioral paradigm must first be able to differentiate task-related variations in brain activity in individual regions. Such variations must be task-specific and reflect the relevant variable responsible for the behavioral change. For example, in a learning study where a sound is paired with a reward, the sound becomes a meaningful signal that elicits a behavioral change, such as a conditioned response. The relevant variable for behavioral change in this example is the learned relationship between the sound and the subsequent reward. Therefore, the neuroimaging study must be based on a comparison of tasks with identical number and kind of stimuli (i.e., sounds and rewards), and differing only on the relevant learned relation between the sounds and rewards. Unless this requirement is met, it is not possible to unequivocally interpret any variation in regional activity in the brain as specifically correlated with the relevant variable (e.g., auditory learning) responsible for the behavioral change.

The second condition is linked to the realization that behavioral change is brought about by the integrative action of multiple regions in the brain. Thus, for the analysis of functional brain imaging data, it is an advantage to examine task-related covariations in the activities of multiple brain regions. The alternative view of expecting only one or a few brain regions to be exclusively responsible for a behavioral change is based on an equivocal interpretation of brain functioning, namely the view of the brain as a collection of somewhat independent "organs"—each one with a specialized cognitive function. One among many examples of this view may be the extreme "localizationist" position that the hippocampus or the medial temporal lobe is the site for a particular type of memory function in the brain (Squire, Knowlton, & Musen, 1993). On the contrary, brain operations mediating behavioral change rely on the intercommunications between distributed regions in the brain that operate like functional networks in any given task, as will be explained here (see also reviews by Gonzalez-Lima & McIntosh, 1994; McIntosh & Gonzalez-Lima, 1994b).

It follows from the foregoing conceptual framework that if behavioral change is an emergent (i.e., system-level) property of interacting brain regions, understanding it using neuroimaging requires a functional network analysis of the patterns of interactions between multiple regional activations in the brain. The experimental designs, analytical approach, and theoretical interpretations proposed in this chapter are not in agreement with lesion-based "localizationist" views of behavioral change, as restricted to a local activity change limited to "higher order" regions or some specialized neuroanatomical system responsible for behavioral change. Examples from our neuroimaging studies of auditory learning will be used to illustrate how brain activity linked to behavioral change follows two basic principles of brain functioning: (1) the spatial segregation of stimulus–response information in distributed regions of the brain (i.e., topographic representational maps); and (2) the integration of spatially-segregated information into functional networks that are task-specific, but that may participate in multiple brain functions when their interactions change (i.e., computational network maps). The terms "brain functioning" and "behavioral change" are meant to emphasize our concern, not so much for "cognitive operations" that try to explain "the mind," but for understanding integrative patterns of brain activity that can be observed with modern functional imaging techniques. These patterns may provide insights into the neurophysiological substrates of information processing underlying the modification of behavior in humans as well as other mammals.

II. Experimental Designs to Relate Behavioral Changes with Brain Activity

Brain activity is modified depending on the requirements for behavioral change in any given experimental design. Neural activity correlates of behavioral change can be analyzed designing neuroimaging experiments in which associative and nonassociative behavioral effects of stimuli can be separated. Below we provide specific examples of within- and between-subject designs from our work with fluorodeoxyglucose (FDG) autoradiography in rats (see Gonzalez-Lima & McIntosh, 1994; McIntosh & Gonzalez-Lima, 1994b, for reviews).

A. Within-Subjects Designs

An obvious approach is the use of repeated measures of the same subject using different testing conditions or activation paradigms. This approach is commonly used in positron emission tomography (PET) studies and referred to as the "subtraction" method. This method relies on the assumption that the subtraction between the levels of activation produced by a less-demanding control task and a more complex experimental task reflects brain activity specifically involved in the experimental task. But, whether or not the sequence of behavioral tasks reflects some monotonic increase in complexity and corresponding brain activations is a difficult issue that has not been adequately addressed in most imaging studies.

The goal of our within-subjects designs is to use the neural principle of topographic representational maps to visualize the behavioral effects of stimuli in terms of changes in brain activity patterns. A key concept here is that of *feature maps versus meaning maps* (Scheich et al., 1992). In brief, the hypothesis tested is that a conditioned stimulus (CS) leading to a given behavioral change has acquired a specific *meaning* to the subject, and that this acquired meaning is represented by neural maps in a manner analogous to other physical *features* of the stimulus. Neuroimaging techniques are ideally suited to reveal the spatial maps of brain activity that represent the specific attributes of a given stimulus. In the case of signal learning, such as in studies of habituation (Gonzalez-Lima, Finkenstädt, & Ewert, 1989a, 1989b), sensitization, and conditioning (Gonzalez-Lima, 1989 for review), our brain imaging studies suggest a model of learning involving the interactions between the neural maps that represent the stimulus attributes, that is, learning as interacting maps of attributes. These stimulus attributes include both physical features and behavioral meaning (Gonzalez-Lima, 1992).

In the case of FDG autoradiographic studies in animals, a repeated measures design is not possible because the animals are killed to obtain the autoradiographs. However, it is possible to take advantage of the segregated topographic representation of stimuli in the brain to develop a within-subjects design. For example, the differential conditioning paradigm implemented by Gonzalez-Lima and Agudo (1990) takes advantage of the tonotopic representation of sounds of different frequencies in different (spatially-segregated) locations of auditory system structures. This organizing principle of segregated representations of sensory information in the auditory system has been demonstrated in neuroimaging studies with animals using 2-deoxyglucose (2DG) autoradiography (Ryan, Zabrina, Nigel, & Keithley, 1988), and in humans using PET (Lauter, Herscovitch, Formby, & Raichle, 1985).

An emphasis in our research has been to use within-subjects designs to overcome intersubject variability in neuroimaging measures and to eliminate any need for absolute measures, avoiding in this manner any issues surrounding calculation of absolute units. For example, a within-subjects design was implemented to study the neural correlates of sounds that were reinforced or nonreinforced using a differential conditioning paradigm with two tones (Gonzalez-Lima & Agudo, 1990). Since tones of different frequencies activate separate regions of auditory structures (tonotopic mapping), it becomes possible to compare differential

neural activities produced by the associative (reinforced versus nonreinforced) effects of high and low frequency tones within tonotopically organized regions of the same subject (Gonzalez-Lima, 1992).

Gonzalez-Lima and Agudo (1990) trained rats with two sounds used as CSs. Presentation of these CSs to untrained rats produced two discrete tonotopic regions of activation corresponding to the representation of low and high sound frequency (Hz), as shown in *Figure 1*, with dorsal and ventral bands of activation in the inferior colliculus. In a trained group of animals, the low frequency sound was always reinforced with the aversive unconditioned stimulus (US), making this sound a CS^+ (reinforced CS). In contrast, the high frequency sound was randomly or explicitly nonreinforced, making this sound a CS^- (nonreinforced CS). In another group of trained rats, the reverse was done, so that the high sound was the CS^+ and the low sound the CS^-. This counterbalanced design was used to determine if the neural representational maps of the same sounds changed as a function of US reinforcement. That is, each tonotopically organized neural region can be used as its own control to compare the CS^+ versus CS^- effects of the same physical stimuli. This design allowed the demonstration of differences in FDG uptake within the same structure of the same subjects as a function of CS^+ or CS^- training of the sound. A ratio of functional activation such as FDG uptake of CS^+/CS^- can be measured for each subject. This can be used for a direct neuroimaging comparison of activational differences in the representation of sounds based on their learned behavioral significance. Within-subjects ratios of FDG uptake changes in the differentially conditioned rats showed that the individual ratio of CS^+/CS^- labeling was greater than the corresponding CS^-/CS^+ ratio. In the inferior colliculus, the mean uptake ratios demonstrated significantly larger metabolic activity of 17% for the dorsal band and 18% for the ventral band when tones served as CS^+ during training. The perimeter of the band of FDG uptake was also significantly greater when the tone was paired with the US. The mean perimeter of the dorsal band when reinforced (CS^+) was 35% greater than when not reinforced (CS^-). The ventral band showed a 24% increase when reinforced as compared to when not reinforced.

Besides subjects with paired CS and US, four other control groups of rats were examined in terms of FDG uptake. It was found that progressively larger FDG uptake values in the inferior colliculus were produced as expected, that is increasing as a function of CS presentation in untrained as compared to unstimulated rats, followed by unpaired and paired CS–US groups. However, differential effects between the two tones

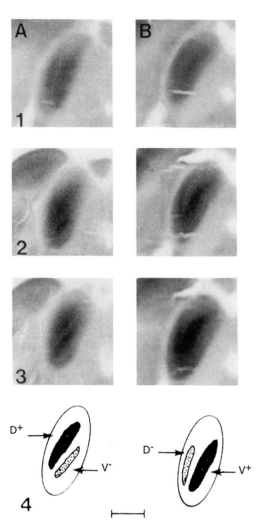

Figure 1 Effects of differential conditioning on FDG uptake in the rat left inferior colliculus. (A) Effect of low tone (D$^+$ band) paired with aversive reinforcer and high tone (V$^-$ band) unpaired. (B) Effect of high tone (V$^+$ band) paired with aversive reinforcer and low tone unpaired (D$^-$ band). The tonotopic bands of the reinforced tone (+) were always greater than the unreinforced tone (−), independent of whether the reinforced tone was the low or the high tone. Rows 1–3 are autoradiographs at anterior, middle, and posterior levels of the inferior colliculus where individual comparisons were made in each image. These levels corresponded to the central nucleus of the inferior colliculus, as no separated bands could be discriminated in more anterior and posterior ends. Row 4 is a highly schematic diagram of the differential effects between the dorsal (D) and ventral (V) tonotopic bands as a function of paired (+) and unpaired (−) differential conditioning of the tones. Bar = 2 mm. (From Gonzalez-Lima & Agudo, 1990. Reprinted with permission.)

in each subject were found only with pairing. This provided a rather clear dissociation between reinforced and nonreinforced sound effects. The differential metabolic responses depended on the learned reinforcing value of the sound as opposed to its purely sensory effects.

These findings in the inferior colliculus, differentiating the CS$^+$ versus CS$^-$ spatial patterns of activation of the same stimuli, provided for the first time a direct (within–structure) anatomical comparison of the modification of the functional maps that represent a sensory stimulus as a result of associative learning. This neuroimaging demonstration contributed to a new perspective in the field of neural substrates of learning, pioneered by numerous electrophysiological studies of behavior-dependent changes in the brain's responses to sensory stimuli (for a review see Weinberger, 1995). These findings support a concept of *sensory learning* that postulates a functional reorganization of sensory maps in the brain depending on the acquired behavioral significance of stimuli (Gonzalez-Lima & Agudo, 1990; Gonzalez-Lima, 1992). Therefore, in the design and interpretation of studies involving behavioral change, it should be considered that learning and related behavioral changes are not simply a function of some specialized "higher order" cerebral structures such as neocortex or hippocampus. Learning effects responsible for behavioral change affect regions of the brain traditionally viewed as devoted to sensory processing.

B. Between-Subjects Designs

It is also possible to implement valid between-subjects designs, if adequate attention is given to the issue of control groups in such a way as to account for the variables present in each task. For example, in neuroimaging studies of Pavlovian conditioning involving a CS and a US, it is fundamental to have controls exposed to the same kind and amount of CS and US present in the conditioning group (Gonzalez-Lima & Scheich, 1984a, 1984b, 1986a, 1986b).

The goal of our between-subjects designs is to use groups with the same kind and number of stimuli, differing only on the learned relationship between the stimuli. A key concept here is that of *low versus high joint probability* of events happening together (Rescorla, 1968). Brain activity differences between the effects of the same stimuli in the groups are interpreted as resulting from the predictive informational relation between events. This is the key associative variable represented by the differences in brain activity between otherwise comparable presentations of the same stimuli in the control groups (Gonzalez-Lima, 1992).

Therefore, between-subjects control procedures should be designed to separate associative from nonassociative effects in conditioning studies. Rescorla (1968, 1988) has proposed that for conditioning studies aimed at determining the associative effects of a CS, the CS should not be explicitly unpaired with the US;

rather the CS and the US should be presented randomly or pseudorandomly in such a way that the CS has a low probability of predicting US onset. In practice, a pseudorandom control is normally used, rather than a truly random control, because most studies give a limited number of CS and US presentations. This pseudo-randomly unpaired condition may be more preferable as an associative control than an explicitly unpaired condition, because the pseudorandom CS has a low predictive value of the US, whereas the explicitly unpaired CS reliably predicts the absence of the US. The adopted convention is to regard events with a joint probability of less than .05 as occurring at random, and not reflecting a significant associative value, as compared with events that always occur jointly in the case of CS–US pairing. Conversely, explicitly unpaired events that always occur separately should be regarded as leading to associative negative correlations between CS and US. This constitutes a form of inhibitory conditioning, as opposed to simply the failure to learn a positive relation (see Miller & Spear, 1985, for a review).

Both conditioned and random groups should involve an identical number of the same stimuli, with the only difference being the joint probability of the CS–US, that is, the predictive informational relation as the key associative component of conditioning (Rescorla, 1988). To compare conditioning groups with other groups without the same kind and number of stimuli presented during testing (as has been done in some studies of brain metabolic activity) is inadequate to separate associative learning effects from nonassociative effects of the stimuli. Such conditioning studies cannot be regarded as adequate studies of learning functions because they cannot provide any information on the specific associative learning effects involved in a given conditioning paradigm. For example, a study by Bryan and Lehman (1988) using ^{14}C-glucose does not incorporate any unpaired control groups (whether explicitly or randomly unpaired) to compare with the conditioned rats. Instead conditioned (CS–US) and unconditioned animals (without US), in different contexts during the ^{14}C-glucose administration session are compared. It is impossible from such a design to separate any associative learning effects due to conditioning, because none of the control groups can be equated in terms of history of stimulus presentations with the conditioned rats. Thus, the general nonspecific decrease in metabolic activity found in all the structures investigated in one of their groups cannot possibly be interpreted in terms of associative conditioning effects. Associative effects leading to a CR can only be isolated in relation to a control condition showing no CRs and containing all other elements of the conditioning procedure, with

the exception of the temporal pairing between CS and US. The between-subjects interpretation of associative effects is relative to the comparison between a paired CS–US conditioning group with an adequate unpaired CS–US control group that involved the same kind and number of stimuli used in the conditioning group. Without such a relative control comparison, it is meaningless to refer to an *absolute* associative effect on brain activity.

Gonzalez-Lima and Scheich (1984a, 1984b, 1986a, 1986b) investigated various aspects of associative learning in the auditory system using a between-groups classical conditioning paradigm. This approach allows the study of the interaction of two stimuli in paired and unpaired presentations. Therefore, the learned behavioral meaning of a stimulus (CS) can be discriminated from its physical parameters. Arousal-related versus learning-related processes can also be discriminated by the use of sensitization groups receiving the same amount of stimulation but not developing conditioned responses to the CS.

Electrophysiological studies of unit activity during learning indicate that auditory responses of awake, behaving animals to acoustic stimuli are dependent not only on the physical properties of a stimulus, but also on its learned significance (Birt & Olds, 1982; Weinberger & Diamond, 1987). Therefore, the FDG method was used to analyze the effects of an aversive learning experience on the response of the auditory system to an acoustic stimulus. The experiment involved freely behaving rats in a Pavlovian conditioning paradigm in which a sound CS (4–5 kHz frequency modulated tone) was temporally paired with aversive reticular stimulation (US). The unconditioned response (UCR) was a rapid decrease in heart rate evoked by the US. The conditioned response (CR) was a bradycardiac response (criterion: 1 beat/s reduction of heart rate) following onset of the sound CS. Eight groups of rats were subjected to: (1) the tone CS without conditioning, (2) the aversive US alone, (3) the paired CS–US (acquisition), (4) the tone CS after conditioning (extinction), (5) the US prior to the CS (sensitization), (6) the unpaired CS–US (pseudoconditioning), (7) the CS after pseudoconditioning, and (8) no stimulation (Gonzalez-Lima & Scheich, 1984a, 1984b, 1986a, 1986b).

One major finding was the differential effect produced by the same tone before (Fig. 2, Row 1) and after (Fig. 2, Row 4) conditioning. The results also showed that reticular mechanisms interact with incoming acoustic stimuli and modulate the response of auditory structures (Fig. 2; compare Row 1 with the sound alone with Rows 5 and 6 with the sound plus reticular stimulation). Within each auditory structure, from cochlear nucleus to auditory cortex, the regions of

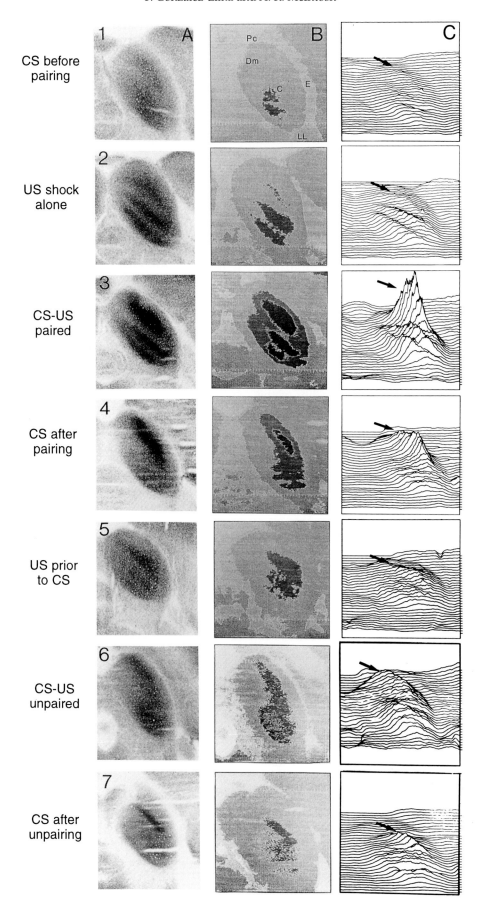

overlap of the spatial representations of CS and US developed an enhanced metabolic response during conditioning (Fig. 2; indicated by arrow in Row 3). The learned motivational value of the tone CS was represented in its tonotopically defined neuronal maps throughout the auditory pathway. These FDG studies provided the first anatomical demonstration of the effects of sensitization and learning on a sensory system (Gonzalez-Lima & Scheich, 1984a, 1984b). These observations support the concept that auditory responses are dependent both on the *physical* and the *behavioral* parameters of a stimulus (Weinberger, 1995).

The FDG findings in the auditory system also supported the concept that associative learning represents a *distributed property* of neuronal maps, which may be demonstrated in any structure which meets the appropriate requirements of time and space convergence of CS and US inputs (Gonzalez-Lima, 1989). The question remained of how classical conditioning would modify neural activity in nonauditory forebrain structures. This question is particularly relevant in view of the extensive literature available on the role of some cortical and limbic structures in mammalian learning (Rosenzweig & Bennett, 1976). In an attempt to answer this question, the uptake of FDG during and after auditory Pavlovian conditioning was examined in all telencephalic and diencephalic structures of the rat brain (Gonzalez-Lima & Scheich, 1986b).

The most important outcome of this study was the identification of forebrain structures which showed significant metabolic changes during conditioning, namely prefrontal cortex, posterior parietal cortex, medial thalamus, lateral habenula, caudal striatum, and hippocampal formation. The prefrontal cortex showed discrete regions with enhanced FDG uptake during conditioning and pseudoconditioning. The medial thalamus was greatly activated in all groups subjected to reticular stimulation. The dorsomedial nucleus showed its largest activation during conditioning. The caudal portion of the caudate-putamen and the fundus

striati, corresponding to a projection field from the medial geniculate, showed an overall increase in FDG uptake during conditioning. A columnar organization was well-defined in the posterior parietal cortex of rats subjected to CS–US pairing. Significant FDG changes in parietal cortex and lateral habenula were found mainly in the right hemisphere. These changes, revealed by FDG, were the first demonstration of forebrain structures with localized metabolic alterations related to learning and reticular sensitization.

It is likely that nonsensory structures metabolically activated by presentation of a CS after Pavlovian conditioning form part of a distributed neural system involved in the memory representation of that particular CS in mammalian brains. The idea of a distributed representation is further substantiated by the FDG study of John, Tang, Brill, Young, and Ono, (1986). They showed that all the nonauditory structures activated during and after Pavlovian conditioning in our experiments were involved also in a visually guided task performed by operantly conditioned split-brain cats. However, they found a considerably larger number of structures involved in operant performance of a runaway task for food reward than we found using a simple classical conditioning of heart rate. Our combined results of FDG studies of auditory conditioning (Gonzalez-Lima & Scheich, 1984a, 1984b, 1985, 1986a, 1986b; McIntosh & Gonzalez-Lima, 1994a, 1994b) support the concept that sensory learning resulting from Pavlovian conditioning constitutes an anatomically *distributed property* of neuronal maps. This property is functionally represented in the brain throughout the specific sensory maps of the stimuli used as CS, as well as in integrative structures outside of the conventional sensory systems. Relevant discrete regions with high metabolic activity during classical conditioning are part of association cortex, thalamus, striatum, and limbic structures. These structures may be part of systems serving various different functions involved in classical conditioning.

Figure 2 Incorporation of FDG in the right inferior colliculus of rats from groups 1–7 of Gonzalez-Lima and Scheich (1984b). The effects of the stimulus regimes are compared in three ways. (A) FDG autoradiographs from comparable anteroposterior locations. (B) Computer-generated densitometric plots of the autoradiographs divided into five relative intensity classes; the boundary of each class division is indicated by a contour line of white dots. (C) Densitometric profiles corresponding to the same areas shown in Column B. The 4–5 kHz FM tones produced a light band of high FDG in the dorsal region of the central nucleus (Row 1, see arrow). Reticular stimulation produced three bands of high FDG uptake (Row 2). The paired CS–US produced an increase in the three bands of high FDG uptake evoked by the US alone, with a very clear selective enhancement of the dorsal region (Row 3). The tone CS presented alone after training produced a large increase in FDG uptake in the dorsal region (Row 4). The region of highest FDG uptake corresponded to the site of overlap between the independent effects of the CS and US (see arrows). Presentation of the tone immediately after reticular stimulation resulted in a selective (dorsal band) as well as a general increase in labeling (Row 5); note that the three-band pattern of reticular activation is not well defined in Row 5. Note the smaller changes in FDG uptake produced by the CS–US unpaired (Row 6) and after unpairing (Row 7). Pc: paracentral cortex; E: external nucleus; C: central nucleus; Dm: dorsomedial division of C; LL: lateral lemniscus. (From Gonzalez-Lima and Scheich, 1984. Reprinted with permission.)

C. Optimization of Parameters

The first successful neuroimaging studies of classical conditioning (Gonzalez-Lima & Scheich, 1984a, 1984b, 1986a, 1986b) and of behavioral habituation (Gonzalez-Lima et al., 1989a, 1989b) revealed that the parameters that produced the best learning curves were not the most suitable for our functional imaging methods. One way we verified this issue was by replicating behavioral paradigms using optimal behavioral acquisition parameters in conjunction with the FDG method. For example, a one minute intertrial interval was used in conditioning studies with FDG, and basically no reliable effects were obtained. Other experimenters have similarly followed optimal behavioral parameters and also followed the 2DG method for calculation of glucose utilization rates as developed by Sokoloff, Reivich, Kennedy, Des Rosiers, Patlak, Pettigrew, et al. (1977).

From these early experiments it became apparent that some compromises were needed on the behavioral parameters, as well as on the imaging parameters, to obtain the best results. On the behavioral side, a larger number of stimulus presentations was better suited to activate neural systems. We have also used, in the case of auditory stimuli, frequency-modulated (FM) sounds as short sweeps (e.g., upward linear sweeps of 500 msec each, between 4–5 kHz, for several seconds). Instead, the behavioral literature is dominated by the use of pure tones. But, in fact, in nature there are no such things as pure tones in an animal's environment. It is not surprising then that periodic sweeps of FM tones produce better 2DG and FDG labeling than pure tones in forebrain auditory structures (Scheich & Bonke, 1981; Gonzalez-Lima & Scheich, 1986a), because one would expect a larger number of neurons responding to FM tones. To avoid acoustic startle and cardiovascular effects produced by loud stimuli, the intensity of the sound was 60–65 dB in our imaging studies. To minimize any effect of head orientation on sound intensity, whole field sound stimulation was always delivered in a sound-attenuated chamber. While it is important to drive neural activity using FM tones, this kind of activation is specific to the sound stimulus. In contrast, loud stimuli (80 dB and over), as used in most of the behavioral literature, lead to nonspecific changes in neural activity that detract from the sound being a "neutral" stimulus (i.e., without behavioral effects) and from the specificity of the neural activation evoked.

Many behavioral neuroscientists have neglected the use of FDG and other imaging techniques, claiming that they are not sensitive enough to visualize behavioral changes. One of the reasons for this misconception has been because they have not optimized the behavioral parameters for the particular imaging technique. Our work shows that it is quite feasible to visualize behavioral changes in terms of brain activity patterns if one is willing to follow the behavioral parameters and conditions that will optimize the probability of obtaining a positive finding.

On the imaging side, it is important to acknowledge that behavioral effects are not strong as compared to other conditions (e.g., drug-induced or disease states). If subjects are not in the appropriate context, the behavioral value of the stimulus may not be clearly separated as a large signal in the imaging data. It must be absolutely clear for the experimenter that the goals of brain imaging studies of behavioral change are different from those for measuring cerebral metabolic rates. In the case of FDG studies of learning, the goal is to detect a change in a quantitative functional index of brain activity related to behavioral change; that is, to obtain evidence for the involvement of a brain structure in a learning paradigm relative to its activity in a control condition that differs only on the learned relation between the stimuli present. Isolating the biochemical metabolic processes used for quantifying the neural functional change related to learning is not, therefore, central to the goal of these experiments. For example, if blood flow and glucose metabolism both contribute to the functional change produced by learning in a brain region, determining the relative contribution of these metabolic processes is not a goal of these experiments. However, if isolation of blood flow versus glucose utilization rates is of interest, then the reader is referred to the methods described by Sokoloff et al. (1977). Our goals are to visualize neural activity changes related specifically to a learning condition, and not isolating the underlying metabolic processes. Similarly, since a goal of FDG autoradiography is to map activity changes at the regional and system levels, a good resolution is needed, but cellular resolution is not required for this analysis. However, if cellular resolution is of interest then the reader is referred to the methods of Duncan (1992).

Imaging neural activity linked to behavioral change with FDG autoradiography involves the administration of a suitable glucose analog; its transport and uptake by blood flow and brain cells; the adequate stimulation of the brain to produce a detectable activity change; the cumulative trapping of the tracer in brain tissue during the postinjection stimulation period; the postmortem preservation of a diffusible tracer during tissue processing; the autoradiographic visualization of tissue tracer concentrations into detectable labeling; and imaging procedures to prepare the film for data analysis. When appropriate care is given to the contribution of these various factors, FDG autoradiography can become a convenient technique that can be used alone or in combination with other metabolic and histologic procedures, for mapping functional neural pathways modified by a wide variety of behavioral conditions in intact, behaving animals.

In order to achieve the full potential of FDG mapping, it is imperative to consider the specific aims in each stage of an experiment. First, attention must be given to the mode of FDG administration so that the sensitive uptake period is extended beyond the first 15 minutes usually obtained by single bolus intravenous (iv) injections. Second, it is desirable to obtain maximum uptake by increasing the number of stimulus presentations to detect learning-related changes in evoked activity. Third, it is necessary to choose a postinjection survival period that allows sufficient time for FDG uptake and subsequent accumulation in responsive regions. Fourth, cryosectioning must provide adequate section thickness to maximize the amount of radioactive tracer in the tissue without excessive loss of morphological detail. Fifth, autoradiographic procedures should provide a high level of resolution, sensitivity, and specificity for the tracer. Finally, the subsequent procedures in preparing the film for image analysis should preserve the location and regional uptake patterns of the tracer. Therefore, the selection of glucose analog, mode of administration, stimuli presentations, postinjection survival time, cryosectioning procedures, autoradiographic methods, and densitometric procedures influence the success of experiments where FDG or 2DG are used to map functional neural pathways. While each of these components may be changed by the experimenter, overlooking their contributions may lead to inaccurate examinations of neural systems related to behavioral change (Gonzalez-Lima, 1992).

For example, the mode of administration of the tracer is relevant for the success of FDG and 2DG studies of behavioral change. Glucose analogs can be effectively administered via iv, intraperitoneal (ip), subcutaneous (sc), or intramuscular (im) injections based on observations with rodents, primates, cats, amphibians, reptiles, and birds (Gonzalez-Lima et al., 1992). Results using iv or ip injections in rodents are indistinguishable in the labeling of control brains. However, during acquisition or extinction phases of learning paradigms, the ip injected rats show more well-defined changes. This important difference, in the case of learning studies, may be due presumably to the more gradual ip absorption of FDG throughout training trials, as opposed to a single bolus injected iv that results in rapid absorption reflecting mainly the initial portion of the training session. Also, the cumulative effects of

repeated learning trials are shortened to a narrower sensitive period following an iv bolus. In our experience, this is a clear disadvantage when FDG is administered during learning paradigms, because optimal effects are always obtained with more repeated trials that enhance cumulative evoked effects. Furthermore, the point is not whether surgically implanted animals can be freely moving with chronic iv catheters as modified for the 2DG method (Room, Tielemans, De Boer, Tonnaer, Wester, Van den Broek et al., 1989). Rather, it is that an ip injection is preferred to any iv injection (single bolus or slow infusion) for learning studies with FDG, because intact animals without catheters and prior surgical experiences can be used with the ip approach.

Since our goal for FDG autoradiography is to visualize functional changes in brain activity related to behavioral change, rather than to determine rates of glucose utilization, arterial blood sampling throughout the experiment is not needed to measure plasma radioactivity and glucose concentrations. These parameters are needed for the operational equations used to calculate rates per minute of glucose utilization, but they are not required to perform a quantitative autoradiographic evaluation of FDG uptake in brain regions during learning in order to determine functional alterations. A major argument for measuring arterial glucose levels in the 2DG method is that the operational equation of Sokoloff et al. (1977) suggests that brain concentrations of unphosphorylated 2DG vary with changes in plasma glucose concentration. However, overnight fasting and subsequent bleeding for monitoring the levels of plasma glucose appear of no utility in the particular case of FDG autoradiography in normal conscious rats, such as those involved in learning paradigms. Hargreaves, Planas, Cremer, and Cunningham, (1986) found that cerebral regional rates of glucose influx are maintained at similar levels in normal conscious rats, despite almost twofold differences in plasma glucose concentration between rats fed or fasted overnight. Rates of brain glucose phosphorylation were also similar in these two groups, despite wide variations in plasma glucose levels. Repeated withdrawals of arterial blood are not insignificant physiological events for animals such as rats during learning studies. According to Sokoloff, Kennedy, and Smith (1989), "Unless attention is paid to limiting the amount of blood removed in the course of sampling and clearing the dead space, shock can readily be induced in small animals" (p. 167). In the FDG method, we avoid the blood sampling throughout the postinjection survival period and thereby avoid its associated distress to the animal during the critical period for testing the learning effects. Since no surgery or bleeding are involved, intact, undisturbed animals can be used.

D. Developmental Issues

In infant subjects, other factors must be considered for the success of imaging neural activity linked to behavioral change. For example, in developing brains and young subjects it is even more likely that the dynamic regulation of representational maps in sensory systems plays a greater role in behavioral modification (for review see Kossut, 1992). However, immature brains offer a unique opportunity that is not available with adult brains. This is the possibility to assess noninvasively the question of *essential* neural circuitry for particular forms of behavioral change. Immature animals have limited learning capabilities at different ages. One age group may not be capable of succeeding in a learning or memory task, while the same task may be accomplished in older animals (Amsel, 1986, for review).

For example, since rats quickly acquire new learning capabilities as they mature, we could monitor brain activities at various days after birth. These days will correspond to developmental stages characterized by progressively more sophisticated memory capabilities. Specific brain activity changes linked to the various learning and memory capabilities may provide an exciting new approach to map brain–behavior relationships in intact subjects. This could be done to answer the question of *essential* brain systems for a particular behavioral change without the use of invasive methods, such as lesions, to ascertain whether some brain regions are necessary for a given behavioral task.

In infant rats, the period of most rapid brain growth is between 5 to 7 days postnatally (Dobbing & Sands, 1979). The types of learning capabilities seen in infant rats also develop relatively early after birth. For example, habituation to tactile stimulation eliciting limb withdrawal is seen in 3-day-old pups (Campbell & Stehouwer, 1979). Afterwards, only small differences in the speed and size of the habituation response occur between 3 to 15 days postnatally (Campbell & Stehouwer, 1979). Pavlovian conditioning of odor conditioned stimuli paired with aversive (lithium poisoning) unconditioned stimuli is seen in 2-day-old pups (Rudy and Cheatle, 1979). Taste aversion conditioning has been observed in rats by 5 days of age (Rudy & Cheatle, 1979). However, learning tasks such as patterned alternation, that impose a progressive increase in working memory span, can be documented to develop progressively as the rat matures (Green & Stanton, 1989). For example, Amsel and collaborators (Diaz-Granados, Greene, & Amsel, 1992) have used

patterned single alternation (PSA) with milk reward to train pups to run alleys. Learning is expressed as running speed on rewarded trials as compared to slow responding on nonrewarded trials. For PSA learning, the rewarded and nonrewarded trials are alternated. The pattern of high running speed to rewarded trials (but not to nonrewarded trials) is based on the memory of the outcome of the previous trial during the alternation sequence. The memory span can be assessed by progressively increasing the time between trials. Rats of 11 days of age learn PSA when the intertrial interval is 8 sec, but not 30 sec. Rats of 14 days learn PSA with 30 sec intervals, but not with 60 sec, while 17-day-old rats learn PSA with 60 sec intervals (Diaz-Granados et al., 1992). Therefore, the brain activity patterns of rats of different ages can be compared to ascertain the changes linked to the progressive memory span capabilities during the same PSA learning task.

Given the foregoing development of behavioral capabilities in infant rats, it is also likely that the same brain regions may have different functional contributions at different ages resulting from the maturation of connections. As will be explained below, functional connectivity is a key concept to interpret how neural network interactions organize behavioral changes.

III. Neural Network Interactions in the Neuroimaging of Brain–Behavior Relationships

The concept that brain connectivity influences brain functioning guided the development of our structural modeling approach to quantify functional interactions mediated by specific neural connections (McIntosh and Gonzalez-Lima, 1991, 1992a, 1992b, 1993, 1994a, 1994b). In developing our approach, we have kept in mind a basic neurophysiological principle of neural interactions. It states that if neural regions are synaptically connected, the disturbance in the postsynaptic action potentials of a region is passed on to another. That is, brain regions do not merely act locally, they interact with one another in complex neural networks. Hence, brain activity is interdependent on the actions and reactions of the components that form the neural networks. We can now monitor the operations of many neural regions simultaneously using brain imaging methods. The modeling technique presented here, and similar analyses of network interactions, may help us to understand the combined actions of these neural regions and how this activity is related to behavior.

The investigation of network interactions in brain studies may be traced back to the Gerstein, Perkel, and Subramanian (1978) analysis of multiunit electrical recordings and the Gevins, Doyle, Cutillo, Schaffer, Tannehill, and Bressler (1985) analysis of electroencephalographic waves. The first applications of covariance analysis to brain imaging data were reported in Clark, Kessler, Buchsbaum, Margolin, and Holcomb (1984), Horwitz, Duara, and Rapoport (1984), and Metter, Riege, Kuhl, and Phelps (1984). They demonstrated the importance of functional interactions in neural systems by the use of interregional Pearson product–moment correlation coefficients to quantify metabolic mapping data. This method of covariance analysis has provided a major advance in the effort to determine which brain regions are functionally associated with one another during a particular experimental condition. However, when one wants to examine interactions in a multistructure system, interpretations based on pairwise correlations can become complicated. Other approaches that can provide information about neural system interactions are the various multivariate techniques such as discriminant analysis, factor analysis, principal components analysis, and canonical correlation. Some of these techniques have been applied successfully to PET metabolic data from humans (Clark, Ammann, Martin, Ty, & Hayden, 1991; Friston, Frith, Liddle, & Frackowiak, 1993; Friston, 1994), and optical recordings from cortex (Shoham, Ullman, & Grinvald, 1991). One commonality between these techniques is the assumption that brain regions that function together have correlated activities (Horwitz, Soncrant, & Haxby, 1992). These techniques determine patterns of regional interrelations independent of influences mediated by specific neuroanatomical pathways. However, brain functions related to learning and behavioral changes are likely to be highly dependent on the specific connectivity between brain regions (Gonzalez-Lima, 1989, 1992; McIntosh and Gonzalez-Lima, 1994a, 1994b).

A. Structural Equation Modeling

We have shown (McIntosh and Gonzalez-Lima, 1991, 1992a, 1992b, 1993, 1994a, 1994b) how covariance structural equation modeling (Bentler, 1985; Berry, 1984; Bollen, 1989; Davis, 1985; Hayduk, 1987; Jöreskog and Sörbom, 1989; Loehlin, 1987; Long, 1983) (also known as path analysis) could be used to quantify simultaneously the interactions between interconnected brain regions. When applied to neural systems, structural equation modeling uses information about the anatomical pathways and the correlation coefficients between brain regions to determine the functional pathways in a given experiment. Structural modeling uses algorithms that attempt to account for an observed pattern of correlations based on the causal

structure of a system defined by the neuroanatomical connections. The models use interregional correlations of activity to quantify the pairwise pattern of interactions that take place between brain regions.

The application of structural equation modeling to neural data uses the basic assumption that the observed pattern of correlations between brain regions is due, at least in part, to either common influences to both regions or direct anatomical connections between them. By combining the correlations between brain regions and their anatomical connections (causal order), parameters are estimated for all influences in the system. This structural equation modeling application is a logical extension of the interregional correlational approach, since the solutions for the models are derived from correlation coefficients. It adds to the analysis of imaging data, in that instead of looking at regions that are functionally associated in a pairwise manner, the models can demonstrate how specific pathways in entire neural systems interact in different experimental paradigms. Our structural modeling approach has also been recently applied to PET studies of human brain function (McIntosh, Grady, Ungerleider, Haxby, Rapoport, & Horwitz, 1994) and dysfunction (Grafton, Sutton, Couldwell, Lew, & Waters, 1994).

With the increasing application of covariance-based analyses, new terminology has also been introduced. It is useful to clarify these terms and define their relation to the terms we use to describe neural structural equation models. The term *functional connections (connectivity)* refers to the correlations of activity between neural elements in both electrophysiology (Aertsen, Gerstein, Habib, & Palm, 1989) and brain imaging (Friston et al., 1993). To say that two neural elements (neurons or brain regions) have a functional connection is to say that these elements show statistically significant correlated activity without reference to how that correlation is mediated. *Effective connectivity* is a logical progression from functional connectivity, and can be defined as the influence or effect one neural element has on another (Aertsen et al., 1989; Friston et al., 1993). The term *functional network* has been applied to the pattern of covariances among evoked potential sites (Gevins and Cutillo, 1993), but could also be applied to a pattern of covariances obtained through other measures of neural activity. For our application of structural equation modeling to neural systems, we have applied the terms *anatomical* model and *functional* model (McIntosh and Gonzalez-Lima, 1993; McIntosh et al., 1994). The *anatomical model* represents the neuroanatomical connections between brain regions used in the structural equation models. The interregional correlations of activity are used to assign numerical weights to the connections in the anatomical model, leading to the functional model. A *functional model* represents the influences of regions within the model on each other through the anatomical connections. The functional model is closer to the notion of effective connectivity, since it depicts the influence of one region on another. The difference, as will be illustrated below, is that the influences in the functional model are depicted as direct and indirect effects through the anatomical model. Effective connections are not expressed in this manner.

Figure 3 illustrates the basic features of structural equation models. The system, made up of four variables, has a causal structure indicated by the arrows [Fig. 3(A)]. The regions and connections define the *anatomical model* (McIntosh & Gonzalez-Lima, 1993; McIntosh et al., 1994). By using this anatomical model, the correlation matrix [i.e., standardized covariances, Fig. 3(B)] can be decomposed to assign functional weights or *path coefficients*—given by letters v–z—to each of the arrows. The addition of the path coefficients defines the *functional model* (McIntosh and Gonzalez-Lima, 1993; McIntosh et al., 1994). The path equations [Fig. 3(C)] and structural equations [Fig. 3(D)] are mathematically equivalent, but the structural

equations provide a more computationally efficient method to solve for the path coefficients.

Therefore, in our application of structural modeling to study brain–behavior relationships, the analysis began by construction of an *anatomical* model linking the regions of interest through their known anatomical connections. Then, *functional* models for the various groups were constructed using structural equation modeling. In the models, activity correlations were decomposed to calculate numerical weights, or path coefficients, for each anatomical path. These path coefficients were then used to compare the network interactions for the different group models. Therefore, the application of structural modeling to analyze functional interactions in the brain involves five major steps: (1) construction of the anatomical model or path diagram of the neural system; (2) computation of the correlation matrix of activity between the relevant regions that form the model; (3) creation of the structural equations for the system to express mathematically the variance in activity in each region, as a function of the variance of other brain regions and some residual influence; (4) solving the equations in the model to find optimal solutions for path coefficients and residuals in agreement with the observed correlations matrix of activity; and (5) statistical evaluation of the various functional models to determine significant differences due to group treatments.

These steps have been explained in detail in a paper (McIntosh & Gonzalez-Lima, 1994b) where we presented the general application of structural equation modeling to brain imaging, providing the methodological background needed for a better understanding of the present section. In the next section, we review a specific application of structural equation modeling to functional brain data from Pavlovian conditioning experiments.

B. Network Analysis of Pavlovian Conditioning

Gonzalez-Lima and Scheich (1984a, 1984b, 1986a, 1986b) provided the initial visualization of the anatomically distributed activity changes in Pavlovian conditioning using a brain-imaging approach. Other metabolic mapping techniques applied to the study of Pavlovian conditioning also have revealed multiple regions with activity changes (Trusk & Stein, 1988). Similarly, operant conditioning studies using FDG in rats (Hock & Scheich, 1986) and cats (John et al., 1986), or using 2DG in monkeys, (Friedman & Goldman-Rakic, 1988; Matsunami, Kawashima, & Satake, 1989) have also revealed activity changes widely distributed in the brain. This distributed change is comparable with

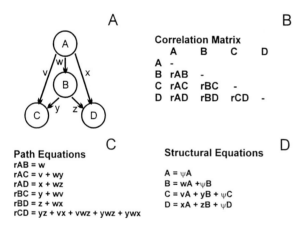

Figure 3 Schematic representation of methods involved in structural equation modeling of a neural system. (A) Path diagram of a simple network with four brain regions (A, B, C, D) and their anatomical connections (indicated by arrows). (B) The information about the correlations of activities between regions is used in conjunction with the path diagram (A) to calculate the strength of influences through the connections, known as the path coefficients (*v, w, x, y, z*). (C) Path equations show how the correlations between regions can be decomposed to solve for the path coefficients. (D) Structural equations show the variance in activity in each region as a function of the weighted variance of other brain regions and a residual influence (indicated by ψ). These residuals are not shown in A and C for simplicity. (From "Structural equation modeling and its application to network analysis in functional brain imaging," A R. McIntosh & F. Gonzalez-Lima, *Human Brain Mapping,* Copyright ©1994 Wiley-Liss, Inc., a subsidiary of Wiley & Sons, Inc.)

prior electrophysiological evidence of distributed learning mechanisms (John & Schwartz, 1978). However, it became apparent that if learning is an emergent property of distributed brain activity, it cannot be fully understood by considering the component parts of the brain individually. Here we review how structural equation modeling may be applied in the study of distributed neuroanatomical networks. The examples used are from animal learning experiments with rats, but the guiding principles and the specific approach presented also apply to the study of neural network interactions in the central nervous systems of humans and other mammals. The focus is on what is gained from application of the structural modeling approach to the understanding of brain–behavior relationships.

Network analysis is illustrated here with the results of a conditioning study whose objective was to examine how opposite learned behavioral responses to the same physical sound were differentiated by the pattern of interactions between extraauditory regions of the rat brain (McIntosh & Gonzalez-Lima, 1994a). This study examined the extraauditory network interactions that reflected the differential associative properties of the same physical tone using the Pavlovian-conditioned inhibition paradigm (LoLordo & Fairless, 1985). Conditioned excitation entails presenting two stimuli with one stimulus (A^+, the conditioned excitor) always paired with another stimulus (reinforcer). The A^+ then predicts the occurrence of the reinforcer, or US. Conditioned inhibition differs in that the stimulus (X^-, the conditioned inhibitor) predicts the absence of reinforcement. There are numerous methods to achieve conditioned inhibition, and the present study used a procedure where X^- was trained by compound presentation with A^+ (Pavlovian-conditioned inhibition, A^+/AX^-). This associative paradigm involves contrasting A^+ trials with trials where stimuli A and X are presented together as a compound that signals the absence of reinforcement. This results in stimulus X acquiring the behavioral properties of a conditioned inhibitor. The same physical tone was trained as a conditioned excitor (A^+) for one group and a conditioned inhibitor (X^-) for another, using a footshock as the unconditioned stimulus (US).

In previous applications of structural equation modeling, a system of interest was defined before analysis [e.g., auditory (McIntosh & Gonzalez-Lima, 1991, 1993)] and visual (McIntosh & Gonzalez-Lima, 1992a)]. For the present study, it was not possible to predict accurately which neural system(s) would be involved in this form of conditioning. Therefore, the neural systems were defined by the data and were constructed based on regions showing significant differences between groups in both univariate and multi-variate statistical examinations. This approach took full advantage of the FDG mapping technique by using objective criteria to select brain areas that were part of a functional network (McIntosh et al., 1994). In essence, this allowed the brain to indicate which neural systems distinguish a tone with different acquired behavioral meaning.

Regional differences in FDG uptake were found in the sulcal frontal cortex (SFC), lateral septum (LS), medial septum–diagonal band (MS–DB), retrosplenial cortex (RS), and dentate-interpositus nuclei of the cerebellum (DEN). Discriminant analysis selected three other regions that significantly discriminated the tone excitor and inhibitor groups: perirhinal cortex (PRh), nucleus accumbens (ACB), and the anteroventral nucleus of the thalamus (AVN).

The final anatomical model consisted of the seven areas presented in Figure 4. The basal forebrain regions were organized in a circuit based on reciprocal anatomic connections between the MS–DB and LS (Luiten, Kuipers, & Schitumaker, 1992), because there does appear to be strong connections between the LS and the vertical diagonal band (Witter, Daelmans, Jorritsma-Byham, Staiger, & Wouterlook, 1992). Reciprocal connections between the MS–DB and ACB also were included (Phillipson & Griffiths, 1985; Powell & Leman, 1976). A unidirectional anatomic connection was placed between the LS and ACB (Phillipson & Griffiths, 1985). Anatomical projections from the MS–DB to the limbic cortical areas PRh and RS were included (Deacon, Eichenbaum, Rosenberg, & Eckmann, 1983). The two limbic cortical regions were also part of an anatomic circuit with the AVN, with a reciprocal connection between the AVN and RS (Domesick, 1972; Sripanidkulchai & Wyss, 1986). Finally, both the RS and PRh received input from the SFC (Deacon et al., 1983). This arrangement allowed for the evaluation of the models in terms of two anatomically defined circuits. One was a basal forebrain circuit containing the two septal regions and ACB. The second was a limbic thalamocortical circuit composed of SFC, RS, PRh, and AVN. The two circuits interacted via the projections from the basal forebrain to the limbic thalamocortical circuit.

Figure 4 presents the functional network models for the effects transmitted through direct anatomic connections. Significant differences in path coefficients between the models for the tone excitor group versus the tone inhibitor group were observed within both the basal forebrain and limbic thalamocortical circuit, and in the connections between circuits.

Most differences between tone excitor and inhibitor models within the two forebrain circuits were in the sign rather than the magnitude of the path coefficients.

Direct Effects
Conditioned Excitor Model

Direct Effects
Conditioned Inhibitor Model

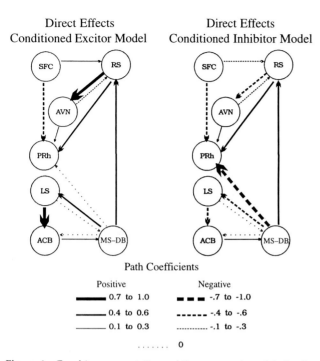

Path Coefficients

Positive		Negative	
━━━	0.7 to 1.0	▬ ▬ ▬	-.7 to -1.0
────	0.4 to 0.6	- - - -	-.4 to -.6
────	0.1 to 0.3	··········	-.1 to -.3
	·······	0	

Figure 4 Graphic representations of the structural models for the basal forebrain and limbic thalamocortical circuits for conditioned excitor and conditioned inhibitor groups. Values represented here are the direct effects of each structure upon all regions that it is anatomically connected to. The magnitude of the direct effect is proportional to arrow width for each path. Values for the width gradient are given in the legend at the bottom of the figure. Positive path coefficients are shown as solid arrows, whereas negative ones are shown as segmented arrows. RS: restrosplenial cortex; AVN: anteroventral nucleus of the thalamus; PRh: perirhinal cortex; MS–DB: medial septum–vertical diagonal band; ACB: nucleus accumbens; SFC: sulcal frontal cortex; LS: lateral septal nucleus. (Adapted from McIntosh & Gonzalez-Lima, *Journal of Neurophysiology,* 1994a. Reprinted with permission.)

In the basal forebrain circuit for the tone excitor model, the effects were transmitted through positive covariance relationships in the model. The main difference in the tone inhibitor model was a change in those relationships to negative. Although there was also a decrease in magnitude in the LS–ACB path, the primary difference between models was in the sign of the effects. A similar sign change was present in the limbic thalamocortical circuit between the RS and AVN, and the SFC and RS, implying a qualitative shift within the circuit. The qualitative change in the interactions among basal forebrain regions may reflect processes distinguishing the opposite affective significance of the conditioned tone.

The neural processes encoding the affective component of the CS in the basal forebrain circuit may have interacted with the limbic circuit by the projections of the MS–DB. The increase in the strength of the

MS–DB–PRh path, a quantitative change, may imply that one site of convergence for information about affective and associative components of the CS was in the limbic cortical circuit through the PRh. In differential conditioning, the PRh was identified as an area that was commonly activated in both paired and explicitly unpaired conditioning, compared to random controls (Gonzalez-Lima, 1992). On the basis of lesion studies, others have suggested that the PRh provides the most important contribution to some memory tasks (Zola-Morgan, Squire, Amaral, & Suzuki, 1989) and is a key structure in the circuit involved in fear-potentiated startle (Rosen, Hitchcock, Miserendino, Falls, Campeau, & Davis, 1992). The models extend these observations to show the functional involvement of the PRh in a larger circuit, involved in coding associative information and receiving convergent affective information from the basal forebrain.

In some cases, the pattern of differences in the path coefficients was consistent with the differences in mean FDG uptake between the two groups. The path coefficient for the corticocortical SFC–RS link differed between models as did mean FDG activity in these regions. The two septal nuclei also demonstrated this relationship, showing both a difference in the path coefficient representing the MS–DB–LS connection and in mean FDG activity. There were path coefficients that differed between models, but where FDG activity did not differ in connected regions (AVN, PRh). This is not an inconsistency, as it is entirely possible for two regions to show changes in covariance without a marked change in regional activity, and it emphasizes the need to examine both mean activity levels and covariances to fully assess brain functioning linked to behavioral changes (Horwitz et al., 1992). Indeed, an electrophysiological study suggests that learning-related plasticity first involves a change in the covariances between neural elements, which then leads to a change in regional activity (Ahissar, Vaadia, Ahissar, Bergman, Arieli, & Abeles, 1992).

IV. Summary and Conclusions

Several of our neuroimaging studies with FDG and auditory learning paradigms served to illustrate that the analysis of brain functions linked to behavioral changes can be guided by the concepts of distributed maps and network interactions in the brain. Distributed maps point to the importance of determining the functional variations in multiple regions of the brain. Network interactions emphasize the necessity of putting together numerous variables of regional activation by determining the covariations in interregional activities. These concepts are fundamental for the interpretation of brain–behavior linkages, because multiple parallel neural systems act together in the brain to achieve an observed behavioral change. Nevertheless, most traditional concepts in behavioral neuroscience, and recently in cognitive neuroscience, are based mainly on evidence obtained concerning the role a particular structure plays in a particular behavior.

For example, research on memory has differentiated between those memory processes that are "hippocampal dependent" and "hippocampal independent" (Squire et al., 1993). These theories incorporate data from animal lesion studies, human clinical studies, and studies that monitor regional activity during tasks of interest (e.g., electrophysiology). On the other hand, if the covariance among neural elements is critical to brain operation, the role of any given region in a particular behavior must be viewed in the context of its interactions with other regions. Network analytic approaches have supported the idea that brain function involves the cooperative interaction among many neural regions, and though it may be that a particular area is critical for a certain function, the performance of any task is a result of the functional interactions of many distributed neural regions (John and Schwartz, 1978; Gonzalez-Lima, 1992; McIntosh & Gonzalez-Lima, 1993).

The study of neural interactions will be important for relating cognitive theories with brain operations. It is highly unlikely that the functional organization of the brain follows the independent modular organization of psychological constructs. Therefore, it is also unlikely that a single brain region has only one cognitive function. Instead, functionally specialized anatomical networks within the brain may be more easily related to cognitive constructs. There may not be a single brain area that represents "attention" for instance, but there are more likely numerous brain areas whose interactions represent attention operations. The important point is that it may be possible for parts of the same anatomical network to be involved in another function when the interactions change. For example, numerous behavioral brain studies have suggested that primary auditory areas show activity related both to the perceptual components of a stimulus and its learned behavioral relevance (Gonzalez-Lima, 1992; McIntosh and Gonzalez-Lima, 1993; Recanzone, Schreiner, & Merzenich, 1992; Scheich et al., 1992; Weinberger, 1995). Thus, the same anatomical network can code, in parallel, the perceptual and behavioral properties of stimuli, depending on the nature of the interactions between the parts of the net-

work. The hippocampus has a role in declarative memory processes (Squire et al., 1993), but its activity has also been related to voluntary motor behavior and sensory processing in high states of arousal (Sainsbury, Heyden, & Montoya, 1987), habituation or motivation (Jarrard, 1993), and conflicting dispositions to approach and avoid (Amsel, 1993). These examples suggest that different brain areas can play important roles in multiple functions beyond their classical distinctions, and this may be a general property of the central nervous system, rather than specific to only a few brain regions.

In the case of the differential conditioning study with two tones serving as CS^+ and CS^- (Gonzalez-Lima & Agudo, 1990), FDG neuroimaging revealed that this form of Pavlovian discrimination learning involves multiple parallel neural pathways acting together in the intact brain to mediate the observed behavioral change. As in the case of long-term habituation (Gonzalez-Lima et al., 1989a, 1989b) the rat brain appears to use a combined strategy to shape behavior. This strategy uses many major functional anatomical systems with associative changes capable of producing a differential conditioned response to the reinforced tone and no response to the nonreinforced tone. The overall brain strategy is similar to the one used for long-term habituation in the sense that multiple pathways are engaged. However, the specific structures and functional changes involved in these general systems are clearly unique for these two forms of learning (Gonzalez-Lima, 1992).

In the case of the same tone conditioned as a Pavlovian excitor or inhibitor (McIntosh & Gonzalez-Lima, 1993, 1994a), the brain's operations that differentiated the behavioral significance of a tone stimulus involved both a change in regional activity and in the interactions of auditory and extraauditory regions. It is concluded that associative learning is an emergent property of distributed neural activity and network interactions. Furthermore this property can be investigated using structural equation modeling to combine information about regional activity, interregional covariance relationships, and anatomic connectivity.

The concept that learning can involve changes in multiple dimensions has been in the behavioral and physiological literature for some time (e.g., Hebb, 1955) and has seen some revival in more contemporary theories of learning (Konorski, 1967; Wagner & Brandon, 1989). Brain imaging with FDG has supported this concept by showing learning-related changes in many neural systems, which presumably reflect different dimensions of the behavioral task. For example, changes related to processing and identification of an acoustic CS have been shown in many levels of the auditory system (Gonzalez-Lima and Scheich 1984a, 1984b, 1986a), whereas activity related to affect coding and associative processing may be related to the basal forebrain or midline thalamus and limbic structures, respectively (Gonzalez-Lima & Scheich, 1986b).

Structural equation modeling, with multivariate statistics, adds another dimension to brain imaging data by uncovering areas forming functional neural circuits and quantifying the interactions within and between these circuits. This combined approach yields a great deal of information about how the brain operates as a unit to modulate behavior based on the requirements of the learning paradigm. Rather than asking the question of whether or not a single brain area is essential for learning, with the use of structural equation modeling and brain mapping techniques like FDG, neuroscientists may investigate the neural systems involved in different learning tasks and examine how the interactions within and between neural systems reflect these learning-related changes.

Together, our auditory learning experiments support the general conclusion that behavioral changes in stimulus significance occur in the auditory system, and influence anatomically linked structures distributed in neural systems with specific functional interactions that mediate the behavioral change produced by a specific form of learning. This conclusion is not compatible with the popular misconception that learning and memory functions take place in a separate critical locus or "cognitive organ" within the brain (e.g., hippocampus or medial temporal lobe "memory system"), where the so-called "engram" resides outside sensory maps. The use of neuroimaging to visualize what is happening to brain activity in different forms of learning provides a more complete picture of all the neural systems involved in learning functions, both on the sides of acquisition of stimulus significance and behavioral performance. Functional neuroimaging leads to a more realistic picture of how the brain works as a unit to modify behavior during learning, rather than destroying it with invasive techniques in the "search for the engram" (Lashley, 1950). Interpreting lesion data as reflecting brain function in the absence of the damaged area is misguided, because the lesion will affect the operation of entire neural systems (Webster, 1973; Kosslyn, Dalley, McPeek, Apert, Kennedy, & Caviness, 1993). A new behavioral neuroscience is emerging from detailed functional imaging of the brain in the intact behaving organism. Of vital importance to this new behavioral neuroscience is discovering the functional neural systems mediating different forms of learning, discovering the functional contribu-tions to behavioral change by different neural pathways, discovering the general brain strategies common to various forms of behavior, and discovering the specific functional networks that are linked to stages of brain development with characteristic learning and memory capabilities.

Acknowledgments

We acknowledge support for this work from National Institute of Mental Health Grant R01 MH-43353 and National Science Foundation Grant IBN9222075.

References

Aertsen, A. M. H., Gerstein, G. L., Habib, M. K., & Palm, G. (1989). Dynamics of neuronal firing correlation: Modulation of "effective connectvity". *Journal of Neurophysiology, 61,* 900–917.

Ahissar, E., Vaadia, E., Ahissar, M., Bergman, H., Arieli, A., & Abeles, M. (1992). Dependence of cortical plasticity on correlated activity of single neurons and on behavioral context. *Science, 257,* 1412–1415.

Amsel, A. (1986). Developmental psychobiology and behavior theory: Reciprocating Influences. *Canadian Journal of Psychology, 40,* 311–342.

Amsel, A. (1993). Hippocampal function in the rat: Cognitive mapping or vicarious trial and error? *Hippocampus, 3,* 251–256.

Bentler, P. M. (1985). *Theory and implementation of EQS, A structural equations program.* Los Angeles: PMDB Statistical Software.

Berry, W. D. (1984). *Nonrecursive Causal Models.* Sage University Paper Series on Quantitative Applications in the Social Sciences. Beverly Hills: Sage Publications.

Birt, D., & Olds, M. E. (1982). Auditory response enhancement during differential conditioning in behaving rats. In C. D. Woody (Ed.). *Conditioning: Representation of involved neural functions* (pp. 483–502). New York: Plenum.

Bollen, K. A. (1989). *Structural equations with latent variables.* New York: Wiley.

Bryan, R. M., & Lehman, R. A. W. (1988). Cerebral glucose utilization after aversive conditioning and during conditioned fear in the rat. *Brain Research, 444,* 17–24.

Campbell, B. A., & Stehouwer, D. J. (1979). Ontogeny of habituation and sensitization in the rat. In N. E. Spear & B. A. Campbell (Eds.), *Ontogeny of learning and memory* (pp. 67–100). Hillsdale, NJ: Earlbaum.

Clark, C. M., Ammann, W., Martin, W. R. W., Ty, P., & Hayden, M. R. (1991). The FDG/PET methodology for early detection of disease: A statistical model. *Journal of Cerebral Blood Flow and Metabolism, 11a,* 96–102.

Clark, C. M., Kessler, R., Buchsbaum, M., Margolin, R., & Holcomb, H. (1984). Correlational methods for determining coupling of regional glucose metabolism: A pilot study. *Biological Psychiatry, 19,* 663–678.

Davis, J. A. (1985). *The Logic of Causal Order.* Sage University Paper Series on Quantitative Applications in the Social Sciences. Beverly Hills: Sage Publications.

Deacon, T. W., Eichenbaum, H., Rosenberg, P., & Eckmann, K. W. (1983). Afferent connections of the perirhinal cortex in the rat. *Journal of Comparative Neurology, 220,* 168–190.

Diaz-Granados, J. L., Greene, P. L., & Amsel, A. (1992). Memory-based learning in preweanling and adult rats after infantile X-irradiation-induced hippocampal granule cell hypoplasia. *Behavioral Neuroscience, 106*, 940–946.

Dobbing, J., & Sands, J. (1979). Comparative aspects of the brain growth spurt. *Early Human Development, 3*, 79–83.

Domesick, V. B. (1972). Thalamic relationships of the medial cortex in the rat. *Brain Behavior and Evolution, 6*, 457–483.

Duncan, G. E. (1992). High resolution autoradiographic imaging of brain activity patterns with 2-deoxyglucose: Regional topographic and cellular analysis. In F. Gonzalez-Lima, T. Finkenstädt, & H. Scheich (Eds.), *Advances in metabolic mapping techniques for brain imaging of behavior and learning functions* (NATO ASI Series, Vol. 68, pp. 151–172). Dordrecht, The Netherlands: Kluwer.

Franz, S. I. (1912). New phrenology. *Science, 35*, 321–328.

Friedman, H. R., & Goldman-Rakic, P. S. (1988). Activation of the hippocampus and dentate gyrus by working-memory: A 2-deoxyglucose study of behaving rhesus monkeys. *Journal of Neuroscience, 8*, 4693–4706.

Friston, K. J. (1994). Functional and effective connectivity in neuroimaging: A synthesis. *Human Brain Mapping, 2*, 56–78.

Friston, K. J., Frith, C. D., Liddle, P. F., & Frackowiak, R. S. J. (1993). Functional connectivity: The principal-component analysis of large (PET) data sets. *Journal of Cerebral Blood Flow and Metabolism, 13*, 5–14.

Gerstein, G. L., Perkel, D. H., & Subramanian, K. N. (1978). Identification of functionally related neural assemblies. *Brain Research, 140*, 43–62.

Gevins, A., & Cutillo, B. (1993). Spatiotemporal dynamics of component processes in human working memory. *Electroencephalography and Clinical Neurophysiology, 87*, 128–143.

Gevins, A. S., Doyle, J. C., Cutillo, B. A., Schaffer, R. E., Tannehill, R. S., & Bressler, S. L. (1985). Neurocognitive pattern analysis of a visuospatial task: Rapidly-shifting foci of evoked correlations between electrodes. *Psychophysiology, 22*, 32–43.

Gonzalez-Lima, F. (1989). Functional brain circuitry related to arousal and learning in rats. In J. P. Ewert & M. A. Arbib (Eds.), *Visuomotor coordination: Amphibians, comparisons, models and robots* (pp. 729–766). New York and London: Plenum.

Gonzalez-Lima, F. (1992). Brain imaging of auditory learning functions in rats: Studies with fluorodeoxyglucose autoradiography and cytochrome oxidase histochemistry. In F. Gonzalez-Lima, T. Finkenstädt, & H. Scheich (Eds.), *Advances in metabolic mapping techniques for brain imaging of behavioral and learning functions* (NATO ASI Series, Vol. 68, pp. 39–109), Dordrecht, The Netherlands: Kluwer.

Gonzalez-Lima, F., & Agudo, J. (1990). Functional reorganization of neural auditory maps by differential learning. *Neuroreport, 1*, 161–164.

Gonzalez-Lima, F., Finkenstädt, T., & Ewert, J. P. (1989a). Neural substrates for long-term habituation of the acoustic startle reflex in rats: A 2-deoxyglucose study. *Neuroscience Letters, 96*, 151–156.

Gonzalez-Lima, F., Finkenstädt, T., & Ewert, J. P. (1989b). Learning-related activation in the auditory system of the rat produced by long-term habituation: A 2-deoxyglucose study. *Brain Research, 489*, 67–79.

Gonzalez-Lima, F., Finkenstädt, T., & Scheich, H. (Eds.) (1992). *Advances in metabolic mapping techniques for brain imaging of behavioral and learning functions* (NATO ASI Series, Vol. 68). Dordrecht. The Netherlands: Kluwer.

Gonzalez-Lima, F., & McIntosh, A. R. (1994). Neural network interactions related to auditory learning analyzed with structural equation modeling. *Human Brain Mapping, 2*, 23–44.

Gonzalez-Lima, F., & Scheich, H. (1984a). Classical conditioning enhances auditory 2-deoxyglucose patterns in the inferior colliculus. *Neuroscience Letters, 51*, 79–85.

Gonzalez-Lima, F., & Scheich, H. (1984b). Neural substrates for tone-conditioned bradycardia demonstrated with 2-deoxyglucose. I. Activation of auditory nuclei. *Behavioural Brain Research, 14*, 213–233.

Gonzalez-Lima, F., & Scheich, H. (1985). Ascending reticular activating system in the rat: a 2-deoxyglucose study. *Brain Research, 334*, 70–88.Gonzalez-Lima, F., & Scheich, H. (1986a). Neural substrates for tone-conditioned bradycardia demonstrated with 2-deoxyglucose. II. Auditory cortex plasticity. *Behavioural Brain Research, 20*, 281–293.

Gonzalez-Lima, F., & Scheich, H. (1986b). Classical conditioning of tone-signaled bradycardia modifies 2-deoxyglucose uptake patterns in cortex, thalamus, habenula, caudate-putamen and hippocampal formation. *Brain Research, 363*, 239–256.

Grafton, S. T., Sutton, J., Couldwell, W., Lew, M., & Waters, C. (1994). Network analysis of motor system connectivity in Parkinson's disease: Modulation of thalamocortical interactions after pallidotomy. *Human Brain Mapping, 2*, 45–55.

Green, R. J., & Stanton, M. E. (1989). Differential ontogeny of working memory and reference memory in the rat. *Behavioral Neuroscience, 103*, 98–105.

Hargreaves, R. J., Planas, A. M., Cremer, J. E., & Cunningham, V. J. (1986). Studies on the relationship between cerebral glucose transport and phosphorylation using 2-deoxyglucose. *Journal of Cerebral Blood Flow and Metabolism, 6*, 708–716.

Hayduk, L. A. (1987). *Structural Equation Modeling with LISREL: Essentials and Advances.* Baltimore, MD: John Hopkins Univ. Press.

Hebb, D. O. (1955). Drives and the C. N. S. (conceptual nervous system). *Psychological Review, 62*, 243–254.

Hock, F. J., & Scheich, H. (1986). Functional activity in the brain of socially deprived rats produced by an active avoidance test after Razobazam (Hoe 175) treatment: A 2-deoxyglucose study. *Behavioral and Neural Biology, 4*, 398–409.

Horwitz, B., Duara, R., & Rapoport, S. I. (1984). Intercorrelations of glucose metabolic rates between brain regions: Application to healthy males in a state of reduced sensory input. *Journal of Cerebral Blood Flow and Metabolism, 4*, 633–678.

Horwitz, B., Soncrant, T. T., & Haxby, J. V. (1992). Covariance analysis of functional interactions in the brain using metabolic and blood flow data. In F. Gonzalez-Lima, T. Finkenstädt, & H. Scheich (Eds.), *Advances in metabolic mapping techniques for brain imaging of behavioral and learning functions* (NATO ASI Series, Vol 68, pp. 189–218). Dordrecht, The Netherlands: Kluwer. Publishers

Jarrard, L. E. (1993). On the role of the hippocampus in learning and memory in the rat. *Behavioral and Neural Biology, 60*, 9–26.

John, E. R., & Schwartz, E. L. (1978). The neurophysiology of information processing and cognition. *Annual Review of Psychology, 29*, 1–29.

John, E. R., Tang, Y., Brill, A. B., Young, R., & Ono, K. (1986). Double-labeled metabolic maps of memory. *Science, 233*, 1167–1175.

Jöreskog, K. G., & Sörbom, D. (1989). *LISREL 7 user's reference guide.* Mooresville, IN: Scientific-Software.

Konorski, J. (1967). *Integrative activity of the brain.* Chicago, IL: Univ. of Chicago Press.

Kosslyn, S. M., Dally P. F., McPeek, R. M., Apert, N. M., Kennedy, D. N., & Cavines, V. S., Jr. (1993). Using locations to store shape: An indirect effect of a lesion. *Cerebral Cortex, 29*, 567–582.

Kossut, M. (1992). Plasticity of the barrel cortex neurons. *Progress in Neurobiology, 39*, 389–422.

Lashley, K. S. (1950). In search of the engram. *Symposium of the Society of Experimental Biology, 4*, 454–482.

Lauter, J. L., Herscovitch, P., Formby, C., & Raichle, M. E. (1985). Tonotopic organization in human auditory cortex revealed by positron emission tomography. *Hearing Research, 20*, 199–205.

Loehlin, J. C. (1987). *Latent variable models: An introduction to factor, path and structural analysis.* Hillsdale, NJ: Erlbaum.

LoLordo, V. M., & Fairless, J. L. (1985). Pavlovian conditioned inhibition: The literature since 1969. In R. R. Miller & N. E. Spear (Eds.), *Information processing in animals: Conditioned inhibition* (pp. 1–49). Hilssdale, NJ: Erlbaum.

Long, J. S. (1983). *Covariance structural models, an introduction to LIS-REL.* Sage University Paper Series on Quantitative Applications in the Social Sciences. Beverly Hills: Sage Publications.

Luiten, P. G. M., Kuipers, F., & Schitumaker, H. (1982). Organization of diencephalic and brainstem projections of the lateral septum in the rat. *Neuroscience Letters, 30,* 211–216.

Matsunami, K., Kawashima, T., & Satake, H. (1989). Mode of [^{14}C]2-deoxy-D-glucose uptake into retrosplenial cortex and other memory-related structures of the monkey during a delayed response. *Brain Research Bulletin, 22,* 829–838.

McIntosh, A. R., & Gonzalez-Lima, F. (1991). Structural modeling of functional neural pathways mapped with 2-deoxyglucose: Effects of acoustic startle habituation on the auditory system. *Brain Research, 547,* 295–302.

McIntosh, A. R., & Gonzalez-Lima, F. (1992a). The application of structural modeling to metabolic mapping of functional neural systems. In F. Gonzalez-Lima, T. Finkenstädt, & H. Scheich (Eds.), *Advances in metabolic mapping techniques for brain imaging of behavioral and learning functions* (NATO ASI Series, Vol 68, 219–255). Dordrecht, The Netherlands: Kluwer.

McIntosh, A. R., & Gonzalez-Lima, F. (1992b). Structural modeling of functional visual pathways mapped with 2-deoxy-glucose: Effects of patterned light and footshock. *Brain Research, 578,* 75–86.

McIntosh, A. R., & Gonzalez-Lima, F. (1993). Network analysis of functional auditory pathways mapped with fluorodeoxyglucose: Associative effects of a tone conditioned as a Pavlovian excitor or inhibitor. *Brain Research, 627,* 129–140.

McIntosh, A. R., & Gonzalez-Lima, F. (1994a). Network interactions among limbic cortices, basal forebrain and cerebellum differentiate a tone conditioned as a Pavlovian excitor or inhibitor: Fluorodeoxyglucose mapping and covariance structural modeling. *Journal of Neurophysiology, 72,* 1717–1733.

McIntosh, A. R., & Gonzalez-Lima, F. (1994b). Structural equation modeling and its application to network analysis in functional brain imaging. *Human Brain Mapping, 2,* 2–22.

McIntosh, A. R., Grady, C. L., Ungerleider, L. G., Haxby, J. V., Rapoport, S. I., & Horwitz, B. (1994). Network analysis of cortical visual pathways mapped with PET. *Journal of Neuroscience, 14,* 656–666.

Merzenich, M. M., & Sameshima, K. (1993). Cortical plasticity and memory. *Current Opinions on Neurobiology, 3,* 187–196.

Metter, E. J., Riege, W. H., Kuhl, D. E., & Phelps, M. E. (1984). Cerebral metabolic relationships for selected brain regions in healthy adult. *Journal of Cerebral Blood Flow and Metabolism, 4,* 1–7.

Miller, R. R., & Spear, N. E. (1985). *Information processing in animals: Conditioned inhibition.* Hillsdale, NJ: Erlbaum.

Pascaul-Leone, A., Grafman, J., & Hallett, M. (1992). Modulation of cortical motor output maps during development of implicit and explicit knowledge. *Science, 263,* 1287–1289.

Phillipson, O. T., & Griffiths, A. C. (1985). The topographic order of inputs to nucleus accumbens in the rat. *Neuroscience, (Oxford), 16,* 275–296.

Powell, E. W., & Leman, R. B. (1976). Connections of the nucleus accumbens. *Brain Research, 105,* 389–403.

Recanzone, G. H., Schreiner, C. E., & Merzenich, M. M. (1992). Plasticity in the frequency representation of primary auditory cortex following discrimination training in adult owl monkeys. *Journal of Neuroscience, 13,* 87–103.

Rescorla, R. A. (1968). Probability of shock in the presence and absence of CS in fear conditioning. *Journal of Comparative and Physiological Psychology, 66,* 1–5.

Rescorla, R. A. (1988). Behavioral studies of Pavlovian conditioning. *Annual Review of Neuroscience, 11,* 329–352.

Roland, P. E. (1993). *Brain activation.* New York: Wiley-Liss.

Room, P., Tielemans, A. J. P. C., De Boer, T., Tonnaer, J. A. D. M., Wester, J., Van den Broek, J. H. M., & Delft, A. M. L. (1989). Local cerebral glucose uptake in anatomically defined structures of freely moving rats. *Journal of Neuroscience Methods, 27,* 191–202.

Rosen, J. B., Hitchcock, J. M., Miserendino, M. J. D., Falls, W. A., Campeau, S., & Davis, M. (1992). Lesions of perirhinal cortex but not frontal, medial prefrontal, visual, or insular cortex block fear-potentiated startle using a visual conditioned stimulus. *Journal of Neuroscience, 12,* 4624–4633.

Rosenzweig, M. R. & Bennett, E. L. (1976). *Neural mechanisms of learning and memory.* Cambridge, MA: MIT Press.

Rudy, J. W., & Cheatle, M. D. (1979). Ontogeny of associative learning: Acquisition of odor aversions by neonatal rats. In N. E. Spear & B. A. Campbell (Eds.), *Ontogeny of learning and memory* (pp. 157–188). Hillsdale, NJ: Earlbaum.

Ryan, A. F., Zabrina, F., Nigel, K. W., & Keithley, E. M. (1988). The spatial representation of frequency in the rat dorsal cochlear nucleus and inferior colliculus. *Hearing Research, 36,* 181–190.

Sainsbury, R. S., Heynen, A., & Montoya, C. P. (1987). Behavioral correlates of hippocampal type 2 theta in the rat. *Physiology and Behavior, 39,* 513–519.

Scheich, H., & Bonke, B. A. (1981). Tone versus FM-induced patterns of excitation and suppression in the 2-deoxy-[^{14}C]glucose labeled auditory "cortex" of the Guinea fowl. *Experimental Brain Research, 44,* 445–449.

Scheich, H., Simonis, C., Ohl, F., Thomas, H., & Tillen, J. (1992). Learning-related plasticity of gerbil auditory cortex: Feature maps versus meaning maps. In F. Gonzalez-Lima, T. Finkenstädt, & H. Scheich (Eds.), *Advances in metabolic mapping techniques for brain imaging of behavioral and learning functions,* (NATO ASI Series, Vol. 68, pp. 447–475). Dordrecht, The Netherlands: Kluwer.

Shoham, D., Ullman, S., & Grinvald, A. (1991). Characterization of dynamic patterns of cortical activity by a small number of principal components. *Abstracts of the Society of Neuroscience, 17,* 1089.

Sokoloff, L., Reivich, M., Kennedy, C., Des Rosiers, M. H., Patlak, C. S., Pettigrew, K. D., Sakurada, O., & Shinohara, M. (1977). The [^{14}C]deoxyglucose method for measurement of local cerebral glucose utilization: Theory, procedure and normal values in conscious and anesthetized albino rats. *Journal of Neurochemistry, 28,* 897–916.

Sokoloff, L., Kennedy, C., & Smith, C. B. (1989). The [^{14}C]deoxyglucose method for measurement of local cerebral glucose utilization. In A. A. Boulton, G. B. Baker, & R. F. Butterworth (Eds.), *Neuromethods: Carbohydrates and energy metabolism* (pp. 155–193). Totowa, NJ: Humana Press.

Squire, L. R., Knowlton, B., & Musen, G. (1993). The structure and organization of memory. *Annual Review of Psychology, 22,* 453–495.

Sripanidkulchai K., & Wyss, M. (1986). Thalamic projections to retrosplenial cortex in rat. *Journal of Comparative Neurology, 254,* 143–165.

Trusk, T. C., & Stein, E. A. (1988). Effect of heroin-conditioned auditory stimuli on cerebral functional activity in rats. *Pharmacology, Biochemistry and Behavior, 30,* 983–993.

Wagner, A. R., & Brandon, S. E. (1989). Evolution of a structured connectionist model of Pavlovian conditioning (AESOP). In S. B. Klein & R. R. Mower (Eds.), *Contemporary learning theories: Pavlovian conditioning and the status of learning theory* (pp. 149–189). Hillsdale, NJ: Erlbaum.

Webster, W. G. (1973). Assumptions, conceptualizations, and the search for the functions of the brain. *Physiological Psychology, 1,* 346–350.

Weinberger, N. M. (1995). Dynamic regulation of receptive fields and maps in the adult sensory cortex. *Annual Review of Neuroscience, 18,* 129–158.

Weinberger, N. M., & Diamond, D. M. (1987). Physiological plasticity in auditory cortex: rapid induction by learning. *Progress in Neurobiology, 29,* 1–55.

Weiskrantz, L. (1968). Treatments, inferences, and brain function. In L. Weiskrantz (Ed.), *Analysis of Behavioral Change.* New York: Harper & Row.

Witter, M. P., Daelmans, H. E. M., Jorritsma-Byham, B., Staiger, J. F., & Wouterlook, F. G. (1992). Restricted origin and distribution of projections from the lateral to the medial septal complex in rat and guinea pig. *Neuroscience Letters, 148,* 164–168.

Zohary, E., Celebrini, S., Britten, K. H., & Newsome, W. T. (1994). Neuronal plasticity that underlies improvement in perceptual performance. *Science, 263,* 1289–1292.

Zola-Morgan, S., Squire, L. R., Amaral, D. G., & Suzuki, W. A. (1989). Lesions of perirhinal and parahippocampal cortex that spare the amygdala and hippocampal formation produce severe memory impairment. *Journal of Neuroscience, 9,* 4355–4370.

17

Measurement Issues in the Interpretation of Behavior–Brain Relationships

Jack M. Fletcher,*,† Karla K. Stuebing,* Bennett A. Shaywitz,§, ‖
Michael E. Brandt,*,‡ David J. Francis,** and Sally E. Shaywitz§

Departments of *Pediatrics, †Neurosurgery, ‡Psychiatry and ¶Behavioral Sciences, University of Texas–Houston
Medical School, Houston, Texas 77030; Departments of §Pediatrics and ‖Neurology, Yale University School of
Medicine, New Haven, Connecticut 06510; and **Department of Psychology, University of Houston,
Houston, Texas 77004

I. Introduction

The purpose of this chapter is to discuss measurement issues that influence the interpretation of relationships between indices of cognitive and behavioral functioning and brain status. These measurement issues are important for studies that incorporate both structural and functional neuroimaging modalities. In a structural neuroimaging study, a subject typically receives a battery of cognitive and neuropsychological tests. Either before or after the psychometric evaluation, the subject also receives a neuroimaging study of the brain, such as a magnetic resonance imaging (MRI) scan. Specific areas of the brain are usually measured based on an algorithm for separating different tissue and fluid types for comparison with the behavioral tasks.

In a functional imaging study, the assessments of cognitive and brain status are obtained virtually simultaneously. For example, the subject may be asked to perform a task, such as deciding whether or not two words rhyme. While the subject performs the task, assessments of the metabolic functioning of the brain are made through position emission tomography (PET) or functional MRI (fMRI) modalities. For both functional and structural neuroimaging studies, the goal is to relate behavioral performance on the cognitive tasks to specific areas of the brain hypothesized to be related to task performance.

Establishing these relationships involves a number of study design and measurement issues. Sample sizes are typically small because of the difficulties and expense of these types of investigations. The difficulties occur not only in acquiring the neuroimaging study, but in processing the brain images that have been acquired. When samples are small, the investigator must guard against sources of variability that generally distort estimates of the relationship of behavior and brain.

A related issue concerns the measurement of the psychological constructs of interest. If the construct is not measured at a level where the *latent variable* can be specified, surplus sources of variability that represent measurement error will operate to distort the estimate of the relationship of the psychological variable to the brain measurement. An additional problem is that a poorly measured or multifactorial construct may provide misleading information concerning relationships with the brain. For example, a significant correlation of the Full Scale IQ score from the Wechsler Intelligence Scale for Children (WISC-R; Wechsler, 1974) with a measurement of a particular brain structure should not be taken to indicate that IQ is localized in this brain area, because the Full Scale IQ score is determined by multiple verbal and nonverbal cognitive skills. Although few investigators would make such an interpretation with a measure such as Full Scale IQ, the inference is no better than those underlying interpretations of tests such as the Wisconsin Card Sorting Test

(Heaton, 1981) or the Tower of London (Shallice, 1982) as measures of frontal lobe functions. Such tests are fractionally confounded because they measure multiple abilities (see Levin, Fletcher, Kufera, Harwood, Lilly, Mendelsohn, 1996). Interpretation of how these measures relate to brain function requires a more analytic approach that attempts to break down such tests into component operations for comparison with a measure of brain function.

These study design and measurement issues occur at the level of behavior and brain. In the remainder of this chapter, we will focus on these study design and measurement issues, which involve (a) subject identification, and (b) construct identification. In discussing these two measurement issues, additional problems involving statistical inference will also be highlighted.

II. Subject Identification Issues

There are three primary problems that involve the selection and grouping of subjects for an investigation. These problems involve (a) definition of a sample or population; (b) influence of outliers, particularly in relation to estimates of the strength of an association between behavioral and biological measures; and (c) the influence of subtypes within a sample. Each of these issues has significant influence on the validation of inferences about behavior and brain, particularly on statistical inferences. In discussing these issues, the examples that will be used involve children with developmental disabilities, largely in relation to structural MRI. However, the same issues apply to studies of adults and to other neuroimaging modalities.

A. Statistical Inference

It is important to keep in mind the nature of most neuroimaging investigations of behavior–brain relationships. The *independent* variable is often a variable in the behavioral domain, such as the presence or absence of dyslexia, while the *dependent* variable is the brain measurement. For neuroimaging studies, the inference is often that any difference in the brain measurement "causes" the variation in the independent variable (e.g., presence or absence of dyslexia). This is a reversal of the nature and logic of the traditional (lesion-based) design of brain–behavior studies, where the central nervous system (CNS) variable (lesion location) is the independent variable and some behavioral response is the dependent variable.

Inferring "causal" relationships from neuroimaging studies is difficult to support (Kenney, 1979). The underlying statistical design is quasiexperimental, be-

cause the subjects are not randomly assigned nor are they actively manipulated, as in a treatment study (Cook & Campbell, 1979). More importantly, it is possible to obtain a significant group difference on the brain measurement that is fundamentally unrelated to the independent variable. This situation occurs because (a) there are other unmeasured variables unrelated to the independent variable (e.g., age, gender) that are related to the brain measurement and the dependent variable; and/or (b) the size of the effect, while statistically significant, is not very robust.

The former problem will be discussed in the section on subject identification issues. The latter problem can be addressed by computing various indices of the strength of association. The most common approach is to simply correlate the brain measurement with some index of the independent variable. For example, if dyslexics are studied, the brain measurement can be correlated with a test of reading ability. However, when the sample size is small, estimates of the strength of association may be unduly influenced by the presence of outliers and/or by the presence of group mean differences (i.e., subtypes) in the data. Both of these factors lead to distorted estimates of the strength of association. In the next sections, issues involving subject identification, outliers, and subtypes will discussed.

B. Sample Definition

There is rarely any major interest in studying only one subject for behavior–brain investigations. Although single subject studies are certainly valuable, most investigators form groups according to some independent variable. The use of groups permits aggregation of data and provides for the possibility of assessing the variability in the dependent variables (behavioral responses, brain activation) based on the classification provided by the independent variable (group).

When clinically defined groups are used for a study which evaluates relationships of behavioral responses and neuroimaging assessments, the sample is typically small and there is considerable variability in the dependent variable. Increasing the sample size usually reduces the standard error of the mean and increases power. Smaller effect sizes achieve a specified level of significance, indicating that the relationship is not due to chance. Another influence on effect sizes and statistical significance is variability at the level of the independent variable. This variability may lead to statistically significant relationships that reflect spurious or uncontrolled associations of the independent and dependent variables.

Recent structural neuroimaging investigations of dyslexia provide examples of this problem. These studies have shown that a variety of brain structure measurements are different in individuals with dyslexia relative to some type of comparison group. However, the samples tend to be small. In addition to variations in how subjects were selected (i.e., the definition of dyslexia), there is often substantial variability across subjects and groups in other characteristics. Controlling for this variability may alter the pattern of group differences across dependent variables, analogous to blocking on the independent variable, or an analysis of covariance (Maxwell & Delaney, 1990).

Table 1 summarizes six studies that compared dyslexic and nondyslexic groups on brain measurements. The groups varied in age, gender, and handedness. In none of studies did the group differences on these three variables achieve statistical significance. However, the power for rejecting the null hypothesis is low because of small samples sizes and high variability within groups on the three variables. This variability across studies is of particular concern, because measurements of brain structures are clearly related to age, gender, and handedness (Filapek, 1995; Steinmetz, Volkmann, Jancke, & Freund, 1991), variables that are not obviously related to dyslexia.

The influence of age and gender was assessed by Schultz, Cho, Staib, Kier, Fletcher, Shaywitz, et al. (1994). Although the groups appear closely matched on these variables, covarying for either age or gender significantly reduced the between-groups effect sizes for the brain structure measurements. Many structural measures that significantly differentiated the groups no longer did so when variability due to age and gender was partialled from the MRI measurements. Hence, even minor variations in variables such as age and gender influence the magnitude of group differences in studies with small sample sizes. This is important because each of these studies tended to implicate a

different brain area as critically important for reading disability.

C. Outliers

An *outlier* is a subject who falls outside some defined distribution of observations. In any study, outliers can exercise undue influence on estimates of variability, and interfere with accurate estimates of statistical tests of significance. In correlational studies, outliers exercise undue influence on estimates of the strength of association.

Figure 1 provides an example of the influence of outlier observations. This figure compares WISC-R Performance IQ scores and an area measurement of the corpus callosum from a midsagittal MRI slice in 10 subjects. The observations were randomly generated. The Pearson correlation (*r*) for these two measures is .68, implying a fairly strong relationship. However, there is one observation with a large corpus callosum measurement and very high Performance IQ (see arrow). The effect of this subject is to angle the regression line in a positive direction. Eliminating this subject reduces the correlation to .37, which is not statistically significant in a small sample.

As this example shows, extreme values of individual observations exercise excessive influence on the strength of the relationship of two variables. *Leverage* is dependent on the value of the predictor value (X axis), while the *influence* of a data point on a correlation depends on its values on both the X and Y axes (Hamilton, 1992). Leverage typically ranges from 1/N, where N = sample size, to 1.0. A commonly employed rule of thumb based on Huber (1981) is as follows (Hamilton, 1992): Maximum leverage ≤ .2 = Safe; 0.2 ≤ Maximum leverage ≤ .5 = Risky; Maximum leverage > .5 = Avoid if possible.

The leverage and influence of a data point can be estimated. When the leverage of any given point is

Table 1   Age, Gender, and Handedness Differences across Structural Neuroimaging Studies of Children with Dyslexia and Normal Readers

Study	Age Dyslexic/normal	Gender (M:F) Dyslexic/normal	Handedness (LH:RH) Dyslexic/normal
Larsen et al. (1990)	15.1/15.4	15:4/15:4	4:15/2:17
Hynd et al. (1990)	9.9/11/8	8:2/8:2	3:7/0:10
Jernigan et al. (1991)	8.9/9.0	13:7/8:4	1:19/2:10
Duara et al. (1991)	39.1/35.3	12:9/15:4	0:21/0:29
Leonard et al. (1993)	15–65/14–52	7:2/5:7	0:9/0:12
Schultz et al. (1994)	8.7/9.0	10:7/7:7	0:14/0:17

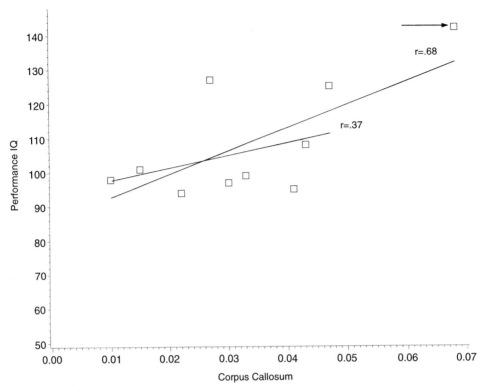

Figure 1. Hypothetical plot of Wechsler Intelligence Scale for Children-Revised (WISC-R, Wechsler, 1974) Performance IQ scores and area measures of the corpus callosum from a midsagittal MRI slice (relative to brain area). The results show that the outlier subject (see arrow) inflates the correlation of these measures.

>.2, too much of the information may be coming from one data point, rather than from the data set as a whole. This relationship is illustrated in Table 2, which shows the effect of changing the Performance IQ value for one high leverage data point (corpus callosum value of .068 in Figure 1; leverage = 0.56). The leverage of the data point stays the same (0.56), regardless of the value of Performance IQ. The influence changes, as does the correlation between the corpus callosum and Performance IQ in the data set as a whole as

the value of Performance IQ changes. When Performance IQ = 119, influence = 0, producing what is likely a more accurate estimate of the correlation of Performance IQ and the corpus callosum (.49). A correlation of .50 was actually found in Fletcher et al. (1996) in an actual sample of children with hydrocephalus.

The key is the need to plot and visualize the data, and not simply accept the computer output without scrutiny. In the next section, similar points will be made concerning the influence of group differences on correlational estimates of strength of association.

D. Subgroups

The presence of group differences within a set of data may also distort estimates of the strength of association. To illustrate, Willerman, Schultz, Rutledge, and Bigler (1991) evaluated the relationship of MRI measures of brain size (adjusted for body weight) and psychometric intelligence in a sample of college students with higher (≥1350) and lower (≤940) Scholastic Achievement Test (SAT) scores. This approach to sample selection introduces an explicit group structure

Table 2 Estimates of Influence and Effects on the Correlation Coefficient for Hypothetical Values of Performance IQ Based on a Corpus Callosum Area Measurement Value with High Leverage

Corpus callosum	Performance IQ	Leverage	Influence	Correlation
.068	142	.56	0.88	.68
.068	119	.56	0.00	.49
.068	93	.56	1.06	.03
.068	70	.56	2.45	−.29

into the data. A prorated WAIS-R IQ score correlated significantly ($r = .51$) with the measurement of brain size. However, as the authors acknowledged, the sampling strategy produced extremes in the distribution of IQ scores, which inflate the correlation. Application of a statistical correction reduced the magnitude of the correlation to a more modest $r = .35$. Basically, any situation involving nonimpaired and impaired subjects may overestimate the strength of association if the groups differ on one of the variables being correlated (Maxwell & Delaney, 1990).

It is also possible to inappropriately conclude that the strength of association is generalizable because of the presence of subgroups in the data. For example, Table 3 shows Pearson correlations for Verbal IQ and Performance IQ with the area measurement of the corpus callosum from a sample composed of children with several etiologies producing hydrocephalus. The correlation for the total sample is higher for Performance IQ than for Verbal IQ. However, as the correlations for each subgroup show, the relationships are largely obtained for the two groups with shunted hydrocephalus (aqueductal stenosis and meningomyelocele), not for the groups as a whole. The correlation of Performance IQ and the corpus callosum in neurologically normal children is negligible (Fletcher et al., 1996). The relationship emerges largely in children who have shunted hydrocephalus, and does not reflect more general relationships of corpus callosum and Performance IQ.

E. Recommendations

These comments about the estimation of strength of association in small samples should not be taken in a discouraging tone. Rather, investigators must carefully investigate the data to understand the basis for the results. It is essential to plot the data and look for outliers and subgroups. If outliers are apparent, some

Table 3 Correlations of WISC-R Verbal and Performance IQ with Corpus Callosum/Brain Ratio

	N	Verbal IQ	Performance IQ
Total sample	53	.24	.41*
Aqueductal stenosis	8	−.09	.36**
Meningocele	6	.42	.41
Meningomyelocele	18	.21	.33**
Premature	21	.05	.27

*$p<.01$
**$p<.05$

form of influence analysis should be completed (Hamilton, 1992). Exploratory data analysis methods that involve graphing and visualization of data are entirely acceptable and highly useful (Chambers, Cleveland, Kleiner, & Tukey, 1983; Tukey, 1977). Similarly, subgroup differences may imply that the relationships of certain variables lie in the group structure, not in the covariance of the variables. Simply reporting the group difference may be as strong a statement as possible. Alternatively, the use of nonparametric statistics, such as Spearman's rho, or statistics that are highly suited for small samples, such as odds ratios (Bates & Appelbaum, 1994), may better represent the extent to which the variables of interest are related. The most important point is to graph and visualize the data before statistically analyzing the data.

III. Construct Definition Issues

The issues involved in construct definition revolve around an analytic specification of the latent variables underlying performance on a task. When the goal is to assess performance on a particular measure, the psychometric issues underlying the specification of the latent variables from a construct validity perspective are well-understood (Fletcher, Francis, Stuebing, Shaywitz, Shaywitz, Shankweiler et al., 1996; Nunnally & Bernstein, 1994). Similar issues pertain to adaptations of tasks for brain activation studies using functional neuroimaging modalities. The problems in construct identification have generally not been addressed from a psychometric perspective.

A. Construct Validity

To develop tasks for activation studies, the approach to task development must proceed from a construct validity perspective. In this respect, the validity characteristics of the tasks should be demonstrated independently of the activation procedure. Such development should take advantage of information from the cognitive neurosciences and use tasks where the measurement characteristics can be clearly operationalized. As Cook and Campbell (1979) stated, the "basic problem in construct validity is the possibility that the operations which are meant to represent a particular cause or effect construct can be constructed in terms of more than one construct (p. 52)." Cronbach and Meehl (1955) indicated in the classic treatment of construct validity that the primary problem of the investigator is "What constructs account for variance in test performance?" (p. 282). If an investigator cannot specify these constructs *at a cognitive or behavioral level,* there is no basis for validating a behavior–brain relationship.

The contemporary approach to construct validation asks what *latent variables* underlie performance on a measure of performance. In activation studies, the underlying construct, or latent variables, are inferred on the basis of some observed behaviors (test performance) that presumably reflect an underlying construct. However, observed performance does not fully operationalize the latent variable. For example, a subject's score on the Wisconsin Card Sorting Test (Heaton, 1981) is not fully interchangeable with the construct of "executive function." This is because the score only imperfectly reflects the construct of "executive function." Test performance also reflects the influence of other variables, such as motivation, sustained attention, and the environment in which performance occurs. The construct of executive function only accounts for a portion of variance in the score on the Wisconsin Card Sorting Test. Even more remote is the notion of the Wisconsin Card Sorting Test as a measure of "frontal lobe" function. Performance may activate the frontal lobes, but when a test measures multiple psychological processes, one must question what aspects of the test are related to brain functions.

The task of construct validation research is to determine the degree to which a test measures the construct of interest relative to other latent and observed variables. Specific tests are never direct measures of a construct. Performance on a test is often treated in this fashion, but there are few tests that are pure analytic measures of single constructs. Test performance and latent variables are often treated synonymously, without the careful work on construct validation necessary to specify the degree to which a test measures the latent variables presumed to underlie performance. A consequence of relying solely on observed variables is that imperfect measurement may distort relationships among variables because of correlated errors of measurement.

B. Validating Tasks for Activation Studies

Table 4 outlines 10 steps that should be considered when developing tasks for brain activation studies. These steps are generally self-explanatory, but some elaboration may be helpful.

In order to avoid extensive research and development work, investigators should attempt to select tasks and measures that have some basis in the cognitive and experimental literature (Step 1 in Table 4). It is not necessary to directly replicate a particular measure. However, if a set of tests exists for which the la-

Table 4 Ten Steps in Developing Cognitive and Behavioral Tasks for Brain Activation Studies

1. Cognitive and behavioral measures must have an established basis in experimental research. Select measures that permit analytic decoupling of the underlying latent variables.

2. The measure must possess validity characteristics that exceed face validity—in particular, studies of criterion and construct validity must have been completed that support the measurement characteristics of the task *solely* in the behavioral domain.

3. Temporal reliability must be demonstrable, particularly over time, since repeated assessments are usually obtained.

4. Modifications necessary to adapt the procedure to a brain measurement modality must be shown not to change validity and reliability characteristics (1, 2, & 3 constant).

5. Task adaptation must fit the limitations of the activation technique.

6. A major issue is the specificity of the brain activation pattern; whenever possible, convergent validity must be shown. The strongest example is across brain activation measurement paradigms.

7. It should be possible to modify presentation or stimulus characteristics and deactivate the activating capacity of the task and paradigm.

8. Whenever possible, the double dissociation principle should be used to show selectivity of the activation procedure at the level of the brain. The test should selectively activate different brain areas.

9. Studies must be hypothesis-driven. Exploratory procedures are not desirable except under conditions where no rationale exists for designing tasks or interpreting results from the activation paradigm.

10. Directionality from behavior to brain.

tent variables are fairly well understood, adapting procedures that should operationalize these latent variables should facilitate the activation study. Such an approach permits the investigator to relate findings to a broader body of literature in the behavioral realm. This does not mean that investigators should simply select measures that have been used in psychometric studies. For example, measures such as the Wisconsin Card Sorting Test or the Tower of London Test are clearly factorially confounded and measure multiple constructs. It would be possible to have a subject perform the task during a functional neuroimaging study. However, interpretation of results will be difficult because of the inadequate specification of latent variables. An analytic approach, in which these different operations are identified and successively evaluated, usually in a subtraction methodology, is more likely to yield results that are replicable.

In developing more analytic tasks, the second step in Table 4 is particularly important. The measure should be studied at a behavioral level independently of the activation paradigm. For example, if a measure is presumed to isolate a latent variable such as phonological processing, then the measure should relate to other tests that have demonstrable relationships with the construct of phonological processing.

The need for the measure to reliably measure the latent variable is also an obvious point (Step 3). For example, if a measure depends heavily on novelty for its activation properties, the capacity of the measure to activate a certain brain area may diminish for the repeated administrations. Since most functional neuroimaging studies require repeated administrations, the influence of the task on the activation pattern will vary depending on the number of repetitions. It is generally desirable to train the subject in the task prior to administration. This is a major limitation of tasks such as the Wisconsin Card Sorting Test or the Tower of London, where substantial learning typically occurs by virtue of exposure to the task.

Any modifications of a particular procedure to fit into a brain imaging modality should also be shown not to change the measurement characteristics of the task independently of the activation procedure (Step 4). Again, Steps 1 and 2 are particularly critical. At the same time, it must be possible to do the task under activation conditions (Step 5). Adapting a task such as the Tower of London for an fMRI study may fundamentally alter the task, because the motor manipulations that seem to be an important component at the Tower of London performance may lead to movement artifact in certain types of neuroimaging studies. Simply having the subject visualize moves may not involve the same measurement operations as actual manipulation of the beads in the Tower of London.

There are several issues that involve the relationship of the task to the emerging activation pattern. These are described in Steps 6 through 8. Basically, it should be possible to manipulate the measurement characteristics of the tasks and vary the activation properties. It should also be possible to demonstrate specific activation by a task and to modify the activation results by modifying the measurement operations of the tasks. Finally, Steps 9 and 10 support the need to develop hypotheses that guide the investigation of behavior–brain relationships. In particular, it is important to recognize that directionality is from behavior into the brain. Specifically, a behavioral operation is being measured and then studied in relationship to the brain. The task measures psychological constructs. The brain measurements occur in a different modality in a different area of measurement. The goal of the study is to establish relationships between these two domains of measurement.

The types of recommendations made in Table 4 fit well into the types of subtraction paradigms commonly employed in brain activation studies. A general recommendation is to conceptualize tasks from a very analytic perspective. It is generally useful to layer tasks so that the different operations are carefully specified, and so that tasks can be successively arranged to isolate the operations of interests. In this manner, more complicated tasks that may involve several latent variables can be used. However, the relationship of each of these different latent variables to the brain activation pattern can be specified (Shaywitz et al., this volume).

IV. Conclusions

Inferring and validating relationships of behavior and brain is a complicated process because the domains of measurement are quite different. However, the measurement issues that underlie both domains are similar. Since small samples are inevitable in this type of research, investigators must take care to ensure that they have not introduced unwarranted heterogeneity into the sample, particularly when clinical groups are involved. Similarly, it is very important to examine issues that underlie statistical inference, particularly outliers and subgroups. Another source of measurement error involves construct misspecification. Task development is critical for cognitive neuroscience investigations of behavior and brain. More generally, small samples make it relatively easy to confirm hypotheses, but hard to disconfirm hypotheses. Since hypotheses must be falsifiable in order to be tested, it is critically important to carefully evaluate the data before rejecting the null hypothesis. In this respect, investigators are encouraged to plot and visualize data and to avoid the types of deceptions that are possible when statistical inferences are based on small samples. This is particularly true for correlational studies that are inevitable in behavior–brain investigations. Such studies are inherently quasi-experimental and correlational. Careful and systematic evaluation of the measurement characteristics of the tasks, as well as design and sample selection issues, are usually critical to ensure that the null hypothesis is critically evaluated.

Acknowledgments

Supported in part by NICHD grants P01 21889, Psycholinguistic and Biological Mechanisms in Dyslexia, P5O 25802, Center for Learning and Attention Disorders, and NINDS grant R01 NS25368, Neurobehavioral Development of Hydrocephalic Children. We acknowledge the assistance of Rita Taylor in manuscript preparation.

References

Bates, E., & Appelbaum, M. (1994). Methods of studying small samples: Issues and examples. In S. H. Broman & J. Grafman (Eds.) *Atypical cognitive deficits in developmental disorders: Implications for brain function* (pp. 245–280). Hillsdale, NJ: Erlbaum.

Chambers, J. M., Cleveland, W. S., Kleiner, B., & Tukey, P. A. (1983). *Graphical methods for data analysis.* Belmont, CA: Wadsworth.

Cook, T. D., & Campbell, D. A. (1979). *Quasi-experimentation: Design and analysis issues for field settings.* Chicago: Rand McNally.

Cronbach, L. J., & Meehl, P. E. (1955). Construct validity in psychological tests. *Psychological Bulletin, 52,* 281–302.

Duara, R., Kushch, A., Gross-Glenn, K., Barker, W., Jallad, B., Pascal, S., Lowenstein, D. A., Sheldon, J., Rabin, M., Levin, B., & Lubs, H. (1991). Neuroanatomic differences between dyslexic and normal readers on magnetic resonance imaging scans. *Archives of Neurology, 48,* 410–416.

Filipek, P. A. (1995). Neurobiologic correlates of developmental dyslexia: How do dyslexics' brains differ from those of normal readers. *Journal of Child Neurology, 10* (Suppl. 1), 562–569.

Fletcher, J. M., Bohan, T. P., Brandt, M. E., Kramer, L. A., Brookshire, B. L., Thorstad, K., Davidson, K. C., Francis, D. J., McCauley, S., & Baumgartner, J. E. (1996). Morphometric analysis of the hydrocephalic brain: Relationships with cognitive development. *Child's Nervous System, 12,* 192–199.

Fletcher, J. M., Francis, D. J., Stuebing, K. K., Shaywitz, B. A., Shaywitz, S. E., Shankweiler, D. P., Katz, L., & Morris, R. (1996). Conceptual and methodological issues in construct definition. In G. R. Lyon & N. Krasnegor (Eds.), *Attention, memory, and executive functions.* (pp. 17–42). Baltimore: Paul H. Brookes.

Hamilton, L. C. (1992). *Regression with graphics: A second course in applied statistics.* Pacific Grove, CA: Brookes–Cole.

Heaton, R. K. (1981). *A manual for the Wisconsin Card Sorting Test.* Odessa, FL: Psychological Assessment Resources.

Huber, P. J. (1981). *Robust statistics.* New York: Wiley.

Hynd, G. W., Semrud-Clikeman, M., Lorys, A., Novey, E. S., & Eliopulos, D. (1990). Brain morphology in developmental dyslexia and attention deficit disorder/hyperactivity. *Archives of Neurology, 47,* 919–926.

Jernigan, T. L., Hesselink, J. R., Sowell, E., & Tallal, P. A. (1991). Cerebral structure on magnetic resonance imaging in language- and learning-impaired children. *Archives of Neurology, 48,* 539–545.

Kenny, D. A. (1979). *Correlation and Causality.* New York: Wiley.

Larsen, J. P., Hoien, T., Lundberg, I., & Odegaard, H. (1990). MRI evaluation of the size and symmetry of the planum temporale in adolescents with developmental dyslexia. *Brain and Language, 39,* 289–301.

Leonard, C. M., Voeller, K. K. S., Lombardino, L. J., Morris, M. K., Hynd, G. W., Alexander, A. M., Anderson, H. G., Garofalakis, M., Honeyman, J. C., Mao, J., Agee, O. F., & Staab, E. V. (1993). Anomalous cerebral morphology in dyslexia revealed with MR imaging. *Archives of Neurology, 50,* 461–469.

Levin, H. S., Fletcher, J. M., Kufera, J. A., Harward, H., Lilly, M. A., Mendelsohn, D., Bruce, D., & Eisenberg, H. M. (1996). Dimensions of cognition measured by the Tower of London and other cognitive tasks in head injured children and adolescents. *Developmental Neuropsychology, 12,* 17–34.

Maxwell, S. E., & Delaney, H. D. (1990). *Designing experiments and analyzing data: A model comparison perspective.* Belmont, CA: Wadsworth.

Nunnally, J. C., & Bernstein, I. N. (1994). *Psychometric theory* (3nd ed.). New York: McGraw-Hill.

Schultz, R. T., Cho, N. K., Staib, L. H., Kier, L. E., Fletcher, J. M., Shaywitz, S. E., Shankweiler, D. P., Katz, L., Gore, J. C., Duncan, J. S., & Shaywitz, B. A. (1994). Brain morphology in normal and dyslexic children: The influences of sex and age. *Annals of Neurology, 35,* 732–742.

Shallice, T. (1982). specific impairments of planning. *Philosophical Transactions of the Royal Society of London, 298,* 199–209.

Steinmetz, H., Volkmann, J., Jancke, L., & Freund, H. J. (1991). Anatomical left–right asymmetry of language-related temporal cortex is different in left- and right-handers. *Annals of Neurology, 29,* 315–319.

Tukey, J. W. (1977). *Exploratory data analysis.* Reading, MA: Addison-Wesley.

Wechsler, D. (1974). *Wechsler intelligence scales for children—revised.* New York: Psychological Corporation.

Willerman, L., Schultz, R., Rutledge, J. N., & Bigler, E. D. (1991). *In vivo* brain size and intelligence. *Intelligence, 15,* 223–228.

18

Dynamic Growth Cycles of Brain and Cognitive Development

Kurt W. Fischer* and Samuel P. Rose[†]

*Harvard University, Cambridge, Massachusetts 02138; and [†]University of Colorado, Denver, Colorado

I. Introduction

A basic assumption of modern biopsychology is that growth of the brain relates closely to growth of action and thought, yet knowledge of the specific relations between brain and behavior in development has remained limited. In recent decades, research on neural systems has uncovered close relations between a few specific brain components and a few developing behaviors, especially for the visual system (for example, Hubel & Wiesel, 1977; Movshon & Van Sluyters, 1981; Neville, 1991), but there have not been comparable discoveries about connections between brain changes and development of action and thought.

On the other hand, recent research has brought substantial new knowledge about development of both the nervous system by itself and behavior by itself. With this knowledge comes the opportunity to begin to understand how brain and behavior develop together. A key finding of this research is that development in both arenas shows complex patterns, with many growth functions demonstrating nonlinear, dynamic patterns rather than monotonic growth (Fischer & Rose, 1994; Lampl & Emde, 1983; Lampl, Veldhuis, & Johnson, 1992; Rakic, Bourgeois, Eckenhoff, Zecevic, & Goldman-Rakic, 1986; Thatcher, 1994; Thelen & Smith, 1994). These complex patterns, together with novel tools for analysis of dynamic growth functions (Fischer, Bullock, Rotenberg, & Raya, 1993; Grossberg,

1987a; van der Maas & Molenaar, 1992; van Geert, 1994a), open new possibilities for analyzing relations between growth processes in brain and behavior.

Many of the growth patterns for brain and behavior are strikingly similar, fitting into a family of nonlinear dynamic growth curves that suggest common developmental processes. We will first present a few straightforward hypotheses for a model of dynamic development of brain and behavior based on these common growth patterns. Then we will explicate the model, outline the evidence for it, describe guidelines for doing research on dynamic growth, and sketch the more general theory of dynamic skill development.

II. Model of Concurrent Nonlinear Dynamic Growth in Brain and Behavior

Both brain activity and optimal cognitive functioning develop in fits and starts, as shown in Figure 1. Contrary to standard assumptions, growth is not linear or even monotonic, but instead speeds up periodically and then slows down or falls, showing spurts, plateaus, and drops, not smooth change (Fischer & Silvern, 1985; Rakic, et al., 1986; Thatcher, 1994). For many types of growth, the spurts and drops may be disorderly rather than systematic, because dynamic systems often produce numerous fluctuations when there are many different factors affecting growth.

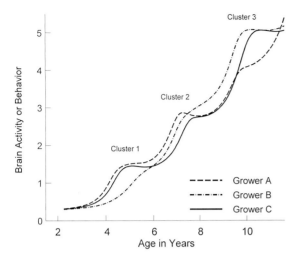

Figure 1 Development of three "independent" growers showing parallel, concurrent growth. These three growth curves were produced by a nonlinear, dynamic, hierarchical mathematical model based on assumptions that the three growers are mostly independent, with only weak links (Fischer & Rose, 1994; van Geert, 1994b, chap. 8). Their growth processes as well as the long-term effects of their weak links produce similarities in growth curves A, B, and C, including three clusters of spurts.

For growth of brain activity and development of cognition as well as emotion (Fischer, Shaver, & Carnochan, 1990), however, the spurts and drops are remarkably systematic. They do not occur in a disorderly fashion but instead seem to group together to form clusters of discontinuous changes at particular age periods, as illustrated in Figure 1. Based on a broad array of evidence, we hypothesize that there is a specific sequence of such clusters of discontinuities in brain and behavior development (Fischer & Rose, 1994).

PROPOSITION 1: BRAIN/BEHAVIOR GROWTH CLUSTERS. *Development of brain activity and behavior moves through a sequence of major reorganizations called levels, each marked by a cluster of spurts, drops, and other discontinuities.*

Brain, cognitive, and emotional development move through a systematic, predictable series of clusters of discontinuities, reflecting basic growth processes of brain and behavior. We will describe the series of changes and a model of the brain and cognitive processes that produce them.

Because developmental processes are multiply determined and dynamic, growth patterns across behaviors and brain characteristics are never identical, with large variability in the shapes of the curves and the ages of discontinuities. At the same time, the dynamics include regulatory processes that produce families of curves with important regularities. Evidence to date indicates that growth curves for behavioral and brain

development show strong regularities in the form of clusters of concurrent discontinuities, as illustrated in Figure 1. The three independent (weakly linked) growers there develop through three such concurrent clusters at approximately 4–5, 6–7, and 9–11 years. These growth curves were produced by a nonlinear dynamic mathematical model of cognitive growth based on the dynamic skill theory of development (Fischer et al., 1993; van Geert, 1994a, Chap. 8). In general, a grower is any characteristic of brain or behavior that shows systematic change with age or some other index of development. In our model, a grower is a skill or brain activity that shows logistic growth and simultaneously has dynamic, weak links to other growers that include prerequisite relations, competition, and support between growers. Although Figure 1 is based on a mathematical model, the growth curves there look remarkably similar to a number of empirical growth curves, as we will illustrate.

PROPOSITION 2: CONCURRENCE OF INDEPENDENT GROWERS. *Concurrent discontinuities in growth occur commonly, even when developing behaviors and brain activities are largely independent. Dynamic properties of the growing organism produce concurrent changes in many independent systems.*

A metaphor for development helps to illuminate how these clusters occur. A person normally grows along multiple independent strands in a developmental web, as shown in Figure 2. Even though the strands are mostly independent, they can show clusters of spurts, such as the concurrent discontinuities marked by the box in Figure 2. Discontinuities are evidenced

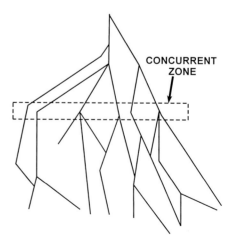

Figure 2 A web of development showing concurrent discontinuities along separate developmental strands. In this developmental web, separate developmental strands show discontinuities (branching or changes in direction) within a common zone of concurrence.

by changes in direction or branching. Dynamic growth regulation processes produce such discontinuities across diverse, largely independent domains or strands.

The relative independence of growth curves is also illustrated in Figure 3 by a close-up view of the three growers that show clusters of discontinuities in Figure 1. When small portions of the three growth curves are viewed up close, long-term clusters become less salient and the independence of the growers becomes evident. Most research reflects the short-term, close-up view in Figure 3 rather than the long-term, distanced view of Figure 1. When viewed up close, many concurrent growth curves show substantial independence, with (weak) linkages being evident only in the longer view.

What is the significance of these clusters of discontinuities? An inference that many researchers wish to draw, in our experience, is that a cluster indicates some single underlying mechanism, such as development of a brain module that controls all the changing growers. The evidence does not support such a single-process explanation, however. By most criteria, growers that cluster are independent of each other (Bidell & Fischer, 1992; Fischer, 1980; Fischer & Rose, 1994; Flavell, 1982; Rakic et al., 1986). Dynamic organismic regulatory processes, as specified by skill theory, can produce such clusters of discontinuities among independent growers.

The concurrence in mostly independent growers arises from the dynamics of growth, not from a single common cognitive or neural process. Many theories of

cognitive development assume that a single mechanism of short-term or working memory serves as a bottleneck that limits all development (Case, 1985; Halford, 1987; Pascual-Leone, 1970). No such mechanism is needed, however, to explain concurrent spurts or drops in development of brain and behavior. For example, rhesus monkeys show concurrent spurts and later drops in synaptic density across diverse cortical regions in the early postnatal period, despite the separation and relative independence of the regions (Rakic et al., 1986). There are many different processes that can produce concurrent discontinuities, and inferences about the meaning of concurrence require both deliberate investigation of growth under diverse assessment conditions and careful mathematical modeling of the processes. Fischer and Farrar (1987) describe some guidelines for investigating relations between developmental discontinuities in order to disentangle various processes that can produce concurrent discontinuities.

Indeed, contrary to common assumptions, concurrence is not at all contradictory with localization and domain specificity, but instead understanding the processes underlying concurrent discontinuities demands analysis of the localization of brain functions and the domain specificity of behaviors. By most criteria, distinct brain activities are localized in different regions of cortex or other brain structures while at the same time they show concurrent discontinuities. Likewise, actions or thoughts are domain-specific and task-specific (Fischer, 1980) even while they show concurrent discontinuities, as illustrated in Figure 2.

PROPOSITION 3: DOMAIN SPECIFICITY AND LOCALIZATION OF GROWERS.   *Developing behaviors and brain activities that undergo concurrent discontinuities are often independent by other criteria, belonging to different domains or strands and localized in different brain regions. Relations between such growers can only be understood through careful analysis of domain specificity of behaviors and localization of brain functions, as well as concurrence of growth functions.*

Behaviors typically involve parallel concurrent distributed brain processes with localization in several brain regions. When two behaviors show common discontinuities at a given age, such as spurts at 8 months of age, they will often belong to distinct domains, such as spatial versus verbal skills, and involve different brain regions, such as parietal and temporal cortices. For example, infants usually show spurts in several spatial skills at about 8 months, as reflected in Piaget's (1937/1954) object-permanence tasks and other spatial tasks (Campos & Bertenthal, 1987); at about the same age they also demonstrate spurts in vocal imitation

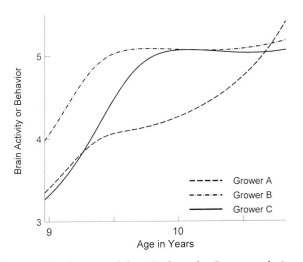

Figure 3 Development of three "independent" growers during a relatively short developmental period. These three growers seem to show vastly different growth curves even though they reflect a cluster of spurts at 9 to 10 years of age. Figure 1 provides a more long-term perspective on these curves.

skills (McCall, 1979; Petitto & Marentette, 1991; Uzgiris, 1976). That is, at roughly 8 months, many infants begin to search skillfully for objects hidden successively in different places, and they begin to expressly imitate simple sounds (intonation contours and syllables) made by their care-givers.

Although these two sets of skills show spurts at the same approximate age, they involve distinct domains and different brain regions. Bell and Fox (1994) have demonstrated that when infants show a spurt in search skills at 8 months, they simultaneously show a spurt in relative power in frontal cortex as measured by electroencephalogram (EEG), as well as increases in frontal–occipital coherence. Changes in most other cortical regions do not relate to the infants' changing search skills, and changes in other skill domains, such as vocal imitation, do not seem to relate to frontal–occipital changes. Object search and vocal imitation belong to different domains (McCall, Eichorn, & Hogarty, 1987; Uzgiris, 1976) and different neural regions (Mills, Coffey-Corina, & Neville, 1994; Petitto & Marentette, 1991; Yakovlev & Lecours, 1967).

How can the combination of concurrence of discontinuities with independence of growth functions be explained? A strong possibility is that similar growth processes occur across independent developmental domains or strands, such as concurrent emergence of a new kind of behavioral control system and neural network in each domain or strand.

PROPOSITION 4: EMERGENCE OF NEW NEURAL NETWORKS AND BEHAVIORAL CONTROL SYSTEMS. *Each new developmental level of behavior marks the emergence of a new kind of behavioral control system, which is supported by growth of a new type of neural network across diverse brain regions. This type of network facilitates construction of control systems at the new level. Similar (but independent) new networks and control systems emerge concurrently in different brain regions and skill domains, and are reflected in clusters of discontinuities in brain growth and cognitive development.*

After the new networks emerge, they are then gradually tuned to form efficient neural and cognitive control systems at the new level. After a lengthy period of consolidation of a network/control system, another new type of network/control system begins to grow for the next developmental level, and so another cluster of discontinuities begins.

PROPOSITION 5: CYCLES OF SUCCESSIVE CLUSTERS OF DISCONTINUITIES. *Development moves through cycles of successive coordinations among simpler networks and control systems to form more complex ones. There are thus a series of clusters of discontinuities reflecting the emergence of*

each new type of control system and network. These cycles have some of the properties of stages, although they arise from dynamic properties and are therefore much more variable than classic characterizations of developmental stages (Fischer et al., 1993; Fischer, Pipp, & Bullock, 1984; van Geert, 1994b). Each cluster of discontinuities is called a level. In addition, the levels form groups called tiers, which reflect higher-order recurring cycles of growth.

The cycles of network growth can arise from many different neural processes, including concurrent growth and pruning of synapses across brain areas during infancy and early childhood (Huttenlocher, 1994; Rakic et al., 1986), myelination of neurons to produce faster neural impulses and thus allow greater coordination (Benes, 1994; Case, 1992; Yakovlev & Lecours, 1967), and other mechanisms that support faster or more effective communication among neural regions. Unlike conventional notions of stage, the cycles do not involve all-or-none changes, occurring everywhere at once. Instead there is a cascade of changes that move through brain areas systematically and cyclically (Thatcher, 1994), as we will describe.

III. Levels and Tiers in Development of Behavior and Brain

Evidence for clusters of discontinuities in behavior and brain development indicates that 13 successive levels develop between birth and 30 years of age, as shown in Table 1. After outlining the levels and the higher-order cycles called tiers, we will review the evidence for discontinuities.

The ages in Table 1 mark the emergence of each level—the time when a person can first control a number of skills at that level and, by hypothesis, the time when a new kind of neural network is emerging in diverse brain regions. Of course, there is variation across individuals and domains in exact age of emergence. Dynamic skill theory provides a framework for describing the structures of skills (control systems) in any task domain (Fischer, 1980) and the conditions and designs for detecting clusters of discontinuities (Fischer et al., 1993; Fischer & Farrar, 1987). The skill structures form a developmental scale of control systems for coordination of increasingly complex sources of variation in behavior.

Developmental changes can be described in three different grains of detail. At the finest grain, skills develop through a sequence of small, microdevelopmental steps, taking place across relatively short time intervals. Skill theory provides a set of rules for predicting and explaining these small steps in skill coordination

Table 1 Levels of Development of Behavior and Brain

Level	Tier				Age[a]
	Reflex	Sensorimotor	Representational	Abstract	
Rf1: Single Reflexes	$\begin{bmatrix} A \end{bmatrix}$ or $\begin{bmatrix} B \end{bmatrix}$				3–4 wk
Rf2: Reflex Mappings	$\begin{bmatrix} A \text{ —— } B \end{bmatrix}$				7–8
Rf3: Reflex Systems	$\begin{bmatrix} A^E_F \longleftrightarrow B^E_F \end{bmatrix}$				10–11
Rf4/Sm1: Single Sensorimotor Actions	$\begin{bmatrix} A^E_F \longleftrightarrow B^E_F \\ \Updownarrow \\ C^G_H \longleftrightarrow D^G_H \end{bmatrix} \equiv \begin{bmatrix} \mathbf{I} \end{bmatrix}$				15–17
Sm2: Sensorimotor Mappings		$\begin{bmatrix} \mathbf{I} \text{ —— } \mathbf{J} \end{bmatrix}$			7–8 mo
Sm3: Sensorimotor Systems		$\begin{bmatrix} \mathbf{I}^M_N \longleftrightarrow \mathbf{J}^M_N \end{bmatrix}$			11–13
Sm4/Rp1: Single Representations		$\begin{bmatrix} \mathbf{I}^M_N \longleftrightarrow \mathbf{J}^M_N \\ {}^O_P \Updownarrow {}^O_P \\ \mathbf{K} \longleftrightarrow \mathbf{L} \end{bmatrix} \equiv \begin{bmatrix} Q \end{bmatrix}$			18–24
Rp2: Representational Mappings			$\begin{bmatrix} Q \text{ —— } R \end{bmatrix}$		3.5– 4.5 yr
Rp3: Representational Systems			$\begin{bmatrix} Q^U_V \longleftrightarrow R^U_V \end{bmatrix}$		6–7
Rp4/Ab1: Single Abstractions			$\begin{bmatrix} Q^U_V \longleftrightarrow R^U_V \\ {}^W_X \Updownarrow {}^W_X \\ S \longleftrightarrow T \end{bmatrix} \equiv \begin{bmatrix} \mathscr{Y} \end{bmatrix}$		10–12
Ab2: Abstract Mappings				$\begin{bmatrix} \mathscr{Y} \text{ —— } \mathscr{Z} \end{bmatrix}$	14–16
Ab3: Abstract Systems				$\begin{bmatrix} \mathscr{Y}^{\mathscr{C}}_{\mathscr{D}} \longleftrightarrow \mathscr{Z}^{\mathscr{C}}_{\mathscr{D}} \end{bmatrix}$	18–20
Ab4: Principles				$\begin{bmatrix} \mathscr{Y}^{\mathscr{C}}_{\mathscr{D}} \longleftrightarrow \mathscr{Z}^{\mathscr{C}}_{\mathscr{D}} \\ {}^{\mathscr{C}}_{\mathscr{D}} \Updownarrow {}^{\mathscr{C}}_{\mathscr{D}} \\ \mathscr{A}^{\mathscr{C}}_{\mathscr{D}} \longleftrightarrow \mathscr{B}^{\mathscr{C}}_{\mathscr{D}} \end{bmatrix}$	23–25

Note: In skill structures, each letter denotes a skill component, with each large letter designating a main component (set) and each subscript or superscript a subset of the main component. Plain letters designate components that are reflexes, in the sense of innate action-components. Bold letters designate sensorimotor actions, italic letters representations, and script letters abstractions. Lines connecting sets designate relations forming a mapping, single-line arrows designate relations forming a system, and double-line arrows relations forming a system of systems.

[a]Ages given are modal ages at which a level first emerges according to research with middle-class American or European children. They may well differ across social groups.

and differentiation. Most steps do not involve developmental discontinuities but are simply points along a pathway of skill construction—that is, along a strand in a developmental web as in Figure 2.

Certain steps in a sequence mark the emergence of a new developmental level, a capacity to construct a new type of control system or skill. It is at these steps that clusters of discontinuities occur for behavior and brain development. As the person enters a new level, he or she shows stage-like spurts in optimal performance and concurrent discontinuities in growth of brain activity, probably reflecting cycles of growth of cortical networks. Assessment of fine-grained steps greatly facilitates detection of discontinuities, because it provides tools for detection of amount and speed of change at a grain finer than levels themselves.

At the broadest grain, levels group into cycles called tiers, which involve a series of four successive levels, as shown in Table 1. Tiers involve cycles of growth in skill complexity, from single units, to mappings, to systems, and finally, to systems of systems. With the fourth level of systems of systems, a radically new type of unit for controlling behavior emerges—reflexes, actions, representations, or abstractions, respectively. Consequently, development of the first level of a new tier is an especially strong type of discontinuity, evident in radical changes in both behavior and brain development. For example, the emergence of the representational tier late in the second year produces the onset of complex language and a host of other changes that radically transform children's behavior. Because a new tier involves building a new kind of unit through melding together systems of systems, there is a need for neural glue to cement the components together. This glue seems to be provided by the frontal cortex, which plays a major role in holding components on line so that they can be coordinated. The beginning of each new tier is marked, we hypothesize, by a large surge in EEG relative power in the frontal area, reflecting strong frontal participation in formation of the new tier. We expect that cycles of other kinds of cortical change are evident for each tier as well, and we will present some hypotheses about such cycles.

One task of brain–behavior research is to determine how tiers and levels connect with cycles of brain change, but before we present our model of these cycles, we will review briefly the evidence for clusters of discontinuties at 13 levels of development.

A. Evidence for Levels in Behavior Development

For all 13 levels in Table 1, there is evidence for clusters of discontinuities in development of action, thought, and emotion. Evidence is reviewed by Fischer and Rose (1994), more extensively by Fischer and Silvern (1985), and by Fischer and Hogan (1989) for infancy. For all levels, there is evidence of the emergence of new capacities and clusters of discontinuities in growth curves at approximately the ages listed in Table 1. Of course, the exact ages and the shapes of the growth curves vary dynamically as a result of the plethora of factors contributing to behavior development.

Although there is supportive evidence for every level, the evidence is especially strong for the fourth through twelfth levels, Sm1 through Ab3, because there has been much more relevant research between 3 months and 20 years of age than for earlier or later ages. Figure 4 shows discontinuities at three points in infancy, from an analysis by McCall, Eichorn, and Hogarty (1977), using data from the Berkeley Growth Study. Longitudinal test performance demonstrated marked drops in stability at approximately 8, 13, and 21 months of age; the authors interpret the rise from low stability at 4 months as evidence for another discontinuity. Drops in stability are an index of clusters of discontinuities in growth (Fischer et al., 1984). Many other studies have shown spurts in performance and/or drops in stability at these approximate ages for most infants (for example, Bell & Fox, 1994; Corrigan, 1983; Pipp, Fischer, & Jennings, 1987; Reznick & Goldfield, 1992; Uzgiris, 1976).

The levels during childhood and adolescence are illustrated by data from a study of the development of reflective judgment in Figure 5 (Kitchener, Lynch, Fischer, & Wood, 1993). Adolescents and young adults

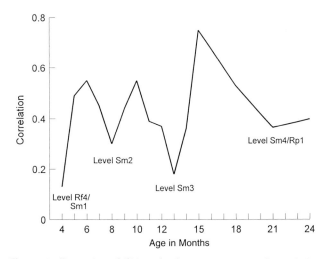

Figure 4 Drops in stabilities of infant test scores in the Berkeley Growth Study. Infants evidenced drops in stability at approximately 8, 13, and 21 months, as well as a major increase in stability at 4–5 months. These discontinuities mark the four developmental levels indicated on the graphs. This graph shows longitudinal data for girls as reported by McCall et al. (1977).

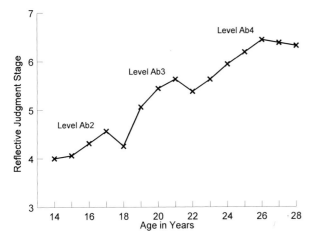

Figure 5 Spurts in development of reflective judgment. Growth cycles (marked by spurts) occurred at approximately ages 14–17, 18–21, and 22–26 years, marking three levels in the development of abstractions. Data are from a study of American youth in Denver by Kitchener et al. (1993).

were asked how to deal with complex, ill-defined knowledge dilemmas, such as determining whether chemical additives to food are helpful or harmful. The complexity of their arguments fell into seven levels of development, as documented in earlier research by Kitchener and King (1990). (Kitchener and King use the word "stages" instead of "levels," but the research indicates that the sequence fits the criteria outlined here for levels.) The sophistication of people's arguments showed general increases in level between 14 and 28 years, with spurts centered at approximately 16, 20, and 25 years of age. Many other studies have shown similar discontinuities in performance at similar ages across diverse domains (Fischer & Kennedy, 1996; Harter & Monsour, 1992; Kennedy, 1994; Lamborn, Fischer, & Pipp, 1994; Martarano, 1977; Moshman & Franks, 1986).

It is important *not* to take these findings to mean that all behaviors show developmental discontinuities at these ages. The levels are evident primarily for behaviors (a) that increase in complexity with development and (b) that are measured under assessment conditions that support optimal performance (at the upper limit of a person's capacity).

B. Evidence for Levels in Brain Development

There is also substantial evidence for successive discontinuities for developmental levels in brain growth, although the evidence is less extensive than for behavior development. Many of the findings about discontinuities, especially for brain activity, head growth, and synaptic density, are reviewed in Fischer and Rose (1994). Although scores of studies contribute relevant

evidence, most of them do not sample age often enough to provide precise descriptions of growth functions. The several studies with appropriate age sampling uniformly show cyclicity in brain growth.

Combining all these data sources, we find evidence for discontinuities associated with the first twelve levels from Table 1. For the thirteenth level, we have not yet found any appropriate data on brain growth. Like most body organs, the brain grows in fits and starts (Lampl & Emde, 1983; Lampl et al., 1992; Thatcher, 1994; Yakovlev & Lecours, 1967), and those discontinuities generally match the ages for the first twelve levels listed in Table 1. Of course, for individual children, the fits and starts vary around the particular ages listed, and different brain regions and characteristics show different growth functions and different exact ages for discontinuities.

For very early infancy, the few relevant studies support the existence of the levels. For example, Fischer and Rose (1994) found that head circumference in American infants measured during routine medical visits showed spurts during four successive age periods—at approximately 3–4, 7–8, 10–11, and 15–18 weeks of age.[1] Head circumference is not the best measure of brain growth, because it is not a direct measure of a brain property and because growth changes are small relative to error of measurement. For early infancy, however, measurement problems are less severe because the amount of growth is so large.

For later infancy the brain data are much more substantial, showing discontinuities clustered at ages similar to those for cognitive development: approximately 3–4, 6–8, and 11–13 months, and 2 years (Bell & Fox, 1994; Chugani & Phelps, 1986; Hagne, Persson, Magnusson, & Petersén, 1973; Ohtahara, 1981). Figure 6 shows spurts at approximately 4, 8, and 12 months of age in development of relative power for occipital EEG in a study of Japanese children (Mizuno, Yamauchi, Watanabe, Komatsushiro, Takagi, Iinuma, et al., 1970).

During childhood and adolescence, discontinuities in brain growth cluster at approximately 2, 4, 7, 11, 15, and 20 years (Chugani, Phelps, & Mazziotta, 1987; Dustman & Beck, 1969; Hartley & Thomas, 1993; Somsen & Klooster, 1994; Stauder, Molenaar, & van der Molen, 1993; Thatcher, 1994; see also Huttenlocher, 1994). A classic study of relative power in the EEG in Figure 7 shows spurts at approximately 2, 4, 8, 12, 15, and 19 years (Hudspeth & Pribram, 1992; John, 1977; Matousek & Petersén, 1973). Thatcher (1994) reported discontinuities at 3–4, 5–7, and 9–10 years of age, when

---

[1] These data were collected by Bonnie Camp of the University of Colorado Health Sciences Center, who kindly shared them with us.

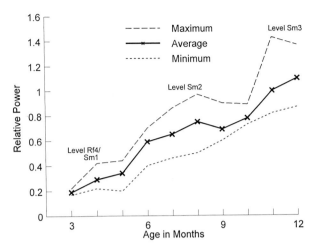

Figure 6 Development of relative power in occipital EEG in infants. Relative power is the ratio of power for the band from 7.17 to 10.3 Hz to power for the band from 2.4 to 3.46 Hz. Growth cycles (marked by spurts) occurred at approximately ages 3–5, 6–8, and 9–12 months, marking three developmental levels. Data are from a study of Japanese infants by Mizuno et al. (1970).

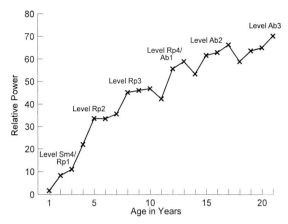

Figure 7 Development of relative power in alpha EEG in occipital-parietal (O-P) area in childhood and adolescence. Relative power is the percentage of amplitude in microvolts of absolute energy in the alpha band divided by the sum of the amplitudes in all bands. Growth spurts occurred at approximately ages 1–2, 3–5, 6–10, 11–13, 14–17, and 18–21 years, indicating six successive developmental levels. Data are for Swedish subjects and were originally reported by Matousek and Petersén (1973) and subsequently by John (1977).

the pattern of cyclical variation in coherence shifts in what he suggests are cusp catastrophes (van der Maas & Molenaar, 1992). The rate and amplitude of oscillation in coherence shifts at each of these ages, and thus, by hypothesis, at the ages for other levels as well.

C. A Model of Brain–Behavior Relations for Levels and Tiers

In addition to the series of clusters of discontinuities, brain development seems to show more detailed cycles of change in specific brain regions and functions; these cycles relate to both developmental tiers and levels (Fischer & Rose, 1994). At the broadest grain, shifts between tiers appear to be marked by a long-term cycle of frontal EEG power growth. Within each tier, movement from one level to the next seems to involve spurts in power over most cortical areas, with especially strong growth in a different cortical region for each level. Within each level, cortical coherence seems to show a systematic growth cycle, with distinct patterns for left and right hemispheres.

A fundamental function of the frontal cortex is to sustain information over time about some activity, even while other activities are occurring (Case, 1992; Goldman-Rakic, 1986; Pennington, 1994). This function is exactly what is required for coordinating two activities—taking them from independence or competition to co-occurrence (being held on line at the same time) and then coordination, which is the basic process for developing from one level to the next.

The frontal cortex may be involved in most major cognitive–developmental advances, as suggested by the Thatcher (1991, 1994) research on development of coherence in the EEG. In his large study of brain-activity development, Thatcher found that the frontal cortex was involved in over 90 percent of the coherence patterns that showed systematic development between birth and 20 years. No other cortical area was so prominent. He inferred that the frontal area leads most brain development, in some sense guiding or directing the formation of cortical network connections.

Examining a more specific developmental achievement, Bell and Fox (1994) found frontal involvement in development of the ability to search for hidden objects (often called "object permanence"). When 8-month-olds showed a spurt in this search ability, they also showed a spurt in frontal power as well as increased coherence between the frontal and occipital areas. These findings suggest an increased capacity for the frontal area to hold spatial information online from the occipital area.

The apparent specialization of the frontal cortex for holding information on line, which is so central to coordination of components, seems to make it pivotal in many large-scale developmental changes. We hypothesize that the frontal cortex provides the foundation for the largest developmental reorganization—the emergence of a new tier—which produces a new kind of unit of activity, such as the emergence of representation and complex language at about 2 years, and the emergence of abstractions at about 10 years.

HYPOTHESIS A: ROLE OF FRONTAL CORTEX IN DEVELOPMENTAL TIERS AND LEVELS.   The frontal cortex plays a central role in cementing together skill systems to form a new unit at the beginning of a new tier. This role is reflected in an increase in frontal EEG power with the transition to a new tier. In addition, emergence of each new developmental level within a tier is marked by a cluster of discontinuities in cortical connections as measured by EEG coherence, with most of these discontinuities involving connections between frontal and other cortical areas. This cluster reflects formation of the new kind of neural network for each level.

More specific cycles of cortical growth also characterize development, as diagrammed in Table 2. The growth cycle characteristic of a tier shows systematic changes in the location and extent of EEG power at each successive level in the tier. There is also a second growth cycle characteristic of a level, in which the connectivity of cortical regions cycles through specific locations and then repeats the cycle for every level. The shift between levels is also marked by a general change in the pattern of cycling (period and amplitude) for many regions. The model of these cycles is based primarily on findings from the two largest, most relevant studies of development of human EEG—the classic Swedish investigation by Matousek and Petersén (1973; Hudspeth & Pribram, 1992; John, 1977) and Thatcher's (1991, 1994) more recent American investigation. Both of these studies assessed a very wide age range with cross-sectional assessment at annual increments.

HYPOTHESIS B: CYCLE OF EEG POWER FOR EACH TIER. The start of a new tier is marked by a spurt in frontal EEG power, followed by spurts in other areas moving generally from the back to the front of the brain. Each level is marked by a cluster of spurts across areas and an especially strong spurt in one area: first the occipital-parietal, followed by the temporal, then the central, and finally the frontal again as another tier emerges.

The cycle is outlined in Table 2, and Figure 8 shows an example of it for the representational and abstract tiers based on the Hudspeth and Pribram (1992) reanalysis of the data of the Swedish study. They combined power across the four EEG frequency bands to derive a single growth index for each cortical region. Just at the age when one tier ended and a new tier began (at about 1 to 1½ years for the representational tier and 9 years for the abstract tier), relative EEG power spurted in the frontal-temporal area. Then a little later, at the age when the tier was fully under way (at about 2 and 11 years, respectively), there was an unusually

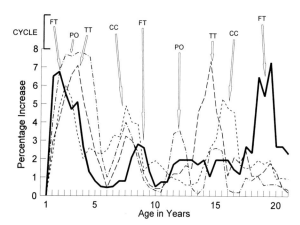

Figure 8 Growth cycle for representational and abstract tiers of relative EEG power across cortical regions. The end of one developmental tier and the beginning of the next is marked by a spurt in frontal-temporal power, as shown by the dark solid line. Each developmental level within a tier involves a cluster of spurts as well as a cycle in the size of the spurt from back to front: parietal-occipital (PO) to temporal-temporal (TT) to central-central (CC) to frontal-temporal (FT). The cyclical components are marked at the top of the figure. Data are from Hudspeth and Pribram's reanalysis of the Matousek and Petersén data by combining data across the four frequency bands to create a single growth index. They also estimated half-year EEG levels. Data are plotted as change scores, as in the original research report.

large power spurt in the occipital-parietal region at the back of the cortex, accompanied as well by spurts in other areas. As children progressed through the levels of each tier, power growth gradually moved from the occipital-parietal (Level 1 in Table 2) forward to the temporal (Level 2) and central (Level 3) areas. The fourth level brought the return of a frontal-temporal spurt with the end of one tier and the beginning of another (recall that the last level of one tier is the first level of the next, as shown in Table 1). Although Hudspeth and Pribram have data for only the ages of the representational and abstract tiers, we predict that the pattern will occur for the reflex and sensorimotor tiers as well. In those cases, the first signs of frontal-temporal followed by occipital-parietal spurts will occur at approximately 2–4 weeks and 3 months, respectively.

The data in the Swedish study did not distinguish between left and right hemispheres, and it was therefore not possible to analyze hemispheric differences, which would surely be expected. For example, there may be more right frontal and left occipital–parietal growth in power at the beginning of a tier (see Segalowitz, 1994). The Swedish study also did not distinguish between males and females, and there are probably important gender differences in the details of the cycle.

Table 2   Model of How Skill Levels in a Tier Relate to EEG Development

Level	Skill structure	Hemisphere coherence cycle[a]	Front-to-back power spurt cycle[b]
1. Single sets	[A] or [B]	Right global to local ⇓ Left local to global ⇓ Both global ⇓	Frontal spurt ⇓ Spurts over broad area, especially occipital-parietal ⇓
2. Mappings	[A — B]	Right global to local ⇓ Left local to global ⇓ Both global ⇓	Spurts over broad area, especially temporal ⇓
3. Systems	[$A^E_F \longleftrightarrow B^E_F$]	Right global to local ⇓ Left local to global ⇓ Both global ⇓	Spurts over broad area, especially central ⇓
4. Systems of systems	[$A^E_F \longleftrightarrow B^E_F$ ⇕ $C^G_H \longleftrightarrow D^G_H$]	Right global to local ⇓ Left local to global ⇓ Both global	Frontal spurt ⇓ Spurts over broad area, especially occipital-parietal

[a]Based on Thatcher's findings as described in his chapter, coherence changes cycle systematically through the hemispheres. One cycle of these changes is hypothesized to involve movement through one developmental level or stage.

[b]Based on the analyses of Hudspeth and Pribram (1992; John, 1977; Matousek & Petersén, 1973), EEG power seems to spurt in the frontal area at the very beginning of a new tier (emergence of actions, representations, or abstracts in Table 1). Then power spurts over broad areas of the cortex for each level. The highest spurts for each level tend to move from back to front as a child develops through the four levels.

HYPOTHESIS C: CYCLE OF GROWTH AND CORTICAL CONNECTIVITY FOR EACH LEVEL. Each skill level is marked by both a discontinuity in the nature of the cortical connection and a cycle of growth in connections between cortical areas, as reflected in changes in EEG coherence (Thatcher, 1994). Coherence for a pair of cortical regions typically oscillates in a regular fashion, and that pattern of oscillation shifts with the emergence of a new level, showing changes in period and amplitude. At the same time, coherence growth also cycles systematically through a series of cortical regions. At the start of the transition to a new level, both cortexes show growth of long-distance, global connections, which mostly tie frontal with occipital and parietal cortex. Then, growth sites in the right hemisphere move from global, long-distance connections to local, adjacent ones. Next, growth sites in the left hemisphere move from local to global connections. Finally, both hemispheres again show growth of long-distance connections as another new level emerges.

Table 2 shows how this cycle repeats across the four levels in a tier. In general at each level, connectivity in the right hemisphere contracts during the cycle, moving from distant connections to local ones (from integration to differentiation, in Thatcher's terms). Connectivity in the left hemisphere expands, moving from local connections to distant ones (from differentiation to integration).

This hypothesized cycle is conceptually compelling because it provides an appropriate mechanism for the growth of new neural networks at each developmental level. The point of maximal growth moves systematically through cortical regions until networks all around the cortex are encompassed. This is how there can be independent neural networks that show concurrent growth spurts in the same age period.

Also, Thatcher's (1994) data for ages of the cycles correspond reasonably well with the ages for three of the developmental levels inferred from behavior development and EEG power growth: approximately 4, 7, and 10 years. Of course, further research will be required to replicate the cycle beyond Thatcher's study and to determine how well the cycles correspond to skill levels. Research will need to address several key questions besides replication. The skill framework requires two levels and cycles in the preschool years (Levels Rp1 and 2 emerging at approximately ages 2 and 4 years). Thatcher's current data are ambiguous with respect to these two levels, perhaps because detection requires more than one assessment per year. In addition, a similar cycle is predicted to occur for every level in Table 1, including several in the first two years and two in late adolescence and early adulthood, which existing data do not address.

In addition to the general growth cycles in Table 2, there are of course developments specific to domains and ages and not common across levels or tiers. For example, in Thatcher's study, coherence for the cortical areas most centrally involved in language (the regions that include Broca's and Wernicke's areas) demonstrated dramatic increases in later infancy and the early preschool years, both within and between hemispheres (Greenfield, 1991; Thatcher, 1991, 1992). These are the ages when children's language is developing through some of the most dramatic spurts in all of human development. Also, in early development, there may be more involvement of nonfrontal areas than in later development, in that early levels involve more overt actions and perceptions, whereas later levels involve more internal, abstract thinking, which presumably requires greater frontal involvement. Data from the Swedish study indicate that frontal power shows especially prominent growth in adolescence (Hudspeth & Pribram, 1992). Similarly, many developments specific to domains and ages are to be expected. Localization and specificity of function work with the general growth cycles, not in opposition to them.

IV. A Framework for Developmental Research: Control Systems Involving Both Brain and Behavior

Developmental regularities can be found at several levels of analysis: in different structures or functions of the brain and in constituent elements of behavior. But in analyzing these developmental regularities, it is important to avoid a common mistake. The regularities that we have described for brain and behavior development do not apply to all developing characteristics of brain and behavior. On the contrary, the same developmental regularities will not be found everywhere. Development has many different shapes! Some behaviors and brain characteristics show one set of developmental regularities, such as continuous growth, and others show another set of developmental regularities, such as series of discontinuities.

The lesson of these differences in regularities is to search for the kinds of growth patterns one seeks in the places they are most likely to be found. Effective research should be built on a developmental framework that encompasses variations in growth patterns. The dynamic skill model is designed to deal with a wide array of kinds of growth patterns and to provide concepts and methods for determining where to find them. Research to test or elaborate upon the models and hypotheses we have put forth must be designed to take account of these issues of variability, or it is doomed to fail.

Our framework for understanding different shapes of development is based on the hypothesis that many major developmental changes involve the coordination of lower-order components into higher-order control systems (Schore, 1994; Thelen & Smith, 1994; van Geert, 1994b). We call these control systems "dynamic skills" (Fischer et al., 1993; Fischer & Rose, 1994; Fischer, Kenny, & Pip, 1990). The components of these control systems are *both* neurological and behavioral, for the obvious reason that our brains do not function autonomously from behavior. Moreover, they are also contextual, with elements of the body and the immediate perceived context participating directly in the control systems. Of course, brains function in the service of producing a behavior in a context, and different behaviors and contexts organize brain functioning differently. What brings brain, behavior, and context together is the momentary purpose toward which they are directed. This purpose is expressed through the construction of a control system (dynamic skill) from a repertoire of preexisting skills. In the next moment, a different goal will require the construction of a different or modified control system.

Moment by moment we construct, modify, and elaborate control systems, and moment by moment our neurological states change as our behavior varies. The context and goal of the moment has dramatic effects on the nature and complexity of our control systems. Effective research on development, especially research on relations between brain and behavior, must deal directly with the facts of variation. Research must be designed to deal with the wide range of shapes of development that occur for different characteristics of brain and behavior and under different assessment conditions.

A. Mechanisms of Variation and Developmental Range

The maturity or complexity of people's behavior and their neurological functioning varies widely and systematically from moment to moment and across contexts and states. A 4-year-old boy watches his preschool teacher acting out a pretend story with dolls: The patient doll tells the doctor doll he has a cold, and the doctor doll examines him and gives him medicine to make him feel better. The boy promptly acts out a similar story, demonstrating understanding of the roles of doctor and patient in interaction.

Ten minutes later, the teacher asks the boy to show her the best story he can about a doctor and a patient, like the one he did before. Instead of producing the complex story he did earlier, however, he produces a much simpler story, making the doctor doll simply walk around the doctor's office carrying a thermometer, with no interaction between doctor and patient. Repeated efforts to get him to show his "best story" produce similar results.

Is the boy capable of acting out a doctor–patient interaction, or is he not? Different contexts for assessment produce radically different, replicable results. People show different levels of competence under different conditions, even when the conditions assess the same content domain, such as acting out a story about a doctor and a patient.

As this and many other possible examples demonstrate, the developmental level of behavior varies with assessment context, state of arousal, emotional state, and goal, just to name a few of the most obvious sources of variation. Some researchers have argued that these variations demonstrate an absence of general developmental stages (Brainerd, 1978; Flavell, 1982; Thelen & Fogel, 1989), but these arguments are flawed because they overlook the order in the variability. The organization of behavior develops systemati-

cally, and it also varies from moment to moment. These facts are contradictory only for overly simple concepts of stage and variation. Real behaviors—and real neural networks—function not at a single level but in a range or zone (Brown & Reeve, 1987; Bullock, Carpenter, & Grossberg, 1991; Fischer et al., 1993; Grossberg, 1987b). Research on developmental levels must take into account the existence of this range, and focus on the parts of the variation that show stage-like characteristics.

Our framework begins with the assumption that brain and behavior develop through control systems that integrate person and context together. From the behavioral side, we use the concept of skill to characterize control systems because in English usage, skill suggests a combination of person and context (Bruner, 1973; Fischer, 1980). A skill is a characteristic neither of a person nor of a context, but of a person-in-a-context, and likewise a neural network includes the context as part of its functioning. People (children and adults) function at different skill levels for different tasks, states, and situations, and under certain conditions their development through a level will show stage-like properties.

One of the principles of order underlying the variability is what we call *developmental range*, the difference between a person's optimal and functional levels. The concept both specifies an important dimension of variability in brain and behavior development, and provides a set of tools for analyzing the shapes of developmental functions. Optimal-level behaviors typically demonstrate clusters of discontinuities in their growth functions at the ages listed in Table 1, while functional-level behaviors typically show no such discontinuities (Fischer et al., 1984).

Figure 9 illustrates this difference in a study of development of concepts of self-in-relationships in Seoul, Korea (Fischer & Kennedy, 1996; Kennedy, 1994). Adolescents and young adults were interviewed about how they conceived themselves in their important relationships (with their mother, father, teacher, best friend, sibling, and so forth). Under a low-support condition that assessed functional level, they described what they were like in those relationships and answered some general questions about how their various conceptions of themselves related to each other. Under a high-support condition that assessed optimal level, the same adolescents used a technique to help themselves keep in mind their various conceptions and relate them to each other: They wrote each self-description on a small piece of paper, placed all the papers in a self-diagram, and then answered a series of structured questions about the diagram.

These adolescents showed vastly different developmental patterns for optimal and functional levels. The

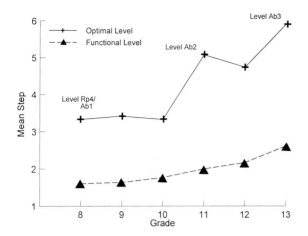

Figure 9 Development of conceptions of self-in-relationships in adolescents in Seoul, Korea. Optimal-level growth shows spurts for two developmental levels, while functional-level growth shows no such spurts, only slow gradual increase.

curve for optimal level showed much higher performance as well as two spurts in level, one for abstract mappings and a second for abstract systems. On the other hand, the curve for functional level showed much lower performance and no discontinuities; indeed, there was only modest evidence of any improvement over the 6 year period. The different conditions thus produced radically different conclusions about the nature of development of self-conceptions in Korean adolescents. A focus on the optimal condition leads to the conclusion that Korean adolescents show sophisticated self-understanding and that it includes two successive spurts in performance. A focus on the functional condition leads to the conclusion that Korean adolescents have unsophisticated self-understanding and show hardly any developmental advance between grades 8 and 13. We argue that both of these conclusions are correct, since both conditions reflect real findings about Korean adolescents' self-understandings.

The optimal level specifies the most complex skills that the person can consistently control under optimal conditions, including an alert state, a familiar context, practice with the task, contextual support for high-level performance, and the absence of interfering conditions such as conflicting emotions. The 4-year-old boy showed his optimal level for doctor-patient roles when his teacher primed a high-level story for him. The Korean adolescents showed their optimal level for understanding self-in-relationships when they were interviewed with a technique that supported and primed their remembering and connecting various self-concepts.

Without optimal conditions, people usually perform at lower steps on a developmental scale. Their

activities still show an upper limit, but one that is much lower than the optimal level. This limit is the functional level for the context, the highest level beyond which the person's skills do not go without optimal support. The removal of contextual support for high-level performance often causes an immediate drop to the person's functional level. Without support, the 4-year-old boy no longer produced a story about doctor-patient interaction but instead simply made a doctor doll carry around a thermometer. Without support, the Korean adolescents showed low levels of self-understanding and little evidence of development over a period of 6 years.

Reinstitution of appropriate contextual support produces a rapid jump to optimal level, and elimination of the support produces a rapid drop to functional level. A key factor in this robust phenomenon of variation is contextual priming of important elements of the task. Priming of the gist of the task often induces optimal performance, allowing a child to sustain high-level understanding. Neural networks function in the same way, with a match between external priming and internal organization producing resonance and movement to a higher level of functioning. In this way, a single neural network produces different levels of behavior depending upon context and state, in exactly the manner demonstrated by the behavioral research on developmental range (Bullock et al., 1991; Fischer et al., 1993; Grossberg, 1987b).

B. Methodological Guidelines for Research

Studying relations between brain and behavior development must take account of the wide variability of behavior as well as the complexities of measuring brain function. Much neuroscientific research places primary emphasis on measurement of neural functions and uses extremely limited assessments of behavior, even when behavior is an explicit focus of investigation. Most studies use a single behavioral task, sometimes with a few parametric variations. A single task cannot provide an adequate ruler for measuring development, and it cannot capture the variations between optimal and functional levels.

The hypothesized relations between discontinuities in development of brain and behavior require assessments that can capture the shapes of developmental functions for both brain and behavior. The designs most commonly used for developmental studies are rarely sensitive enough to allow comparison of the shapes of development or the timing of discontinuities in the two domains. Consequently, most prior developmental studies have not provided adequate data for determining the shapes of developmental functions or relating them across domains. Several articles provide good, detailed reviews of specific methods for studying developmental discontinuities (Fischer & Canfield, 1986; Fischer et al., 1984; van der Maas & Molenaar, 1992).

In general, the power of a study for detecting discontinuities and relating brain and behavioral development is enhanced by four features of research design. First, good developmental rulers are used—in particular, multiple-step assessments rather than the single tasks so popular with neuroscientists. Second, good developmental clocks are used, with the ages of subjects spread continuously and evenly across the range in which development is being measured. Third, more than one domain of skill is assessed, because performance in one task domain is no more representative of behavioral development in general than activity in one part of the cortex is representative of brain activity or neurological development in general. Fourth, assessment conditions are varied because developmental discontinuities will be found primarily under optimal conditions, and not under ordinary spontaneous assessment conditions (optimal versus functional levels). With the framework we have suggested for predicting relations between discontinuities in brain and behavioral development, it is possible to use these guidelines to design powerful studies of brain–behavior relations in development.

V. Conclusion: Detecting and Explaining Developmental Levels in Brain and Behavior

As our sketch of the 13 developmental levels indicates, each level requires a new type of control system to coordinate component skills, and each produces a cluster of discontinuities in brain and behavioral growth. Our simple proposition is that each of these levels is founded in development of a new type of control system, which is composed of both a neural network and a set of behaviors in a particular context. The key new capacity at each level is the coordination of components to form a more complex control system incorporating previous skills, and a key cortical region for that capacity for most levels is probably the frontal area, which seems to be specialized for holding information on line from various cortical regions while other activities occur.

The convergence is remarkable between the ages of brain-growth spurts evident in EEG and head-growth findings and the ages of growth spurts for cognitive and emotional developments (summarized in Table 1). These periods of growth spurts are prime candidates

for descriptive research to test for the predicted developmental levels and to begin to unravel how brain and behavior develop together. Unfortunately, almost all relevant studies have investigated either brain growth or behavior development, not both. There are hardly any studies that assess development of both brain and behavior in the same people, so most of the specific connections between brain-growth discontinuities and developmental levels still have not been tested.

An important part of research on our model of brain–behavior relations will be testing the co-occurrence of discontinuities for brain and behavior for each developmental level. According to our argument, the optimal level shifts abruptly at certain periods in development, showing stage-like change. Within some limited age periods, spurts or other discontinuities in development of both behavior and brain activity can be detected in a wide range of different domains. For example, there are spurts at approximately 8 months of age in object permanence, vocal imitation, crawling, fear of heights, EEG power in the frontal cortex, and EEG coherence between the frontal and occipital cortexes (Campos & Bertenthal, 1987; Bell & Fox, 1994; McCall et al., 1977; Mizuno et al., 1970; Schore, 1994; Seibert, Hogan, & Mundy, 1984; Uzgiris, 1976). At about 15 years, there are spurts in arithmetic concepts, judgments about the bases for knowledge, Piagetian formal-operations tasks, constructs about social relationships, conflicts about the self, EEG power in the temporal region, and EEG coherence between the frontal and occipital regions (Fischer et al., 1990; Harter & Monsour, 1992; Hudspeth & Pribram, 1992; Kitchener et al., 1993; Lamborn et al., 1994; Martarano, 1977; Thatcher, 1994).

Of course, the various spurts for emergence of a new optimal level are not instantaneous but are spread over a limited time interval, forming a cluster of changes that are similar but different. They do not all occur at exactly the same age, nor do they produce exactly the same developmental growth function. Infants, for example, do not suddenly metamorphose on the first day of their eighth month. There is only an approximate synchrony of discontinuities within a definable time interval.

Likewise, the cluster of discontinuities does not reflect a single, coherent mental mechanism or neural module like the powerful, general competences hypothesized by Piaget (1957) and Chomsky (1965). They reflect concurrent, largely independent developments of different but similar capacities to build skills at a given level of complexity. This change in capacity is not unitary, and it does not automatically eventuate in skill changes. Instead, people must take time and effort to actually build the changed skills that the capacities and networks make possible, and factors such as state and task contribute to the actual skills produced. Even when people have constructed a new skill at optimal level, they typically require optimal contextual support to produce it. Discontinuities in level are consistently evident only under optimal assessment conditions. Most conditions where researchers have traditionally assessed development are nonoptimal and produce slow, gradual, continuous growth, even when people are performing the same tasks that show discontinuities under optimal conditions.

Explaining the series of developmental levels will require new concepts beyond those currently available. It will be essential to describe the neurological components that contribute to control systems at each developmental level and to analyze how those components work together to produce an emerging behavioral level, including their network properties. We have suggested a first simple model of how these components may develop for each psychological level and tier in terms of EEG power and coherence. We have also suggested how neural networks may be coordinated to form more complex control systems (Fischer et al., 1993; Fischer & Rose, 1994). However, these models are only beginnings. At this point, the developmental framework will need to move beyond the limits of current models of cortical functioning and neural networks. To grow and learn, people must somehow organize their control systems and networks into a long series of successively more complex levels, a developmental sequence of reorganizations. Explaining these changes will require new visions of how the brain works and how neural networks are formed.

Acknowledgments

Preparation of this chapter was supported by a fellowship from the Center for Advanced Study in the Behavioral Sciences for the first author, and grants from Harvard University, the MacArthur Network on Early Childhood, Mr. and Mrs. Frederick P. Rose, and the Spencer Foundation. Portions of the chapter were adapted from Fischer and Rose (1994). The authors thank Diane Beals, Daniel Bullock, Bonnie Camp, Robbie Case, Geraldine Dawson, Eric Fischer, Jerome Kagan, Bruce Kennedy, Karen Kitchener, Peter Molenaar, A. H. Parmelee, Han van der Maas, Robert Thatcher, Paul van Geert, and Sheldon White for their contributions to the concepts and data presented.

The chapter is dedicated to the memory of the late Samuel P. Rose.

References

Bell, M. A., & Fox, N. A. (1994). Brain development over the first year of life: Relations between EEG frequency and coherence and cognitive and affective behaviors. In G. Dawson & K. W. Fischer (Eds.), *Human behavior and the developing brain* (pp. 314–345). New York: Guilford.

Benes, F. (1994). Development of the corticolimbic system. In G. Dawson & K. W. Fischer (Eds.), *Human behavior and the developing brain* (pp. 176–206). New York: Guilford.

Bidell, T. R., & Fischer, K. W. (1992). Beyond the stage debate: Action, structure, and variability in Piagetian theory and research. In R. Sternberg & C. Berg (Eds.), *Intellectual development* (pp. 100–140). New York: Cambridge Univ. Press.

Brainerd, C. J. (1978). The stage question in cognitive-developmental theory. *The Behavioral and Brain Sciences, 1*, 173–182.

Brown, A. L., & Reeve, R. (1987). Bandwidths of competence: The role of supportive contexts in learning and development. In L. S. Liben (Ed.), *Development and learning: Conflict or congruence?* Hillsdale, NJ: Erlbaum.

Bruner, J. S. (1973). Organization of early skilled action. *Child Development, 44*, 1–11.

Bullock, D., Carpenter, G. A., & Grossberg, S. (1991). Self-organizing neural network architectures for adaptive pattern recognition and robotics. In P. Antognetti & V. Milutinovic (Eds.), *Neural networks: Concepts, applications, and implementations* (Vol. 1, pp. 33–53). Englewood Cliffs, NJ: Prentice-Hall.

Campos, J. J., & Bertenthal, B. I. (1987). Locomotion and psychological development in infancy. In F. Morrison, K. Lord, & D. Keating (Eds.), *Advances in applied developmental psychology* (Vol. 2, pp. 11–42). New York: Academic Press.

Case, R. (1985). *Intellectual development: Birth to adulthood.* New York: Academic Press.

Case, R. (1992). The role of the frontal lobes in the regulation of human development. *Brain and Cognition, 20*, 51–73.

Chomsky, N. (1965). *Aspects of the theory of syntax.* Cambridge, MA: MIT Press.

Chugani, H. T., & Phelps, M. E. (1986). Maturational changes in cerebral function in infants determined by ^{18}FDG Positron Emission Tomography. *Science, 231*, 840–843.

Chugani, H. T., Phelps, M. E., & Mazziotta, J. C. (1987). Positron emission tomography study of human brain functional development. *Annals of Neurology, 22*, 487–497.

Corrigan, R. (1983). The development of representational skills. In K. W. Fischer (Ed.), *Levels and transitions in children's development. New directions for child development, 21*, 51–64. San Francisco: Jossey–Bass.

Dustman, R. E., & Beck, E. C. (1969). The effects of maturation and aging on the waveform of visually evoked potentials. *Electroencephalography and Clinical Neurophysiology, 265*, 2–11.

Fischer, K. W. (1980). A theory of cognitive development: The control and construction of hierarchies of skills. *Psychological Review, 87*, 477–531.

Fischer, K. W., Bullock, D., Rotenberg, E. J., & Raya, P. (1993). The dynamics of competence: How context contributes directly to skill. In R. H. Wozniak & K. W. Fischer (Eds.), *Development in context: Acting and thinking in specific environments* (pp. 93–117). Hillsdale, NJ: Erlbaum.

Fischer, K. W., & Canfield, R. L. (1986). The ambiguity of stage and structure in behavior: Person and environment in the development of psychological structures. In I. Levin (Ed.), *Stage and structure: Reopening the debate* (pp. 246–267). Norwood, NJ: Ablex.

Fischer, K. W., & Farrar, M. J. (1987). Generalizations about generalization: How a theory of skill development explains both generality and specificity. *International Journal of Psychology, 22*, 643–677.

Fischer, K. W., & Hogan, A. (1989). The big picture for infant development: Levels and variations. In J. Lockman & N. Hazen (Eds.), *Action in social context: Perspectives on early development* (pp. 275–305). New York: Plenum.

Fischer, K. W., & Kennedy, B. (in press). Dynamics of cognitive development: Variability and limits. In E. Amsel & K. A. Renninger (Eds.), *Development and change.* Hillsdale, NJ: Erlbaum.

Fischer, K. W., Kenny, S. L., & Pipp, S. L. (1990). How cognitive processes and environmental conditions organize discontinuities in the development of abstractions. In C. N. Alexander, E. J. Langer, & R. M. Oetzel (Eds.), *Higher stages of development* (pp. 162–187). New York: Oxford Univ. Press.

Fischer, K. W., Pipp, S. L., & Bullock, D. (1984). Detecting discontinuities in development: Method and measurement. In R. Emde & R. Harmon (Eds.), *Continuities and discontinuities in development* (pp. 95–121). New York: Plenum.

Fischer, K. W., & Rose, S. P. (1994). Dynamic development of coordination of components in brain and behavior: A framework for theory and research. In G. Dawson & K. W. Fischer (Eds.), *Human behavior and the developing brain* (pp. 3–66). New York: Guilford.

Fischer, K. W., Shaver, P., & Carnochan, P. G. (1990). How emotions develop and how they organize development. *Cognition and Emotion, 4,* 81–127.

Fischer, K. W., & Silvern, L. (1985). Stages and individual differences in cognitive development. *Annual Review of Psychology, 36,* 613–648.

Flavell, J. (1982). On cognitive development. *Child Development, 53,* 1–10.

Goldman-Rakic, P. (1986). Circuitry of the prefrontal cortex and the regulation of behavior by representational knowledge. In F. Plum & V. Mountcastle (Eds.), *Handbook of physiology.* Bethesda, MD: American Physiological Society.

Greenfield, P. M. (1991). Language, tools, and brain: The ontogeny and phylogeny of hierarchically organized sequential behavior. *Behavioral and Brain Sciences, 14,* 531–551.

Grossberg, S. (1987a). *The adaptive brain* (2 vols.). Amsterdam: Elsevier/North-Holland.

Grossberg, S. (1987b). Competitive learning: From interactive activation to adaptive resonance. *Cognitive Science, 11,* 23–63.

Hagne, I., Persson, J., Magnusson, R., & Petersén, I. (1973). Spectral analysis via fast Fourier transform of waking EEG in normal infants. In P. Kellaway & I. Petersén (Eds.), *Automation of clinical electroencephalography* (pp. 103–143). New York: Raven.

Halford, G. S. (1987). A structure-mapping approach to cognitive development. *International Journal of Psychology, 22,* 609–642.

Harter, S., & Monsour, A. (1992). Developmental analysis of conflict caused by opposing attributes in the adolescent self-portrait. *Developmental Psychology, 28,* 251–260.

Hartley, D., & Thomas, D. G. (1993). Brain electrical activity changes and cognitive development. Paper presented at the meetings of the Society for Research in Child Development. New Orleans, LA.

Hubel, D. H., & Wiesel, T. N. (1977). Functional architecture of macaque monkey visual cortex. *Proceedings of the Royal Society, London, Series B, 193,* 1–59.

Hudspeth, W. J., & Pribram, K. H. (1992). Psychophysiological indices of cerebral maturation. *International Journal of Psychophysiology, 12,* 19–29.

Huttenlocher, P. (1994). Synaptogenesis in human cerebral cortex. In G. Dawson & K. W. Fischer (Eds.), *Human behavior and the developing brain* (pp. 137–152). New York: Guilford.

John, E. R. (1977). *Functional neuroscience. Volume 2: Neurometrics.* Hillsdale, NJ: Erlbaum.

Kennedy, B. (1994). *The development of self-understanding in adolescents in Korea.* Unpublished doctoral dissertation, Harvard University.

Kitchener, K. S., & King, P. M. (1990). Reflective judgment: Ten years of research. In M. L. Commons, C. Armon, L. Kohlberg, F. A. Richards, & J. D. Sinnott (Eds.), *Adult development 3.* New York: Praeger.

Kitchener, K. S., Lynch, C. L., Fischer, K. W., & Wood, P. K. (1993). Developmental range of reflective judgment: The effect of contextual support and practice on developmental stage. *Developmental Psychology, 29,* 893–906.

Lamborn, S. D., Fischer, K. W., & Pipp, S. L. (1994). Constructive criticism and social lies: A developmental sequence for understanding honesty and kindness in social interactions. *Developmental Psychology, 30,* 495–508.

Lampl, M., & Emde, R. N. (1983). Episodic growth in infancy: A preliminary report on length, head circumference, and behavior. In K. W. Fischer (Ed.), *Levels and transitions in children's development. New Directions for Child Development, 21,* 21–36. San Francisco: Jossey-Bass.

Lampl, M., Veldhuis, J. D., & Johnson, M. L. (1992). Saltation and stasis: A model of human growth. *Science, 258,* 801–803.

Martarano, S. C. (1977). A developmental analysis of performance on Piaget's formal operations tasks. *Developmental Psychology, 13,* 666–672.

Matousek, M., & Petersén, I. (1973). Frequency analysis of the EEG in normal children and adolescents. In P. Kellaway & I. Petersén (Eds.), *Automation of clinical electroencephalography* (pp. 75–102). New York: Raven Press.

McCall, R. (1979). Qualitative transitions in behavioral development in the first years of life. In M. H. Bornstein & W. Kessen (Eds.), *Psychological development from infancy.* New York: Erlbaum.

McCall, R. B., Eichorn, D. H., & Hogarty, P. S. (1977). Transitions in early mental development. *Monographs of the Society for Research in Child Development, 42*(3, Serial No. 171).

Mills, D. L., Coffey-Corina, S. A., & Neville, H. J. (1994). Variability in cerebral organization during primary language acquisition. In G. Dawson & K. W. Fischer (Eds.), *Human behavior and the developing brain* (pp. 427–455). New York: Guilford.

Mizuno, T., Yamauchi, N., Watanabe, A., Komatsushiro, M., Takagi, T., Iinuma, K., & Arakawa, T. (1970). Maturation of patterns of EEG: Basic waves of healthy infants under 12 months of age. *Tohoku Journal of Experimental Medicine, 102,* 91–98.

Moshman, D., & Franks, B. A. (1986). Development of the concept of inferential validity. *Child Development, 57,* 153–165.

Movshon, J. A., & Van Sluyters, R. C. (1981). Visual neural development. *Annual Review of Psychology, 32,* 477–522.

Neville, H. J. (1991). Neurobiology of cognitive and language processing: Effects of early experience. In K. R. Gibson & A. C. Petersen (Eds.), *Brain maturation and cognitive development: Comparative and cross-cultural perspectives* (pp. 355–380). New York: Aldine de Gruyter.

Ohtahara, S. (1981). Neurophysiological development during infancy and childhood. In N. Yamaguchi & K. Fujiwasa (Eds.), *Recent advances in EEG and EMG data processing* (pp. 369–375). Amsterdam: Elsevier/North Holland.

Pascual-Leone, J. (1970). A mathematical model for the transition rule in Piaget's developmental stages. *Acta Psychologica, 32,* 301–345.

Pennington, B. F. (1994). The working memory function of the prefrontal cortices: Implications for developmental and individual differences in cognition. In M. M. Haith, J. B. Benson, R. J. Roberts Jr., & B. F. Pennington (Eds.), *Development of future-oriented processes* (pp. 243–289). Chicago: Univ. of Chicago Press.

Petitto, L. A., & Marentette, P. F. (1991). Babbling in the manual mode: Evidence for the ontogeny of language. *Science, 251,* 1493–1496.

Piaget, J. (1954). *The construction of reality in the child* (M. Cook, Transl.). New York: Basic Books. (Originally published, 1937).

Piaget, J. (1957). Logique et équilibre dans les comportements du sujet. *Études d'Épistémologie Génétique, 2,* 27–118.

Pipp, S. L., Fischer, K. W., & Jennings, S. L. (1987). The acquisition of self and mother knowledge in infancy. *Developmental Psychology, 22*, 86–96.

Rakic, P., Bourgeois, J.-P., Eckenhoff, M. F., Zecevic, N., & Goldman-Rakic, P. (1986). Concurrent overproduction of synapses in diverse regions of the primate cerebral cortex. *Science, 232*, 232–235.

Reznick, J. S., & Goldfield, B. A. (1992). Rapid change in lexical development in comprehension and production. *Developmental Psychology, 28*, 406–413.

Schore, A. N. (1994). *Affect regulation and the origin of the self: The neurobiology of emotional development.* Hillsdale, NJ: Erlbaum.

Segalowitz, S. J. (1994). Developmental psychology and brain development: A historical perspective. In G. Dawson & K. W. Fischer (Eds.), *Human behavior and the developing brain* (pp. 67–92). New York: Guilford.

Seibert, J. M., Hogan, A. E., & Mundy, P. C. (1984). Mental age and cognitive stage in young handicapped and at-risk children. *Intelligence, 8*, 11–29.

Somsen, R. J. M., & van't Klooster, B. J. (1994). *Effects of age, sex, task, and retest condition on eyes open and eyes closed background EEG spectral indices in school-aged children.* Unpublished Research Report, University of Amsterdam.

Stauder, J. E. A., Molenaar, P. C. M., & van der Molen, M. W. (1993). Scalp topography of event-related brain potentials and cognitive transition during childhood. *Child Development, 64*, 768–788.

Thatcher, R. W. (1991). Maturation of the human frontal lobes: Physiological evidence for staging. *Developmental Neurospychology, 7*, 397–419.

Thatcher, R. W. (1992). Cyclic cortical reorganization during early childhood development. *Brain and Cognition, 20*, 24–50.

Thatcher, R. W. (1994). Cyclic cortical reorganization: Origins of human cognitive development. In G. Dawson & K. W. Fischer (Eds.), *Human behavior and the developing brain* (pp. 232–266). New York: Guilford.

Thelen, E., & Fogel, A. (1989). Toward an action-based theory of infant development. In J. Lockman & N. Hazan (Eds.), *Action in social context: Perspectives on early development* (pp. 23–63). New York: Plenum.

Thelen, E., & Smith, L. B. (1994). *A dynamic systems approach to the development of cognition and action.* Cambridge, MA: MIT Press.

Uzgiris, I. C. (1976). Organization of sensorimotor intelligence. In M. Lewis (Ed.), *Origins of intelligence: Infancy and early childhood.* New York: Plenum.

van der Maas, H., & Molenaar, P. (1992). A catastrophe-theoretical approach to cognitive development. *Psychological Review, 99*, 395–417.

van Geert, P. (1994a). A dynamic systems model of cognitive growth: Competition and support under limited resource conditions. In E. Thelen & L. Smith (Eds.), *Dynamical systems in development: Applications.* Cambridge, MA: MIT Press.

van Geert, P. (1994b). *Dynamic systems of development: Change between complexity and chaos.* London: Harvester Wheatsheaf.

Yakovlev, P. I., & Lecours, A. R. (1967). The myelogenetic cycles of regional maturation of the brain. In A. Minkowsky (Ed.), *Regional development of the brain in early life* (pp. 3–70). Oxford: Blackwell.

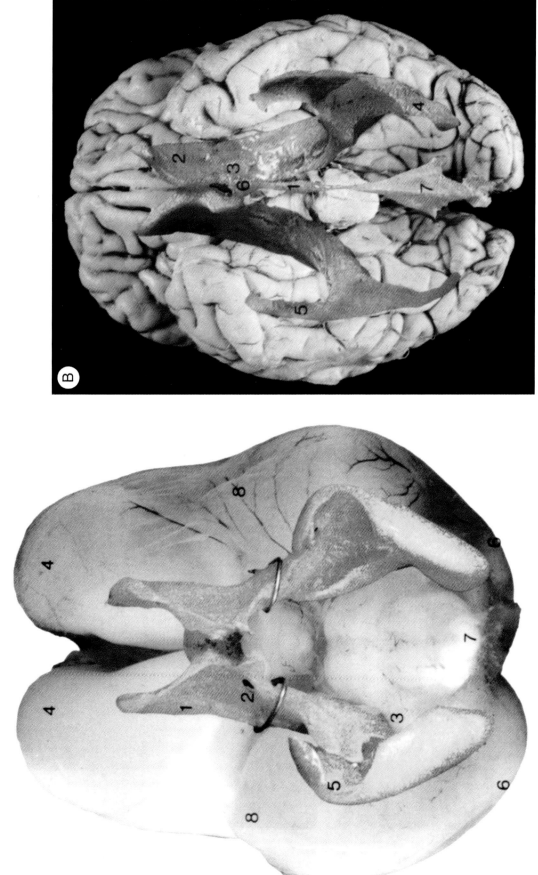

Plate 1A The base of the brain of a 130-mm crown-rump length fetus with latex casts of the lateral ventricles superimposed. [From *Atlas of the Human Brain and Spinal Cord* (p. 26), by M. England and J. Wakely. Copyright 1991 by Mosby-Yearbook, Inc. Reprinted with permission.]

Plate 1B The base of an adult brain with latex casts of the lateral ventricles superimposed. [From *Atlas of the Human Brain and Spinal Cord* (p. 71), by M. England and J. Wakely. Copyright 1991 by Mosby-Yearbook, Inc. Reprinted with permission.]

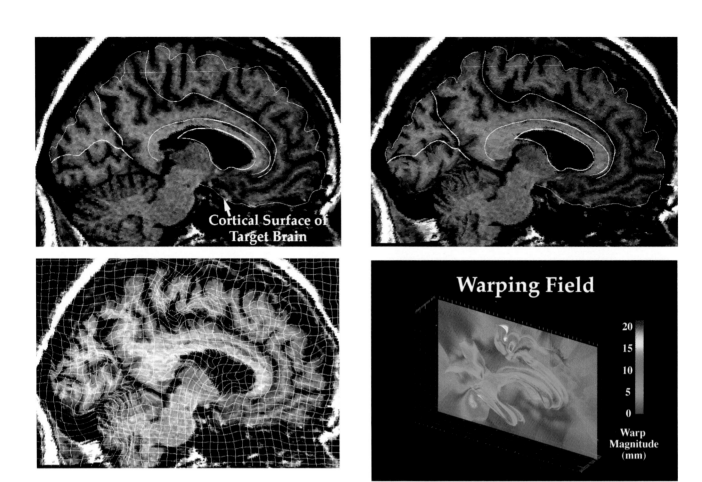

Plate 2   Quantification and mapping of local anatomic changes. 3D warping algorithms offer several advantages for quantifying complex patterns of local anatomic change. The top panels show a T_1-weighted MR sagittal brain slice image from (left) an elderly normal subject, and (right) the result of warping this reference anatomy into structural correspondence with a target scan from a patient with Alzheimer's disease. Cortical, ventricular, and cerebellar surface boundaries in both images were digitized, converted to parametric mesh form, and used to constrain the 3D deformation of the reference image onto the target. The lower left panel shows the transformation applied to a regular grid in the reference coordinate system. The magnitude of the 3D deformation field is also shown (lower right) on the surface anatomy of the target brain, as well as on a parasagittal plane 7 mm into the right hemisphere. This plane slices orthogonally through many of the surfaces driving the transformation. Note the smooth continuation of the warping field from the complex anatomic surfaces into the surrounding brain architecture and the highlighting of the severe deformations in the pre-marginal cortex, ventricular, and cerebellar areas. Warping algorithms may also be applied to developmental image data, in order to highlight and quantify dilation and contraction patterns in the anatomy at a very local level. (Data from Thompson and Toga, in preparation.)

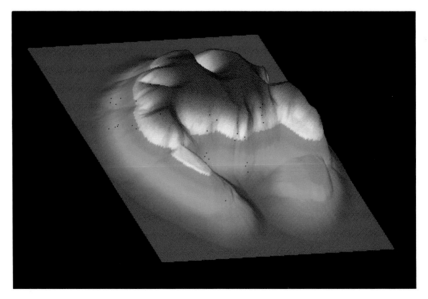

Plate 3   Slice from a distance field. A polyhedral mesh surface model of the cortex has been used to construct the distance field, a volume which encodes the distance to the nearest surface point from each location in space. A single slice from the field is shown, with the distance value shown as height and color-coded. The surface boundary corresponds to the green/yellow boundary.

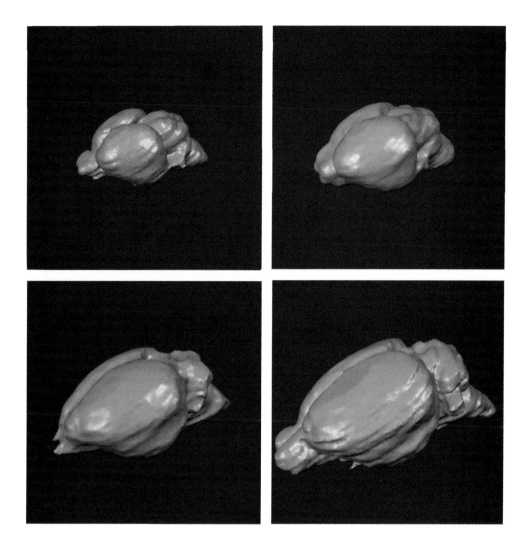

Plate 4 Distance fields applied to developmental modeling. Surface models of rat cortex at two developmental stages have been used to form distance fields. Weighted averaging of the distance fields followed by isosurface creation creates intermediate surfaces. Images shown are frames from an animation sequence at time-points 0, 1/3, 2/3, and 1.

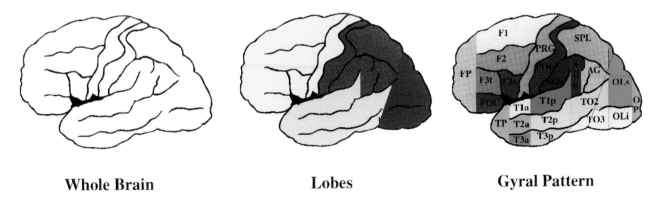

Whole Brain   **Lobes**   **Gyral Pattern**

Plate 5 Schematic representation of some of the spatial scales of brain morphometry. The scales shown range from hemisphere to systems-level gyral topology.

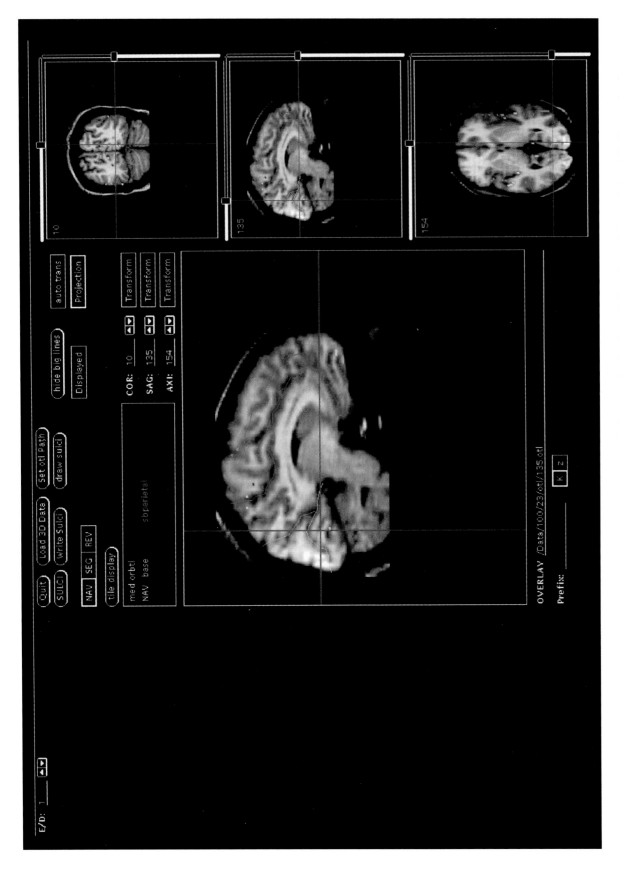

Plate 6 The identification of landmarks, nodes, and fissures requires multiplanar navigation through the volumetric image data set. Optimum visualization and identification of each of these features require positional normalization and the ability to navigate and interact with the image data from all cardinal image orientations (coronal, sagittal, and axial). Each view is cross-referenced with the others, and any editing or segmentation which occurs in one view is cross-referenced to the others.

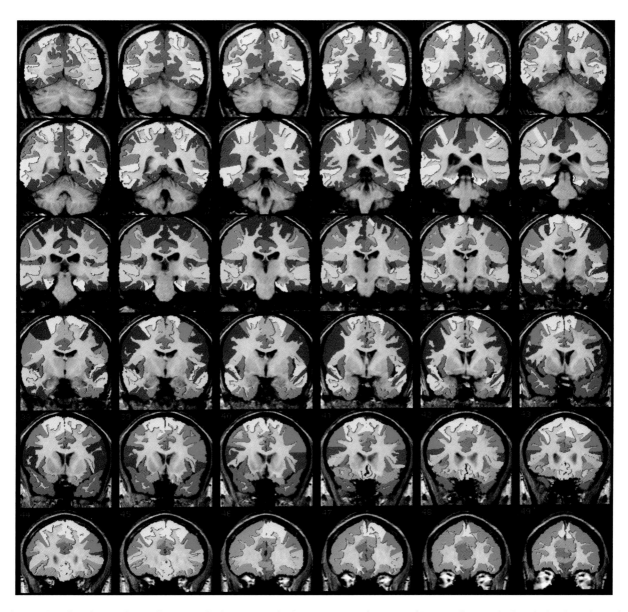

Plate 7 Results of cortical parcellation applied to a normal subject. A series of 36 coronal images shown which includes the colorized results of the cortical parcellation.

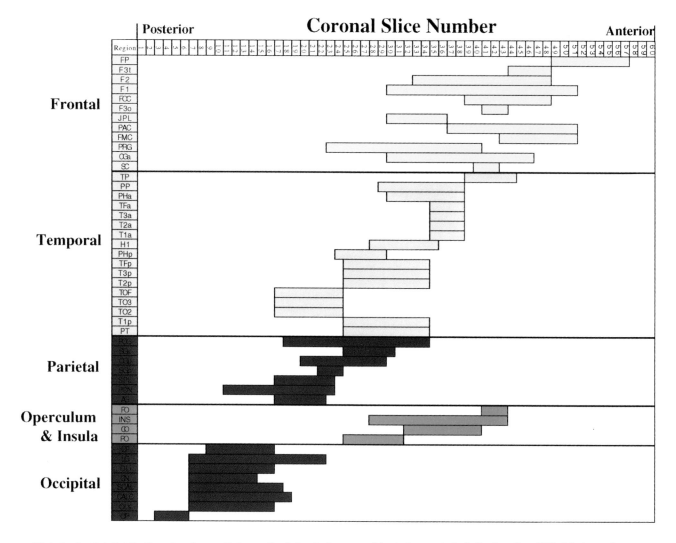

Plate 8 Spatial distribution of each parcellation unit relative to the coronal (anterior–posterior) slice location. With this type of presentation, the entire relative layout of the parcellation units can be appreciated at a glance.

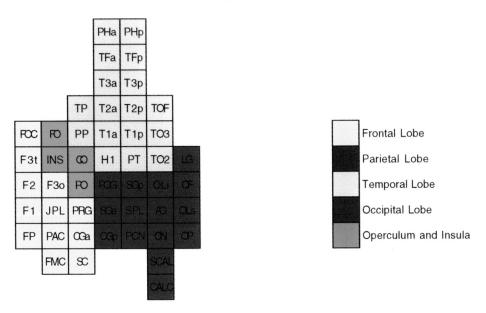

Plate 9 Schematic representation of the cortical parcellation system where each parcellation unit is given a unit size representation. The relative topology of the brain is *not* maintained in this representation, but it provides a standard form upon which to codify regional results, and facilitate intersubject comparison. In this example, each parcellation unit is color-coded by its lobe.

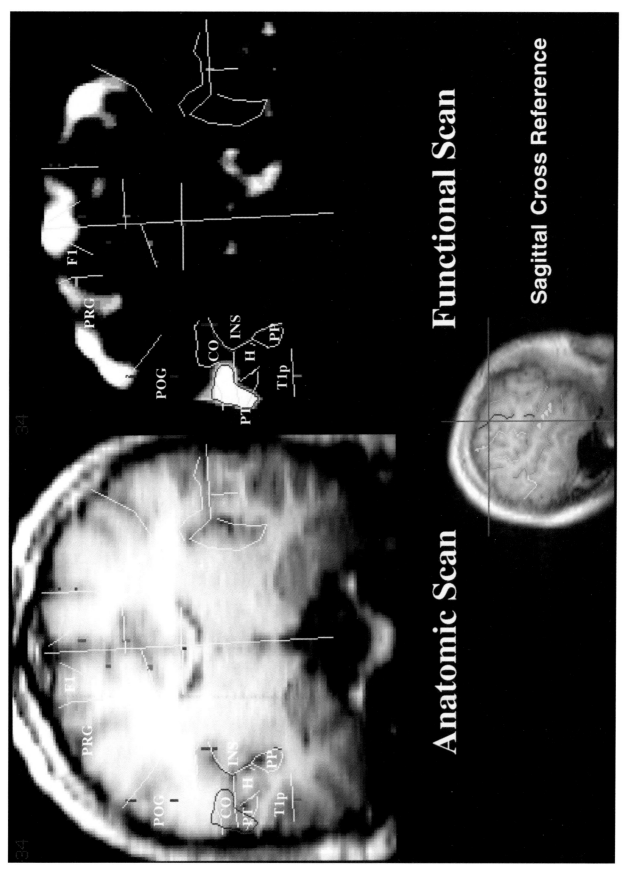

Plate 10 An example slice showing the correspondence between the functional statistical map and the anatomic image from a verb generation fMRI activation study. The images include the results of sulcal identification, and permit interpretation in terms of the cortical parcellation system.

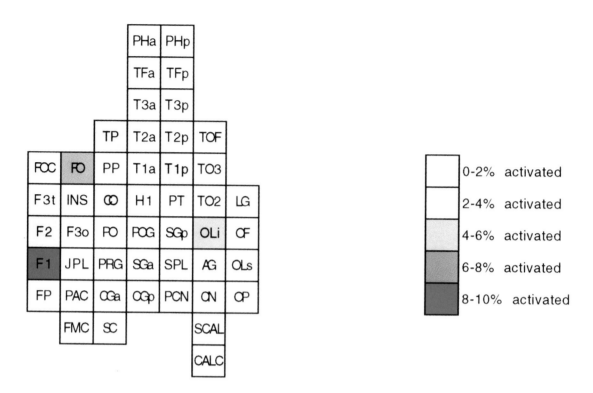

Plate 11 Idealized cortical parcellation map where each unit is given a grayscale intensity that is proportional to the percentage of the parcellation unit, which is activated above the $p < .0001$ level. This is demonstrated for the left hemisphere only from a passive word reading paradigm.

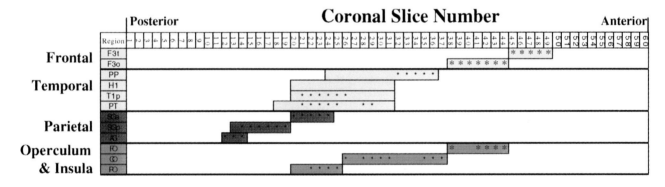

Plate 12 The location of the parcellation units and the presence of activation (*) for a verb generation task viewed for the 13 perisylvian language-related parcellation units. This view elucidates some details of the spatial distribution of activation foci for this task.

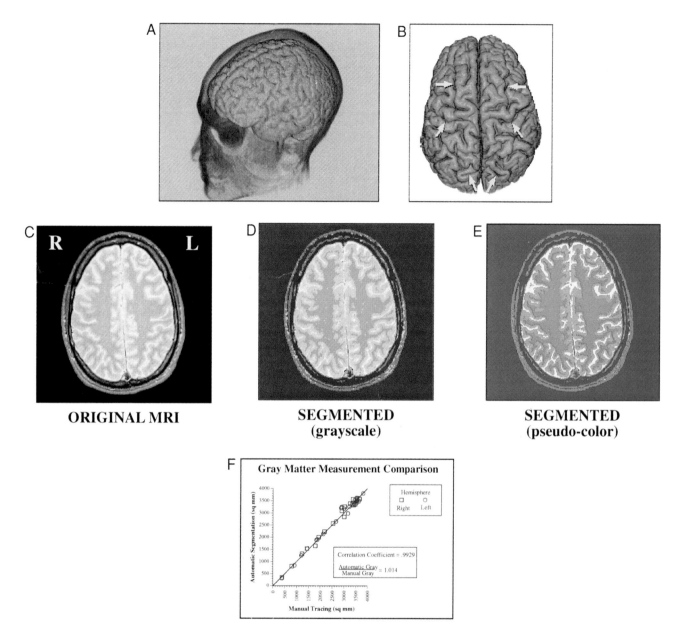

ORIGINAL MRI

SEGMENTED (grayscale)

SEGMENTED (pseudo-color)

Plate 13 (A) and (B): Two examples of high-resolution 3D brain reconstructions. On the left, to orient the viewer, the subject's brain is seen through the skull which is made semitransparent. Use of 3D brain images allows identification of surface landmarks used in subdividing the cerebrum into frontal, parietal, temporal, and occipital lobes according to classical anatomical conventions. For example, in the brain on the right, arrows point to several surface structures that are easily seen in such 3D reconstructions. (C), (D), and (E): Fully automated tissue segmentation. Pixels are classified according to both global and local characteristics. Shown are (C) an original (*PD+T2*) MRI image, (D) a segmented image rendered in a grayscale similar to the original, and (E) a pseudo-color version which highlights the different tissues (CSF and partial volume CSF = white, gray matter = orange, white matter = green). (F) Comparison between manual tracing and the automatic computer algorithm on 20 slices through the cerebral cortex shows a high correlation and only a 1.4% difference in total gray matter volume. [Adapted from Egaas, 1995.]

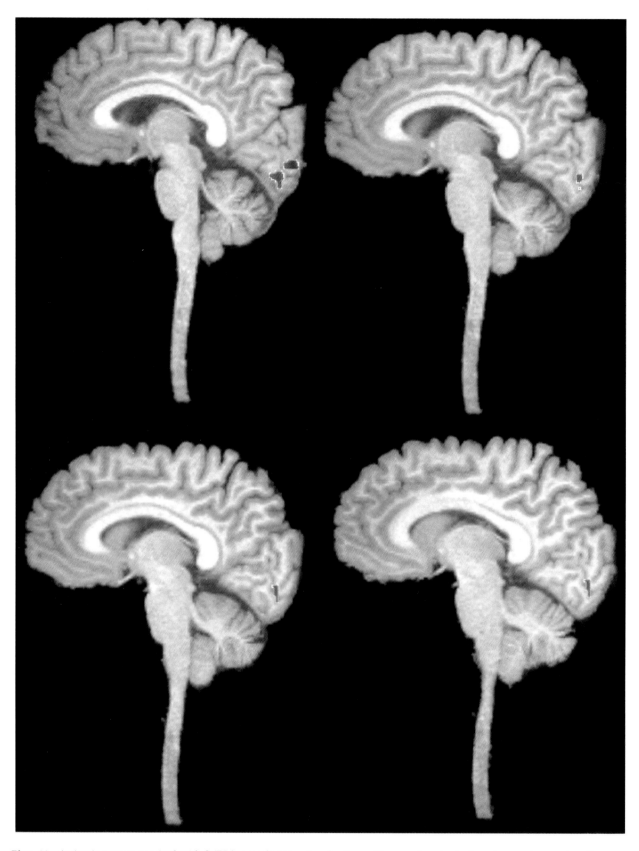

Plate 14 Activation maps acquired with fMRI (z-maps) contrasting fixation with reversing checkerboard, superimposed on the same subject's high-resolution structural MRI.

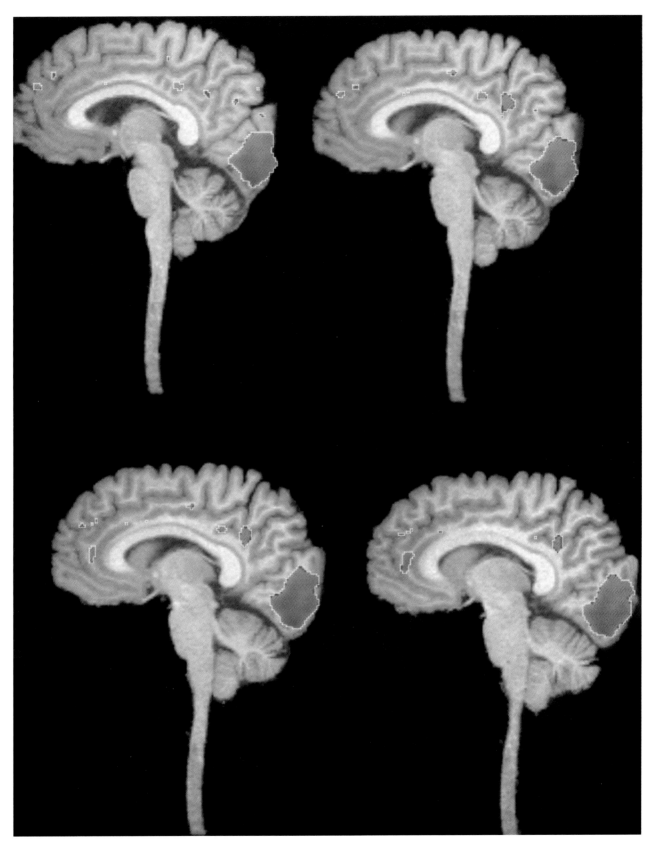

Plate 15 PET results contrasting fixation with reversing checkerboard (activation maps represent 20% increase), superimposed on the same subject's high-resolution structural MRI.

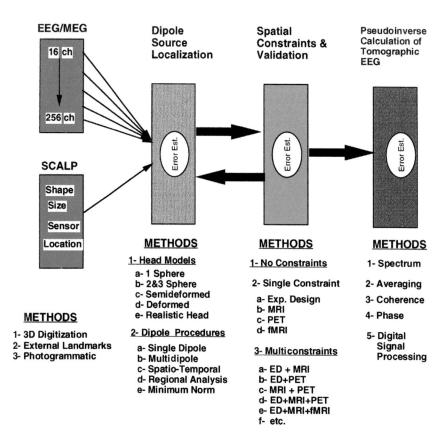

Plate 16 Diagrammatic illustration of some of the concepts, issues, and procedures involved in dipole source localization and multimodal registration of EEG to PET and MRI. ED = experimental design.

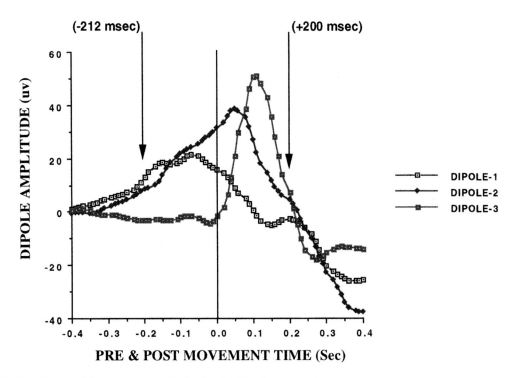

Plate 17 The time history of the moment magnitude of each of the three equivalent dipole sources. (For further details on the methods and model see Toro et al., 1993.) [Adapted from Eckhorn et al., 1988.]

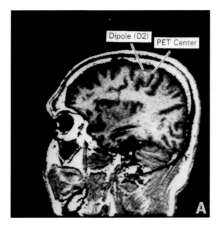

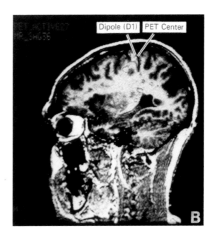

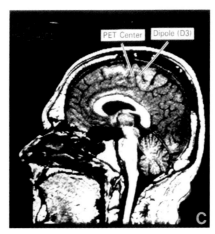

Plate 18 (A) Multimodal sagittal image of the ipsilateral right hemisphere (sagittal slice no. 74). The rCBF PET image registered with the corresponding sagittal MRI was obtained after averaging of three images obtained during the execution of self-paced right index finger movements after the injection of H_2O^{15} and subtraction from averaged rest scans. The location of source 2 (i.e., D2, see Fig. 3, Chapter 9) in the spherical head model in the same subject executing the same task has been projected into the PET and MRI images (open cross) after the appropriate coordinate transformations and rotations (see Wang et al., 1994, for more details of the technique). Both the dipole source and the active PET region are located near the ipsilateral hand region in the anterior bank of the central sulcus. The distance between the dipole source location (left arrow) and the center of the active PET region (right arrow) is approximately 10 mm. The Talairach and Tournoux (1988) atlas coordinates of the registered PET and dipole source 2 are approximately c, 3, and E_2 in the right hemisphere (x, y, z coordinates are + 1.4 cm for horizontal, + 4.1 cm for medial–lateral slice, + 5.0 cm for top to bottom).

(B) Multimodal sagittal image of the contralateral left hemisphere (sagittal slice no. 36). The location of source 1 (i.e., D1, see Fig. 3, Chapter 9) in the spherical head model in the same subject executing the same task has been projected into the PET and MRI images (white cross) after the appropriate coordinate transformations and rotations (see Wang et al., 1994). Both the dipole source and the active PET region are located near the hand region in the anterior bank of the central sulcus. The distance between the dipole source location (left arrow) and the center of the active PET region (right arrow) is less than 3 mm. The Talairach and Tournoux (1988) atlas coordinates of the registered PET and dipole source 1 are approximately c, 3, E_2 in the left hemisphere (x, y, z coordinates are + 1.4 cm for horizontal, + 4.1 cm for medial–lateral slice, + 5.0 cm for top to bottom).

(C) Multimodal sagittal image of the contralateral left hemisphere (sagittal slice no. 51). The location of source 3 (i.e., D3, see Fig. 1, Chapter 9) in the spherical head model in the same subject executing the same task has been projected into the PET and MRI images (white cross) after the appropriate coordinate transformations and rotations (see Wang et al., 1994). Both the dipole source and the active PET region are located in the anterior bank of the supplemental motor cortical region. The distance between the dipole source location (left arrow) and the center of the active PET region (right arrow) is approximately 6 mm. The Talairach and Tournoux (1988) atlas coordinates of the registered PET and dipole source 3 are approximately a, 3–4, and E_1 in the left hemisphere (x, y, z coordinates are + .4 cm for horizontal, + .5 cm for medial–lateral slice, + 4.6 cm for top to bottom). [Adapted from Eckhorn et al., 1988.]

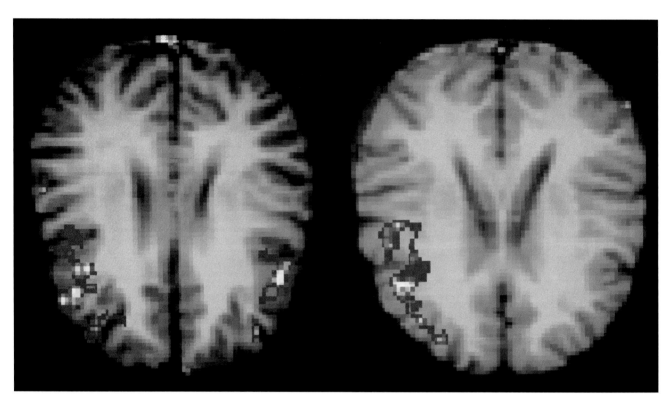

Plate 19 Composite images of the distribution of activations comparing rhyme–case tasks (phonological processing) for 19 males (left) compared to 19 females (right). Color dots represent pixels for which the mean value of the split *t* statistic from averaging the 19 subjects was higher than .4 (dark red dots are close to .4 while yellow approaches 1). Activations are shown for levels 6–7 of the Talairach system (Atlas of Talairach and Tournoux, 1988, p. 114). Males show unilateral activation, primarily in the left inferior frontal gyrus, with minor activation of the left middle frontal gyrus. In females, phonological processing activates both the left and right inferior frontal gyri. There is smaller activation of the left and right middle frontal gyri.

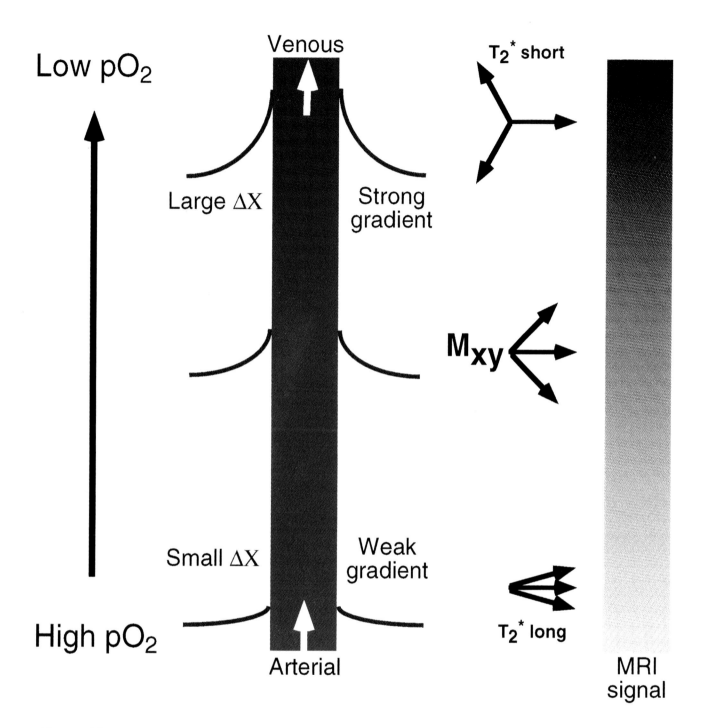

Plate 20 Schematic representation of the *blood oxygen level dependent* (BOLD) contrast mechanism. Arterial blood contains oxyhemoglobin which has similar magnetic susceptibility (X) to surrounding tissue. At lower oxygen tension, deoxyhemoglobin in red cells has marked paramagnetism and induces magnetic field gradients both within and immediately exterior to the vasculature. MRI signal is derived from tissue water, which experiences a nonuniform magnetic field in the presence of deoxygenated blood. The transverse decay rate of the nuclear magnetization is faster in an inhomogeneous field and thus the signal is lower. If, as a result of activation, the flow increase exceeds the additional oxygen usage, then oxygen tension in the venous side increases, the field becomes more uniform, and the signal increases.

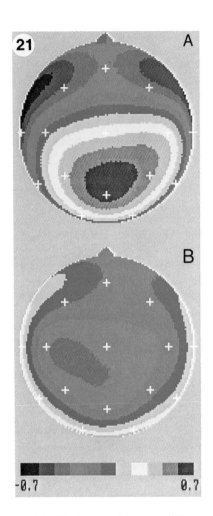

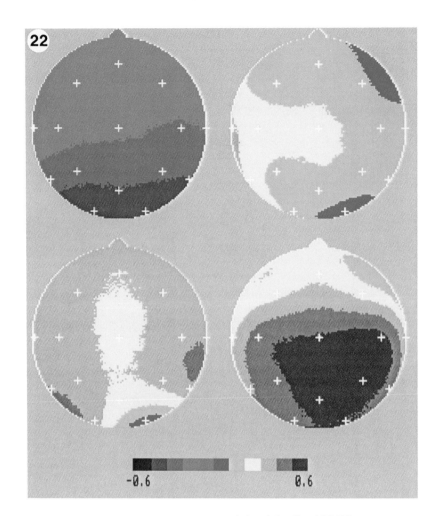

Plate 21   Topographic maps of the principal component loadings for the P3, 400 ms component (A) and the "late N," 900 ms component (B).

Plate 22   Maps of the correlation between the PET glucose metabolism measured at left and right Brodmann's area 37 and the loadings for the P3, 400 ms component (top) and the "late N," 900 ms component (bottom). The correlations are partialled, covarying total gray matter metabolism and age.

19

Functional Specialization and Integration in the Brain: An Example from Schizophrenia Research

Karl J. Friston

*The Wellcome Department of Cognitive Neurology, Institute of Neurology and the MRC
Cyclotron Unit, Hammersmith Hospital
London, W12 OHS United Kingdom*

I. Introduction

The brain appears to adhere to two principles of functional organization: *functional segregation* and *functional integration,* where the integration within and between functionally segregated areas is mediated by functional or effective connectivity. The characterization of functional segregation, integration, and connectivity is an important theme in many areas of neuroscience, especially in functional imaging.

This chapter reviews ideas and techniques that are commonly used to make inferences about how the brain is organized. There are two basic approaches: The first depends on detecting focal differences using a functional segregation or specialization view of the brain. The second is based on correlated changes in different parts of the brain and emphasizes the interactions within, and integration of, distributed brain systems. This chapter is divided into two halves that discuss (1) the role of *statistical parametric mapping* in making inferences about regionally specific effects, and (2) *eigenimage analysis* and related multivariate approaches that are used to characterize functionally connected systems and interactions between brain areas. Both halves consider the conceptual and mathematical foundations of the approaches and focus on the brain regions implicated in word generation and the interactions between these regions in schizophrenia.

Studies of functional specialization usually rely on some form of statistical parametric mapping. Statistical parametric mapping refers to the construction of spatially extended statistical processes to test hypotheses about regionally specific effects. Statistical parametric maps, or SPMs, (e.g., *t* maps) are image processes with voxel values that are, under the null hypothesis, distributed according to a known probability density function. The success of statistical parametric mapping is largely due to the simplicity of the idea: Namely, one analyzes each and every voxel using any standard (univariate) statistical test. The resulting statistical parameters are assembled into an image—the SPM. The SPM is then interpreted as a spatially extended statistical process by referring to the probabilistic behavior of stationary Gaussian fields. "Unlikely" excursions of the SPM are interpreted as regionally specific effects, attributable to the sensorimotor or cognitive process that has been manipulated experimentally. This characterization of physiological responses appeals to functional segregation as the underlying model of brain function. In this sense, one could regard all applications of statistical parametric mapping as testing some variant of the functional segregation hypothesis.

Statistical parametric mapping has been used very successfully to establish functional specialization as principle of organization in the human brain. More recent work has focussed on the integration of functionally specialized areas. One framework (Friston, Frith,

Liddle, & Frackowiak, 1993; Friston, Firth, & Frakowiak, 1993b) makes a key distinction between *functional connectivity*, the temporal correlations between remote neurophysiological events, and *effective connectivity*, the influence one neural system exerts over another. These concepts were originally elaborated upon in the analysis of separable neural spike trains from multiunit electrode recordings (Gerstein and Perkel, 1969). A powerful use of functional connectivity is in the characterization of distributed brain systems: The functional connectivity (covariance) matrix, obtained from a time-series of images, is subject to principal component analysis (PCA) or singular value decomposition (SVD). The resulting eigenimages (principal components or spatial modes) each identify a distributed system, comprising regions that are jointly implicated by virtue of their functional interactions. This analysis of neuroimaging time-series is predicated on established techniques in electrophysiology, both electroencephalogram (EEG) and multiunit recordings. For example, in the analysis of multichannel EEG data, the underlying spatial modes that best characterize the observed spatiotemporal dynamics are identified with a Karhunen Loeve expansion (Friedrich, Fuchs, & Haken, 1991). Commonly, this expansion is in terms of the eigenvectors of the covariance matrix associated with the time-series. The spatial modes are then identical to the principal components identified with a PCA. SVD is a related technique (Golub and Van Loan, 1991) which has been used, with the Karhunen Loeve expansion, to identify spatial modes in multiunit electrode recordings (Mayer-Kress, Barezys, & Freeman, 1991).

The PCA, or equivalently SVD, of a neuroimaging time-series uses functional connectivity as its conceptual basis. Functional connectivity is, however, an operational definition and makes no comment on the causal mediation of the observed correlations. *Effective connectivity* is closer to the intuitive notion of a connection and relies on some model of the influence one cortical region exerts over another. The applications and theory of effective connectivity and related techniques such as structural equation modeling and path analysis (McIntosh, Grady, Ungerleider, Haxby, Rapoport, & Horwitz, 1993) are probably the least developed, but represent one of the most exciting, areas in imaging neuroscience.

In summary, two distinct themes have emerged in the analysis of functional imaging data: (1) testing some variant of the functional segregation hypothesis by assessing the significance of regionally specific effects, and (2) a descriptive approach to characterizing neurophysiological changes, or dynamics, in terms of distributed systems (eigenimages or spatial modes).

Spatiotemporal dynamics imply a time-series, and the latter techniques are likely to enjoy an increasing role in data analysis as the trend to repeated scans in single subjects gains momentum (particularly in functional magnetic resonance imaging, fMRI).

II. Functional Segregation

A. Conceptual Foundations

These sections introduce the notion of functional segregation from a neuroreductionist viewpoint and introduce a useful taxonomy of experimental design and analysis.

1. Functional Segregation in the Brain

The functional role played by any elemental component (e.g., neuron) of a "connected" system (e.g., brain) is largely defined by its connections. Certain patterns of cortical projections are so common that they could amount to rules of cortical connectivity. "These rules revolve around one, apparently, overriding strategy that the cerebral cortex uses—that of functional segregation" (Zeki, 1990). Functional segregation demands that cells with common functional properties be grouped together. This in turn necessitates both convergence and divergence of cortical connections. The extrinsic connections between cortical regions are not continuous but occur in patches or clusters. This patchiness has, in some instances, a clear relationship to functional segregation. For example, V2 has a distinctive cytochrome oxidase architecture, consisting of thick stripes, thin stripes, and interstripes. When recordings are made in visual area 2 (V2), directionally selective (but not wavelength or color selective) cells are found exclusively in the thick stripes. Retrograde labeling of cells in V5 is limited to these thick stripes. All the available physiological evidence suggests that V5 is a functionally homogeneous area that is specialized for motion. Evidence of this nature supports the notion that patchy connectivity is the anatomical correlate of functional segregation and specialization (see Zeki, 1990 for a full discussion).

If it is the case that neurons in a given cortical area share a common responsiveness (by virtue of their extrinsic connectivity) to some sensorimotor or cognitive attributes, then *this functional segregation is also an anatomical one*. Challenging a subject with the appropriate sensorimotor attribute or cognitive process should lead to increased activity in, and only in, the area of interest. This is the model upon which subtraction is predicated.

2. Cognitive and Sensorimotor Subtraction

The tenet of this approach is that the difference between two tasks can be formulated as a separable cognitive or sensorimotor component, and that the regionally specific differences in brain activity identify the corresponding functionally specialized area. Early applications of subtraction range from the functional anatomy of word processing (Petersen, Fox, Posner, Mintun, & Raichle, 1989) to functional specialization in extrastriate cortex (Lueck, Zeki, Friston, Deiber, Cope, Cunningham, et al., 1989). The latter studies involved presenting visual stimuli with and without some specific sensorial attribute (e.g., color, motion, etc.). The areas highlighted by subtraction were identified with homologous areas in monkeys that showed selective electrophysiological responses to equivalent visual stimuli.

Cognitive subtraction is conceptually simple and represents a well-established and powerful device in functional mapping. It is, however, predicated on possibly untenable assumptions about the relationship between brain dynamics and the functional processes that ensue (and where these assumptions may be tenable, they are not demonstrated to be so). The main concerns with subtraction and additive factors logic can be reduced to the relationship between neural dynamics and cognitive processes. For example, even if, from a functionalist perspective, a cognitive component could be added without interaction among preexisting components, the brain's implementation of these processes is almost certainly going to show profound interactions. This follows from the observation that neural dynamics are nonlinear. Indeed, nearly all theoretical and computational neurobiology is based on this observation. The possible fallibility of the fundamental assumption behind subtraction has prompted the exploration of other approaches.

3. Parametric Designs

The premise here is that regional physiology will vary monotonically and systematically with the amount of cognitive or sensorimotor processing. Examples of this approach include the experiments of Grafton, Mazziotta, Presty, Friston, Frackowiak, and Phelps (1992), who demonstrated significant correlations between regional cerebral blood flow (rCBF) and the performance of a visually guided motor tracking task (using a pursuit rotor device) in the primary motor area, supplementary motor area, and pulvinar thalamus. The authors associated this distributed network with early procedural learning. On the sensory side Price, Wise, Ramsay, Friston, Howard, Patterson, et al. (1992) have demonstrated a remarkable linear relationship between rCBF in periauditory regions and frequency of aural word presentation. Significantly, this correlation was not observed in Wernicke's area, where rCBF appeared to correlate, not with the discriminative attributes of the stimulus, but with the presence or absence of semantics.

Parametric approaches avoid many of the philosophical and physiological shortcomings of "cognitive subtraction" in testing for systematic relationships between neurophysiology and sensorimotor, psychophysical, pharmacologic, or cognitive parameters. These systematic relationships are not constrained to be linear or additive and may show very nonlinear behavior. The fundamental difference between subtractive and parametric approaches lies in treating a cognitive process, not as a categorical invariant, but as a dimension or attribute that can be expressed to a greater or lesser extent. It is anticipated that parametric designs of this type will find an increasing role in psychological and psychophysical activation experiments.

Time dependent changes in physiology are clearly central in studies of learning and memory. Many animal models of procedural learning depend on habituation and adaptation, either at a behavioral or electrophysiological level. In the context of functional imaging, physiological adaptation to a challenge is simply the change in rCBF activation with time. This is an interaction.

4. Factorial Designs

At its simplest, an interaction is basically a change in a change. Interactions are associated with *factorial* designs, where two *factors* are combined in the same experiment. The effect of one factor on the effect of the other is assessed by the interaction term (two factors interact if the level of one factor affects the effect of the other). Factorial designs have a wide range of applications. The first positron emission tomography (PET) experiment of this sort was perhaps the simplest imaginable, and examined the interaction between motor activation (sequential finger opposition paced by a metronome) and time (rest–performance pairs repeated 3 times) (Friston, Frith, Passingham, Liddle, & Frackowiak, 1992). Significant adaptation was seen in the cerebellar cortex (ipsilateral to hand moved) and cerebellar nuclei. These results are consistent with the electrophysiological studies of Gilbert and Thach (1977), who demonstrated a reduction in simple and complex spike activity of Purkinje cells in the cerebellum during motor learning in monkeys. Psychopharmacological activation studies are examples of a factorial design (Friston, Grasby, Bench, Frith, Cowen, Little, et al., 1992). In these studies subjects perform a series of baseline-activation pairs before and after the administration of a centrally acting drug. The interaction term reflects the modulatory drug effect on the task-dependent physiological response. These studies provide an exciting insight into the relationship between cognition and neurotransmitter function in human (Friston, Grasby, et al 1992; Grasby, Friston, Bench, Cowen, Frith, Liddle, et al., 1992).

B. Statistical Parametric Mapping

All the examples cited in the previous sections used statistical parametric maps. SPMs are spatially extended statistical processes that are used to test hypotheses about regionally specific effects in neuroimaging data. The most established sorts of statistical parametric maps (e.g., Friston, Frith, Liddle, & Frackowiak, 1991a; Worsley, Evans, Marrett, & Neelin, 1992) are based on linear models, for example analysis of covariance (ANCOVA), correlation coefficients, and t tests. These are all special cases of the *general linear model.* Statistical parametric mapping represents the convergence of two well-established bodies of theory (the general linear model and the theory of Gaussian fields) to provide a complete and simple framework for the analysis of imaging data.

The general linear model is used to assess the effect that one is interested in, in terms of a t value at each and every voxel. The resulting image of t values constitute the SPM. Statistical inferences based on this SPM are complicated by the enormous number of univariate tests performed and the fact that these test are not independent. These special considerations have prompted the development of distributional approximations pertaining to the height of maxima in the SPM (u) and the spatial extent (k) of thresholded regions. This development has been in the context of the theory of Gaussian fields (Friston et al., 1991a; Worsley et al., 1992; Friston, Worsley, Frackowiak, Mazziotta, & Evans, 1994), in particular, the theory of level-crossings (Friston et al., 1991a) and differential topology (Worsley et al., 1992). Using these theoretical results, one can assign a p value to an activated region based either on its maximal height $P(Z_{\max} > u)$ or its spatial extent $P(n_{\max} > k)$. These p values can be considered "corrected" for the volume of the SPM analyzed and its inherent nonindependence or smoothness.

C. An Example Using Word Generation in Normal Subjects

1. The Data

The data were obtained from 5 subjects scanned 12 times (every 8 minutes) while performing one of two verbal tasks. Scans were obtained with a CTI PET cam-

era (model 953B). ^{15}O was administered intravenously as radiolabeled water infused over 2 minutes. Total counts per voxel during the buildup phase of radioactivity served as an estimate of rCBF. Subjects performed two tasks in alternation. One task involved repeating a letter presented aurally at one per 2 seconds *(word shadowing).* The other was a paced verbal fluency task, where the subjects responded with a word that began with the letter presented *(intrinsic word generation).* To facilitate intersubject pooling, the data were realigned and spatially [stereotactically] normalized and smoothed with an isotropic Gaussian kernel (full width at half maximum (FWHM) of 16mm). The confounding effect of global activity was removed by designating global activities as covariates of no interest. This example is equivalent to a one way ANCOVA with a blocked design (c.f. Friston, Frith, Liddle, Lammertsma, Dolan, & Frackowiak, 1990). There are 12 condition specific effects, 5 subject effects, and a covariate effect (see the corresponding design matrix in Fig. 1).

2. The Functional Anatomy of Word Generation: A Subtractive Approach

In this section we assess the activations associated with cognitive components in word generation that are not in word shadowing (e.g., the intrinsic generation of word representations and the "working memory" for words already produced). Following the philosophy of cognitive subtraction, these effects were obtained after subtracting the word shadowing from the verbal fluency conditions. The results of this analysis are presented in Figure 1, which shows the design matrix, the contrast, and the resulting SPM{Z}. The results demonstrate significant activations in the left anterior cingulate, left dorsolateral prefrontal cortex (DLPFC), operculum and related insula, thalamus, and left extrastriate (among others). These results suggest that the anterior cingulate, left DLPFC (including Broca's area), and thalamic regions are strongly implicated in the intrinsic generations of words. The corresponding deactivations (not shown) were most pronounced in the temporal regions, including Wernicke's area.

3. The Relevance to Schizophrenia

Underlying the design and interpretation of this experiment is an assumption that the prefrontal cortices are necessary for intrinsically generated behavior. The evidence for this association derives from studies of patients with neurological problems, unit recording studies in behaving primates, and functional imaging studies during cognitive activation. *Psychomotor poverty* in schizophrenia is closely related to psy-

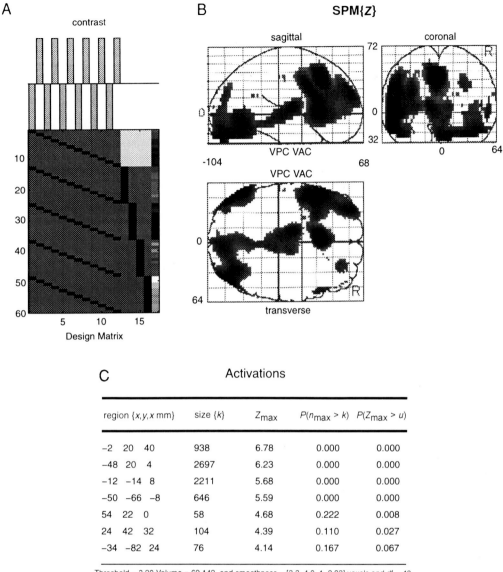

Figure 1 Functional anatomy of word processing. (A) Design matrix: This is an image representation of the design matrix used to model the various effects. Because elements of this matrix can take negative values, the gray scale is arbitrary and has been scaled to the minimum and maximum. The form of the design matrix is as follows: Condition effects, subject effects, and confounding (global) covariates. Contrast: This is the contrast or vector defining the linear compound of parameters tested with the *t* statistic. The contrast is displayed over the corresponding columns (effects) of the design matrix. The contrast can be seen to test for differences between the verbal fluency (even) and word shadowing (odd) conditions. (B) SPM{Z}: This is a maximum intensity projection of the thresholded SPM{t} following transformation to the Z score. (C) Tabular data are presented of "significant" regions. The location of the maximal voxel in each region is given with the size of the regions *(k)*, and the peak Z score. For each region the significance is assessed in terms of $P(Z_{max} > u)$ and $P(n_{max} > k)$. These represent *p* values that have been corrected for the volume of the SPM.

chomotor retardation (Benson, 1990), which includes decreased spontaneous movement, decreased communication, flatness of vocal inflection, unchanging facial expression, and social withdrawal. Among the most common causes of psychomotor retardation is damage to the frontal lobes and Parkinson's disease. In particular, patients with damage to the anterior cingulate and/or supplementary motor area (SMA) tend to become mute and show decreased spontaneous movement (Damasio & Van Hoesen, 1983). Passingham, Chen, and Thaler (1989) have demonstrated that SMA and anterior cingulate lesions in monkeys impair responses when the movement is self-initiated, but have little effect when the movement is extrinsically cued.

Largely akinetic patients with Parkinson's disease, can show a dissociation between movements which are self-initiated and extrinsically cued [e.g., paradoxical kinesis (Marsden, Parkes, & Quinn, 1982)]. In functional mapping it is now well-established that the prefrontal cortex is concerned with intrinsically generated behavior, that is, implicitly mnemonic (e.g., Frith, Friston, Liddle, & Frackowiak, 1991a, 1991b; Friston et al., 1991b).

On the basis of this evidence, prefronto-cortical dysfunction such as hypofrontality (Ingvar and Franzen, 1974) may appear to be a sufficient explanation for the negative signs of schizophrenia. However, the argument developed in this chapter is that prefronto-cortical function cannot be divorced from its integration into remaining brain systems, either at a physiological or a cognitive level. The second half of this chapter introduces some techniques that have been developed to look at coordinated and distributed interactions in the brain.

III. Functional Integration

The next sections review the basic distinction between functional and effective connectivity (as the terms are used in neuroimaging) and their role in addressing several aspects of functional organization (e.g., the topography of distributed systems, integration between cortical areas, and regional interactions). In particular, we focus on fronto-temporal integration in schizophrenia.

A. Conceptual Foundations

A landmark meeting, that took place on the morning of August 4th, 1881, highlighted the difficulties of attributing function to a cortical area, given the dependence of cerebral activity on underlying connections (Phillips, Zeki, & Barlow, 1984). Goltz (1881), although accepting the results of electrical stimulation in dog and monkey cortex, considered the excitation method inconclusive, in that the movements elicited might have originated in related pathways, or currents could have spread to distant centers. The principle of correlating a behavior with cerebral excitation is still employed today. With modern methods, this excitation is usually endogenous and measured with functional imaging. Despite advances over the past century, the question remains. Are the physiological changes elicited by sensorimotor or cognitive challenges explained by functional segregation, or by integrated and distributed changes mediated by neural connections? The question itself has important implications

for data analysis and interpretation that are now considered.

1. Origins and Definitions

In the analysis of neuroimaging, time-series functional connectivity is defined as the temporal correlations between spatially remote neurophysiological events (Friston, Frith, Liddle, et al., 1993). This definition is operational and provides a simple characterization of functional interactions. The alternative is to refer explicitly to effective connectivity (i.e., the influence one neuronal system exerts over another) (Friston, Frith, & Frackowiak, 1993b). These concepts were originated in the analysis of separable spike trains obtained from multiunit electrode recordings (Gerstein and Perkel, 1969; Gerstein, Bedenbaugh, & Aertsen, 1989; Aertsen and Preissl, 1991). Functional connectivity is simply a statement about the observed correlations; it does not provide any direct insight into how these correlations are mediated. For example, at the level of multiunit microelectrode recordings, correlations can result from *stimulus-locked transients*, evoked by a common afferent input, or reflect *stimulus-induced oscillations*, phasic coupling of neural assemblies, mediated by synaptic connections (Gerstein et al, 1989). To examine the integration within a distributed system, defined by functional connectivity, one turns to *effective connectivity*.

Effective connectivity is closer to the intuitive notion of a connection and can be defined as the influence one neural system exerts over another, either at a synaptic (cf. synaptic efficacy) or cortical level. In electrophysiology, there is a close relationship between effective connectivity and synaptic efficacy. "It is useful to describe the effective connectivity with a connectivity matrix of effective synaptic weights. Matrix elements $[C_{ij}]$ would represent the effective influence by neuron j on neuron i" (Gerstein et al., 1989). It has also been proposed that "the [electrophysiological] notion of effective connectivity should be understood as the experiment and time-dependent, simplest possible circuit diagram that would replicate the observed timing relationships between the recorded neurons" (Aertsen & Preissl, 1991).

Although functional and effective connectivity can be invoked at a conceptual level in both neuroimaging and electrophysiology, they differ fundamentally at a practical level. This is because the time-scales and nature of the neurophysiological measurements are very different (seconds versus milliseconds and hemodynamic versus spike trains). In electrophysiology, it is often necessary to remove the confounding effects of stimulus-locked transients (that introduce correlations *not* causally mediated by direct neural interactions) in order to reveal the underlying connectivity. The confounding effect of stimulus-evoked transients is less problematic in neuroimaging, because the promulgation of dynamics from primary sensory areas onwards *is* mediated by neuronal connections (usually reciprocal and interconnecting). However, it should be remembered that functional connectivity is not necessarily due to effective connectivity (e.g., common neuromodulatory input from ascending aminergic neurotransmitter systems or thalamo-cortical afferents) and, where it is, effective influences may be indirect (e.g., polysynaptic relays through multiple areas).

2. The Relationship between Functional Connectivity in Imaging and Electrophysiology

Clearly there is an enormous difference between the correlations in rCBF measured over many seconds and the fast phasic dynamics that mediate neural interactions. The purpose of this section is to suggest a fundamental relationship between functional connectivity at a large-scale physiological level and at a neural level.

Functional connectivity between two areas (in terms of functional imaging) implies that their pool activity goes up and down together. Is it reasonable to suppose that two regions with high pool activity will share a significant number of neurons whose dynamic interactions occur within a time frame of milliseconds? We suggest it is. There are two lines of evidence in support of a relationship between fast dynamic interactions and slower variations in pool activity: (1) Aertsen and Preissl (1991) have investigated the behavior of artificial networks, analytically and using simulations. They concluded that *short term effective connectivity varies strongly with, or is modulated by, pool activity.* Pool activity is defined as the product of the number of neurons and their mean firing rate. The mechanism is simple: the efficacy of subthreshold excitatory postsynaptic potentials (EPSPs) in establishing dynamic interactions is a function of postsynaptic depolarization, which in turn depends on the tonic background of activity. (2) The second line of evidence is experimental and demonstrates that the presence of fast interactions is associated with intermediate or long term correlations between distant neurons. Nelson, Salin, Munk, Arzi, and Bullier (1992) have characterized effective connections between neurons or small groups of neurons, in Brodmann's area (BA) 17 and BA 18 of cat extrastriate cortex. By cross-correlating activity, they demonstrated that the most likely temporal relationship between spikes was a synchronous one. Furthermore, the cross-correlograms segregated into three nonoverlapping groups with modal widths of 3 ms, 30 ms, and 400 ms. The short term correlation structures

(3 and 30 ms) were almost always associated with the intermediate (400 ms) correlations. These observations suggest an interaction between short term (<100 ms) and intermediate (100–1000 ms) correlations.

In summary, the idea is that coactivated regions will have increased (correlated) rCBF and neuronal pool activity. Higher background discharge rates augment postsynaptic depolarization and susceptibility to fast dynamic interactions at a neural level, both within and between the regions coactivated. This susceptibility may correspond to enhanced functional and effective connectivity at a neural level.

B. Eigenimage Analysis

1. Measuring a Pattern of Correlated Activity

In this section we introduce a simple way of measuring the amount a pattern of activity (representing a connected brain system) contributes to the functional connectivity or variance–covariances observed. Functional connectivity is defined in terms of correlations or covariances (correlations are normalized covariances). The point to point functional connectivity between one voxel and another is not usually of great interest. The important aspects of the covariance structure are the patterns of correlated activity, subtended by (the enormous number of) pairwise covariances. In measuring these patterns, it is useful to introduce the concept of a *norm*. Vector and matrix norms serve the same purpose as absolute values for scalar quantities. In other words, they furnish a measure of distance. One frequently used norm is the 2-norm, which is simply the length of the vector. The vector 2-norm can be used to measure the degree to which a particular pattern of brain activity contributes to the covariance structure. If a pattern is described by a column vector (p), with an element for each voxel, then the contribution of that pattern to the covariance structure can be measured by the 2-norm of $M \cdot p = |M \cdot p|_2$. M is a (mean corrected) matrix of data with one row for each successive scan and one column for each voxel (^{T} denotes transposition):

$$|M \cdot p|_2^2 = p^T \cdot M^T \cdot M \cdot p \qquad (1)$$

Put simply the 2-norm is a number that reflects the amount of variance-covariance or functional connectivity that can be accounted for by a particular distributed pattern. If the time-dependent changes occur predominantly in the regions described by the pattern (p), then the correlation between the pattern of activity and p *over space* will vary substantially *over time*. The 2-norm measures this temporal variance in the spatial correlation. It should be noted, of course, that the 2-

norm only measures the pattern p that one is interested in. There may be many other important patterns of functional connectivity even if the 2-norm for a particular pattern is very small. This begs the question "what are the most prevalent patterns of coherent activity?" To answer this question, one turns to eigenimages or spatial modes.

2. Eigenimages and Spatial Modes

In this section the concept of eigenimages or spatial modes is introduced in terms of the patterns of activity (p) in the previous section. In this section we show that the spatial modes are simply those patterns that account for the *most* variance-covariance (i.e., have the largest 2-norm).

Eigenimages or spatial modes are most commonly obtained using singular value decomposition (SVD). SVD is an operation that decomposes the original time-series (M) into two sets of orthogonal vectors (patterns in space and patterns in time), u and v where

$$[u \; s \; v] = \text{SVD}\{M\}$$

such that

$$M = u \cdot s \cdot v^{\text{T}}, \tag{2}$$

where u and v are unitary orthogonal matrices (the sum of squares of each column is unity and all the columns are uncorrelated), and s is a diagonal matrix (only the leading diagonal has nonzero values) of decreasing singular values. A rearrangement of Eq. (2) shows v to be the eigenvectors of the functional connectivity matrix ($C = M^{\text{T}}M$):

$$M^{\text{T}}M \cdot v = C \cdot v = v \cdot s^2. \tag{3}$$

The columns of $v = [v^1 \ldots v^n]$ correspond to the eigenimages or spatial modes. The corresponding eigenvalues are given by the leading diagonal of s^2. Referring back to Eq. (1) shows that the singular value of each eigenimage is simply its 2-norm. Because SVD maximizes the largest singular value, the first eigenimage is the pattern that accounts for the greatest amount of the variance-covariance structure. In summary, SVD and equivalent devices are powerful ways of decomposing an imaging time-series into a series of orthogonal patterns than embody, in a stepdown fashion, the greatest amounts of functional connectivity. Each eigenvector defines a distributed brain system that can be displayed as an image. The distributed systems that ensue are called *eigenimages* or *spatial modes* and have been used characterize the spatiotemporal dynamics of neurophysiological time-series from several modalities, including multiunit electrode recordings (Mayer-Kress et al., 1991), EEG (Friedrich et al., 1991), magne-

toencephalography (MEG) (Fuchs, Kelso, & Haken, 1992), PET (Friston, Frith, Laddle, et al 1993), and functional MRI (Friston, Jezzard, Frackowiak, & Turner, 1993).

One might ask what the column vectors of u in Eq. (2) correspond to. These vectors are the time-dependent profiles associated with each eigenimage. They reflect the extent to which an eigenimage is expressed in each experimental condition or over time. These vectors play an important role in the functional attribution of the distributed systems defined by the eigenimages. This point and others will be illustrated in the next section.

3. An Eigenimage Analysis of the Word Generation Study

Voxels were selected from the verbal fluency activation data described above [using the omnibus F ratio to identify voxels significant at $p < .05$ (uncorrected)] The time-series from each of these voxels formed a mean corrected data matrix M with 12 rows (one for each condition) and 69,142 columns (one for each voxel).

M was subject to SVD as described in the previous section. The distribution of eigenvalues (Fig. 2C) suggested only two spatial modes are required to account for most of the observed variance-covariance structure. The first mode accounted for 60% of the variance. The first eigenimages (v^1) had negative loadings (Fig. 2B) in the anterior cingulate (BA 24, 32), the left DLPFC (BA 46), Broca's area (BA 44), the thalamic nuclei, and in some extrastiate regions. Positive loadings (Fig. 2A) were seen bitemporally, in the posterior cingulate and medial prefrontal cortex. The post hoc functional attribution of these spatial modes is usually based on their time-dependent profiles (u^i). According to u^1 (Fig. 2D), the first mode is (negatively) prevalent in the verbal fluency tasks with positive scores in word shadowing and may represent an *intentional* system critical for the intrinsic generation of words (compare this eigenimage with the equivalent SPM analysis in Fig. 1). The second mode (not shown) corresponded to a highly nonlinear, monotonic time effect with greatest prominence in the earlier conditions.

The implications of this analysis are that word generation involves profound negative interactions between prefrontal and temporal regions. In other words, we can consider this study as evoking substantial prefronto-temporal functional connectivity. The remaining sections of this chapter concentrate on characterizing this particular functional interaction in schizophrenia (Friston, Liddle, & Frith, 1994).

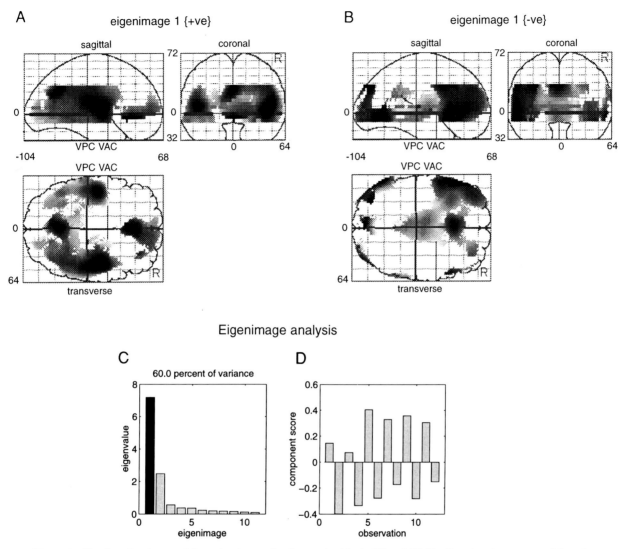

Figure 2 The first eigenimage of the activation study of normal subjects. (A) and (B): The first eigenimage or spatial mode corresponding to the first eigenvector of the functional connectivity matrix. This mode is the first eigenvector of $M^T M$. The eigenimage is displayed as a maximum intensity projection in standard SPM format with positive parts on the left and negative parts on the right. (C) Eigenvalue spectrum. (D) Time-dependent expression of the first spatial mode (u^1) or alternatively, eigenvectors of the distribution of points in a functional space (i.e., eigenvector of MM^T). The attribution of the corresponding spatial mode, or direction in a functional space, depends on relating this vector to the tasks employed during the activation. This vector is clearly related to the difference between word generation (even-numbered conditions) and word shadowing (odd-numbered scans). This difference is the intentional or intrinsic generation of word representations.

C. An Example Using Word Generation in Schizophrenia

1. Background

The central thesis of the remaining sections is that although localized pathophysiology of cortical areas (e.g., the DLPFC) may be a sufficient explanation for some signs of schizophrenia, it does not suffice as a rich or compelling explanation for the symptoms of schizophrenia. The conjecture we review here is that symptoms such as hallucinations and delusions are better understood in terms of abnormal interactions or integration between different cortical areas. This dysfunctional integration is expressed at a physiological level as abnormal functional connectivity, and at a cognitive level as a failure to integrate perception and action that manifests as clinical symptoms. The distinction between a regionally specific pathology and a pathology of interaction can be seen in terms of a first order effect (e.g., hypofrontality) and a second order effect that only exists in the relationship between activity in the prefrontal cortex and some other (e.g., temporal) region. In a similar way, psychological abnormalities can be regarded as first order (e.g., a poverty of intrinsically cued behavior in psychomotor poverty) or second order (e.g., a failure to integrate intrinsically cued behavior and perception in reality distortion).

The notion that schizophrenia represents a disintegration or fractionation of the psyche is as old as its name, introduced by Bleuler (1913) to convey a "splitting" of mental faculties. Many of Bleuler's primary processes, such as "loosening of associations" emphasize a fragmentation and loss of coherent integration. In what follows, we suggest this mentalistic "splitting" has a physiological basis, and furthermore, that both the mentalistic and physiological disintegration have precise and specific characteristics that can be understood in terms of functional anatomy.

The evidence for structural and functional abnormalities in both the prefrontal cortices and temporal lobes is strong, particularly in the left hemisphere. This evidence ranges from abnormal quantitative cytoarchitecture (Benes, Davidson, & Bird, 1986) to gross morphological changes evident on MRI scans (Bogerts, Ashtari, Degreef, Alvir, Bilder, & Liberman, 1991) and postmortem (Brown, Colter, Coreslis, Crow, Frith, Jagoe, et al., 1986). Functional abnormalities have been demonstrated using PET (Liddle, Friston, Frith, Jones, Hirsch, & Frackowiak, 1992) and electrophysiology (McCarley, Shenton, Odennell, Faux, Kikinis, Nestor, et al., 1993).

Abnormal integration of prefrontal neural activity and activity in subcortical, limbic, and temporal structures is a common theme, found in many neurobiological accounts of schizophrenia. For example, neurodevelopmental models of schizophrenia (Weinberger, 1987; Murray & Lewis, 1987) refer to the concurrent maturation of the frontal lobes, in terms of myelination, and the emergence of schizophrenic phenomena. In adolescence there is evidence for progressive changes in the nature of cortical interactions (as measured by the EEG), particularly between the left prefrontal and temporal regions (Buchsbaum, Mansour, Teng, Zia, Seigel, & Rice, 1992). The pathophysiological basis of abnormal cognitive processing in schizophrenia has been discussed in terms of abnormal fronto-striatal and fronto-temporal integration (Frith, 1987; 1992).

Although there is less direct evidence for an abnormal integration of prefrontal and temporal activity, there are some intriguing and suggestive observations. For example, psychotic symptoms, including complex auditory hallucinations and delusions, are a prominent feature of metachromatic leukodystrophy presenting in early life (Hyde, Ziegler, & Weinberger, 1992). The pathology of metachromatic leukodystrophy is demyelination affecting many systems but particularly the subfrontal white matter. The possibility that the pathophysiology of schizophrenia leads to a similar prefronto-temporal functional "disconnection" suggests that functional connectivity between these two brain systems should be demonstrably abnormal.

2. The Data

The data were acquired from four groups of 6 subjects with a PET camera (CTI model 93108) using a fast dynamic ^{15}O technique. Each subject was scanned six times during the performance of three word production tasks. The order of the tasks was balanced for time effects (A B C C B A). Task A was a verbal fluency task, requiring subjects to respond with a word that began with a heard letter. Task B was a semantic categorization task where the subject responded "man-made" or "natural," depending on the heard noun. Task C was a word shadowing task where the subject simply repeated what was heard. All the images were stereotactically normalized and mapped into a standard anatomical space (Talairach & Tournoux, 1988). Differences in rCBF due simply to whole brain differences were removed using ANCOVA (Friston et al., 1990). A mean rCBF estimate for each voxel, for each of the six conditions (scans), for each group, was obtained by averaging over the 6 subjects in each group. A subset of voxels was selected, for subsequent analysis, if the differences between any of the six scans accounted for a significant amount of variance (ANCOVA F > 3.9 p < .001 df 5, 24) in one or more of the four groups. The result was a large mean corrected matrix (M) of rCBF estimates for each of the four groups, comprising six rows (one for each scan) and 4802 columns (one for each voxel).

The four groups comprised one group of 6 normal subjects and three groups of 6 schizophrenic patients [DSMIII-R (1987)]. The patients were all relatively chronic, medicated, stable, and middle-aged. The schizophrenic groups were categorized according to their performance on a series of verbal fluency tasks. The first group (poverty) produced less than 24 words on a standard (one minute) FAS verbal fluency task. The other groups all produced more than 24 words. The second schizophrenic group (odd) produced neologisms and/or words not in the semantic category specified and/or five or more unusual words. Unusualness was defined using the Battig and Montague (1969) category norms. The third group was unimpaired according to the above criteria. Although this categorization is explicitly in terms of performance on psychological tests germane to the activation paradigm employed, the three groups can be loosely identified with the three dimensions commonly found in clinical ratings of schizophrenia (Liddle, 1987; Bilder, Mukherjee, Reider, & Pandurangi, 1985; Mortimer, Lund, & McKenna, 1990; Arndt, Alliger, & Andreason, 1991): (1) *psychomotor poverty,* characterized by reduced speech, spontaneous movement, and flattened affect; (2) *disorganization,* associated with inappropriate affect, thought disorder, incoherence, and poverty of content of speech; and (3) *reality distortion,* with hallucinations and delusions but less neuropsychological impairment (Liddle & Morris, 1991).

3. Differences in Functional Connectivity and the Generalized Eigenvector Solution

In this section we present a direct analysis of the differences between the patterns of correlated activity between normal subjects and schizophrenic patients. This is achieved by identifying the eigenimage that reflects the functional connectivity in the normal subjects, not expressed in a schizophrenic group (d_1). This eigenimage is obtained by using the generalized eigenvector solution

$$C_n \cdot d_1 = C_p \cdot d_1 \cdot \lambda_1$$

or

$$C_p^{-1} \cdot C_n \cdot d_1 = d_1 \cdot \lambda_1 \tag{4}$$

where C_p and C_n are the poverty schizophrenic and normal functional connectivity matrices respectively. It can be seen that d_1 is the eigenvector of $C_p^{-1} \cdot C_n$ In other words, the eigenimage that maximizes the ratio of the 2-norms in normals and the poverty group $\| d_1 \cdot C_n \cdot d_1 \| / \| d_1 \cdot C_p \cdot d_1 \|$. More intuitively, this eigenimage is the pattern that dominates in normal subjects *relative* to the schizophrenics.

The results of this analysis are presented in Figure 3. The pattern (Fig. 3 A and B) that best captures the differences is similar to the pattern seen in previous sections (Fig. 2), namely negative correlations between left DLPFC and bilateral superior temporal regions. The amount to which this pattern was expressed in each individual group is shown in Figure 3 (C), using the appropriate 2-norm $\| d_1 \cdot C \cdot d_1 \|$. This measure simply reflects the degree d_1 contributes to the variance-covariance structure C (cf. the eigenvalue). It is seen that this eigenimage, while prevalent in the normal subjects, is virtually absent in all the three schizophrenic groups. Equivalently, the substantial prefronto-temporal functional connectivity within the system portrayed in Figure 3 is not found in the schizophrenics. It is important to note that only one of the schizophrenic groups (the poverty group) was used to define this eigenimage, and yet it is absent in the remaining schizophrenic groups.

Figure 4 shows the complementary analysis, where the eigenimage was chosen to show functional connectivity prevalent in the poverty schizophrenic group that was minimally expressed in the normal group. The main feature of this functional connectivity pattern was a positive left prefronto-left middle temporal interaction. Again, although the data from the odd and unimpaired group were not used to constrain the eigenvector solution, this pattern is also found in these groups.

4. Implications

In summary, compared to normal subjects, the schizophrenic groups showed a very different pattern of distributed cerebral interactions. The nature of this difference was remarkably consistent across the groups of schizophrenia analyzed. The main differences between normal subjects and patients was a double dissociation in terms of regionally specific prefronto-temporal functional connectivity: (1) Profound left prefronto-superior temporal interactions were seen in normal subjects but not in schizophrenia; and (2) marked left prefronto-left infero-middle temporal correlations were marked in the schizophrenic groups, but less so in normal subjects. A further qualitative difference was that the fronto-temporal covariances were negative in normals but positive in patients. These results indicate not only regionally specific and consistent differences in functional connectivity, but a complete reversal in the nature of the large scale prefronto-temporal interactions. This reversal can be regarded as a failure of prefrontal cortex to suppress activity in the temporal lobes (or vice versa).

The coherent temporal succession of self-initiated action and perception depends on a continuous dialogue between neural systems responsible for executing motor behavior and sensory systems that register the consequences. This dialogue may be mediated by connections between prefrontal cortex and appropriate sensory systems to integrate the sensed and expected consequences of acting. An extremely useful metaphor for this sort of neuronal interaction is found in the occulomotor system (cf. Feinberg, 1978). Helmholtz (1866) pointed out that when we move our eyes the image slips across the retina, and yet we perceive the world as stationary. This phenomenon can be accounted for by corollary discharge or reafference copy (Sperry, 1950; von Holst & Mittelstaedt, 1950). Robinson and Wurtz (1976) identified cells in the superficial layers of the superior colliculus that respond to moving stimuli but do not respond when the eye is moved across a stationary target. At that time, they tentatively identified the frontal eye fields (in the prefrontal cortex) as the source of modulating corollary

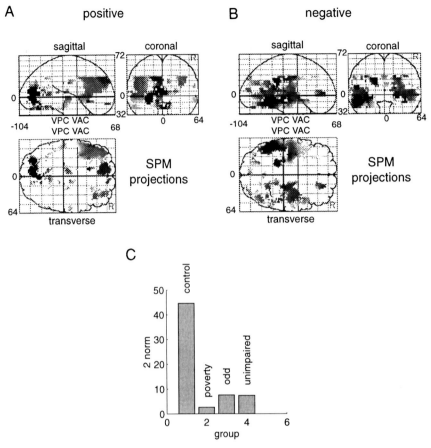

Figure 3 (A) and (B): Eigenimage analysis of the differences between normal subjects and (poverty) schizophrenic patients. The SPMs depict positive and negative components of the eigenimage that is maximally expressed in the normal group and minimally expressed in the poverty group. In fact, this pattern is virtually absent in all the schizophrenic data. This point is made by expressing the amount of functional connectivity attributable to this eigenimage in each of the four groups, using the appropriate 2-norm (C).

discharge. Similar selectivity of unit responses for extrinsically and intrinsically caused sensory changes is found in the auditory system. Muller-Preuss and Jurgens (1976) identified cells in the auditory cortex of squirrel monkeys that respond to extrinsically generated sounds, but not to self-generated vocalization. Ploog (1979) concluded that the inhibition of these cells is caused by corollary discharges associated with vocalization, possibly from the anterior cingulate (in the prefrontal cortex). The anterior cingulate projects not only to Broca's area but also auditory areas, including Brodmann's area 22.

The picture that emerges is of modulatory interactions between prefrontal cortex and posterior sensory cortex that serve to integrate perception and action. A failure of this integration, or at a neurophysiological level, dysfunctional prefronto-temporal connectivity, may compromise (1) intrinsically generated action,

secondary to disintegration between (prefrontal and premotor) intentional and (discriminative and proprioceptive) sensory systems, and (2) aberrant perception resulting from misattribution of a self-induced sensory change to the external agencies. All of these are sequelae that are very pertinent to schizophrenia.

In conclusion, intrinsically generated behavior and the integration of that behavior into the perceptual domain depends on coherent interactions between prefrontal cortices and those devoted to perceptual representations. Of the many interactions among these systems, we have focused on efferents from the prefrontal cortex to sensory systems and their role in modulating target activity. This modulatory role may be as simple as suppressing responsiveness to self-induced sensory changes [for which electrophysiological evidence exists (Muller-Preuss & Jurgens, 1976)], or they may reflect dynamic interactions that are less easy

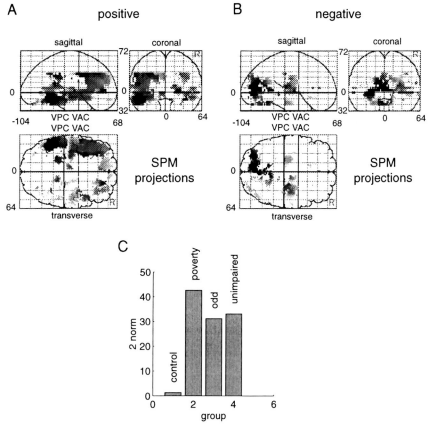

Figure 4 As for Figure 3, but here the eigenimage identified was maximally expressed in the poverty group and minimally expressed in the normal subjects.

to characterize. Many signs and experiential symptoms of schizophrenia impinge on the relationship of self to others as mediated by language and expression (or absence of it) (e.g., poverty of speech, inappropriate or flat affect, incoherent speech, decreased content of speech, auditory hallucinations, and paranoid delusions). The functional anatomy of language-related perceptual representations centers on the temporal regions It follows that there might be something quite specific about fronto-temporal disconnection and schizophrenia. In this regard, structural MRI studies of schizophrenic brains have found abnormalities in the superior temporal gyrus and underlying white matter with some consistency (McCarley et al., 1993).

IV. Conclusion

This chapter has reviewed the basic distinction between approaches based on functional segregation (statistical parametric mapping) and functional integration (eigenimage analysis). There are many ways to make inferences about functional segregation in the brain us-

ing SPMs. Three important classes of experimental design are subtractive, parametric, and factorial. Each of these is associated with a particular instance of the general linear model. Statistical inferences about the resulting SPM are made using distributional approximations from the theory of Gaussian fields.

Functional integration is mediated by anatomical, functional, and effective connections. In neuroimaging, functional connectivity forms the basis for characterizing patterns of correlations using eigenimages or spatial modes. Although a purely descriptive approach, eigenimage analysis has allowed us to make some provisional but intriguing observations regarding the integrity of functional connectivity between prefrontal and temporal regions in schizophrenia.

Acknowledgments

KJF was funded by the Wellcome Trust during part of this work. I would like to thank all my colleagues for help in the development of this work, particularly those at the Wellcome Department of Cognitive Neurology, UK.

References

Aertsen, A., & Preissl, H. (1991). Dynamics of activity and connectivity in physiological neuronal networks. *Non-linear dynamics and neuronal networks* (pp. 281–302). New York: Ed Schuster HG VCH.

American Psychiatric Association (1987). *Diagnostic and statistical manual of mental disorders* (3rd eds., revised). Washington, D.C.: American Psychiatric Press.

Arndt, S., Alliger, R. J., & Andreasen, N. C. (1991). The distinction of positive and negative symptoms: The failure of a two dimensional model. *British Journal of Psychiatry, 158,* 317–322.

Battig, W. F., & Montague, W. E. (1969). Category norms of verbal items in 56 categories: A replication and extension of the Connecticut norms. *Journal of Experimental Psychology, 80,* 1–46.

Benes, F. M., Davidson, J., & Bird, E. D. (1986). Quantitative cytoarchitectural studies of the cerebral cortex of schizophrenics. *Archives of General Psychiatry, 43,* 31–35.

Benson, D. F. (1990). Psychomotor retardation. *Neuro-psychiatry, Neuropsychology and Behavioral Neurology, 3,* 36–47.

Bilder, R. M., Mukherjee, S., Reider, R. O., & Pandurangi, A. A. K. (1985). Symptomatic and neuropsychological components of defect states. *Schizophrenia Bulletin, 11,* 409–419.

Bleuler, E. (1913). Dementia Praecox or the group of schizophrenias: Translated into English 1987. In J. Cutting & M. Shepherd (Eds.), *The clinical routes of the schizophrenia concept.* Cambridge, UK: Cambridge Univ. Press.

Bogerts, B., Ashtari, M., Degreef, G. J., Alvir, J., Bilder, R. M., and Leiberman, J. A. (1991). Reduced temporal limbic structure volumes on magnetic resonance images in first episode schizophrenia *Psychiatric Research on Neuroimaging, 35,* 1–13.

Brown, R., Colter, N., Coreslis, J. A. N., Crow, T. J., Frith, C. D., Jagoe, Johnstone, E. C., & Marsh, L. (1986). Postmortem evidence of structural brain changes in schizophrenia: differences in brain weight, temporal horn area, and parahippocampal gyrus compared with affective disorder. *Archives of General Psychiatry, 43,* 36–42.

Buchsbaum, M. S., Mansour, C. S., Teng, D. G., Zia, A. D., Seigel, B. V., & Rice, D. M. (1992). Adolescent developmental changes in topography of EEG amplitude. *Schizophrenia Research, 7,* 101–107.

Damasio, A. R., & Van Hoesen, G. W. (1983). Emotional disturbances associated with focal lesions of the frontal lobe. In K. Heilman & P. Satz (Eds.), *Neuropsychology of human emotion.* New York: Plenum.

Feinberg, I. (1978). Efference copy and corollary discharge: Implications for thinking and its disorders. *Schizophrenia Bulletin, 4,* 636–640.

Friedrich, R., Fuchs, A., & Haken, H. (1991). Modelling of spatiotemporal EEG patterns. In I. Dvorak & A. V. Holden (Eds.), *Mathematical approaches to brain functioning diagnostics.* New York: Manchester Univ. Press.

Friston, K. J., Frith, C. D., Liddle, P. F., Lammertsma, A. A., Dolan R. D., & Frackowiak, R. S. J. (1990). The relationship between local and global changes in PET scans. *Journal of Cerebral Blood Flow and Metabolism, 10,* 458–466.

Friston, K. J., Frith, C. D., Liddle, P. F., & Frackowiak, R. S. J. (1991a). Comparing functional (PET) images: The assessment of significant change. *Journal of Cerebral Blood Flow and Metabolism, 11,* 690–699.

Friston, K. J., Frith, C. D., Liddle, P. F., & Frackowiak, R. S. J. (1991b). Investigating a network model of word generation with positron emission tomography *Proceedings of the Royal Society, London B, 244,* 101–106.

Friston, K. J., Frith, C., Passingham, R. E., Liddle, P. F., & Frackowiak, R. S. J. (1992). Motor practice and neurophysiological adaptation in the cerebellum: A positron tomography study. *Proceedings of the Royal Society, London B, 248,* 223–228.

Friston, K. J., Grasby, P., Bench, C., Frith, C., Cowen, P., Little, P., Frackowiak, R. S. J., & Dolan, R. (1992). Measuring the neuromodulatory effects of drugs in man with positron tomography. *Neuroscience Letters, 141,* 106–110.

Friston, K. J., Frith, C. D., Liddle, P. F., & Frackowiak, R. S. J. (1993). Functional connectivity: The principal component analysis of large (PET) data sets. *Journal of Cerebral Blood Flow and Metabolism, 15,* 5–14.

Friston, K. J., Frith, C. D., & Frackowiak, R. S. J. (1993). Time-dependent changes in effective connectivity measured with PET. *Human Brain Mapping, 1,* 69–80.

Friston, K. J., Jezzard, P., Frackowiak, R. S. J., & Turner, R. (1993). Characterizing focal and distributed physiological changes with MRI and PET. *Functional MRI of the brain,* (pp. 207–216). Berkely, CA: Society of Magnetic Resonance in Medicine.

Friston, K. J., Worsley, K. J., Frackowiak, R. S. J., Mazziotta, J. C., & Evans, A. C. (1994). Assessing the significance of focal activations using their spatial extent. *Human Brain Mapping, 1,* 214–220.

Friston, K. J., Liddle, P. F., & Frith, C. D. (1994). Dysfunctional frontotemporal integration in schizophrenia. *Neuropsychopharmacology, 10,* 538S.

Frith, C. D. (1987). The positive and negative symptoms of schizophrenia reflect impairments in the initiation and perception of action. *Psychological Medicine, 134,* 225–235.

Frith, C. D. (1992). *The cognitive neuropsychology of schizophrenia.* Sussex, U. K.: Erlbaum.

Frith, C. D., Friston, K. J., Liddle, P. F., & Frackowiak, R. S. J. (1991a). Willed action and the prefrontal cortex in man. *Proceedings of the Royal Society, London B, 244,* 241–246.

Frith, C. D., Friston, K. J., Liddle, P. F., & Frackowiak, R. S. J. (1991b). A PET study of word finding. *Neuropsychologia, 28,* 1137–1148.

Fuchs, A., Kelso, J. A. S., & Haken, H. (1992). Phase transitions in the human brain: Spatial mode dynamics *International Journal of Bifurcation and Chaos, 2,* 917–939.

Gerstein, G. L., & Perkel, D. H. (1969). Simultaneously recorded trains of action potentials: Analysis and functional interpretation. *Science, 164,* 828–830.

Gerstein, G. L., Bedenbaugh, P., & Aertsen, A. M. H. J. (1989) Neuronal assemblies *IEEE Transactions on Biomedical. Engineering, 36,* 4–14.

Gilbert, P. F. C., & Thach, W. T. (1977). Purkinje cell activity during motor learning. *Brain Research, 128,* 309–328.

Goltz, F. (1881). In W. MacCormac (Ed.), *Transactions of the 7th international medical congress* (Vol. 1, pp. 218–228). London: Kolkmann.

Golub, G. H., & Van Loan, C. F. (1991). *Matrix computations* (2nd ed., pp. 241–248). Baltimore and London: Johns Hopkins Univ. Press.

Grafton, S., Mazziotta, J., Presty, S., Friston, K. J., Frackowiak, R. S. J., & Phelps, M. (1992). Functional anatomy of human procedural learning determined with regional cerebral blood flow and PET. *Journal of Neuroscience, 12,* 2542–2548.

Grasby, P., Friston, K. J., Bench, C., Cowen, P., Frith, C., Liddle, P., Frackowiak, R. S. J., & Dolan, R. (1992). Effect of the 5-HT1$_A$ partial agonist buspirone on regional cerebral blood flow in man. *Psychopharmacology, 108,* 380–386.

Helmholtz, H. (1866). *Handbuch der Physiologischen Optik.* Leipzig, Germany: Voss.

von Holst, E., & Mittelstaedt, H. (1950). Das reafferenzprinzip. *Naturwissenschaften, 37,* 464–476.

Hyde, T. M., Ziegler, J. C., & Weinberger, D. R. (1992). Psychiatric disturbances in metachromatic leukodystrophy—Insights into the neurobiology of psychosis. *Archives of Neurology, 49,* 401–406.

Ingvar, D. H., & Franzen, G. (1974). Abnormalities of cerebral blood flow distribution in patients with chronic schizophrenia. *Acta Psychiatrica Scandinavia, 50,* 425–436.

Liddle, P. F. (1987). The symptoms of chronic schizophrenia: A re-examination of the positive–negative dichotomy *British Journal of Psychiatry, 151,* 145–151.

Liddle, P. F., & Morris, D. L. (1991). Schizophrenic syndromes and frontal lobe performance. *British Journal of Psychiatry, 158,* 340–345.

Liddle, P. F., Friston, K. J., Frith, C. D., Jones, T., Hirsch, S. R., & Frackowiak, R. S. J. (1992). Patterns of cerebral blood flow in schizophrenia. *British Journal of Psychiatry, 160,* 179–186.

Lueck, C. J., Zeki, S., Friston, K. J., Deiber, N. O. Cope, P., Cunningham, V. J., Lammertsma, A. A., Kennard, C., & Frackowiak, R. S. J. (1989). The colour centre in the cerebral cortex of man. *Nature (London), 340,* 386–389.

Marsden, C. D., Parkes, J. D., & Quinn, N. (1982). Fluctuations of disability in Parkinson's disease: Clinical aspects In C. D. Marsden & S. Fahn (Eds.), *Movement disorders* (pp. 459–467). London: Butterworth.

Mayer-Kress, G., Barczys, C., & Freeman, W. (1991). Attractor reconstruction from event-related multi-electrode EEG data. In I. Dvorak & A. V. Holden (Eds.), *Mathematical approaches to brain functioning diagnostics.* New York: Manchester Univ. Press.

McCarley, R. W., Shenton, M. E., Odonnell, B. F., Faux, S. F., Kikinis, R., Nestor, P. G., & Jolesz, F. A. (1993). Auditory P300 abnormalities and left posterior superior temporal gyrus volume reduction in schizophrenia. *Archives of General Psychiatry, 50,* 190–197.

McIntosh, A. R., Grady, C. L., Ungerleider, L. G., Haxby, J. V., Rapoport, S. I., & Horwitz, B. (1993). Network analysis of cortical visual pathways mapped with PET. *Journal of Neuroscience, 14,* 655–666.

Mortimer, A. M., Lund, C. E., & McKenna, P. J. (1990). The positive-negative dichotomy in schizophrenia. *British Journal of Psychiatry, 157,* 41–49.

Muller-Preuss, P., & Jurgens, U. (1976). Projections from the 'cingular' vocalization area in the squirrel monkey. *Brain Research, 103,* 29–43.

Murray, R. M., and Lewis, S. R. (1987). Is schizophrenia a developmental disorder? *British Medical Journal, 295,* 681–682.

Nelson, J. I., Salin, P. A., Munk, N. M. J., Arzi, M., & Bullier, J. (1992). Spatial and temporal coherence in cortico–cortical connections: A cross-correlation study in areas 17 and 18 in the cat. *Visual Neuroscience, 9,* 21–37.

Passingham, R. E., Chen, Y. C., & Thaler, D. (1989). Supplementary motor cortex and self initiated movement. In M. Ito (Ed.), *Neural programming* (pp. 13–24). Tokyo: Japan Scientific Societies Press.

Petersen, S. E., Fox, P. T., Posner, M. I., Mintun, M., & Raichle, M. E. (1989). Positron emission tomographic studies of the processing of single words *Journal of Cognitive Neuroscience, 1,* 153–170.

Phillips, C. G., Zeki, S., Barlow, H. B. (1984). Localization of function in the cerebral cortex. Past present and future. *Brain 107,* 327–361.

Ploog, D. (1979). Phonation, emotion, cognition: With reference to the brain mechanisms involved. *Brain and mind CIBA Foundation symposium 69* (pp. 79–86). Elsevier: Amsterdam.

Price, C., Wise, R. J. S., Ramsay, S., Friston, K. J., Howard, D., Patterson, K., & Frackowiak, R. S. J. (1992). Regional response differences within the human auditory cortex when listening to words. *Neuroscience Letters, 146,* 179–182.

Robinson, D. L., and Wurtz, R. H. (1976). Use of an extraretinal signal by monkey superior colliculus neurons to distinguish real from self induced movement. *Journal of Neurophysiology, 39,* 832–870.

Sperry, R. W. (1950). Neural basis of the spontaneous opticokinetic response produced by visual inversion: *Journal of Comparative Physiological Psychology, 43,* 482–489.

Talairach, J., & Tournoux, P. (1988). *A Co-planar stereotaxic atlas of a human brain.* Stuttgart, Germany: Thieme.

Weinberger, D. R. (1987). Implications of normal brain development for the pathogenesis of schizophrenia *Archives of General Psychiatry 44,* 660–669.

Worsley, K. J., Evans, A. C., Marrett, S., & Neelin, P. (1992). A three-dimensional statistical analysis for rCBF activation studies in human brain. *Journal of Cerebral Blood Flow and Metabolism, 12,* 900–918.

Zeki, S. (1990). The motion pathways of the visual cortex. In C. Blakemore (Ed.), *Vision: Coding and efficiency* (pp. 321–345). Cambridge, UK: Cambridge Univ. Press.

20

Self-Regulation and Cortical Development: Implications for Functional Studies of the Brain

Phan Luu* and Don M. Tucker*,[†]

*Department of Psychology, University of Oregon, Eugene, Oregon; and [†]Electrical Geodesics, Inc.,
Eugene, Oregon*

I. Introduction

"Development is an ongoing, dynamic process. The anatomical method is a static one, providing a glimpse of only one point in time for any given case" (Huttenlocher, 1990, pp. 523–524).

To understand neuropsychological development is to confront the fact that the brain is mutable, such that its structural organization reflects the history of the organism. Moreover, this structure reflects both what is most important to the organism and what the organism is capable of at that particular time. It has become apparent that the brain is highly plastic and capable of structural reorganization (Jenkins & Merzenich, 1987; Recanzone, Merzenich, Jenkins, Grajski, & Dinse, 1992). The now classic work by Merzenich and colleagues with monkeys showed that the boundaries of cortical representation of the hands and digits are highly dependent upon their use (Recanzone, Merzenich, Jenkins, et al., 1992; Recanzone, Merzenich, & Schreiner, 1992). The implication from these studies is that the cortex is capable of organizational changes throughout the organism's life span. Indeed, recent electroencephalogram (EEG) studies have shown that the period of cortical organization may be very protracted in humans (Thatcher, 1992, 1994). From these EEG studies, cortical organization proceeds in stages, which are repeated periodically. This cyclic recapitulation reflects the constant shaping of cortical wiring throughout an individual's life span.

II. Concepts of Self-Organization

Cortical development and organization should not be viewed as passive processes that are solely dependent upon genetics and environmental input. Rather, they should be regarded as processes of self-organization guided by self-regulatory mechanisms. Even before evidence for cortical plasticity existed, Jackson remarked on the importance of self-organization and brain evolution: "We develop as we must, that is, according to what we are by inheritance; and also as we can, that is, according to external conditions. There is something more: there is what I will call Internal Evolution, a process which goes on the most actively in the highest centers" (Jackson, 1931, p. 71).

Jackson believed that internal evolution results in lasting rearrangements of cortical representations, some of which may not actually correspond to any specific experience with the environment nor to any behavioral consequences. Rather, these representations are the result of self-organizing processes that are relatively free of environmental influence. To restate Jackson's proposal, cortical development is also a self-regulating processes. Thus, a functional understanding of cortical organization and development requires an understanding of how cortical organization and development are motivated. Particularly illustrative is evidence showing that a stimulus' influence on cortical reorganization is dependent upon attentional processes (Merzenich & Sameshima, 1993; Recanzone, Merzenich, & Schreiner, 1992a). Attentional mechanisms may be primitive as well as sophisticated and they are tightly coupled to motivational mechanisms.

Neuroimaging techniques such as positron emission tomography (PET), functional magnetic resonance imaging (fMRI), and high density EEG recording have revealed new insights into the structures of the brain and their related functions under normal and abnormal functioning. However, to proceed beyond the static, descriptive, anatomical level, researchers using these new techniques must address the questions and frame the results in a manner that is consistent with the dynamic nature of cortical organization and self-regulation.

In this chapter we outline a framework of development and cortical organization that is appreciative of the dynamic nature of development, representation, and regulation. Of fundamental importance to these processes are mechanisms of self-regulation. To understand the influence and control of these mechanisms we look to the organizational structure of the brain. We emphasize vertical organization because we believe it provides a key to understanding self-regulatory processes, and that the top of this hierarchy of self-regulation is the frontal lobe. Development within this vertical organization is seen as proceeding from the inside out, to the level of the association areas, importantly the prefrontal cortex, and from the outside in, also to the level of the association areas and, again, more specifically the prefrontal cortex. These two gradients can be conceived as gradients that converge centrally onto the prefrontal cortex. Within this framework, the prefrontal cortex may be the latest to develop but, along with its connections with limbic and paralimbic areas, this region may be the most influential to overall cortical organization (Thatcher, 1994).

III. Vertical Organization

Drawing upon his observations and the evidence at the turn of the century, Jackson (1931) formulated a system in which disorders of the brain can be understood. Jackson believed that brain evolution is an ascending process in which new structures are superordinate to older structures. The developmental trend from this perspective is a shift away from the most determined and specialized to the least organized, from the automatic to the voluntary, and from the simplest to the most complex. In this model, the pathology observed after cerebral lesions can be understood in terms of the remaining older structures; that is, the dissolution of the brain. If not explicit in Jackson's formulation, it is at least implicit that cerebral evolution is characterized by a vertical arrangement of structures. The vertical organization and development of the central nervous system reflects the addition of more specialized functions. The more recent structures serve a regulatory role to those structures that are subordinate to it.

This framework has been used to understand the multiple levels of thermal regulation (Satinoff, 1978) in which higher centers of thermal regulation are considered to regulate and coordinate lower thermal regulation centers through facilitation and inhibition. Other examples of this hierarchical control can be seen in infant development. It is well known that during infant development certain reflexes seen at birth disappear with the maturation of the child (e.g., the Babinski sign). These same reflexes can be observed in the adult after brain damage. For Jackson, these reflexes are seen as positive symptoms that reflect functioning of the remaining cerebral structure(s); these remaining structures are released from the control of more recently evolved cortical areas. This approach, emphasizing ontogenetic recapitulation of phylogenetic development, has also been used to explain the various manifestation of social interaction as the infant matures (Konner, 1991). For example, the social smile of the infant is similar to the social display behaviors of animals that are controlled by subcortical mechanisms. The manifestation of more complex social behaviors such as attachment, fear of separation, and fear of strangers is dependent upon limbic structures. Indeed, maternal behaviors that appear to be specific to mammals have been attributed to cortical structures that are absent in the reptilian brain (MacLean, 1987)

A. Cortical Regulation as a Vertical Process

For modern neuroscience, the discovery of the brainstem reticular activating system by Moruzzi and Magoun reintroduced the notion of vertical cortical organization (Luria, 1973). This discovery showed that centers controlling the state of cortical arousal are not in the cortex, but rather that they are situated in brainstem areas. The effect was that the cortex was no longer the sole focus of attention; structures that lie below the cortex were now seen to be important, if not critical, to mental functioning. However, it is difficult to account for the attentional control and activity of the brain with a unidimensional construct of arousal (Tucker, Luu, & Pribram, 1995; Tucker & Williamson, 1984).

Tucker and Williamson (Tucker & Williamson, 1984) proposed a system of arousal and activation, controlled by brainstem nuclei, that provide the foundation for qualitative changes in attention and cognition. The activation system is centered on dopaminergic pathways. This system produces a tonic form of activation that provides a redundancy bias that routinizes action and focuses attention. The arousal system is regulated by norepinephrine. This system operates in an opposite, yet complementary, manner to the activation system. Attention is broadly allocated and the bias is for habituation. These systems are broadly distributed throughout the cortex, although asymmetrically, so that cortical tone, and thus attention and cognition, is regulated by these two fundamental dimensions of activation and arousal.

Activation and arousal in the Tucker and Williamson model (Tucker & Williamson, 1984) integrate level of activity with typical styles of engagement (e.g., attentional styles) as well as affect. Arousal and activation are not cold but are inherently affective. From the study of the fundamental structure of mood, two underlying dimensions have emerged that are consistent with the activation and arousal systems proposed by Tucker and Williamson. Based upon a comprehensive reanalysis of the literature, Watson and Tellegen (1985) found positive and negative affect to be the fundamental dimensions of mood states. They suggested that these dimensions are not merely descriptive of mood but that they are also descriptive of engagement styles. In other words, each dimension describes affect and the related style of engaging the environment. From a vertical perspective, the grouping of engagement styles, cognition, and affect reflects the functions of the arousal and activation systems at multiple level of the neural axis.

The reticular activation system is now just generally thought of as an ascending system, even though a descending system, centered on the prefrontal cortex, has been described (Luria, 1973; Nauta, 1964; Pribram, 1960). The prefrontal cortex has been shown in both animals (Buchanan & Powell, 1993; Kaada, Pribram, & Epstein, 1949) and humans (Livingston, Chapman, Livingston, & Kraintz, 1947) to be involved in autonomic responses. The prefrontal cortex has been shown to have extensive connections with limbic and brainstem areas, importantly with the reticular network (Nauta, 1964). Consistent with the Jacksonian principle of vertical organization, the prefrontal areas, mainly the medial and ventral surfaces, have been suggested to play a regulatory role, through inhibition and facilitation, over the ascending system, so that it can indirectly regulate the arousal state for the rest of the brain (Luria, 1973).

The prefrontal cortex is thus positioned as an association area for the limbic endbrain (Pribram, 1960) in which it receives information about states and drives and can, in turn, fine-tune and coordinate limbic functions with environmental demands. Pribram argued that the frontal lobe acts as a regulator of internal functions, representing internal regulatory processes and states. The more primitive modes of tonic activation and phasic arousal may be recruited by the prefrontal cortex for self-regulation during both development and social interaction (Tucker et al., 1995). For example, in states of anxiety, the frontal lobe may regulate attentional and cognitive biases through the dopaminergic activation system. The net effect of this regulation is that attention becomes focused and routinized motor actions are facilitated (Tucker & Derryberry, 1992). If chronic anxiety is experienced during development, the effect may be that cortical structures may be configured to operate in a way that maximizes focused and stereotyped actions and cognitions.

B. Cerebral Maturation in the Vertical Dimension

The development of the central nervous system has been described as progressing from the inside out (Pribram, 1960). At the core is the level of the brainstem. Pribram argued that periventricular areas behave in a manner that is similar to peripheral sensory mechanisms. These areas are involved in homeostatic states and are thus sensitive to environmental stimuli. Their sensitivities are not solely dependent upon receiving information from the peripheral receptors. Thus, to the degree that they are independently sensitive to stimuli and that they respond to physiochemical substances, they are very much like sensory receptors. The next ring out is the reticular network. The reticular network, as mentioned previously, is involved in the regulation of cortical states and has close associations with the periventricular areas. Beyond the reticular network is the limbic system. Through its multiple and dense connections with diencephalon and brainstem structures, Pribram argued that the limbic system links and regulates the homeostatic and arousal functions of the brainstem and reticular network, respectively. The concentric organization of development is also seen at cortical levels. In the frontal lobe, the archicortex and paleocortex on the medial and basal surface progress through levels of differentiation that end up on the dorsolateral surface (Pandya & Yeterian, 1990).

This concentric organization should be viewed as additive to the vertical dimension, so that cerebral development and organization through phylogeny proceed in an upward direction as well as outward. Maturation is seen to proceed in a similar manner. That is, brainstem and subcortical structures mature before most cortical structures. This sequence of development has important implications for cortical development and organization, as will be discussed in what follows.

Maturation of cerebral structures can be assessed by a variety of measures. One of the most common measures is the degree of myelin staining observed in sectioned brains. Areas that are darkly stained, reflecting heavy myelination, are assumed to be more mature than lightly stained areas. From myelination-staining studies, brainstem areas, with the exception of the reticular formation, show dark staining at or shortly after birth (Yakovlev & Lecours, 1967). Some have claimed that myelination of the brainstem is mostly completed during infancy (Gibson, 1991). The beginning of myelination and mature myelination occur later in the striatum (e.g., the putamen and globus pallidus) than the brainstem, but before cortical areas such as the frontal and temporal poles (Brody, Kinney, Kloman, & Gilles, 1987). Glucose metabolism in infants also follows this subcortical-cortical gradient (Chugani & Phelps, 1986).

This gradient suggests that at different ages different structures are more involved in the control of behavior. Because the brainstem structures are the first to myelinate and are followed shortly after by midbrain and subcortical forebrain areas, the infant has been described as a subcortical creature (Bronson, 1982). Because these early myelinating structures are comparatively primitive by the Jacksonian principle of evolution and dissolution, their influences on experience and behavior are consequently automatic, simple, and unarticulated. Thus, cortical development in the infant is guided by primitive drives and the need for homeostatic equilibrium.

C. Central Convergence in Maturation

Traditionally, the association areas are believed to be most recent in phylogenetic development (Luria, 1973). However, other evidence suggests that it is the primary motor and sensory areas, rather than the association areas, that are the youngest (Pandya, Seltzer, & Barbas, 1988; Pandya & Yeterian, 1990). Pandya and associates traced the development of the primary motor and sensory areas back to the limbic cortices on the basomedial surface of the hemispheres. It is interesting that the most recent and the most primitive central nervous system structures are sensory areas; both the core and the shell are dedicated to sensory functions. However, the sensory core and shell have different sensory properties. The core is dedicated to diffuse, unarticulated sensory functions that are related to

homeostatic states (Pribram, 1960, 1981). Pribram refers to the nonlocalized distributed sensory functions as protocritic and as cortically represented in the frontal lobe. The shell, with its fine topographic maps, is the complete opposite and is referred to as epicritic by Pribram. The epicritic system involves the posterior association areas.

The outline of maturation from the inside-out and from the bottom-up applies up to the level of the cortex. However, at the level of the cortical hemispheres the pattern reverses so that the primary sensorimotor areas myelinate and reach a mature level of myelination before the association, paralimbic, and limbic structures (Brody et al., 1987; Gibson, 1991).

All of the cortical gyri show some myelination at birth except for the frontal and temporal association areas (Gibson, 1991). The pre- and postcentral gyri are the first to myelinate, and mature myelination occurs well in advance of the prefrontal and temporal poles (Brody et al., 1987). The association areas and limbic system show little myelination at birth, and mature myelination in these areas is only achieved after extensive postnatal development (Brody et al., 1987; Gibson, 1991). In cerebral metabolic studies, the pre- and postcentral gyri are associated with the highest level of glucose utilization at 5 weeks of age (Chugani & Phelps, 1986). Chugani and Phelps showed that the frontal and association areas do not display mature patterns of glucose utilization until approximately 8 months postnatally. Thus, cortically, the gradient of maturation is seen as proceeding from the pre- and postcentral gyri towards the occipital and frontal poles (Kinney, Brody, Kloman, & Gilles, 1988), with the frontal and temporal poles maturing later than the occipital poles (Brody et al., 1987; Huttenlocher, 1990). The gradient of cortical maturation is an inward fanning from the sensory specific areas to the association areas. The "inward" direction used to describe the maturation gradient is in relation to the tracing of cortical evolution by Pandya and colleagues (1988).

Subcortically, the brainstem projections and thalamus also show this fanning-in maturation gradient. Brainstem fiber-systems mediating sensory functions mature earlier than brainstem fiber-systems that mediate integrative functions. At an early age, sensory-specific and motor thalamic nuclei show darker staining in their projections to cortical areas than nonspecific, thalamic nuclei (Yakovlev & Lecours, 1967).

Not only do cortical and subcortical maturation follow the same gradient, they also appear to be sychronized. Yakovlev and LeCours (1967) observed that fibers projecting from the nonspecific nuclei of the thalamus to cortical sites appear to be coincident in their sequence of myelination with the limbic–

paralimbic and association cortical projections to subcortical areas. Furthermore, the reticular network shows a protracted maturation rate that is not seen for other subcortical projections. This extended period of maturation for the reticular network coincides with the maturation of the frontal to subcortical projections.

In the vertical dimension, the brain is organized (Pribram, 1960) and matures from the inside out. At the level of the cerebral hemispheres the pattern reverses, such that the gradient of maturation is from the outside in. These two gradients are synchronized so that cerebral maturation can be described as a process that converges upon limbic and frontal association areas. Before we turn to the topic of limbic and frontal lobe regulation of cortical organization, it is worthwhile to distinguish between two types of cortical plasticity and their relevance to the late maturing cortical areas.

IV. Experience–Expectant versus Experience–Dependent Organization

Because Hughlings Jackson believed that the frontal lobe is positioned at the top of the neural hierarchy and is thus the least determined, it may be the most responsive to the processes of internal evolution. By myelination (Brody et al., 1987), synaptic density (Huttenlocher, 1979), and metabolism standards (Chugani & Phelps, 1986), the frontal lobe and the related limbic and paralimbic structures are protracted in their maturation. Because of this prolonged developmental period, the implication for self-regulatory sculpting of cortical organization is greatest in these areas. In the terms of modern neuroscience, the cortical shaping that occurs beyond time-limited, critical periods and is less dependent upon specific sensory stimuli is referred to as "experience–dependent," to distinguish it from the more elementary "experience–expectant" cortical plasticity (Greenough & Black, 1992).

Experience-expectant plasticity depends upon the overproduction of synapses in anticipation of particular experiences necessary for synaptic maintenance and elimination (Greenough & Black, 1992). The overproduction of synapses in anticipation of environmental input is a result of environmental events, which provide the bases for synaptic pruning, reliably occurring throughout the phylogeny of the species. Once pruning has occurred in these experience–expectant networks, they remain extremely stable. Prototypical examples of this form of plasticity are the ocular dominance columns of the visual cortex. The brief interval displayed by experience–expectant plasticity is consistent with the notion of critical periods.

In contrast, Greenough and Black (1992) argue that experience-dependent plasticity encodes information that is idiosyncratic, as opposed to being common to the species (e.g., visual input at a prespecified time), and not limited by critical periods. The basic mechanisms underlying both types of plasticity may be the same, but the events initiating each are fundamentally different. Experience-expectant plasticity is characterized by a single burst of synaptic overproduction. In contrast, "experience-dependent processes have a quiltwork of small blooms that may further regress on individual schedules" (Greenough & Black, 1992, p. 175). EEG evidence has proven to be consistent with this notion of cyclic reorganization (Thatcher, 1992, 1994). Thus, experience-dependent processes are mechanism by which the Jacksonian concept of internal evolution is achieved. However, the self-regulatory mechanism needs to be delineated.

V. The Limbic Forebrain and Prefrontal Cortex as Central Regulators of Development

A. Frontal Lobe Representations

The concepts of vertical organization, central convergence, and experience-dependent plasticity can be used to describe the representations taking shape within the frontal lobe. From the study of embryogenesis, the concept of developmental induction argues that preceding structures can influence the course of maturation and organization for subsequent structures (Greenough & Black, 1992). It is now well known that cortical organization is a competitive processes (Edelman, 1989; Jenkins & Merzenich, 1987) in which cortical space is at a premium. The resulting cortical representation reflects the state at which competing inputs have settled. Disruption of the equilibrium can occur, for example, through deafferentation (Pons, Garraghty, & Mishkin, 1988) or extensive use of the afferent pathways (Recanzone, Merzenich, Jenkins, et al., 1992), thereby inducing reorganization of cortical maps.

In the sequential maturation of the central nervous system, the lack of intersensory competition has been argued to be important to cortical development and functioning (Turkewitz & Kenny, 1982). Turkewitz and Kenny suggested that staggered maturation of sensory systems provides minimal intersensory competition, allowing for the corresponding cortical areas and behavior to be easily organized. This form of early development lays down a foundation for subsequent development. Greenough and Black (Greenough & Black,

1992) reviewed evidence suggesting that as simple, sensory, experience-expectant maps develop, they provide the experience necessary for succeeding maps. With increasing maturation of the association areas and fibers, competition emerges between intercortical areas and causes disequilibration, providing the opportunity for cortical reorganization (Turkewitz & Kenny, 1982). Reorganization of sensory experience may be a fundamental process underlying cortical and cognitive processes (Edelman, 1989). However, to be consistent with the self-regulatory nature of the brain, brainstem neuromodulator projections must guide cortical reorganization and integration so that they conform to motivational demands.

Cortical organization based upon competition implies that neural activity is sufficient. However, it is important to note that organizational changes do not occur solely from neural activity. Indeed, Greenough and Black (Greenough & Black, 1992) noted that neural activity and cortical plasticity have been dissociated; cortical reorganization appears to be dependent upon attentional process as well as sensory input (Merzenich & Sameshima, 1993; Recanzone, Merzenich, Jenkins, et al., 1992). Evidence suggests that synaptic development, structure, and degeneration may be regulated by neurotransmitters and modulators. Neurotransmitters and modulators have been shown to directly affect synaptic networks by suppressing or facilitating neurite outgrowth (Mattson, 1988). Through this process, transmitter substances may encode information at the network level by shaping its development, in the spirit of connectionist models, as well as encode and transfer information in a traditional, discrete, synapse-to-synapse manner. Of some importance is the fact that the neurotransmitters and modulators affect synaptic growth at the level of the synapse (Mattson, 1988). In this way, local networks may be sculpted and refined independent of where the originating soma is located. On the other hand, catecholamine projections are widespread and thus have the capability to provide coherence in synaptic pruning across broadly distributed networks. For example, Collins and Depue (1992) suggest that dopamine (DA) cells from the ventral tegmental area (VTA) can alter and reinforce the synaptic connectivity between structures that make up behavioral systems, such as the orbitofrontal cortex and the nucleus accumbens.

Neuromodulators like dopamine and norepinephrine make up the activation and arousal systems, respectively, and inherent in the functioning of these systems are biases in cognitive control and affective states (Tucker & Williamson, 1984). It is conceivable that each system influences cortical shaping in a manner that is consistent with its inherent biases, so that organization is consolidated in a like manner up and down the neural axis. Cortical shaping as guided by neuromodulator systems inherently reflects the self-regulating history of the organism, and not just the caprices of environmental input alone.

The late maturation and convergence of information onto association and limbic areas necessitate that organization and representation within limbic and prefrontal cortices involves a negotiation between protocritic and epicritic states; that is, the compromise between environmental and internal demands (Pribram, 1960, 1981). Tucker (1992) has proposed an adaptive network model of control, in which limbic and paralimbic cortices develop and maintain representations of the motivational significance of perceptual and motor patterns. In this sense, Tucker's model is equivalent to Pribram's (Pribram, 1960, 1981) notion of the protocritic system. That is, frontal representations are characterized by experiences that have been constrained by limbic and subcortical structures involved in motivational states.

Frontal and limbic structures represent functional compromises and are involved in regulating brainstem networks. This center not only regulates immediate behavior and cortical functioning, but it also regulates subsequent cerebral organization as well (Thatcher, 1994).

B. Frontal Lobe and Cyclic, Cortical Organization

From a vertical perspective, information must pass up and down the vertical hierarchy to achieve coherence, a form of recurrent reentrant processing (Edelman, 1989). The organization of information through these multiple levels is maintained by limbic and prefrontal networks. At first or second pass through the axis, frontal and cortical networks would resonate in a certain mode based upon the configuration of the representation and the affective state of the organism. The resonance within this network would sustain information on succeeding passes so that sensorimotor patterns are consolidated (Tucker, 1992). A resonating system has been proposed for internal representations following ecological models of perception (Shepard, 1984). Within this model, Shepard proposes that resonance occurs at many levels during perception. Some resonances reflect abstract invariances of perception (e.g., the edibleness of an apple), while others reflect more specific invariances (e.g., orientations of features). According to Shepard, the invariances that these networks resonate to are the result of internalizing invariances that have occurred throughout the evolution of the species. However, there are networks, based upon experience, that resonate to invariances that are idiosyncratic to the organism. In humans, these networks are located in frontal and limbic areas and may be characterized as "personal affordance" networks. The qualities inherent within environmental stimuli and situations that these networks resonate to will be fundamentally different for each individual.

Some EEG work suggests that cortical organization is a cyclic process with clear spatial gradients (Thatcher, 1992, 1994). The cycles are periodically revisited. In this cyclic process, the frontal lobe regulates synaptogenesis of the posterior networks in a manner that resembles a population model that pits predator against prey (Thatcher, 1994); the frontal networks behave in a predatory fashion and the posterior networks play the role of prey. The model suggests that competition for cortical territory in the predator–prey relationship involves direct connections between frontal and posterior areas. However, it cannot be ruled out that the frontal areas also use their privileged connections with brainstem areas (via the descending reticular network) to their competitive advantage. Nevertheless, Thatcher describes this sculpting process as a process that reduces the discrepancy between the microanatomy of the cerebrum and environmental demands. To the extent that each person is endowed with frontal and limbic personal affordance networks that are prepared to resonate to (i.e., ready to support) environmental information in individually specific ways, sculpting of posterior networks will reflect these differences. What is important to one individual, as indicated by representation in his or her frontal and limbic networks, is indirectly manifested in posterior networks. As discrepancies between microanatomy and environmental demands are reduced, differences in network architecture between individuals are increased.

VI. Conclusion

It has been repeatedly suggested in recent years that brain development is an ongoing process that ends only with the death of the organism (Brown, 1994; Turkewitz & Kenny, 1982). In order to understand the function of the brain, we can no longer ignore this fact; theories about brain functioning must incorporate this fundamental process of life. Anatomical perspectives are no longer adequate. This is not meant to imply, however, that they are not useful. Anatomical methods are static and can only tell us what the structure of interest is at the particular moment of study. In contrast, because developmental perspectives are inherently

dynamic, they readily provide a model in which interactions between structures and interactions between structure and environment can be understood. That is, they allow us to frame abnormal processes in terms of deviations from normal system development (Cicchetti & Tucker, 1994).

Anatomical models inherently stress that structure dictates function, but the principles of cortical plasticity and developmental induction argue that the opposite is also true, that function dictates structure (Turkewitz & Kenny, 1982). Indeed, when we look at frontal lobe functioning, this becomes readily apparent. It is of little doubt that the frontal lobe plays a role in self-regulation (an instance in which structure dictates function). However, the nature of this regulation is fundamentally different between individuals. In other words, the personal affordances encoded within frontal lobe networks resonate differently to the same situation for each person. For example, massive frontal lesions can produce symptoms that are collectively referred to as "environmental dependency syndrome" (Lehrmitte, 1986). This syndrome is characterized by the patient's rigid dependence upon the environment to regulate his or her behavior. Lehrmitte describes a patient who upon seeing a bed during the middle of the day changed and proceeded to go to bed, even though no explicit demands by the observer were made. Lehrmitte noted that the nature of the dependence is markedly different between individuals. Its manifestation reflects the history (personal affordance) of the individual. In social situations, a housewife with this disorder will display environmental dependency symptoms that are consistent with her background, whereas an individual with the same disorder but a different background will behave differently under identical social situations (Lehrmitte, 1986). Observations such as this have led some to suggest that an understanding of frontal lobe disorders requires an understanding of the history of the individual (Mesulam, 1986). To the extent that the frontal lobes sculpt subsequent networks of the posterior areas (Thatcher, 1994), we have an instance in which function dictates structure. Moreover, the impositions placed upon posterior networks by frontal lobe mechanisms represent self-regulating processes.

In this chapter, we have outlined a vertical model of cerebral organization, maturation, and development. In this model, vertical integration is a critical feature of fundamental brain functioning, such as regulation of cerebral tone and organization, as well as higher-order processes such as cognition. Cortical organization was discussed from a self-regulatory perspective in which fundamental activation and arousal systems of the brainstem are seen to be critical components. At the top of the vertical hierarchy of regulation and organization are the frontal networks, involving prefrontal and limbic cortices. The frontal and limbic areas are seen as sites of central convergence that support individually specific representation based upon internal and external constraints. The frontal and limbic networks in sculpting posterior networks serve to tailor the organization of the brain to meet the requirements of the world in individually specific ways.

References

Brody, B. A., Kinney, H. C., Kloman, A. S., & Gilles, F. H. (1987). Sequence of central nervous system myelination in human infancy. I. An autopsy study myelination. *Journal of Neuropathology and Experimental Neurology, 46*, 283–301.

Bronson, G. W. (1982). Structure, status, and characteristics of the nervous system at birth. In P. Stratton (Ed.), *Psychobiology of the human newborn* (pp. 99–118). New York: Wiley.

Brown, J. W. (1994). Morphogenesis and the mental process. *Development and Psychopathology, 6*, 551–563.

Buchanan, S. L., & Powell, D. (1993). Cingulothalmic and prefrontal control of autonomic function. In B. A. Vogt & M. Gabriel (Eds.), *Neurobiology of the cingulate cortex and limbic thalamus* (pp. 381–414). Boston: Birkhauser.

Chugani, H. T., & Phelps, M. E. (1986). Maturational changes in cerebral function in infants determined by FDG postiron emission tomography. *Science, 231*, 840–843.

Cicchetti, D., & Tucker, D. M. (1994). Development and self-regulatory structures of the mind. *Development and Pschopathology, 6*, 533–549.

Collins, P. F., & Depue, R. A. (1992). A neurobehavioral systems approach to developmental psychopathology: Implications for disorders of affect. In &. S. L. T. D. Cicchetti (Eds.), *Rochester symposium on developmental psychopathology: developmental perspectives on depression* (pp. 29–101). Rochester: Univ. of Rochester Press.

Edelman, G. (1989). *The remembered present: A biological theory of consciousness.* New York: Basic Book.

Gibson, K. R. (1991). Myelination and behavioral development: A comparative perspective on questions of neoteny, altriciality and intelligence. In K. R. Gibson & A. C. Petersen (Eds.), *Brain maturation and cognitive development* (pp. 29–63). New York: Aldine de Gruyter.

Greenough, W. T., & Black, J. E. (1992). Induction of brain structure by experience: Substrates for cognitive development. In M. Gunnar & C. Nelson (Eds.), *Developmental behavioral neuroscience: Minnesota symposium on child psychology* (pp. 155–200). Hillsdale, NJ: Erlbaum.

Huttenlocher, P. R. (1979). Synaptic density in human frontal cortex. Developmental changes and effects of aging. *Brain Research, 163*, 195–205.

Huttenlocher, P. R. (1990). Morphometric study of human cerebral cortex development. *Neuropsychologia, 28*, 517–527.

Jackson, J. H. (1931). The evolution and dissolution of the nervous system. In *Selected writings of John Hughlings Jackson* (Vol. 2, pp. 45–75). London: Hodder and Stoughton.

Jenkins, W. M., & Merzenich, M. M. (1987). Reorganization of neocortical representations after brain injury: A neuophysiological model of the bases of recovery from stroke. *Progress in Brain Research, 71*, 249–266.

Kaada, B. R., Pribram, K. H., & Epstein, J. A. (1949). Respiratory and vascular response in monkeys from temporal pole, insula, orbital surface and cingulate gyrus. *Journal of Neurophysiology, 12*, 347–356.

Kinney, H. C., Brody, B. A., Kloman, A. S., & Gilles, F. H. (1988). Sequence of central nervous system myelination in human infancy. II. patterns of myelination in autopsied infants. *Journal of Neuropathology and Experimental Neurology, 47*, 217–234.

Konner, M. (1991). Universals of behavioral development in relation to brain myelination. In K. R. Gibson & A. C. Petersen (Eds.), *Brain maturation and cognitive development* (pp. 181–223). New York: Aldine de Gruyter.

Lehrmitte, F. (1986). Human autonomy and the frontal lobes. Part II: Patient behavior in complex and social situations: The "environmental dependency syndrome." *Annals of Neurology, 19*, 335–343.

Livingston, R. B., Chapman, W. P., Livingston, K. E., & Kraintz, L. (1947). Stimulation of the orbital surface of man prior to frontal lobotomy. In J. F. Fulton, C. D. Aring, & B. S. Wortis (Eds.), *Research publications association for research in nervous and mental disease: The frontal lobes* (pp. 421–432). Baltimore: Williams & Wilkins.

Luria, A. R. (1973). *The working brain: An introduction to neuropsychology.* New York: Basic Books.

MacLean, P. D. (1987). The midline frontolimbic cortex and the evolution of crying and laughter. In E. Perceman (Ed.), *The frontal lobes revisited* (pp. 121–141). New York: IRBN Press.

Mattson, M. P. (1988). Neurotransmitters in the regulation of neuronal cytoarchitecture. *Brain Research Reviews, 13*, 179–212.

Merzenich, M. M., & Sameshima, K. (1993). Cortical plasticity and memory. *Current Opinion in Neurobiology, 3*, 187–196.

Mesulam, M. (1986). Frontal cortex and behavior. *Annals of Neurology, 19*, 320–325.

Nauta, W. J. H. (1964). Some efferent connections of the prefrontal cortex in the monkey. In J. M. Warren & K. Akert (Eds.), *The frontal granular cortex and behavior* (pp. 397–409). New York: McGraw-Hill.

Pandya, D. N., Seltzer, B., & Barbas, H. (1988). Input–output organization of the primate cerebral cortex. *Comparative Primate Biology, 4*, 39–80.

Pandya, D. N., & Yeterian, E. H. (1990). Prefrontal cortex in relation to other cortical areas in rhesus monkey: Architecture and connections. *Progress in Brain Research, 85*, 63–94.

Pons, T. P., Garraghty, P. E., & Mishkin, M. (1988). Lesion-induced plasticity in the second somatosensory cortex of adult macaques. *Proceedings of the National Academy of Science, United States of America, 85*, 5279–5281.

Pribram, K. H. (1960). A review of theory in physiological psychology. *Annual Review of Psychology, 11*, 1–40.

Pribram, K. H. (Ed.). (1981). *Emotions.* New York: Wiley.

Recanzone, G. H., Merzenich, M. M., Jenkins, W. M., Grajski, K., & Dinse, H. R. (1992). Topographic reorganization of the hand representation in cortical area 3b of owl monkeys trained in a frequency-discrimination task. *Journal of Neurophysiology, 67*, 1031–1056.

Recanzone, G. H., Merzenich, M. M., & Schreiner, C. E. (1992). Changes in the distributed temporal response properties of SI cortical neurons reflect improvement in performance on a temporally based tactile discrimination task. *Journal of Neurophysiology, 67*, 1071–1091.

Satinoff, E. (1978). Neural organization and evolution of thermal regulation in mamals. *Science, 201*, 16–22.

Shepard, R. N. (1984). Ecological constraints on internal representation: Resonant kinematics of perceiving, imagining, thinking, and dreaming. *Psychological Review, 91*(4), 417–447.

Thatcher, R. W. (1992). Cyclic cortical reorganization during early childhood. *Brain and Cognition, 20*, 24–50.

Thatcher, R. W. (1994). Psychopathology of early frontal lobe damage: dependence on cycles of development. *Development and Psychopathology, 6,* 565–596.

Tucker, D. M. (1992). Developing emotions and cortical networks. In M. Gunnar & C. Nelson (Eds.), *Developmental behavioral neuroscience: Minnesota symposium on child psychology* (pp. 75–127). Hillsdale, NJ: Erlbaum.

Tucker, D. M., & Derryberry, D. (1992). Motivated attention: Anxiety and the frontal executive functions. *Neuropsychiatry, Neuropsychology, and Behavioral Neurology, 5,* 233–252.

Tucker, D. M., Luu, P., & Pribram, K. H. (1995). Social and emotional self-regulation. *Annals of the New York Academy of Sciences, 769,* 213–239.

Tucker, D. M., & Williamson, P. A. (1984). Asymmetric neural control systems in human self-regulation. *Psychological Review, 91,* 185–215.

Turkewitz, G., & Kenny, P. A. (1982). Limitations on input as a basis for neural organization and perceptual development: A preliminary theoretical statement. *Developmental Psychobiology, 15,* 357–368.

Watson, D., & Tellegen, A. (1985). Toward a consensual structure of mood. *Psychological Bulletin, 98*(2), 219–235.

Yakovlev, P. I., & Lecours, A. R. (1967). The myelinogenetic cycles of regional maturation of the brain. In A. Minkowski (Ed.), *Regional development of the brain in early life* (pp. 3–70). Oxford: Blackwell.

Index